Advances in Oncological Medicine

Advances in Oncological Medicine

Edited by Maria Walters

hayle medical

New York

Hayle Medical,
750 Third Avenue, 9th Floor,
New York, NY 10017, USA

Visit us on the World Wide Web at:
www.haylemedical.com

ISBN: 978-1-63241-703-9

The publisher's policy is to use permanent paper from mills that operate a sustainable forestry policy. Furthermore, the publisher ensures that the text paper and cover boards used have met acceptable environmental accreditation standards.

Printed in China.

Cataloging-in-Publication Data

Advances in oncological medicine / edited by Maria Walters.
p. cm.
Includes bibliographical references and index.
ISBN 978-1-63241-703-9
1. Oncology. 2. Cancer. 3. Cancer--Treatment. 4. Tumors. I. Walters, Maria.
RC254 .A78 2019
616.994--dc23

Table of Contents

Preface

Over the recent decade, advancements and applications have progressed exponentially. This has led to the increased interest in this field and projects are being conducted to enhance knowledge. The main objective of this book is to present some of the critical challenges and provide insights into possible solutions. This book will answer the varied questions that arise in the field and also provide an increased scope for furthering studies.

Oncology is a branch of medicine which is concerned with the prevention, diagnosis, and treatment of cancer. The term, cancer, refers to the diseases associated with the abnormal cell growth in the body, which have the potential to invade or spread to other parts. A medical practitioner who has specialized in this field is called an oncologist. Smoking or the intake of tobacco in other forms is considered to be the leading cause of cancer. Other risk factors include obesity and alcohol consumption. Cancer can be potentially treated by chemotherapy, radiation therapy, surgery, targeted therapy, hormonal therapy and synthetic lethality. The preferred mode of treatment varies according to the location and stage of the disease. The performance status of the patient is also taken into consideration. Cancer patients experience pain due to the tumor infiltrating or compressing nearby body parts, or due to the treatment or diagnostic procedure performed. Cancer pain management is therefore an essential aspect of cancer care. This book contains some path-breaking studies in the field of oncological medicine. Such selected concepts that redefine oncological medicine have been presented in it. The topics covered in this book offer the readers new insights in the field of oncological medicine.

I hope that this book, with its visionary approach, will be a valuable addition and will promote interest among readers. Each of the authors has provided their extraordinary competence in their specific fields by providing different perspectives as they come from diverse nations and regions. I thank them for their contributions.

Editor

1

A Unique Presentation of Occult Primary Breast Cancer

Inaya Ahmed,[1] Kavita Dharmarajan,[2] Amy Tiersten,[3] Ira Bleiweiss,[4] Hank Schmidt,[5] Sheryl Green,[2] and Richard L. Bakst[2]

[1] *Rutgers Robert Wood Johnson Medical School, New Brunswick, NJ 08901, USA*
[2] *Department of Radiation Oncology, Icahn School of Medicine at Mount Sinai Hospital, New York, NY 10029, USA*
[3] *Department of Medical Oncology, Icahn School of Medicine at Mount Sinai Hospital, New York, NY 10029, USA*
[4] *Department of Pathology, Icahn School of Medicine at Mount Sinai Hospital, New York, NY 10029, USA*
[5] *Department of Surgery, Icahn School of Medicine at Mount Sinai Hospital, New York, NY 10029, USA*

Correspondence should be addressed to Richard L. Bakst; richard.bakst@mountsinai.org

Academic Editor: Gianfilippo Bertelli

We are reporting a case of a 34-year-old woman with occult primary breast cancer discovered after initially presenting with neurological symptoms. She was successfully treated with neoadjuvant chemotherapy followed by definitive axillary lymph node dissection and ipsilateral whole breast radiotherapy. The case presented is unique due to the rarity of occult primary breast cancer, especially in light of her initial confounding neurological signs and symptoms, which highlights the importance of careful staging.

1. Introduction

Occult primary breast cancer is defined as histologically proven breast cancer discovered outside the breast in the absence of a primary breast tumor. Occult primary breast cancer was first described in 1907 by Halsted. The incidence of occult primary breast cancer is 0.3–1.0% of all newly diagnosed breast cancers, and due to its rarity, its natural history has not yet been clearly documented [1]. Traditionally occult primary breast cancers were treated with mastectomy and axillary lymph node dissection; however, with the advent of breast MRI and improvement in radiation techniques, the management of this rare entity is changing. Here, we report a case of occult primary breast cancer with a unique initial presentation, and we review the currently available literature on diagnosis, treatment, and prognosis of this rare disease.

2. A Case Report

A 34-year-old woman with a history of headaches, seizure activity, and recently diagnosed breast cancer was initially referred to the Department of Radiation Oncology for irradiation of lesions in the brain concerning for metastases.

One year prior to presenting to our clinic, she developed headaches and altered mental status. Magnetic resonance imaging (MRI) of the brain was suggestive of leptomeningeal enhancement with multiple nodular areas throughout the brain and brainstem (Figure 1). Further workup, including lumbar puncture, was nondiagnostic. While her initial symptoms spontaneously resolved, a similar episode occurred 6 months later. At this time she developed a large, palpable, right axillary node.

Diagnostic workup including an ultrasound imaging of the right axilla exhibited 2 large, adjacent, heterogeneous lymph nodes with loss of the fatty hila. Bilateral mammogram was suspicious for malignancy in the right breast, and follow-up MRI confirmed right axillary lymphadenopathy and also demonstrated extensive patchy enhancement in the right breast, involving the medial breast as well as the upper outer quadrant (Figure 2).

Ultrasound-guided biopsy of a right axillary lymph node revealed invasive ductal carcinoma. Immunohistochemistry was positive for HER2 and negative for estrogen and progesterone receptors. Stereotactic biopsy of the breast resulted in benign findings, demonstrating fibroadenoma, secretory

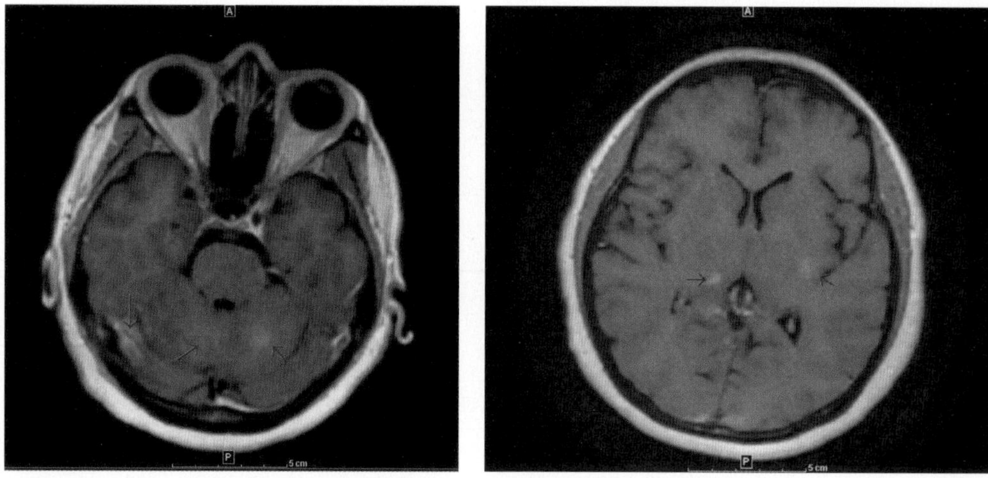

(a) (b)

Figure 1: MRI brain: axial T1 images with contrast (a and b) demonstrating nodular enhancement (red arrows) in multiple areas of the brain.

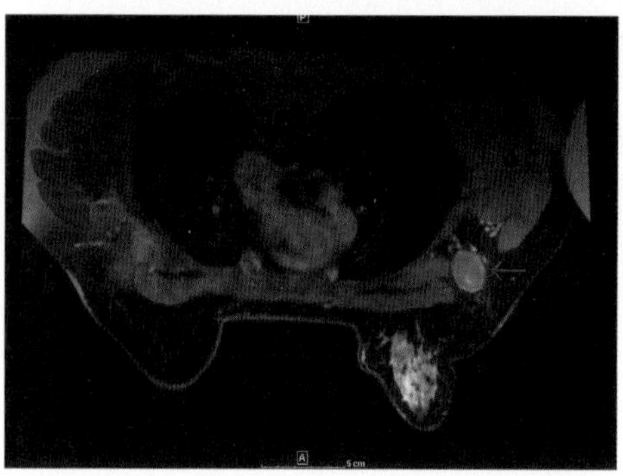

Figure 2: MRI breast: axial T1 image with contrast demonstrating normal breast tissue with right axillary lymphadenopathy (red arrow).

changes, and stromal fibrosis with calcifications. Two subsequent MRI-guided biopsies were consistent with benign tissue. Staging positron emission tomography (PET) scan confirmed disease in the right axilla, with no FDG avidity in any other area, including the right breast and the areas corresponding with the brain lesions seen previously on MRI.

Repeat brain MRI exhibited progression of prior findings. In light of her new cancer diagnosis, it was felt that her MRI findings represented leptomeningeal carcinomatosis. She was therefore referred to the Department of Radiation Oncology for whole brain radiotherapy. However, scrutiny of her MRI and review of her prior imaging with both neurology and neuroradiology lead to a favored diagnosis of a primary granulomatous, rather than a metastatic, process in the brain. No biopsies were performed at the time.

In the absence of metastatic disease, the patient initiated definitive treatment consisting of neoadjuvant chemotherapy, consisting of four cycles of docetaxel, trastuzumab, and pertuzumab, followed by three cycles of 5-fluorouracil, epirubicin, and cyclophosphamide, which she tolerated well with no major toxicities.

In lieu of undergoing mastectomy, the patient elected to undergo breast conserving therapy (BCT), which consists of axillary lymph node dissection and whole breast radiotherapy. All of the 22 lymph nodes dissected were negative for malignancy, though 2 nodes exhibited chemotherapy-related changes (Figure 3). After about 1.5 months of recovery, the patient initiated radiotherapy. She underwent external beam radiotherapy to 50 Gy in 25 daily fractions to the right breast, axilla, and supraclavicular fossa (Figure 4).

Three months after completion of radiotherapy, she was not exhibiting any side effects or residual toxicity and continues to be free of headaches or neurological symptoms.

3. Discussion

Rarely, a breast cancer patient has histologically proven breast cancer found outside the breast without a detectable primary breast tumor. Almost always the site of detected disease is an axillary lymph node. The incidence of axillary breast cancer with occult primary is 0.3–1.0%, with a peak incidence at the age of 55 [1, 2]. Historically, a relatively large proportion of patients (20–30%) with occult primary breast cancer have reported a family history of breast cancer, although this was not the case for our patient [8].

Diagnostic workup for an axillary metastasis must first rule out other primary sites of disease. This may involve history and physical (including full skin exam for melanoma), chest X-ray, mammography, PET scan, hepatic imaging, and serum studies [9]. Dedicated imaging of the breast for occult primary breast cancer includes breast ultrasound and MRI. MRI's high sensitivity for breast tumors may optimize diagnostic accuracy and, in turn, disease management [10]. If a primary site is identified, the patient should undergo appropriate surgical management with a lumpectomy or mastectomy with lymph node evaluation.

Occult primary breast cancer has traditionally been treated with ipsilateral mastectomy and axillary lymph node dissection (ALND). However, practice patterns have steadily

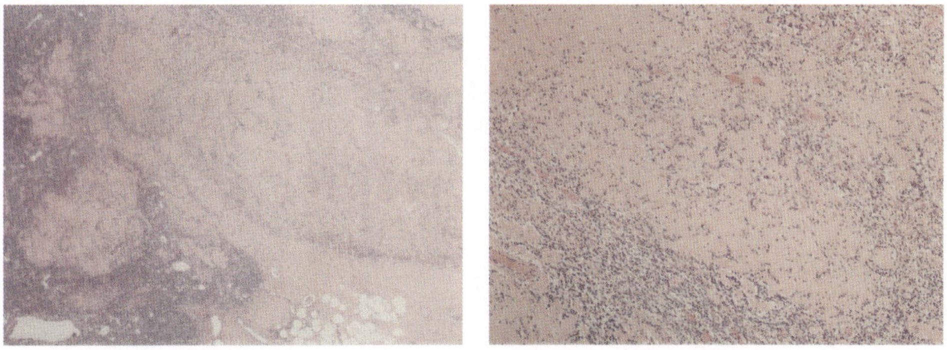

FIGURE 3: Axillary nodal pathology. Hematoxylin and eosin stained tissue slides from axillary lymph node dissection following chemotherapy. Low (a) and high power (b) from her lymph node showing large geographic areas of fibrosis where tumor was before chemotherapy.

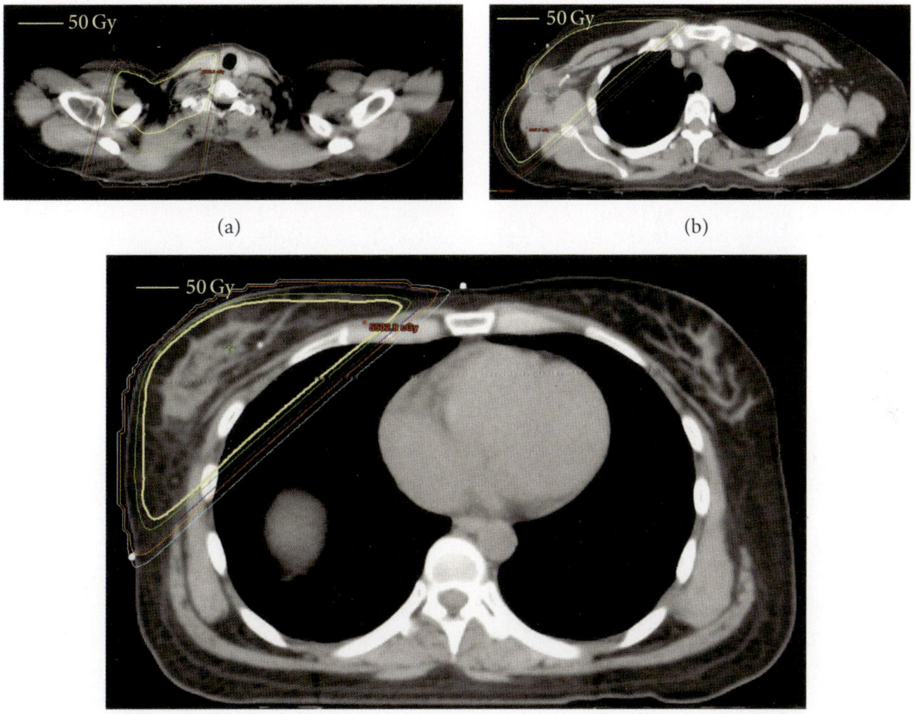

FIGURE 4: 3D conformal radiotherapy plan for our patient: axial dose distribution to the supraclavicular fossa (a), axilla (b), and breast (c).

transformed over the last two to three decades with a push toward BCT [3]. In the case of occult primary breast cancer, BCT entails ipsilateral ALND and radiotherapy to the whole breast. Whole breast radiotherapy and mastectomy have been associated with statistically equivalent outcomes in several studies, with a 10-year overall survival of 65% [1, 3–5]. In comparison, a 2010 SEER database analysis reported that patients treated with ALND only or observation without intervention exhibited diminished survival rates of 58.5% ($P = 0.02$) and 47.5% ($P = 0.04$), respectively [3]. Furthermore, failure to provide any intervention to the ipsilateral breast is unacceptable, as locoregional failure in those cases may exceed 80% [6].

Disease recurrence patterns are also reported to be similar among patients treated with either mastectomy or BCT. In a 2012 retrospective analysis of 95 patients treated with either mastectomy (with ALND), BCT, or ALND only, patients treated with mastectomy or BCT exhibited a 3-year local recurrence-free survival (LRFS) of 88.9–90.0% and overall recurrence-free survival (RFS) of 71.9–81.6%, with no difference between the two cohorts ($P = 0.71$, 0.94) [4]. Patients treated solely with ALND demonstrated significantly diminished 3-year LRFS (70.2%) and overall RFS (52.1%). These results are comparable to those of prior smaller, retrospective studies, reporting similar recurrence rates among patients undergoing mastectomy or BCT and

Table 1: Summary of literature reviewed on occult primary breast cancer.

	Median F/U (yr)	Patients	Overall survival		Recurrence-free survival		Locoregional recurrence	Distant recurrence
			5 yr OS	10 yr OS	5 yr RFS	10 yr RFS		
Vlastos et al. (2001) [1]	7.0	BCT: 32	79%	64%	72%	63%	13%	22%
		Mast: 13	75%	66%	67%	56%	15%	31%
Galimberti et al. (2004) [2]	3.4	50	—	—	—	—	4%	12%
Walker et al. (2010) [3]	4.0	BCT: 202		67.1%	—	—	—	—
		Mast: 268	—	63.5%	—	—	—	—
		ALND: 126	—	58.5%*	—	—	—	—
		Obs: 94	—	47.5%*	—	—	—	—
He et al. (2012) [4]	3.2	BCT: 13	—	—	—	—	8%	15%
		Mast: 64	—	—	—	—	11%	6%
		ALND: 18	—	—	—	—	28%	6%
Campana et al. (1989) [5]	9.0	31	76%	71%	86%	75%	25%	29%
Foroudi and Tiver (2000) [6]	9.2	BCT: 12	—	—	—	—	25%	0%
		Mast: 2	—	—	—	—	0%	0%
		Obs: 6	—	—	—	—	83%	—
Barton et al. (2011) [7]	5.7	BCT: 35	84%	—	64%	—	14%	—
		No RT: 13 (nodal and/or partial breast resection)	85%	—	34%*	—	85%	—

(i) *Statistically significant value.
(ii) BCT: breast conserving therapy, RT: radiotherapy, Mast: mastectomy, ALND: axillary lymph node dissection, and Obs: observation.
(iii) OS: overall survival, RFS: recurrence-free survival, F/U: follow-up period, and mo: month.
(iv) —: not reported.

poor outcomes in patients without any treatment to the ipsilateral breast [1, 7, 11]. Accordingly, local therapy to the ipsilateral breast, either mastectomy or BCT, plays a crucial role in the treatment of occult primary breast cancer. These studies are summarized in Table 1.

From the available retrospective literature, data regarding disease prognosticators remains relatively elusive. Many of the known prognositc factors in primary breast cancer have been investigated, including age, tumor grade, hormone receptor status, HER2/neu status, and nodal stage [1, 3–5]. To date, only nodal status has been consistently associated with survival outcomes in occult primary breast cancer. In the 2010 SEER analysis, Walker et al. found that patients with ≥10 positive lymph nodes had worse overall survival ($P < 0.01$) and cause-specific survival ($P = 0.02$) than those with <10 nodes positive [3]. Smaller retrospective studies have shown a significant improvement in survival when patients have 1–3 versus ≥4 positive lymph nodes [1, 4, 5]. Although extent of nodal disease clearly influences prognosis, the importance of specific nodal sites (i.e., axillary versus infraclavicular) remains unclear.

Due to the rarity of occult primary breast cancer, much about this disease has yet to be fully defined. With the incidence of this presentation too infrequent for prospective study, therapeutic decisions are synthesized utilizing the available retrospective data. In patients with occult primary breast cancer, thorough diagnostic evaluation is crucial in ruling out other primary malignancies, and breast MRI is standard to confirm the absence of a primary breast tumor. In terms of definitive therapy for occult primary breast cancer, BCT or mastectomy with ALND provides equivalent survival and recurrence outcomes, and the practice of BCT is steadily increasing. Furthermore, nodal status serves as the main prognostic factor in these cases. With definitive treatment with BCT and only 2 positive lymph nodes, we expect an excellent prognosis for our patient. Lastly, this case reminds us that careful staging of any patient is critical. If not for a thoughtful diagnostic process and careful interdisciplinary approach to patient management decisions at our institution, our patient may have received unnecessary therapy for presumed brain metastases and have not received definitive treatment.

References

[1] G. Vlastos, M. E. Jean, A. N. Mirza et al., "Feasibility of breast preservation in the treatment of occult primary carcinoma presenting with axillary metastases," *Annals of Surgical Oncology*, vol. 8, no. 5, pp. 425–431, 2001.

[2] V. Galimberti, G. Bassani, S. Monti et al., "Clinical experience with axillary presentation breast cancer," *Breast Cancer Research and Treatment*, vol. 88, no. 1, pp. 43–47, 2004.

[3] G. V. Walker, G. L. Smith, G. H. Perkins et al., "Population-based analysis of occult primary breast cancer with axillary lymph node metastasis," *Cancer*, vol. 116, no. 17, pp. 4000–4006, 2010.

[4] M. He, L. C. Tang, K. D. Yu et al., "Treatment outcomes and unfavorable prognostic factors in patients with occult breast cancer," *European Journal of Surgical Oncology*, vol. 38, no. 11, pp. 1022–1028, 2012.

[5] F. Campana, A. Fourquet, M. A. Ashby et al., "Presentation of axillary lymphadenopathy without detectable breast primary (T_0 N_{ib} breast cancer): experience at Institut Curie," *Radiotherapy & Oncology*, vol. 15, no. 4, pp. 321–325, 1989.

[6] F. Foroudi and K. W. Tiver, "Occult breast carcinoma presenting as axillary metastases," *International Journal of Radiation Oncology Biology Physics*, vol. 47, no. 1, pp. 143–147, 2000.

[7] S. R. Barton, I. E. Smith, A. M. Kirby, S. Ashley, G. Walsh, and M. Parton, "The role of ipsilateral breast radiotherapy in management of occult primary breast cancer presenting as axillary lymphadenopathy," *European Journal of Cancer*, vol. 47, no. 14, pp. 2099–2106, 2011.

[8] S. W. Harrington, "Survival rates of radical mastectomy for unilateral and bilateral carcinoma of the breast," *Surgery*, vol. 19, no. 1, pp. 154–166, 1946.

[9] E. C. Halperin, C. A. Perez, and L. W. Brady, *Perez and Bradys Principles and Practice of Radiation Oncology*, Lippincott Williams & Wilkins, 5th edition, 2008.

[10] National Comprehensive Cancer Network, *Breast Cancer (Version 3.2014)*, 2014, http://www.nccn.org/professionals/physician_gls/PDF/breast.pdf.

[11] R. Varadarajan, S. B. Edge, J. Yu, N. Watroba, and B. R. Janarthanan, "Prognosis of occult breast carcinoma presenting as isolated axillary nodal metastasis," *Oncology*, vol. 71, no. 5-6, pp. 456–459, 2007.

2

Lymphocyte-Predominant Hodgkin's Disease in Children: A Case Study

James R. Stier[1,2] and Robert J. Vasquez[3,4,5]

[1]*Department of Pediatrics, Tulane University School of Medicine, New Orleans, LA 70112, USA*
[2]*Department of Pediatrics, Ochsner Health System, New Orleans, LA 70112, USA*
[3]*Department of Pediatrics, Tulane University School of Medicine, New Orleans, LA 70112, USA*
[4]*Department of Pediatric Hematology-Oncology, Ochsner Health System, New Orleans, LA 70121, USA*
[5]*University of Queensland School of Medicine, Brisbane, QLD 4006, Australia*

Correspondence should be addressed to Robert J. Vasquez; rovasquez@ochsner.org

Academic Editor: Nurdan Tacyildiz

A three-year-old boy presented with an enlarging neck mass. Biopsy demonstrated IgD-positive nodular lymphocyte-predominant Hodgkin lymphoma (NLPHL), which was staged as IIa. The patient received cyclophosphamide, doxorubicin, vincristine, and prednisone (CHOP) with rituximab and had excellent results. NLPHL is a relatively rare disease that is biologically distinct from classic Hodgkin lymphoma (cHL). NLPHL is a B-cell malignancy likely of germinal center origin that has an overall good prognosis and favorable response to treatment. Unlike cHL, NLPHL is ubiquitously CD20-positive. Recent evidence supports the efficacy of targeted anti-CD20 therapy in NLPHL, though prospective data is limited. This case demonstrates several unique features of NLPHL and further supports the use of rituximab in front-line therapy. The clinical characteristics among patients at various ages are discussed with a special focus on the IgD-positive subtype. A thorough literature search demonstrates this to be the youngest patient with NLPHL yet described.

1. Case

A three-year-old boy originally from Saudi Arabia was referred to ENT clinic with a five-week history of an enlarging right neck mass associated with fevers, night sweats, and fatigue. Physical exam revealed a roughly 2.5 × 4 cm slightly tender, mobile, matted lymph node located inferior to the sternocleidomastoid with several smaller cervical lymph nodes palpated bilaterally. The patient was given a course of oral antibiotics and though his systemic symptoms quickly resolved the neck mass persisted. He subsequently underwent excisional biopsy of the mass. Surgical dissection revealed a 6 × 3 × 3 cm node adherent to the internal jugular vein. The node and several surrounding satellite lymph nodes were removed and sent for pathologic analysis.

Flow cytometry was normal with 96% "unremarkable" T-cells and 1.8% blasts. EBV and AFB stains were negative. The specimens were sent to two major pathology centers for further study. Final interpretation from both consulting institutions was consistent with *nodular lymphocyte-predominant Hodgkin lymphoma* (NLPHL) with morphology demonstrating atypical lymphoid cells staining positive for CD20, IgD, CD45, OCT-2, PAX-5, and bcl-6 but negative for CD15 and CD30. Architecturally, the tissue featured nodular areas consisting of a CD21-positive follicular dendritic cell meshwork with areas of more diffuse growth amidst a T-cell-rich background—all features resembling those previously described in typical IgD-positive NLPHL.

PET/CT (Figure 1) demonstrated increased tracer uptake within bilateral cervical lymph nodes (estimated SUV of 4.5) and spleen (estimated SUV of 3.6). Bone marrow biopsies showed no morphologic evidence of metastatic disease. Staging was discussed with several international Hodgkin experts who agreed that splenic disease without involvement of

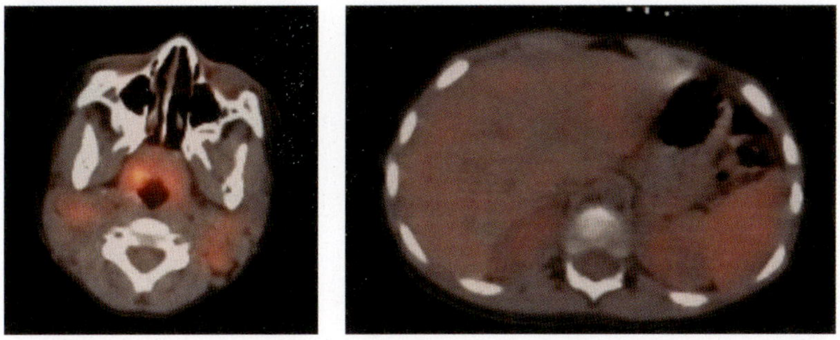

(a) (b)

FIGURE 1: PET/CT demonstrates increased tracer uptake within bilateral cervical lymph nodes and the nasopharyngeal region (often normal in children). Slightly increased uptake in the spleen is seen in the image on the right with no apparent focal lesion.

thoracic or intra-abdominal lymph nodes would be unlikely in NLPHL particularly without focal areas of hypermetabolic activity within the spleen; however, we could not completely discount this finding and it factored into our therapy plan. B-symptoms are unusual in NLPHL and since the patient's systemic symptoms resolved with antibiotics and did not recur in the intervening weeks prior to initiation of chemotherapy, we concluded that the constitutional symptoms were likely due to an unrelated infectious process. The lymphoma was therefore staged as IIa.

The patient underwent three cycles of chemotherapy with cyclophosphamide, doxorubicin, vincristine, and prednisone with rituximab (R-CHOP) at standard dosing (cyclophosphamide 800 mg/m^2, doxorubicin 50 mg/m^2, and vincristine 1.4 mg/m^2 on days 1 and 8, prednisone 40 mg/m^2/day for 7 days, and rituximab 375 mg/m^2). Rituximab was added due to presence of CD20 positivity and as a way of amplifying therapy, given the uncertainty of splenic involvement, while hopefully not increasing risk for late effects. The patient tolerated chemotherapy well with no admissions for fever and neutropenia and no significant toxicities. Repeat PET/CT scans performed at one month and five months following completion of chemotherapy showed complete resolution of all hypermetabolic activity. Eight months after completion of therapy, the family moved back to Saudi Arabia, and a pediatric oncologist in that region subsequently assumed the patient's care. As of this writing, the patient is doing well with no evidence of recurrence at more than 2 years after therapy.

2. Overview

Nodular lymphocyte-predominant Hodgkin lymphoma (NLPHL) accounts for approximately 5% of all cases of Hodgkin lymphoma [1]. Histologic and molecular features of NLPHL demonstrate it to be a unique entity from classic Hodgkin lymphoma (cHL). NLPHL typically has an indolent clinical course often characterized by multiple late relapses. Despite this propensity for relapse, the prognosis of NLPHL following treatment compares favorably to cHL and survival following relapse is also quite high [2]. However, NLPHL has a notable predilection toward developing into diffuse, large B-cell non-Hodgkin's lymphoma (DLBCL) in as many as 12% of cases [3].

3. Presentation

Patients with NLPHL typically present with early-stage disease. In the German Hodgkin Study Group (GHSG), 63% of patients with NLPHL were diagnosed in early stages compared with 22% of cHL patients [4]. Among pediatric patients, NLPHL is more common among preadolescent patients and occurs in an approximate male to female ratio of 5 to 1 [5]. The disease constitutes roughly 10–20% of Hodgkin lymphoma in children 14 years of age or younger compared with 5–8% in patients aged 15–19 [6]. A case series of 55 children with NLPHL found the median age of presentation among pediatric patients to be 13 years (ranging from 4 to 17 years in this particular study) [7].

Nodal involvement tends to be peripheral, most often involving the cervical, inguinal, and axillary regions. Mediastinal involvement is uncommon with an incidence of 8% [8]. Organ involvement is relatively rare as well with 8% of patients having spleen, 6% liver, 2% lung, and 1% skeletal involvement [2].

There is often a long lag between initial detection of an enlarged lymph node and diagnosis of NLPHL [9]. The possible delay in detection may be due to the notable lack of B-symptoms in most patients with NLPHL. Only 9% of NLPHL patients in the GHSG presented with a history of B-symptoms, compared with 40% of patients with cHL [4].

4. Diagnosis

Pathologically, NLPHL is characterized by a nodular proliferation of large neoplastic cells that express CD20. The hallmark of NLPHL is the LP ("lymphocyte-predominant") cell. Previously known as the L&H ("lymphocytic and histiocytic") cell due to the belief that it was of histiocytic origin, the LP cell is now known to be of B-cell lineage [10]. The cell is also occasionally referred to as the "popcorn cell" due to its resemblance to a kernel of popcorn. Malignant LP cells in NLPHL constitute around 1% of the total lymph node mass [11]. The nodular appearance likely represents transformation of germinal centers, and at least a partially nodular pattern is required for diagnosis according to the current WHO definition [12].

IgD expression among LP cells in NLPHL (as noted in our patient) has been rarely described in the literature. One large case series looked at 180 patients with NLPHL, of whom 48 (27%) demonstrated IgD positivity [13]. The IgD-positive cases were more likely to demonstrate LP cells in an extrafollicular distribution (69%) than were IgD-negative cases (13%). The IgD-positive cases also presented at a younger median age (21 versus 44 years) and had an even stronger male predominance (23 to 1 versus 1.5 to 1). None of the IgD-positive cases showed coexpression of IgM or IgG but 93% were positive for the transitional B-cell surface protein CD38. The distribution of affected lymph nodes in this study was cervical > inguinal > axillary in IgD-positive cases versus axillary > inguinal > cervical in IgD-negative disease. This study concluded that cases of IgD-positive NLPHL do not differ from IgD-negative cases regarding cellular derivation and most other immunophenotypic characteristics but do exhibit distinctive clinical features and more often involve the interfollicular region in a background relatively rich in T-cells [13].

Another review of 302 pediatric and adult patients also showed that IgD positivity was significantly more common in pediatric patients (70% versus 38% in adults). The male to female ratio was 16 to 1 in IgD-positive cases with a median age of 14 years for IgD-positive patients versus 21 for IgD-negatives [14]. A match-paired analysis from the GHSG database also supported a strong propensity toward male sex and younger age in IgD-positive patients [15].

5. Prognosis

The overall prognosis of NLPHL compares favorably to cHL. One long-term observational study followed 164 patients in France between 1973 and 2003 [3]. In this study, the 5-year and 10-year progression-free survival (PFS) rates were 81% and 60%, respectively, for the 106 (65%) patients who underwent treatment. Fifty-eight (35%) patients were followed with a watch-and-wait strategy. Among this group of patients, progression-free survival rates were 59% and 41%, respectively. While progression was more common in the watch-and-wait group, overall survival at 5 and 10 years did not differ significantly between the two groups. Limitations of this study include the long 30-year time period for enrollment, which resulted in a wide range of treatment modalities. Furthermore, the median age of participants was 30 years at the time of enrollment (range: 8 to 64 years) possibly decreasing validity in young and elderly patients.

In a large retrospective analysis of 8,298 HL patients treated within 8 prior GHSG studies (performed between 1988 and 2002), NLPHL had a small but statistically significant advantage in overall survival and freedom from treatment failure (OS 96% versus 92%, $P = 0.0116$; FFTF 88% versus 82%, $P = 0.0093$). The included studies enrolled a total of 394 patients with NLPH and 7,904 with cHL and excluded patients younger than 16 [16]. Despite limited data on pediatric outcomes, survival in NLPHL has been generally shown to be excellent with overall survival at or near 100% in most studies [10].

Few histopathologic factors impacting prognosis have been elucidated. A small matched-paired analysis from the GHSG database did not show significant differences in relapse rate with expression of IgD, CD15, p-STAT6, ICOS, or those positive for Epstein-Barr virus. However, there was a slightly lower relapse rate among patients presenting with a pattern of epithelioid cell clusters [15]. Fan and colleagues investigated the pathologic appearance of 77 cases of NLPHL from patients aged 4 to 91 years and showed that a pattern resembling diffuse T-cell-rich B-cell lymphoma was significantly more common in cases of recurrence [17]. A review of 423 NLPHL cases from 9 GHSG trials showed that histopathologic variation characterized by lymphoma cells outside of the B-cell nodules or overall B-cell depletion was associated with advanced disease (29.5% versus 14.6%, $P = 0.0012$) and a higher relapse rate (18.1% versus 6.5% at 5 years, $P = 0.0009$) [18].

6. Treatment

Treatment for NLPHL is evolving and most evidence for therapy is based on retrospective studies. The view of NLPHL as a subtype of cHL has historically led to treatment strategies that have been similar or identical between these two diseases, though they are now increasingly recognized as distinct.

Almost all patients now receive a relatively short (often 6–9 weeks) course of chemotherapy with or without radiation [11]. Therapy of Stage I disease, however, may involve surgical resection of the tumor only, which in two studies had an overall survival rate of 100% but an event-free survival of 57% and 69% at 43 and 70 months, respectively [19, 20].

The current role of low-dose involved-field radiation therapy (LD-IFRT) is an area of ongoing debate and investigation. So far, the relatively few prospective and controlled randomized trials comparing chemotherapy alone to LD-IFRT with chemotherapy have demonstrated a superior event-free survival among the combined modality treatment groups while overall survival has not differed significantly [21].

In fact, overall NLPHL survival with treatment was 100% in each of five prospective studies published between 2007 and 2012. These studies enrolled between 26 and 81 patients, with three comparing chemotherapy to chemotherapy-plus-radiation treatment groups. Length of followup ranged from 5 to 10 years. Chemotherapy regimens used in these studies were diverse and included COPP/ABV, CVP, VAMP, and DBVE [7, 19, 22–24].

There are currently two large ongoing multicenter studies to help elucidate the preferred treatment modality. A German study by Koerholz and colleagues compares three treatment groups—surgery alone, surgery plus CVP, and CVP alone. A Children's Oncology Group study employs a stepwise therapeutic approach involving tumor resection followed by observation for 6-7 weeks. Patients with evidence of residual disease after observation then receive CHOP every three weeks for a total of three cycles. Patients with residual disease following chemotherapy then proceed to involved-field radiation.

A few studies are also investigating the use of rituximab, an anti-CD20 monoclonal antibody, which has shown promise as a therapeutic option in NLPHL and has become near-standard therapy for relapsed disease. In a prior retrospective analysis of 88 cases of NLPHL over a 30-year period, 8 patients received rituximab during the course of their treatment, though none as first-line therapy. There were no cases of relapse in the 4 patients who received rituximab as second-line therapy, while 2 of 4 patients who received rituximab as part of 3rd- through 5th-line therapy ultimately relapsed. The median followup for these 8 patients was 30 months [25].

A prospective study of 15 patients with relapsed or refractory NLPHL demonstrated response in 94% of patients treated with rituximab monotherapy with 8 patients achieving complete remission and 6 achieving partial remission [26]. A prospective study of 28 newly diagnosed patients showed response in 100% with 24 patients achieving complete remission and 4 achieving partial remission with rituximab monotherapy [1].

One study by Advani and colleagues evaluated the time course for treatment with rituximab. This prospective study of 39 patients with NLPHL compared one course of rituximab monotherapy (375 mg/m^2) weekly for 4 weeks with the same dose of rituximab for 4-week cycles repeating every 6 months for a total of 2 years. Twenty-three patients (12 new diagnoses and 11 previously relapsed) in the one-month treatment group were compared to 16 patients (9 new diagnoses and 7 previously relapsed) in the cycled-therapy group. Overall, 67% of all patients achieved complete remission and 33% partial remission after the initial 4 weeks of rituximab monotherapy. At the end of the study, estimated 5-year PFS was 39.1% for the one-month treatment group versus 95.7% for the cycled treatment group. The study supported an approximate 3-year increase in length of PFS by the cycled protocol in both first-line and relapsed settings, though the difference was not statistically significant likely due to the small number of enrolled patients [27].

7. Conclusion

NLPHL remains a relatively rare disease with a good overall prognosis among both children and adults. In this paper, we report the case of a 3-year-old boy with newly diagnosed NLPHL (to our knowledge, the youngest case ever reported in the literature) who achieved complete remission of his Stage IIa disease with combined cytotoxic chemotherapy and the anti-CD20 antibody rituximab.

The outcome of this case supports the use of rituximab with traditional chemotherapy regimens as first-line, upfront therapy for NLPHL—though prospective studies are needed to confirm the added benefit of this combined-treatment approach. The prognosis and clinical significance of IgD-positive disease are another area that warrants further investigation. Answering these clinical questions will take a concerted effort and cooperation of multiple centers given the relatively low incidence of NLPHL.

References

[1] D. A. Eichenauer, M. Fuchs, A. Pluetschow et al., "Phase 2 study of rituximab in newly diagnosed stage IA nodular lymphocytepredominant Hodgkin lymphoma: a report from the German Hodgkin Study Group," *Blood*, vol. 118, no. 16, pp. 4363–4365, 2011.

[2] V. Diehl, M. Sextro, J. Franklin et al., "Clinical presentation, course, and prognostic factors in lymphocyte- predominant Hodgkin's disease and lymphocyte-rich classical Hodgkin's disease: report from the European Task Force on lymphoma project on lymphocyte-predominant Hodgkin's disease," *Journal of Clinical Oncology*, vol. 17, no. 3, pp. 776–783, 1999.

[3] I. Biasoli, A. Stamatoullas, V. Meignin et al., "Nodular, lymphocyte-predominant Hodgkin lymphoma: a long-term study and analysis of transformation to diffuse large B-cell lymphoma in a cohort of 164 patients from the adult lymphoma study group," *Cancer*, vol. 116, no. 3, pp. 631–639, 2010.

[4] L. Nogová, T. Reineke, C. Brillant et al., "Lymphocyte-predominant and classical Hodgkin's lymphoma: a comprehensive analysis from the german Hodgkin study group," *Journal of Clinical Oncology*, vol. 26, no. 3, pp. 434–439, 2008.

[5] C. L. Schwartz, "Special issues in pediatric Hodgkin's disease," *European Journal of Haematology*, vol. 75, supplement 66, pp. 55–62, 2005.

[6] A. Punnett, R. W. Tsang, and D. C. Hodgson, "Hodgkin lymphoma across the age spectrum: epidemiology, therapy, and late effects," *Seminars in Radiation Oncology*, vol. 20, no. 1, pp. 30–44, 2010.

[7] A. Shankar, G. W. Hall, S. Gorde-Grosjean et al., "Treatment outcome after low intensity chemotherapy [CVP] in children and adolescents with early stage nodular lymphocyte predominant Hodgkin's lymphoma—an Anglo-French collaborative report," *European Journal of Cancer*, vol. 48, no. 11, pp. 1700–1706, 2012.

[8] P. M. Mauch, L. A. Kalish, M. Kadin, C. N. Coleman, R. Osteen, and S. Hellman, "Patterns of presentation of Hodgkin disease: implications for etiology and pathogenesis," *Cancer*, vol. 71, no. 6, pp. 2062–2071, 1993.

[9] I. A. Lee and A. S. LaCasce, "Nodular lymphocyte predominant hodgkin lymphoma," *The Oncologist*, vol. 14, no. 7, pp. 739–751, 2009.

[10] A. Shankar and S. Daw, "Nodular lymphocyte predominant Hodgkin lymphoma in children and adolescents—a comprehensive review of biology, clinical course and treatment options," *British Journal of Haematology*, vol. 159, no. 3, pp. 288–298, 2012.

[11] R. Küppers, "Molecular biology of Hodgkin lymphoma," *Hematology/American Society of Hematology. Education Program*, vol. 2009, no. 1, pp. 491–496, 2009.

[12] S. H. Swerdlow, E. Campo, N. L. Harris et al., Eds., *World Health Organization Classification of Tumours of Haematopoietic and Lymphoid Tissues*, World Health Organization, Geneva, Switzerland, 4th edition, 2008.

[13] S. Prakash, T. Fountaine, M. Raffeld, E. S. Jaffe, and S. Pittaluga, "IgD positive L&H cells identify a unique subset of nodular lymphocyte predominant Hodgkin lymphoma," *American Journal of Surgical Pathology*, vol. 30, no. 5, pp. 585–592, 2006.

[14] A. R. Huppmann, A. Nicolae, G. W. Slack et al., "EBV may be expressed in the LP cells of nodular lymphocyte-predominant hodgkin lymphoma (NLPHL) in both children and adults," *The American Journal of Surgical Pathology*, vol. 38, no. 3, pp. 316–324, 2014.

[15] S. Hartmann, D. A. Eichenauer, A. Plütschow et al., "Histopathological features and their prognostic impact in nodular lymphocyte-predominant Hodgkin lymphoma—a matched pair analysis from the German Hodgkin Study Group (GHSG)," *British Journal of Haematology*, vol. 167, no. 2, pp. 238–242, 2014.

[16] L. Nogová, T. Reineke, C. Brillant et al., "Lymphocyte-predominant and classical Hodgkin's lymphoma: a comprehensive analysis from the german Hodgkin study group," *Journal of Clinical Oncology*, vol. 26, no. 3, pp. 434–439, 2008.

[17] Z. Fan, Y. Natkunam, E. Bair, R. Tibshirani, and R. A. Warnke, "Characterization of variant patterns of nodular lymphocyte predominant Hodgkin lymphoma with immunohistologic and clinical correlation," *American Journal of Surgical Pathology*, vol. 27, no. 10, pp. 1346–1356, 2003.

[18] S. Hartmann, D. A. Eichenauer, A. Plütschow et al., "The prognostic impact of variant histology in nodular lymphocyte-predominant Hodgkin lymphoma: a report from the German Hodgkin Study Group (GHSG)," *Blood*, vol. 122, no. 26, pp. 4246–4252, 2013.

[19] C. Mauz-Körholz, S. Gorde-Grosjean, D. Hasenclever et al., "Resection alone in 58 children with limited stage, lymphocyte-predominant Hodgkin lymphoma-experience from the European network group on pediatric Hodgkin lymphoma," *Cancer*, vol. 110, no. 1, pp. 179–185, 2007.

[20] B. Pellegrino, M. J. Terrier-Lacombe, O. Oberlin et al., "Lymphocyte-predominant Hodgkin's lymphoma in children: therapeutic abstention after initial lymph node resection—astudy of the French Society of Pediatric Oncology," *Journal of Clinical Oncology*, vol. 21, no. 15, pp. 2948–2952, 2003.

[21] B. E. Appel, L. Chen, A. Buxton, S. L. Wolden, D. C. Hodgson, and J. B. Nachman, "Impact of low-dose involved-field radiation therapy on pediatric patients with lymphocyte-predominant Hodgkin lymphoma treated with chemotherapy: a report from the Children's Oncology Group," *Pediatric Blood & Cancer*, vol. 59, no. 7, pp. 1284–1289, 2012.

[22] M. L. Metzger, H. J. Weinstein, M. M. Hudson et al., "Association between radiotherapy vs no radiotherapy based on early response to VAMP chemotherapy and survival among children with favorable-risk Hodgkin lymphoma," *Journal of the American Medical Association*, vol. 307, no. 24, pp. 2609–2616, 2012.

[23] S. S. Donaldson, M. P. Link, H. J. Weinstein et al., "Final results of a prospective clinical trial with VAMP and low-dose involved-field radiation for children with low-risk Hodgkin's disease," *Journal of Clinical Oncology*, vol. 25, no. 3, pp. 332–337, 2007.

[24] C. K. Tebbi, N. P. Mendenhall, W. B. London et al., "Response-dependent and reduced treatment in lower risk Hodgkin lymphoma in children and adolescents, results of P9426: a report from the Children's Oncology Group," *Pediatric Blood & Cancer*, vol. 59, no. 7, pp. 1259–1265, 2012.

[25] C. Jackson, B. Sirohi, D. Cunningham, A. Horwich, K. Thomas, and A. Wotherspoon, "Lymphocyte-predominant Hodgkin lymphoma—clinical features and treatment outcomes from a 30-year experience," *Annals of Oncology*, vol. 21, no. 10, pp. 2061–2068, 2010.

[26] H. Schulz, U. Rehwald, F. Morschhauser et al., "Rituximab in relapsed lymphocyte-predominant Hodgkin lymphoma: long-term results of a phase 2 trial by the German Hodgkin Lymphoma Study Group (GHSG)," *Blood*, vol. 111, no. 1, pp. 109–111, 2008.

[27] R. H. Advani, S. J. Horning, R. T. Hoppe et al., "Mature results of a phase II study of rituximab therapy for nodular lymphocyte-predominant Hodgkin lymphoma," *Journal of Clinical Oncology*, vol. 32, no. 9, pp. 912–918, 2014.

3

Malignant Triton Tumors in Sisters with Clinical Neurofibromatosis Type 1

Basnet Alina,[1,2] Jofre A. Sebastian,[1,3] and Capo Gerardo[1,4]

[1] *Trinitas Regional Medical Center, Seton Hall University of Health and Medical Sciences, Elizabeth, NJ 67202, USA*
[2] *Department of Internal Medicine, Trinitas Regional Medical Center, Elizabeth, NJ 67202, USA*
[3] *Touro College of Osteopathic Medicine, 230 W 125th Street No. 1, New York, NY 10027, USA*
[4] *Department of Hematology and Oncology, Trinitas Comprehensive Cancer Center, Elizabeth, NJ 07202, USA*

Correspondence should be addressed to Basnet Alina; basnetalina@hotmail.com

Academic Editor: Yoshihito Yokoyama

Malignant triton tumors (MTTs) are rare and aggressive sarcomas categorized as a subgroup of malignant peripheral nerve sheath tumors (MPNSTs). MTTs arise from Schwann cells of peripheral nerves or existing neurofibromas and have elements of rhabdomyoblastic differentiation. We report the occurrence of MTTs in two sisters. The first patient is a 36-year-old female who presented with left sided chest wall swelling. She also had clinical features consistent with neurofibromatosis type 1 (NF-1). Debulking of the mass showed high-grade malignant peripheral nerve sheath tumor with skeletal muscle differentiation (MTT). The patient was treated with ifosfamide and adriamycin along with radiation. Four years after treatment, she still has no evidence of disease recurrence. Her sister subsequently presented to us at the age of 42 with left sided lateral chest wall pain. Imaging showed a multicompartmental retroperitoneal cystic mass with left psoas involvement. The tumor was resected and, similarly to her sister, it showed high-grade malignant peripheral nerve sheath tumor with rhabdomyoblastic differentiation (MTT). The patient was started on chemotherapy and radiation as described above.

1. Introduction

Malignant triton tumors (MTTs) are a histological subgroup of the malignant peripheral nerve sheath tumors (MPNSTs) with focal component of heterologous skeletal muscle differentiation [1]. MPNSTs are of neuroectodermal origin and arise from the Schwann cells of peripheral nerves or nearby cells, usually through independent perineural differentiation or within preexisting neurofibromas [1–4]. MTTs derive their name from the triton salamander which possesses the ability to develop supernumerary limbs composed of mixed neurogenic and muscular components following sciatic nerve implantation on its dorsal surface [5, 6].

MTTs account for 5–10% of MPNSTs [1, 3] and occur, on average, during the 3rd to 5th decade [1]. Previous studies have reported a 50–70% occurrence of these tumors in the setting of neurofibromatosis type 1 (NF-1) [4]. The tumor behaves very aggressively, with a high rate of local recurrence peaking at 43–50% [1, 7]. The five-year survival rate is reported to be 14% [3] as compared to 34–60% for MPNSTs alone [1]. The median time to progression is 6 months [3]. MTTs pose many diagnostic challenges for pathologists because of the nuanced findings histologically, often resulting in a misdiagnosis to the conventional MPNST [1, 3]. The correct diagnosis relies heavily on histologic criteria, and immunohistochemistry becomes crucial for narrowing the differential diagnosis [8]. MTTs behave more aggressively; these patients have a shorter metastases-free interval and shorter survival as compared to MPNSTs [4, 7]. Thus, MTTs must be differentiated from conventional MPNSTs in order to ensure prompt and aggressive treatment [1, 3].

Once diagnosed, physicians face the difficulty of determining the proper therapeutic regimen. Due to the rarity of this type of tumor; there is no treatment consensus available yet. Wide surgical excision or debulking of the tumor with negative margins and successive radiotherapy is currently often employed [4]. The role of chemotherapy, albeit unproven in efficacy, continues to be used in many cases and it must be noted that this reflects a distinct difference from MPNSTs, where adjuvant chemotherapy is sometimes not used after debulking due to the lack of survival benefit seen as mentioned by Stucky et al. [1, 9, 10]. Moreover, some investigators have employed different combinations of chemotherapy in higher doses in order to achieve a better result in MTT patients [7].

Here we discuss two unique cases describing two sisters who were diagnosed with MTTs only a few years apart. Their presentation stands out from the literature available in their interpatient relationship, gender, and age of presentation. Although MTT is described as an exceedingly rare tumor, the fact that it occurred in two siblings in conjunction with clinical NF-1 is of interest. To our knowledge, no prior cases of MTTs occurring in siblings have been described in the literature. Additionally, MTTs in the setting of NF-1 have been described in a patient population of primarily young males [11]. Our patients are, however, female and slightly older than the age associated with NF-1. Finally, despite the aggressive behavior that characterizes this tumor type and the poor prognosis of this disease, even with rigorous therapeutic regimens, it is worthy of noting that one of the sisters remains disease-free even after 4 years of treatment.

2. Case Report

We describe the presentation of malignant triton tumors in two siblings who are familiar to our cancer center. The first patient is a 36-year-old female with past medical history of asthma who presented to us with complaints of left sided chest wall swelling and mild pain that progressed over a few days. She denied the history of smoking, alcohol, or drugs. Family history was significant for colon cancer in father and maternal aunt. She was not sexually active. On examination, she was found to have axillary freckling, café au lait spots, and mild cognitive impairment. The findings were consistent with NF-1. There was no associated hepatosplenomegaly noted on examination. On imaging, a very large soft tissue mass measuring 15 cm by 15 cm by 13 cm in the left lower anterior lateral chest wall with possible ulceration and axillary lymphadenopathy was seen. The mass infiltrated the adjacent chest wall musculature; however, the ribs and lungs were commented as being intact and clear, respectively (Figure 1). At the time, it was thought to be a possible soft tissue abscess. Thereafter, debridement of the left sided chest mass was undertaken. Due to the rarity of the histologic findings, our pathology department referred this case to Memorial Sloan Kettering for a second opinion. Their findings are quoted as "mainly monotonous undifferentiated spindle cells arranged in intersecting fascicles and vague storiform pattern with high mitotic activity." Immunohistochemical (IHC) stains revealed tumor cells positive for desmin, vimentin, and myogenin as well as focal reactivity for S-100 (Figure 2). On the other hand, markers CD31, CK, EMA, and CD57 were reported to be negative. These results were, thus, consistent with the diagnosis of a high-grade malignant peripheral nerve sheath tumor with focal divergent skeletal muscle differentiation (triton tumor) in the background of fat and fibrous tissue. After discussion in the multidisciplinary round, we decided to give her adjuvant chemotherapy consisting of ifosfamide and adriamycin for four cycles along with pre- and postchemotherapy radiation. She was started on combination chemotherapy of ifosfamide 2 g/m^2 with mesna 2 g/m^2 alternating with adriamycin 75 g/m^2 every other week for first two cycles four weeks apart and then continued with ifosfamide and mesna for the rest of the two cycles without adriamycin. Concomitant radiation was given after the 2nd cycle and continued till the 3rd chemotherapy cycle. The radiation therapy was applied to the left abdominal wall, with a total dose of 65.4 Gy, with initial photon fields, followed by shrinking fields with electrons with 33 dose fractions during the course of two months. She currently follows up in our cancer center and has no evidence of disease recurrence four years after her treatment.

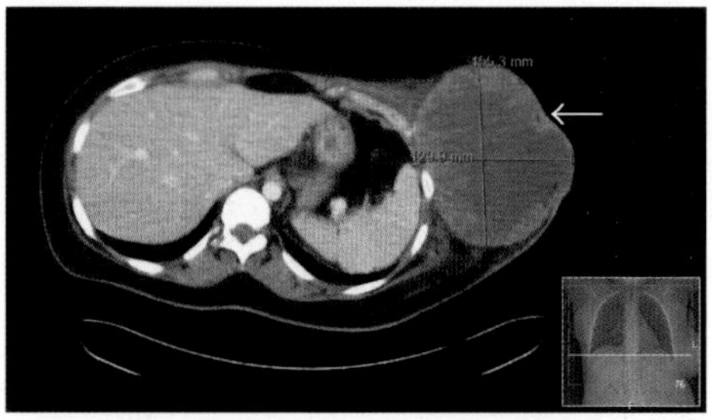

Figure 1: Arrow pointing to the soft tissue mass in the left lateral chest wall with its measurement.

Unfortunately, her younger sister presented to us a few years later at the age of 42 with complaints of pain in the left lateral chest wall with radiation to the left flank that was worsening over 3-4 months. There was no trauma preceding the event. She had no past medical history and was a nonsmoker and nonalcoholic. She was not sexually active. On examination, café au lait spots were also noted on her along with mild cognitive impairment. There was fullness on the left side of the chest underneath the left ribs with some tenderness to palpation but no axillary lymphadenopathy or splenomegaly. On imaging, a multicompartmental retroperitoneal cystic mass in the posterior pararenal space was observed. It extended through the posterior abdominal wall, measuring 10 cm by 7.7 cm by 10.4 cm, and exerted a compressive effect on the left psoas muscle while simultaneously displacing the left kidney anteriorly. Bulky mediastinal and paratracheal lymphadenopathy was additionally observed (Figures 3 and 4). There was no intrathoracic or pleural involvement. She underwent debulking surgery for the mass. Subsequently, histopathological examination of the retroperitoneal mass showed high-grade malignant peripheral nerve sheath tumor with rhabdomyoblastic differentiation (triton tumor) (Figure 5). The tumor was described to have spindle and pleomorphic malignant schwannoma cells, scattered rhabdomyoblasts, and focal areas of necrosis. Immunohistochemical stains are positive with NF-200, desmin, and MyoD. The Ki67 stain demonstrated a proliferative rate of 90%,

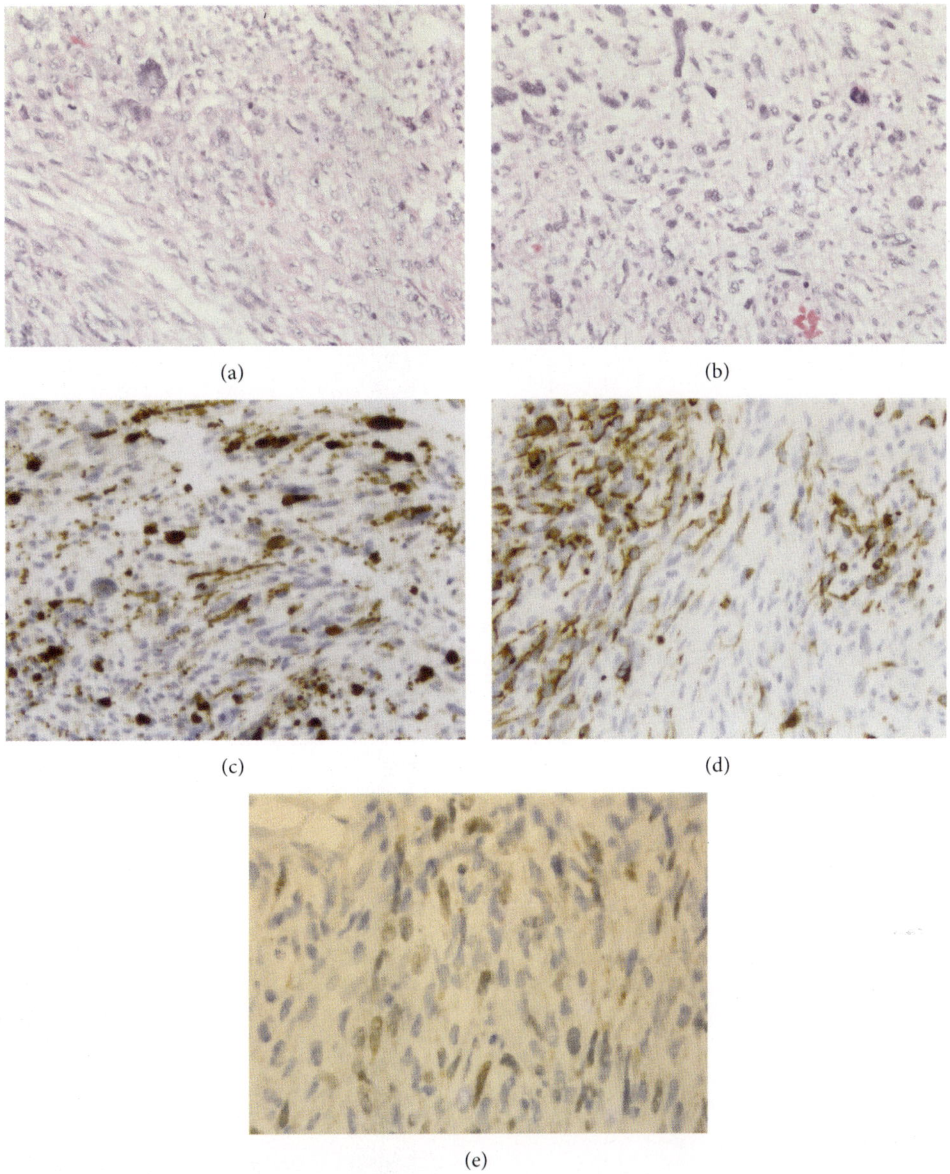

Figure 2: (a) and (b) Malignant triton tumor (MTT) cells. Tumor cellularity and spindle shaped pleomorphic cells are apparent. Interspersed eosinophilic muscle fibers are within the field (H&E). (c) Positive immunohistochemical stain with desmin highlighting presence of striated muscle within tumor. (d) Positive immunohistochemical stain with S-100. This verifies the presence of neural component within the tumor. (e) Positive immunohistochemical stain with MyoD transcription factor demonstrating myogenic component of tumor.

which was also evident by the abundancy of mitotic figures. She is currently undergoing chemotherapy with ifosfamide with adriamycin at the exact same dosing schedule received by her sister. We plan to continue this treatment regimen for four cycles with concurrent radiotherapy.

3. Discussion

MPNSTs with elements of rhabdomyoblastic differentiation are termed as malignant triton tumors (MTTs). MTTs are referred to as a mosaic tumor due to their muscular and neurogenic components [12]. Masson was the first to report the presence of rhabdomyoblasts in this neurogenic tumor and described them as rhabdomyomas of the nerve [13]. It was not until 1973 that Woodruff et al. introduced the term MTT [14].

The incidence of MPNSTs is 1 per 100,000 cases [3]. MTTs account for 5–10% of MPNSTs [1]. NF-1 (von Recklinghausen's disease) has been associated with an increased incidence of MPNSTs and MTTs [2]. MTTs are associated with NF-1 disease in 50–70% of the cases, occurring mainly in young males. The remaining cases are comprised of sporadic growths, occurring mostly in older females. A postradiotherapy manifestation has also been described [6]. Unlike the cases described in the literature, our patients are older female patients with MTTs in association with NF-1.

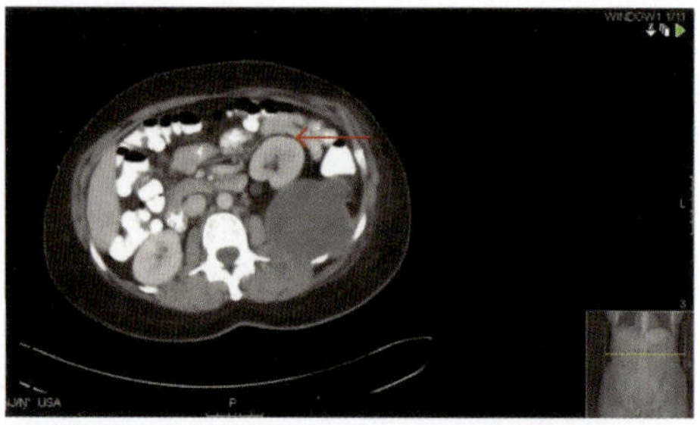

FIGURE 3: Red arrow pointing to the displaced left kidney by the soft tissue mass.

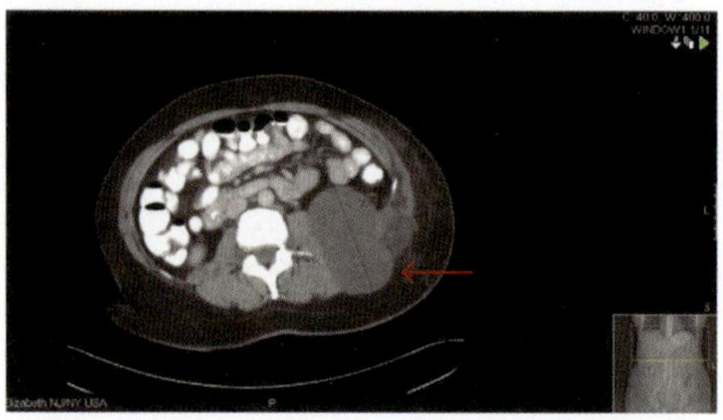

FIGURE 4: Red arrow pointing to the cystic component of the soft tissue mass with its measurement.

The most established theory regarding the histopathogenesis of MTTs is that multipotent neural crest cells of ectomesenchymal origin are capable of divergent differentiation to both nerve and muscle components [3]. It has also been proposed that Schwann cells in neurogenic tumor could be stimulated by motor nerves to differentiate into rhabdomyoblastic components. Alternatively, E. Kamperis et al. demonstrated in a rat model that neoplastic Schwann cells possess the capacity for mesenchymal differentiation into rhabdomyoblasts [6].

In the majority of reported cases, triton tumors are located across peripheral nerves, usually close to the spine, commonly in the head and neck region [3]. Few cases have previously been observed in the mediastinum and extremities [1–3]. Less common sites include buttocks and the retroperitoneum [3]. Cases as rare as intracardiac presentation of MTTs have been reported [15, 16]. MTTs typically present as a rapidly enlarging mass with associated pain and compressive symptoms to adjacent organs.

Woodruff et al. established the original histological criteria for the diagnosis of the malignant triton tumors. He stated that the tumors must arise along the course of a peripheral nerve or in a preexisting neurofibroma in patients with NF-1. Additionally, the tumors must display identical growth characteristics of Schwann cells. Finally, they must contain "bona fide" rhabdomyoblasts originating from the body of peripheral nerve tumor and not from extension or metastasis of an extrinsic rhabdomyosarcoma [14]. Daimaru et al. further broadened the definition to encompass the sporadic forms in patients without NF-1, which, he argued, are microscopically comparable malignant schwannomas with focal rhabdomyoblasts, and tumors consisting predominantly of rhabdomyoblastic differentiation with focal Schwann cell elements occurring within a nerve or in patients with NF-1 [17].

Today, the diagnosis of MTT is generally made according to these criteria as well as immunohistochemical findings for cell origin tracing. Nerve sheath differentiation is confirmed by S-100 protein and Leu-7 (CD57) positivity. Rhabdomyoblastic differentiation is confirmed by immunohistochemical positivity for desmin, actin, and myogenin [3, 12]. Through these findings, the diagnosis of MTT can be positively made and the proper course of treatment can be pursued.

However, one major area of concern for clinicians is the rate of tumor occurrence and regrowth after appropriate treatment. Local recurrence rate varies from 22% to 43% [1, 7, 18] and metastasis has been reported to occur in 20–50% of cases [7, 18]. Recurrence is dependent on several factors, including tumor location, extent of surgical excision, degree of differentiation and growth pattern, and performance status and comorbidities [6]. Tumors originating from head and neck have lower rates of recurrence, whereas tumors originating from the trunk, buttocks, retroperitoneum, and CNS have lower rates of recurrence. Wong et al. reported that MTTs involving nonextremity sites have a higher likelihood to recur.

Lymphatic invasion and lymph node involvement has not been reported in patients with MTT [6]. The most common site of metastasis is lung [1], but common extra pulmonary metastases include bone, liver, peritoneum, and the central nervous system. PET/CT is helpful in detecting distant metastases [1]. Anecdotal views vary regarding the impact of NF-1 status on survival. Zakzouk et al. report that NF-1 is associated with more incidence of metastasis [19], while Kamperis et al. mention, in a literature review, that NF-1 does not affect prognosis [6]. Few reports mention shorter survival in cases of MTT not associated with NF-1 [14].

Currently, there is no consensus regarding the treatment guidelines for malignant triton tumors. Several authors have proposed recommendations, including radical excision, radical excision followed by radiotherapy and chemotherapy, and excision with high dose radiotherapy. However, as for any other sarcoma, resection of the tumor with wide margins followed by radiotherapy is the recommended treatment. The need for chemotherapy has not been clearly defined [19]. Some recent reports suggest that neoadjuvant and adjuvant therapies can eradicate micrometastases [11]. In the case of suboptimal cytoreduction, a second more extensive surgical excision should always be pursued [6]. Proposed chemotherapeutic regimens include PEI (cisplatin, etoposide, and ifosfamide) as first-line chemotherapy and IA (ifosfamide and adriamycin) or MAID (mesna, doxorubicin, ifosfamide, and dacarbazine) as second-line treatment. There have been previously reported cases of MTTs that responded favorably to treatment with isotretinoin (a retinoid analogue) and interferon-α [6]. In conclusion, there are conflicting recommendations in the literature regarding the optimal treatment of MTTs [6, 9, 11, 19]. We can only agree that further investigations and case reports are necessary in order

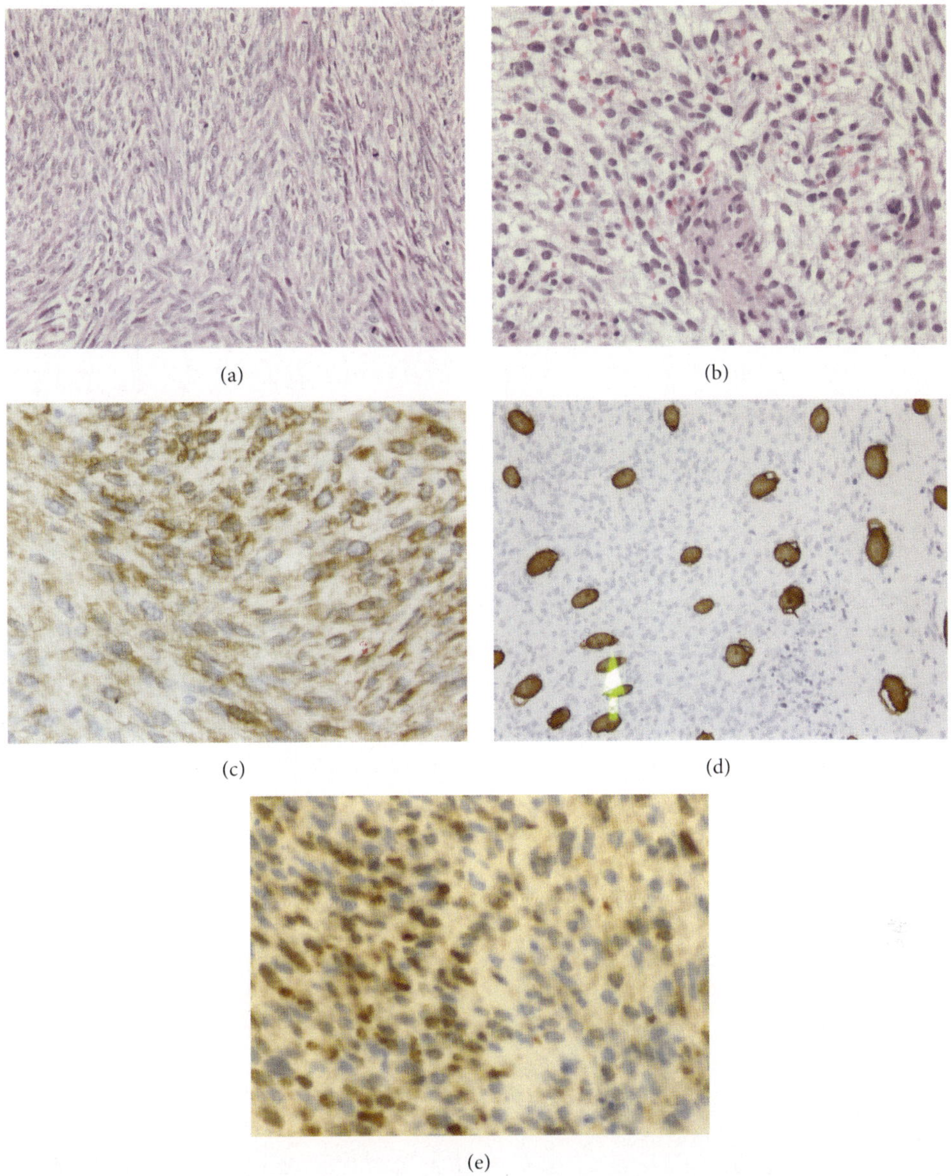

FIGURE 5: (a) Malignant triton tumor (MTT) cells. Spindle, fasciculated, and pleomorphic malignant schwannoma cells are appreciable with numerous mitotic figures in the field. (b) Eosinophilic rhabdomyoblasts within malignant schwannoma cells. (c) Positive immunohistochemical stain with NF-200 highlighting neurofilamentous component of tumor. (d) Positive immunohistochemical stain with desmin. (e) Positive immunohistochemical stain with MyoD transcription factor demonstrating myogenic component of tumor.

to continue contributing to our knowledge of MTTs, their clinical courses, and treatment outcomes.

In our case reports, we treated the first sister with four cycles of adjuvant ifosfamide and adriamycin along with radiotherapy after wide surgical excision and reresection of the tumor. She responded well to it and remains disease-free even after 4 years of initial diagnosis. We are treating the second sister with the same chemotherapy regimen along with concurrent radiotherapy. She is currently responding well to treatment with few side effects. We will continue to monitor her and observe her treatment response.

We present the cases of MTTs in two sisters with clinical neurofibromatosis. Our cases are unique due to their sisterly presentation within a decade of each other. This is in contrast to MPNSTs, which have been previously described in siblings. Additionally, MTTs in the setting of NF-1 have not been seen in our patient demographics: middle-aged females. Given the aggressive nature of this tumor subtype, one of the sisters has remained disease-free for four years after initiation of adjuvant chemotherapeutic therapy. We are hopeful of the treatment potential for her sister. Additionally, the information learned regarding this disease type may help shed light on the role of chemotherapy in care of patients diagnosed with MTTs.

Ethical Aapproval

Written informed consent was obtained from the patient for publication of this case report and accompanying images.

Disclosure

No off-label drug use was disclosed.

Acknowledgments

The authors acknowledge Dr. Leon Isaac and Dr. Heidi Fish, Department of Pathology, Trinitas Hospital, for picture courtesy.

References

[1] S. C. Kamran, A. B. Shinagare, S. A. Howard, J. L. Hornick, and N. H. Ramaiya, "A-Z of malignant peripheral nerve sheath tumors," *Cancer Imaging*, vol. 12, no. 3, pp. 475–483, 2012.

[2] D. S. Nirhale, A. Parasnis, C. Bora, R. Gupta, and P. Aulakh, "Retroperitoneal peripheral nerve sheath tumour of triton type—a case report," *Indian Journal of Surgery*, vol. 75, supplement 1, pp. S12–S14, 2013.

[3] W. Ren, X. Xu, J. Yan, X. Qian, and B. Liu, "Malignant triton tumor of the anterior mediastinum: a case report," *Oncology Letters*, vol. 7, no. 3, pp. 807–810, 2014.

[4] K. Mae, Y. Kato, K. Usui, N. Abe, and R. Tsuboi, "A case of malignant peripheral nerve sheath tumor with rhabdomyoblastic differentiation: malignant triton tumor," *Case Reports in Dermatology*, vol. 5, no. 3, pp. 373–378, 2013.

[5] P. Locatelli, "Formation des memres surnumeraires," *Comptes Rendus de l'Association des Anatomistes*, vol. 20, pp. 279–282, 1925.

[6] E. Kamperis, N. Barbetakis, C. Asteriou, A. Kleontas, and V. Christoforidou, "Malignant triton tumor of the chest wall invading the lung. A case report and literature review," *Hippokratia*, vol. 17, no. 3, pp. 277–280, 2013.

[7] Z. Li, J. Xiang, S. Yan, F. Gao, and S. Zheng, "Malignant triton tumor of the retroperitoneum: a case report and review of the literature," *World Journal of Surgical Oncology*, vol. 10, article 96, 2012.

[8] C. J. Stasik and O. Tawfik, "Malignant peripheral nerve sheath tumor with rhabdomyosarcomatous differentiation (malignant triton tumor)," *Archives of Pathology and Laboratory Medicine*, vol. 130, no. 12, pp. 1878–1881, 2006.

[9] Y. J. McConnell and C. A. Giacomantonio, "Malignant triton tumors—complete surgical resection and adjuvant radiotherapy associated with improved survival," *Journal of Surgical Oncology*, vol. 106, no. 1, pp. 51–56, 2012.

[10] C.-C. H. Stucky, K. N. Johnson, R. J. Gray et al., "Malignant peripheral nerve sheath tumors (MPNST): the mayo clinic experience," *Annals of Surgical Oncology*, vol. 19, no. 3, pp. 878–885, 2012.

[11] P. K. Shetty, S. V. Baliga, and K. Balaiah, "Malignant triton tumor: a rare case," *Indian Journal of Surgery*, vol. 75, supplement 1, pp. S362–S365, 2013.

[12] T. Omar, H. Raslan, S. El-Sheikh, M. Rizq, and A. Draz, "Low-grade malignant triton tumor of the neck: a case report and review of the literature," *Case Reports in Pathology*, vol. 2014, Article ID 674094, 5 pages, 2014.

[13] P. Masson, *Recklinghausen's Neurofibromatosis, Sensory Neuromas and Motor Neuromas*, International Press, New York, NY, USA, 1932.

[14] J. M. Woodruff, N. L. Chernik, M. C. Smith, W. B. Millett, and F. W. Foote Jr., "Peripheral nerve tumors with rhabdomyosarcomatous differentiation (malignant 'triton' tumors)," *Cancer*, vol. 32, no. 2, pp. 426–439, 1973.

[15] Y. Takahashi, Y. Sugita, T. Abe, T. Yuge, T. Tokutomi, and M. Shigemori, "Intraventricular malignant triton tumour," *Acta Neurochirurgica*, vol. 142, no. 4, pp. 473–477, 2000.

[16] S. Kabir, E. I. Kapetanakis, and F. Shabbo, "Intracardiac malignant triton tumor: a first presentation," *Annals of Thoracic Surgery*, vol. 89, no. 3, pp. 968–969, 2010.

[17] Y. Daimaru, H. Hashimoto, and M. Enjoji, "Malignant 'triton' tumors: a clinicopathologic and immunohistochemical study of nine cases," *Human Pathology*, vol. 15, no. 8, pp. 768–778, 1984.

[18] M. Nitsche, M. Reible, K.-H. Pflüger, M. Bergmann, and R. M. Hermann, "Malignant triton tumor of the sciatic nerve as a secondary malignancy after extended field radiotherapy and chemotherapy of Hodgkin's disease," *Case Reports in Oncology*, vol. 7, no. 1, pp. 239–245, 2014.

[19] A. Zakzouk, F. Hammad, O. Langlois, M. Aziz, J. Marie, and O. Choussy, "Malignant triton tumour of the sinonasal tract: case report and literature review," *International Journal of Surgery Case Reports*, vol. 5, no. 9, pp. 608–612, 2014.

Chemotherapy in the Setting of Severe Liver Dysfunction in Patients with Metastatic Colorectal Cancer

Pashtoon Murtaza Kasi, Gita Thanarajasingam, Heidi D. Finnes, Jose C. Villasboas Bisneto, Joleen M. Hubbard, and Axel Grothey

Division of Medical Oncology, Mayo Clinic, Rochester, MN 55905, USA

Correspondence should be addressed to Pashtoon Murtaza Kasi; kasi.pashtoon@mayo.edu

Academic Editor: Jorg Kleeff

The liver is the dominant site of metastases for patients with metastatic colorectal cancer (mCRC). Depending on the timing of diagnosis and the biology of the disease, it is not uncommon for these patients to present with visceral crisis in the form of severe liver dysfunction. Treatment of these individuals is, however, difficult and challenging. The decision to consider chemotherapy in these dire circumstances entails consideration of numerous factors. If we were to focus on just the metabolism of the different drugs and biologic agents available to treat mCRC, both 5-fluorouracil and oxaliplatin alone or in combination with a monoclonal antibody are reasonable choices. Specifically, FOLFOX is a feasible and safe option in patients with mCRC with severe liver dysfunction. Choice of the biologic agent to add to the doublet chemotherapy could be individualized based on the RAS status and the clinical scenario. Based on the divergent experience of treating 2 cases and other prior reports, a summary of recommendations with a model in the form of a "therapeutic triad" is presented. The paper highlights the therapeutic challenges in patients with mCRC and severe liver dysfunction. The choice of chemotherapeutic agents and reports of other cases/series is also presented.

1. Background

The liver is the dominant site of metastases for patients with metastatic colorectal cancer (mCRC). Depending on the timing of diagnosis and the biology of the disease, it is not uncommon for these patients to present with visceral crisis in the form of severe liver dysfunction. The decision to consider chemotherapy in these dire circumstances is challenging and entails consideration of numerous factors. Here we present 2 cases of mCRC with severe liver dysfunction and their discordant outcomes after initiation of chemotherapy alongside a biologic agent. Based on the experience with these cases and other prior reports, a summary of recommendations with a model in the form of a "therapeutic triad" is presented.

2. Case Presentations

2.1. Case 1. Our first case is that of a 43-year-old man who presented with abdominal pain in June 2014. He developed progressive symptoms of night sweats, abdominal pain, weight loss, nausea, and vomiting over the last several weeks. On examination, he was noted to have scleral icterus, a distended abdomen, and hepatomegaly. His performance status (PS) based on the Eastern Cooperative Oncology Group (ECOG) system was 1. Computerized tomography (CT) scan revealed innumerable liver metastases (Figures 1(a) and 1(b)).

Pertinent laboratory findings are summarized in Table 1. Fine needle aspiration (FNA) cytology of a liver lesion confirmed the diagnosis of metastatic moderately differentiated adenocarcinoma. Colonoscopy confirmed the stenosing friable malignancy in the ascending colon with concern for obstruction.

While waiting for diagnostic confirmation, the patient developed fever, tachycardia, leukocytosis, and symptoms of worsening obstruction. He underwent palliative-intent right hemicolectomy. Pathology showed invasive poorly differentiated adenocarcinoma, T4a N2b (18/22) M1 Grade 3 forming a circumferential ulcerated mass in the right colon.

One week postoperatively, he continued to deteriorate clinically and laboratory parameters are shown in Table 1. His

TABLE 1: Pertinent trends in laboratory investigations and clinical parameters for Cases 1 and 2.

	Case 1			Case 2		
	At diagnosis	Postoperative[1]	Postchemo[1]	At diagnosis*	Postoperative[1]	Postchemo[1]
Total bilirubin	1.9	9.4	18.4	—	8.4	3.9
Direct bilirubin	1.4	8.2	16.4	—	6.2	2.4
Aspartate transaminase (AST)	679	1116	1542	—	179	82
Alanine transaminase (ALT)	314	322	—	—	—	—
Alkaline phosphatase (AlkPhos)	379	579	966	—	1708	1167
Carcinoembryonic antigen (CEA)	178.3	271.9	2770	—	0.7	—
ECOG performance status	1	3	5	1	3	0-1

[1]Postoperative and postchemotherapy laboratory investigations were roughly 1 week and 2 weeks apart, respectively.
*At diagnosis, laboratory investigations for Case 2 were reportedly within normal limits.

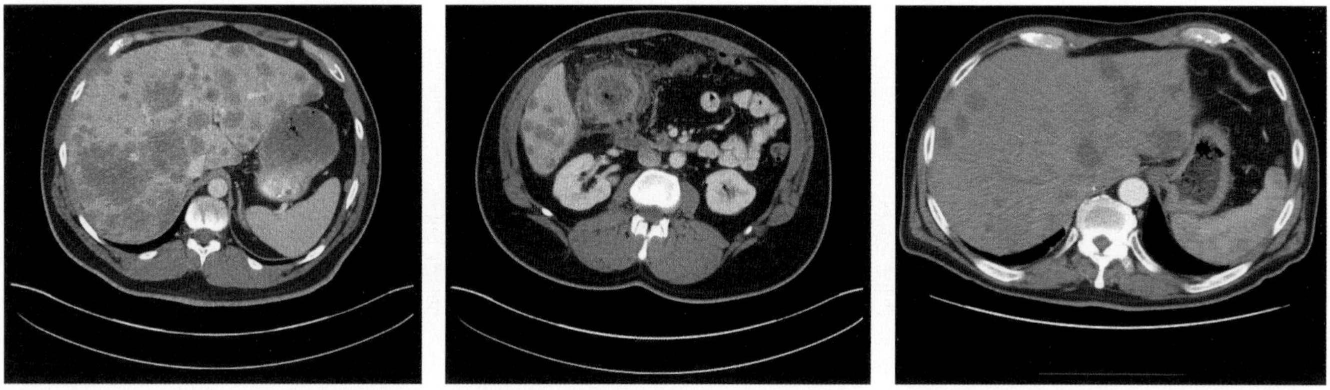

(a) (b) (c)

FIGURE 1: (a) CT scan of the abdomen showing innumerable liver metastases in a patient (Case 1) with colorectal cancer (a) and the primary mass in the ascending colon (b). Image (c) shows a similar scan with multiple liver metastases in another patient (Case 2) with mCRC.

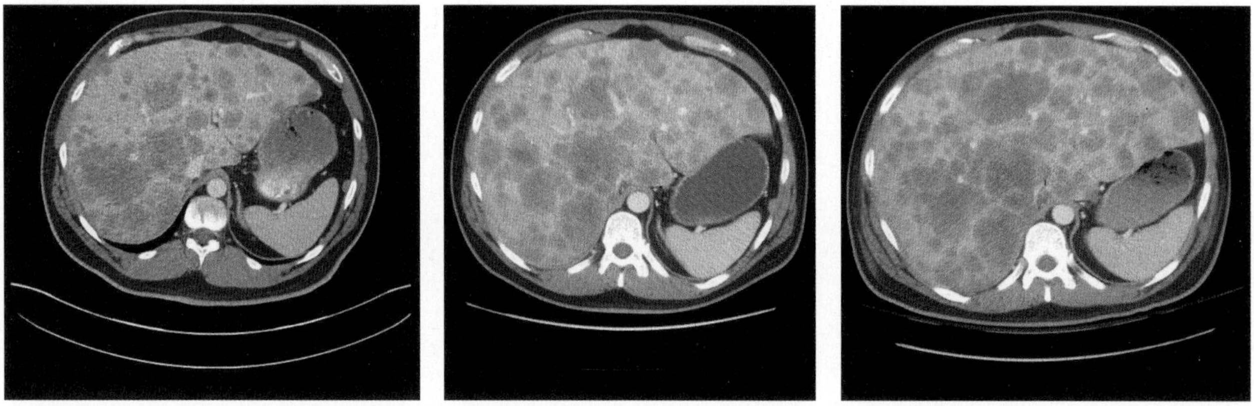

(a) (b) (c)

FIGURE 2: Case 1: CT scan of the abdomen showing rapid progression in both size and number of the previously noted innumerable liver metastases in a patient with mCRC: (a) day 0, (b) day 10, and (c) day 18.

ECOG PS now had declined to 3 from 1 earlier. Updated imaging was obtained and showed dramatic progression of disease as noted in Figure 2.

2.2. Case 2. Our second case is that of a 64-year-old previously healthy man who presented with fatigue and a 45-pound weight loss over three months, ECOG-1. Workup by his primary care physician was notable for iron-deficiency anemia. Colonoscopy revealed a tumor in the ascending colon. CT scan showed extensive liver metastases (Figure 1(c)). He underwent palliative-intent hemicolectomy due to bleeding from the tumor and was noted to have invasive adenocarcinoma, pT3 N2 (15/17) M1 Grade 3 with extensive synchronous liver metastases.

Two weeks later when he presented to our institution, he had developed dark urine. Exam was significant for scleral icterus and hepatomegaly. He had also declined clinically with an ECOG of 3. Pertinent laboratory findings are outlined in Table 1.

2.3. Therapeutic Challenges/Choice: FOLFOX ± Monoclonal Antibody. Both of our cases represented rapidly progressive mCRC with associated visceral crisis in the form of liver dysfunction from innumerable liver metastases. The decision to treat these patients with chemotherapy was complex. However, both of these patients were otherwise healthy prior to rapid clinical deterioration which was attributed in both cases to the disease. Based on consensus and understanding the risks involved, we decided to proceed with chemotherapy alongside a monoclonal antibody since in both patients the tumors were chemotherapy naïve and had not received any prior treatment apart from resection of the primary tumor.

Our first patient was started on modified FOLFOX (mFOLFOX7) with the monoclonal antibody panitumumab added later on once the tumor was noted to be RAS wild-type. Laboratory studies two days later showed significant tumor lysis in the form of hyperkalemia, hyperuricemia, and high lactate dehydrogenase (LDH) (Table 1). The patient subsequently went into renal failure with ongoing worsening liver failure and unfortunately died within 6 weeks.

Our second patient, however, did well with treatment. He was also started initially on modified FOLFOX (mFOLFOX7) with the monoclonal antibody bevacizumab added with cycle 2 of chemotherapy. Within the first cycle of treatment, the patient was noted to have improvement in his signs/symptoms (appetite/jaundice) as well as his laboratory parameters (Table 1). After 5 cycles, his laboratory findings normalized and the hepatomegaly and size of liver metastases decreased. After 10 cycles of mFOLFOX7 with bevacizumab, he was switched to FOLFIRI, followed by FOLFOX and cetuximab, and subsequently single agent cetuximab. The patient survived for 18 months from the time of diagnosis.

The following discussion relates to therapeutic challenges in patients with mCRC and severe liver dysfunction. The choice of chemotherapeutic agents and reports of other cases/series is discussed.

3. Discussion

The occurrence of visceral crisis in the form of liver dysfunction from liver metastases is not an uncommon phenomenon since the liver is the dominant organ of metastases for patients with mCRC. Treatment of these individuals is, however, difficult and challenging in terms of the choice and safety of the different chemotherapies and biologics [1].

These two cases represent rapidly progressive mCRC with significant deterioration within a matter of weeks. Choosing a particular chemotherapy in the setting of organ dysfunction is challenging, especially when there is ongoing decline in the patient's performance status.

If we were to focus on just the metabolism of the different drugs and biologic agents available to treat mCRC, both 5-fluorouracil and oxaliplatin alone or in combination with

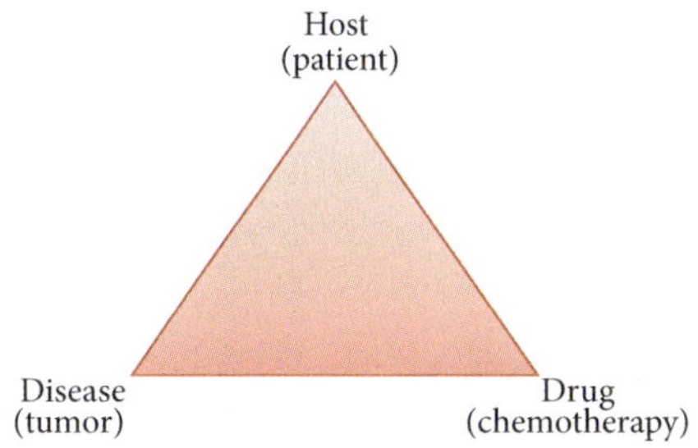

FIGURE 3: "Therapeutic triad" of the host, the drug, and the disease: factors to consider when giving chemotherapy to patients.

a monoclonal antibody are reasonable choices to consider in these patients [2–5]. Table 2 outlines the different agents available to treat mCRC in more detail. FOLFOX is a feasible and safe option in patients with mCRC with severe liver dysfunction (Table 3) [6–9]. In the palliative-intent setting, we typically avoid the 5-FU bolus since it leads to neutropenia, mucositis, and dose delays.

On the other hand, regorafenib and irinotecan would not be recommended in this subset of patients given adverse outcomes reported with respect to hepatic dysfunction (Table 2). TAS-102 is a novel antimetabolite being used for treatment of mCRC; clinical trials to evaluate its safety in patients with hepatic dysfunction are currently ongoing [10]. Mitomycin with capecitabine has also been employed in the palliative setting and does not require dose adjustments for hepatic impairment; however, the regimen is used infrequently [11].

With respect to our two cases, there was rapid deterioration of performance status in these individuals which was attributed to tumor progression. In these situations, an aggressive strategy with doublet based chemotherapy with or without a biologic should be considered. Rapidly progressive, life-threatening disease is a dire now-or-never scenario and if the decision is made to initiate treatment, it would not be appropriate to start with "chemo-light" such as 5-FU single agent.

These cases illustrate two very different extreme outcomes that can be seen in patients with mCRC and concomitant liver dysfunction. While our first patient died within weeks of initiation of chemotherapy, our second patient achieved rapid improvement of symptoms and stabilization of disease for a significant period of time after diagnosis. This is consistent with the 3 other cases reported from Roswell Park Cancer Institute [6]. Outcomes for other patients were somewhat similar with initial response followed by progression later and exposure to multiple lines of chemotherapy approved for mCRC.

These cases open the debate as to if and when systemic chemotherapy with or without biologics is an option for patients with mCRC and liver dysfunction. The decision is not straightforward but can be rationalized along the lines of a "therapeutic triad" incorporating the host, the drug, and the disease, which is usually at the back of our minds when we treat any patient with chemotherapy (Figure 3).

The most important part of the triad is the host (the patient). In our cases and others described in the literature, liver dysfunction was attributed to the metastases, and the

Table 2: List of chemotherapeutic and biologic agents for patients with mCRC.

	Pharmacokinetics	Metabolism	Comments
5-Fluorouracil (5-FU) [13]	$T_{1/2}$ 16 minutes (range 8–20 minutes) Excreted via lung (as CO_2) and urine	Hepatic by dihydropyrimidine dehydrogenase (DPD) to active metabolites 5-fluoroxyuridine monophosphate (F-UMP) and 5-5-fluoro-2'-deoxyuridine-5'-O-monophosphate (F-dUMP)	Limited data in patients with total bilirubin > 5, may be treated with weekly infusion without adjustment [4].
Oxaliplatin [14]	Protein bound $T_{1/2}$ 0.43 to 16.8 hours (distribution) and 391 hours (terminal) Urinary excretion	Nonenzymatic	No apparent alteration in clearance or toxicity in patients with severe liver dysfunction [3, 15, 16].
Irinotecan [17]	SN-38 protein bound $T_{1/2}$ irinotecan 6–12 hours; SN-38 ~10–20 hours Excreted via urine 11–20% and via biliary tract	Hydrolyzed in the liver to active metabolite SN-38 which is further metabolized by glucuronidation by UDP-glucuronosyltransferase 1-1 (also known as UGT1A1)	In patients with varying degrees of liver dysfunction, severe side effects, poor tolerability, and overall worsening of PS were noted. [2, 18, 19]
TAS-102 [10, 20]; combination drug consisting of alpha,alpha,alpha-trifluorothymidine (FTD) and thymidine phosphorylase inhibitor (TPI)	Readily absorbed $T_{1/2}$ FTD 1.4 hours, TPI 1.7–2.1 hours Limited urinary excretion FTD; TPI 29% excreted via urine	FTD undergoes hepatic metabolism, TPI minimal hepatic metabolism	Phase-I studies in patients with hepatic impairment are ongoing.
Regorafenib [21]	$T_{1/2}$ for the drug 28 hours (14 to 58 hours; some metabolites may take longer for excretion, 32 to 70 hours)	Hepatic by CYP3A4 and UGT1A9	Severe drug induced liver injury has been reported with the use of drug; its use in patients with liver dysfunction would generally be avoided and requires close monitoring of liver function tests.
Monoclonal antibodies* [5]	$T_{1/2}$ long: days to weeks	No liver metabolism/clearance	Generally acceptable to use if there are no other contraindications.

*Anti-VEGF antibodies (bevacizumab/aflibercept) and antiepidermal growth factor (EGFR) antibodies (panitumumab/cetuximab) [1].

patients were otherwise healthy and active with a good overall performance status prior to the diagnosis. If these patients already had been declining and had other significant comorbidities, we would have been less inclined to consider any treatment option at all. Both of these patients had palliative-intent surgery to begin with, which signifies overall reasonable clinical status of these patients.

The second consideration is the underlying disease, in this case mCRC. Both of these tumors had no prior exposure to any chemotherapy or biologics; therefore, they were felt to be chemosensitive with potential for response and improvement in organ dysfunction [5]. This is noted in our second case and in other cases described in the literature. In patients with mCRC who develop liver dysfunction from liver metastases after multiple lines of chemotherapy, the odds of further chemotherapy leading to significant organ recovery are low. These patients may actually be harmed with more chemotherapy in the setting of liver dysfunction.

The last consideration is the choice of drug itself. As noted in Table 2, initial considerations should be made towards choosing 5-FU in combination with oxaliplatin. A monoclonal antibody could be considered initially or staggered later as noted in our cases when the RAS status is known. Even though the liver is involved in the turnover of most circulating antibodies, it is not considered rate limiting in this instance. The enzyme dihydropyrimidine dehydrogenase (DPD) metabolizes 5-FU and there are individuals with DPD deficiency that can potentially have severe and potentially

TABLE 3: Previous case reports of patients with mCRC and severe liver dysfunction treated with FOLFOX (reprinted with permission from JNCCN, Journal of the National Comprehensive Cancer Network [7]).

Age (y), sex	mFOLFOX6 (each drug dose: mg/m^2)		Total bilirubin (mg/dL)		CEA (ng/mL)		Response	FOLFOX cycles until disease progression
	1st cycle progression[a]	2nd cycle[a]	Baseline	After 2 cycles	Baseline	After 2 cycles		
Case 1: 63, M [6]	Bolus 5-FU: 300, IV 5-FU: 1800, LV: 200, Ox: 60	Bolus 5-FU: 400, IV 5-FU: 240, LV: 400, Ox: 85	3.5	1.2	188.0	4.8	PR	14
Case 2: 59, F [6]	Bolus 5-FU: 0, IV 5-FU: 2000, LV: 400, Ox: 65	Bolus 5-FU: 0, IV 5-FU: 2400, LV: 400, Ox: 85	5.9	2.1	1.3	895.0	SD	8
Case 3: 37, F [6]	Bolus 5-FU: 0, IV 5-FU: 200, LV: 400, Ox: 85	Bolus 5-FU: 400, IV 5-FU: 2400, LV: 400, Ox: 85	4.2	2.1	3685.0	937.0	PR	≥10
Case 4: 67, M [7]	Bolus 5-FU: 200, IV 5-FU: 1200, LV: 200, Ox: 75	Bolus 5-FU: 200, IV 5-FU: 1200, LV: 200, Ox: 75	9.4	2.4	12.2	4.0	PR	21
Case 5: 58, F [8]	Bolus 5-FU: 0, IV 5-FU: 2400, L-LV: 200, Ox: 85	Bolus 5-FU: 400, IV 5-FU: 2400, L-LV: 200, Ox: 85	3.9	2.2	103.1	96.0	SD	6

CEA: carcinoembryonic antigen; F: female; FOLFOX: 5-FU, leucovorin, and oxaliplatin; IV: infusional; L-LV: levoleucovorin; LV: leucovorin; M: male; Ox: oxaliplatin; PR: partial response; SD: stable disease.
[a]Bolus 5-FU, infusional 5-FU, LV, and oxaliplatin.

lethal side effects [12]. However, genetic assessment for DPD deficiency is not routine practice but can be considered in patients who experience side effects that are out of proportion to those that would ordinarily be seen with 5-FU. With genetic tests, there is typically a long turnaround time that would limit its use in these clinical situations.

The "therapeutic triad" above in combination with other patient specific factors and goals of care can help individualize treatment decisions in patients with severe liver dysfunction and visceral crisis from mCRC.

Abbreviations

ALT: Alanine transaminase
AST: Aspartate transaminase
AlkPhos: Alkaline phosphatase
CEA: Carcinoembryonic antigen
ECOG: Eastern Cooperative Oncology Group
KRAS: Kirsten rat sarcoma oncogene
mCRC: Metastatic colorectal cancer
PS: Performance status
VEGF: Vascular endothelial growth factor.

Disclosure

No writing assistance was utilized in the production of this paper. Table 3 was reprinted with permission from JNCCN, Journal of the National Comprehensive Cancer Network, whose assistance is appreciated.

Acknowledgment

The authors are also deeply indebted to the patients and their families for their trust and for allowing them to utilize their information in the form of a case report.

References

[1] P. M. Kasi, J. M. Hubbard, and A. Grothey, "Selection of biologics for patients with metastatic colorectal cancer: the role of predictive markers," *Expert Review of Gastroenterology & Hepatology*, vol. 9, no. 3, pp. 273–276, 2015.

[2] E. Raymond, V. Boige, S. Faivre et al., "Dosage adjustment and pharmacokinetic profile of irinotecan in cancer patients with hepatic dysfunction," *Journal of Clinical Oncology*, vol. 20, no. 21, pp. 4303–4312, 2002.

[3] J. H. Doroshow, T. W. Synold, D. Gandara et al., "Pharmacology of oxaliplatin in solid tumor patients with hepatic dysfunction: a preliminary report of the National Cancer Institute Organ Dysfunction Working Group," *Seminars in Oncology*, vol. 30, no. 4, pp. 14–19, 2003.

[4] G. F. Fleming, R. L. Schilsky, L. P. Schumn et al., "Phase I and pharmacokinetic study of 24-hour infusion 5-fluorouracil and leucovorin in patients with organ dysfuntion," *Annals of Oncology*, vol. 14, no. 7, pp. 1142–1147, 2003.

[5] K. Shitara, D. Takahari, T. Yokota et al., "Case Series of cetuximab monotherapy for patients with pre-treated colorectal cancer complicated with hyperbilirubinemia due to severe liver metastasis," *Japanese Journal of Clinical Oncology*, vol. 40, no. 3, pp. 275–277, 2010.

[6] M. G. Fakih, "5-Fluorouracil leucovorin and oxaliplatin (FOLFOX) in the treatment of metastatic colon cancer with severe liver dysfunction," *Oncology*, vol. 67, no. 3-4, pp. 222–224, 2004.

[7] R. Elsoueidi, J. Craig, H. Mourad, and E. M. Richa, "Safety and efficacy of FOLFOX followed by cetuximab for metastatic colorectal cancer with severe liver dysfunction," *Journal of the National Comprehensive Cancer Network*, vol. 12, pp. 155–160, 2014.

[8] T. Shimura, H. Kataoka, Y. Hirata et al., "Metastatic colorectal cancer with severe liver dysfunction successfully treated using FOLFOX therapy," *Journal of Gastrointestinal Cancer*, vol. 42, no. 1, pp. 68–72, 2011.

[9] T. Grenader, A. Goldberg, and A. Gabizon, "Combination therapy with oxaliplatin and 5-fluorouracil in a patient with severe hepatic dysfunction associated with metastatic adenocarcinoma of the large bowel," *Anti-Cancer Drugs*, vol. 20, no. 9, pp. 845–847, 2009.

[10] T. Yoshino, N. Mizunuma, K. Yamazaki et al., "TAS-102 monotherapy for pretreated metastatic colorectal cancer: a double-blind, randomised, placebo-controlled phase 2 trial," *The Lancet Oncology*, vol. 13, no. 10, pp. 993–1001, 2012.

[11] G. Chong, J. L. B. Dickson, D. Cunningham et al., "Capecitabine and mitomycin C as third-line therapy for patients with metastatic colorectal cancer resistant to fluorouracil and irinotecan," *British Journal of Cancer*, vol. 93, no. 5, pp. 510–514, 2005.

[12] K. E. Caudle, C. F. Thorn, T. E. Klein et al., "Clinical pharmacogenetics implementation consortium guidelines for dihydropyrimidine dehydrogenase genotype and fluoropyrimidine dosing," *Clinical Pharmacology and Therapeutics*, vol. 94, no. 6, pp. 640–645, 2013.

[13] *Adrucil [Package Insert]*, Teva Parental Medicines, Irvine, Calif, USA, 2007.

[14] *Eloxatin [Package Insert]*, Ben Venue Laboratories, Cleveland, Ohio, USA, 2011.

[15] M. Baur, A. Drescher, M. Gneist, C. Dittrich, and U. Jaehde, "Pharmacokinetics of oxaliplatin in patients with severe hepatic dysfunction," *Cancer Chemotherapy and Pharmacology*, vol. 61, no. 1, pp. 97–104, 2008.

[16] T. W. Synold, C. H. Takimoto, J. H. Doroshow et al., "Dose-escalating and pharmacologic study of oxaliplatin in adult cancer patients with impaired hepatic function: a national cancer institute organ dysfunction working group study," *Clinical Cancer Research*, vol. 13, no. 12, pp. 3660–3666, 2007.

[17] *Camptosar [Package Insert]*, Pfizer, New York, NY, USA, 2014.

[18] C. J. van Groeningen, W. J. F. van der Vijgh, J. J. Baars, H. Stieltjes, K. Huibregtse, and H. M. Pinedo, "Altered pharmacokinetics and metabolism of CPT-11 in liver dysfunction: a need for guidelines," *Clinical Cancer Research*, vol. 6, no. 4, pp. 1342–1346, 2000.

[19] A. P. Venook, C. E. Klein, G. Fleming et al., "A phase I and pharmacokinetic study of irinotecan in patients with hepatic or renal dysfunction or with prior pelvic radiation: CALGB 9863," *Annals of Oncology*, vol. 14, no. 12, pp. 1783–1790, 2003.

[20] *TAS-102: Investigator's Brochure Version G 5.0 14*, Taiho Pharmaceutical, Tokyo, Japan, 2014.

[21] *STIVARGA (Package Insert)*, Bayer Healthcare, 2014.

5

Metastasis of Ciliary Body Melanoma to the Contralateral Eye: A Case Report

Nouritza M. Torossian,[1] Roy T. Wallace,[2] Wen-Jen Hwu,[3] and Agop Y. Bedikian[3]

[1] *Institut Universitaire du Cancer de Toulouse Oncopole, Toulouse, France*
[2] *Retina Consultants of Nashville, Nashville, TN, USA*
[3] *MD Anderson Cancer Center, Houston, TX, USA*

Correspondence should be addressed to Agop Y. Bedikian; abedikia@gmail.com

Academic Editor: Jose I. Mayordomo

Many types of cancers metastasize to the eye. However, uveal melanoma metastasizing to the contralateral choroid is very rare. We report the case of a 68-year-old man with history of treated uveal melanoma of the right eye that developed metastasis to the liver and the choroid of the left eye. Ten years earlier, he was diagnosed to have uveal melanoma of the right eye and was initially treated with plaque radiotherapy. Two years later, upon progression of the disease in the right eye he had enucleation of the eye. We describe the patient's clinical history, the diagnosis of recurrent disease in the contralateral eye, therapy of the left eye, and systemic metastasis. In addition, we reviewed the published medical literature and described the recent advances in the management of uveal melanoma.

1. Introduction

Uveal melanoma is the most common primary intraocular malignant tumor in adults [1]. After cutaneous melanoma, it is the second most common type of primary melanoma, representing about 3% of all melanoma diagnoses [2]. The mean incidence of uveal melanoma in the United States is approximately 5 new cases per million people [2]. There are 4100 new cases of uveal melanoma diagnosed in the United States each year [2]. The peak incidence of uveal melanoma occurs from 65 to 70 years [3]. About 98.8% of the cases occur in Caucasians. Primary uveal melanoma arises from melanocytes located in the uveal tract, which comprises the iris, the ciliary body, and the choroid of the eye [3]. Melanomas of the posterior uveal tract including the ciliary body which usually are diagnosed late in view of location generally are more aggressive, metastasize often, and have the worst prognosis [3, 4]. Symptoms related to locally advanced uveal melanoma depend on the location of the primary. Over 95% of patients have disease limited to the eye at diagnosis [5]. Currently, patients with uveal melanoma often receive eye-preserving plaque radiation therapy and enjoy the same survival as those who undergo enucleation of the eye. Approximately 40% to 50% of patients with primary uveal melanoma ultimately develop systemic metastases [6]. The 5-year and 15-year survival rates from diagnosis of uveal melanoma are 45% and 30%, respectively [6]. Of the patients who die of uveal melanoma, about 60% and 90% do so within 5 and 15 years, respectively [6].

The survival of patients with metastatic uveal melanoma is directly related to the site of metastasis. The liver is involved in as many as 95% of individuals who develop metastatic disease [7, 8] and is the exclusive site of systemic metastasis in about 40% of patients [7]. Other common metastatic sites involved include lung (46%), bone (29%), and skin (17%) [7, 8]. The median survival of patients who develop liver metastasis is reported to be 6 to 7 months, and the 1-year survival rate is estimated to be 10% to 15% [8, 9].

Little progress has been made in the management of systemic metastases [6, 9]. Local, regional and systemic therapies for metastatic uveal melanoma have had little impact on duration of patient survival [9]. Metastatic cancers including melanoma have been reported to spread to the orbit of the eye [10, 11]. Malignancies other than melanoma metastasize to the uveal tract more often. Breast cancer is the most common tumor type to metastasize to the uveal tract and comprise 47% of the cases [12]. Uveal melanoma metastatic to uveal tract of contralateral eye is very rare. Here, we report the case of a 68-year-old man with uveal melanoma of the right eye with metastasis to the choroid of the left eye 10 years after initial treatment of the right eye.

2. Clinical Case

The patient is a 68-year-old white male who was diagnosed to have uveal melanoma of the right eye in June 1995 when he was 58 years old. The primary tumor was a ciliary body and superior choroidal melanoma of the right eye; it was 8 mm in height and 13-14 mm in basal diameter with an early area of neovascularization of the iris. He was treated with Iodine-125 plaque radiotherapy starting on 06/13/1995. It delivered 61.2 Gy at 8 mm depth. Regression of the lesion was observed subsequently. He remained free of the disease for 2 years, and in 1997 he had pain in the right eye due to tumor regrowth. He was treated with enucleation of the eye. In December 2004, he palpated a nodule on the left neck. A fine needle aspirate (FNA) taken from left supraclavicular lymph node on 12/14/2004 showed malignant cells, but definitive diagnosis of melanoma could not be made.

Radiologic staging with CT scan of the chest, abdomen, and pelvis performed in December 2004 showed hepatic metastases. PET scan performed on 12/03/04 detected enlarged lymph nodes in the retroperitoneum, mesenteric area, and the left supraclavicular area in addition to the liver metastases. A CT guided biopsy of the liver metastasis performed on 01/03/2005 showed metastatic melanoma with cells positive for HMB-45 and Melan-A immunohistochemical stains. Review of the pathology slides of the specimens taken from the lymph node and the liver in our institution confirmed the diagnosis of metastatic melanoma. FNA from the left supraclavicular lymph node showed similar findings.

On 01/11/2005 the patient returned with decreased vision in his left eye of 1 week duration. He also complained of seeing black spots and floaters. An MRI of the brain performed on 01/12/2005 showed no evidence of intracranial metastases. On slit lamp fundoscopic examination, multiple small choroidal metastatic lesions were seen in the posterior pole/fundus of the left eye, each measuring about 300 to 500 microns in size, associated with an exudative retinal detachment centrally (Figure 1). Fluorescein angiogram (Figure 2) and Optical Coherence Tomography (Figure 3) confirmed presence of choroidal infiltration with melanoma. The patient's left eye was treated with plaque radiotherapy for palliation. A total activity of 46.67 millicuries was delivered using Iodine-125 plaque that was placed on 01/26/05. Dose was downgraded to 70 Gy from the typical 85 Gy and delivered quickly (in 47 hours) as this was a palliative attempt.

The patient came to M. D. Anderson Cancer Center for a second opinion after seeking advice for therapy at Vanderbilt medical center and Memorial Sloan-Kettering Cancer Center. He was seen in the clinic on 02/08/05. At the time he complained of blurry vision at the left eye in addition

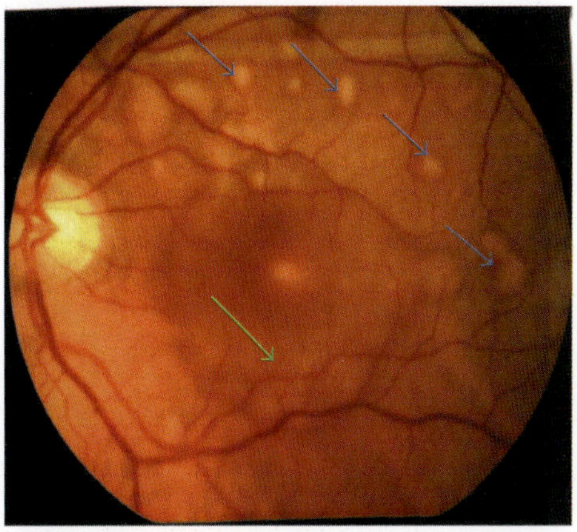

Figure 1: Photograph of the left eye showing creamy yellow choroidal infiltrates with subretinal fluid (blue arrows) extending through the macula (green arrow).

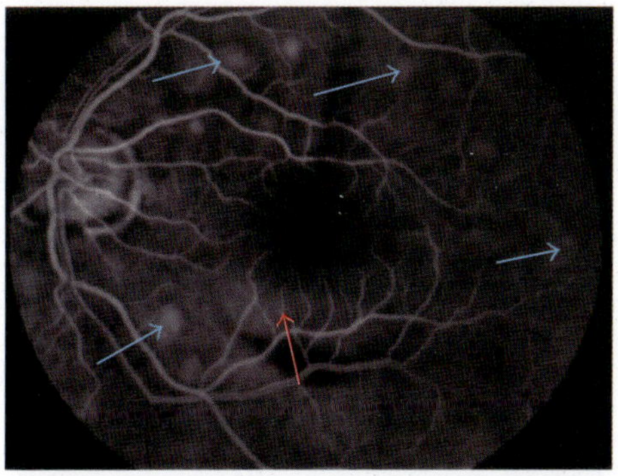

Figure 2: Fluorescein angiogram showing leakage of fluorescein (blue arrows) consistent with areas of choroidal infiltration seen on color photographs and late leakage with subretinal fluid (red arrow).

to abdominal pain. His vital signs were temperature 36.5, pulse 84, respiratory rate 16, and blood pressure 130/86. His Karnofsky performance status was 90%, height 164.5 cm, and weight 84.5 kg. The physical examination findings included right eye prosthesis. Left eye had clear sclera. Extraocular muscles were intact. A 2 cm left supraclavicular lymph node was palpated. Abdomen was soft and obese with the liver edge palpable at 6 cm at the midclavicular line below the costal margin. There were no other palpable abdominal masses. The rest of the physical examination was unremarkable.

The complete blood count was unremarkable. The liver profile and chemistries were normal except for the alkaline phosphatase (210, normal range 38–126 IU/L), ALT (58, normal range 7–56 IU/L), and LDH (1,477, normal range 313–618 IU/L), which were elevated. After radiologic restaging, he was started on temozolomide at 75 mg/m^2/day × 42 days every 8 weeks. Concurrent intrahepatic chemoembolization with cisplatin, doxorubicin, and 300–500 micron PVA particles was done on 2/8/2005 for the treatment of extensive disease in the liver.

A second procedure was performed 4 weeks later. Radiologic restaging on 6/13/2005 showed progression of disease in

TABLE 1: Case reports of uveal melanoma metastatic to the contralateral eye.

Reference	Age in years/sex	Site of primary tumor; therapy	Time[a] to contralateral eye metastasis	Site(s) of extraocular metastasis
Li et al. [13]	75/female	Left eye: enucleation	2 years	Lung, liver
C. L. Shields and J. A. Shields [12]	29/female	Right eye; cobalt 60 plaque radiotherapy, enucleation 9 years later	17 years	Liver, lung, brain
Mitjana et al. [14]	53/male	Left eye	1 year	Skin
Singh et al. [15]	49/female	Left eye; ruthenium 106 plaque radiotherapy	15 years	Liver
Khetan et al. [16]	52/male	Left eye; enucleation	74 months	Abdomen, liver
Shields et al. [17]	52/male	Left eye; enucleation	52 months	Orbit, eyelid, liver
This report	58/male	Right eye; plaque radiotherapy, enucleation 2 years later	10 years	Left cervical, superclavicular, retroperitoneal and mesenteric lymph nodes, liver

[a]From initial presentation.

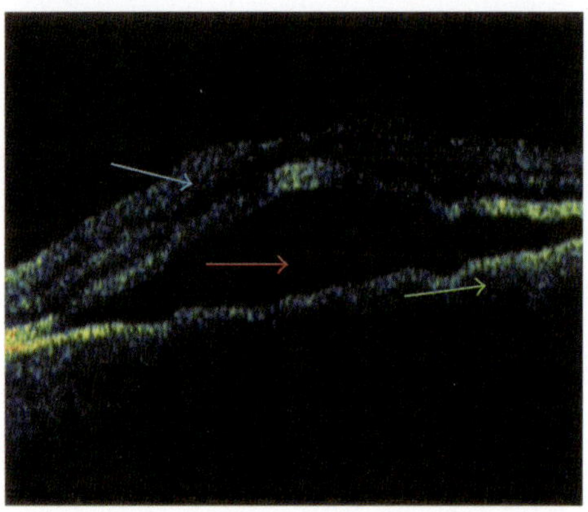

FIGURE 3: Cross-sectional optical coherence tomogram showing cross-sectional image of macula with the retina (blue arrow), subretinal fluid (red arrow), and retinal pigment epithelium and choroid (green arrow).

the liver and at the extrahepatic sites. The patient's systemic therapy was changed to temozolomide, vinblastine, and cisplatin combination. Fundoscopic evaluation on 8/19/2005 showed no active choroidal metastasis. He was stable post-plaque radiotherapy of his left eye. The patient expired on 12/18/2005 in a context of systemic progression.

3. Discussion

Only a few cases of uveal melanoma metastasis to the contralateral choroid have been reported [12–17]. In the 11 cases of skin melanoma metastasized to the uveal tract, the metastases were located in the choroid (5 cases), the iris (4 cases), and the ciliary body (3 cases) [12]. Zografos et al. [18] reported on 20 cases of melanoma metastatic to the eye and the orbit. In fifteen patients with intraocular metastasis the metastases were located in the choroid in 11 cases, in the iris and ciliary body in 2 cases, and in the retina and the vitreous in 2 cases. The primary tumors in the 14 cases of intraocular metastasis were skin melanomas (8 cases), melanomas of the contralateral eye (3 cases), mucosal melanoma (1 case), and melanomas of unknown location (2 cases). The median survival time from diagnosis of uveal tract metastasis was 8.8 (range 1–48) months [18].

In the Collaborative Ocular Melanoma Study (COMS) of primary uveal melanoma only 3 (<1%) of 739 patients with uveal melanoma had metastasis to the contralateral eye or orbit [19]. Case reports of uveal melanoma metastatic to the choroid of contralateral eye are listed in Table 1. Only one of the 7 patients listed in Table 1 did not have liver metastasis. Three patients were found to have metastasis to the choroid of the contralateral eye within 5 years from diagnosis of primary uveal melanoma. Three additional patients were diagnosed to have metastasis to contralateral choroid 10 or more (range 10–17) years after diagnosis of the primary.

In addition to metastasis to the contralateral eye, our case had several uncommon features. The patient's primary melanoma was located in the ciliary body, which is the primary site in only 12% of uveal melanoma cases. The patient also had retinal detachment, which is uncommon at presentation of melanoma of the ciliary body [20]. While most patients with metastatic uveal melanoma present with symptoms related to liver metastasis, our patient presented with left neck lymph node metastasis as the first sign of tumor recurrence. Metastasis to a neck lymph node is very rare and occurs primarily in patients who have invasion of the conjunctiva by the primary tumor. Only 2–4% of patients with advanced uveal melanoma develop lymph node metastasis, and most often the affected lymph nodes are located at the porta hepatis and/or mesentery [6, 21, 22].

While the median time to systemic tumor recurrence in our previously published review of uveal melanoma cases was 3.25 years [21], the patient whose case is described here was diagnosed with metastasis to the contralateral eye 10 years after treatment of the primary tumor, similarly to several other patients with metastasis to choroid of contralateral eye.

A detailed ophthalmoscopic examination by an eye specialist confirmed the presence of multiple choroidal metastases. These findings were confirmed with ultrasonography and angiography. Although we did not biopsy the tumor in the choroid of the contralateral eye to confirm tumor metastasis, in view of concurrent histologically confirmed melanoma metastases in the left supraclavicular lymph node and the liver, the presence of left choroidal metastasis was highly likely.

Plaque radiotherapy significantly alleviated the patient's symptoms related to his recurrent tumor in the contralateral eye and preserved his vision. Lack of control of liver metastasis is associated with poor prognosis [6, 9, 22]; chemoembolization using doxorubicin, cisplatin, and polyvinyl alcohol particles was administered. Unfortunately, the patient's tumor progressed, resulting in the patient's death.

Over the past decade, significant progress has been made in identifying patients at high risk for tumor recurrence and in the use of targeted therapies for management of systemic metastasis based on tumor molecular markers. It has been well established that monosomy 3 is associated with significantly higher risk for systemic metastasis and shorter survival [23, 24]. Certain genes have been identified to be predictive of metastasis in uveal melanoma. A 15-gene microarray assay, which includes 3 control genes, has been successful in discriminating between low-grade and high-grade (class 2) uveal melanomas [25–27]. The multigene expression assay has become a useful tool for selecting patients at high risk for tumor recurrence that may benefit from future adjuvant trials. Inactivation of the *BAP1* gene which codes for an enzyme that binds to BRCA1 and BARD1 in regulating the tumor suppressor complex has been described in up to 84% of class 2 uveal melanomas [28, 29]. Loss of BAP1, as is the case in monosomy 3, may predispose a patient to uveal melanoma for tumor recurrence. In addition, identification of specific genes causing downregulation of tumor suppressor genes on chromosome 3 and upregulation of genes on chromosome 8q has improved our ability to use those genes as potential targets for control of metastatic disease [25–27]. Each of *GNAQ* and *GNA11* has been found in 40% to 45% of patients with metastatic uveal melanoma and, together with several other genes, is associated with systemic spread of uveal melanoma cells [24, 30, 31]. *GNAQ* and *GNA11* mutations cause upregulation of the MAPK pathway, and responses to the MEK inhibitor selumetinib have been reported [32, 33] in early studies. A large study investigating the use of selumetinib for treatment of uveal melanoma is currently in progress.

References

[1] D. H. Abramson, A. C. Schefler, I. J. Dunkel et al., "Neoplasms of the eye," in *Cancer Medicine*, R. Bast Jr., D. Kufe, and R. Pollick, Eds., pp. 1071–1083, BC Decker, London, UK, 7th edition, 2006.

[2] A. D. Singh, M. E. Turell, and A. K. Topham, "Uveal melanoma: trends in incidence, treatment, and survival," *Ophthalmology*, vol. 118, no. 9, pp. 1881–1885, 2011.

[3] A. D. Singh, L. Bergman, and S. Seregard, "Uveal melanoma: epidemiologic aspects," *Ophthalmology Clinics of North America*, vol. 18, no. 1, pp. 75–84, 2005.

[4] M. I. R. Yap-Veloso, R. B. Simmons, and R. J. Simmons, "Iris melanomas: diagnosis and management," *International Ophthalmology Clinics*, vol. 37, no. 4, pp. 87–100, 1997.

[5] E. Kujala, T. Mäkitie, and T. Kivelä, "Very long-term prognosis of patients with malignant uveal melanoma," *Investigative Ophthalmology & Visual Science*, vol. 44, no. 11, pp. 4651–4659, 2003.

[6] A. Y. Bedikian, S. S. Legha, G. Mavligit et al., "Treatment of uveal melanoma metastatic to the liver: a review of the MD Anderson Cancer Center experience and prognostic factors," *Cancer*, vol. 76, pp. 1665–1670, 1995.

[7] R. Kath, J. Hayungs, N. Bornfeld, W. Sauerwein, K. Hoffken, and S. Seeber, "Prognosis and treatment of disseminated uveal melanoma," *Cancer*, vol. 72, no. 7, pp. 2219–2223, 1993.

[8] E. S. Gragoudas, K. M. Egan, J. M. Seddon et al., "Survival of patients with metastases from uveal melanoma," *Ophthalmology*, vol. 98, no. 3, pp. 383–390, 1991.

[9] A. Y. Bedikian, "Metastatic uveal melanoma therapy: current options," *International Ophthalmology Clinics*, vol. 46, no. 1, pp. 151–166, 2006.

[10] J. A. Shields, N. Perez, C. L. Shields, A. D. Singh, and R. C. Eagle Jr., "Orbital melanoma metastatic from contralateral choroid: management by complete surgical resection," *Ophthalmic Surgery and Lasers*, vol. 33, no. 5, pp. 416–420, 2002.

[11] C. Rosenberg and P. T. Finger, "Cutaneous malignant melanoma metastatic to the eye, lids, and orbit," *Survey of Ophthalmology*, vol. 53, no. 3, pp. 187–202, 2008.

[12] C. L. Shields and J. A. Shields, "Choroidal and retinal metastasis," in *Retinal and Choroidal Manifestations of Selected Systemic Diseases*, J. F. Arévalo, Ed., vol. 14, pp. 267–282, Springer Science and Business Media, New York, NY, USA, 2013.

[13] J. Li, K. Resnick, and M. Tso, "Metastasis of malignant melanoma of the choroid and ciliary body to the contralateral choroid," *Graefe's Archive for Clinical and Experimental Ophthalmology*, vol. 231, no. 9, pp. 546–553, 1993.

[14] J. M. C. Mitjana, N. V. Grané, A. A. Civera, N. Sabater, L. A. Barquet, and M. J. R. Caso, "Clinical course of a presumed metastatic uveal melanoma to the contralateral choroid," *Seminars in Ophthalmology*, 2013.

[15] A. D. Singh, J. A. Shields, C. L. Shields, and T. Sato, "Choroidal melanoma metastatic to the contralateral choroid," *The American Journal of Ophthalmology*, vol. 132, no. 6, pp. 941–943, 2001.

[16] V. Khetan, S. Ambatipudi, and L. Gopal, "Presumed metastasis of choroidal melanoma to the contralateral choroid," *Retinal Cases and Brief Reports*, vol. 4, no. 4, pp. 387–389, 2010.

[17] J. A. Shields, C. L. Shields, E. P. Shakin, and L. E. Kobetz, "Metastasis of choroidal melanoma to the contralateral choroid, orbit, and eyelid," *British Journal of Ophthalmology*, vol. 72, no. 6, pp. 456–460, 1988.

[18] L. Zografos, N. Ducrey, D. Beati et al., "Metastatic melanoma in the eye and orbit," *Ophthalmology*, vol. 110, no. 11, pp. 2245–2256, 2003.

[19] Collaborative Ocular Melanoma Study Group, "Development of metastatic disease after enrollment in the COMS trials for treatment of choroidal melanoma," *Archives of Ophthalmology*, vol. 123, no. 12, pp. 1639–1643, 2005.

[20] C. L. Shields, H. Demirci, M. A. Materin, B. P. Marr, A. Mashayekhi, and J. A. Shields, "Clinical factors in the identification of small choroidal melanoma," *Canadian Journal of Ophthalmology*, vol. 39, no. 4, pp. 351–357, 2004.

[21] N. A. Kolandjian, C. Wei, S. P. Patel et al., "Delayed systemic recurrence of uveal melanoma," *American Journal of Clinical Oncology: Cancer Clinical Trials*, vol. 36, no. 5, pp. 443–449, 2013.

[22] E. C. Hsueh, R. Essner, L. J. Foshag, X. Ye, H.-J. Wang, and D. L. Morton, "Prolonged survival after complete resection of metastases from intraocular melanoma," *Cancer*, vol. 100, no. 1, pp. 122–129, 2004.

[23] F. Tschentscher, J. Hüsing, T. Hölter et al., "Tumor classification based on gene expression profiling shows that uveal melanomas with and without monosomy 3 represent two distinct entities," *Cancer Research*, vol. 63, no. 10, pp. 2578–2584, 2003.

[24] S. E. Coupland, S. L. Lake, M. Zeschnigk, and B. E. Damato, "Molecular pathology of uveal melanoma," *Eye*, vol. 27, no. 2, pp. 230–242, 2013.

[25] M. D. Onken, L. A. Worley, J. P. Ehlers, and J. W. Harbour, "Gene expression profiling in uveal melanoma reveals two molecular classes and predicts metastatic death," *Cancer Research*, vol. 64, no. 20, pp. 7205–7209, 2004.

[26] M. D. Onken, L. A. Worley, D. H. Char et al., "Collaborative ocular oncology group report number 1: prospective validation of a multi-gene prognostic assay in uveal melanoma," *Ophthalmology*, vol. 119, no. 8, pp. 1596–1603, 2012.

[27] M. D. Onken, L. A. Worley, M. D. Tuscan, and J. W. Harbour, "An accurate, clinically feasible multi-Gene expression assay for predicting metastasis in uveal melanoma," *Journal of Molecular Diagnostics*, vol. 12, no. 4, pp. 461–468, 2010.

[28] J. W. Harbour, M. D. Onken, E. D. O. Roberson et al., "Frequent mutation of BAP1 in metastasizing uveal melanomas," *Science*, vol. 330, no. 6009, pp. 1410–1413, 2010.

[29] D. E. Jensen, M. Proctor, S. T. Marquis et al., "BAP1: a novel ubiquitin hydrolase which binds to the BRCA1 RING finger and enhances BRCA1-mediated cell growth suppression," *Oncogene*, vol. 16, no. 9, pp. 1097–1112, 1998.

[30] C. D. Van Raamsdonk, K. G. Griewank, M. B. Crosby et al., "Mutations in GNA11 in uveal melanoma," *The New England Journal of Medicine*, vol. 363, no. 23, pp. 2191–2199, 2010.

[31] C. D. van Raamsdonk, V. Bezrookove, G. Green et al., "Frequent somatic mutations of *GNAQ* in uveal melanoma and blue naevi," *Nature*, vol. 457, no. 7229, pp. 599–602, 2009.

[32] A. A. Adjei, R. B. Cohen, W. Franklin et al., "Phase I pharmacokinetic and pharmacodynamic study of the oral, small-molecule mitogen-activated protein kinase kinase 1/2 inhibitor AZD6244 (ARRY-142886) in patients with advanced cancers," *Journal of Clinical Oncology*, vol. 26, no. 13, pp. 2139–2146, 2008.

[33] J. M. Kirkwood, L. Bastholt, C. Robert et al., "Phase II, open-label, randomized trial of the MEK1/2 inhibitor selumetinib as monotherapy versus temozolomide in patients with advanced melanoma," *Clinical Cancer Research*, vol. 18, no. 2, pp. 555–567, 2012.

6

Primary Mediastinal Synovial Sarcoma Presenting as Superior Vena Cava Syndrome: A Rare Case Report

Irappa Madabhavi,[1] Pritam Kataria,[1] Apurva Patel,[1] Swaroop Revannasiddaiah,[2] Asha Anand,[1] Harsha Panchal,[1] Sonia Parikh,[1] Malay Sarkar,[3] Gaurang Modi,[1] Rahul Kulkarni,[1] and Sandip Shah[1]

[1]*GCRI, Civil Hospital Complex, Asarwa, Ahmedabad, Gujarat 830016, India*
[2]*Department of Radiotherapy & Clinical Oncology, Swami Rama Cancer Hospital & Research Institute, Haldwani, Uttarakhand, India*
[3]*Department of Pulmonary Medicine, IGMC, Shimla, Himachal Pradesh, India*

Correspondence should be addressed to Irappa Madabhavi; irappamadabhavi@gmail.com

Academic Editor: Jorg Kleeff

Primary mediastinal sarcomas are aggressive tumors with a very rare incidence. This report describes the case of a 35-year-old male patient who presented with acute symptoms of dyspnoea, facial puffiness, voice-hoarseness, and engorged neck veins. With the clinical picture consistent with the superior vena cava (SVC) syndrome, the patient was investigated with computed tomography of the chest. This revealed a large soft tissue density mass lesion compressing the SVC along with other critical superior mediastinal structures. Histopathological evaluation of the mass revealed features consistent with a soft tissue sarcoma and positive staining was observed for vimentin and S-100. Cytogenetic analysis by fluorescent in situ hybridisation (FISH) demonstrated the t(X:18) translocation. Thus diagnosis was established as primary mediastinal synovial sarcoma. Patient was treated with three cycles of neoadjuvant chemotherapy, to which there was a partial response as per the *RECIST* criteria. Surgical excision of the mediastinal mass was performed, and further postoperative treatment with adjuvant chemoradiotherapy was provided. Patient currently is free of disease. This is to the best of our knowledge the first report in the world literature of a successfully treated case of "primary mediastinal sarcomas presenting as SVC syndrome." Patient is under regular surveillance at our clinic and remains free of recurrence one year after treatment completion.

1. Introduction

Soft tissue sarcomas (STS) are rare malignant tumors comprising less than 1% of all malignant neoplasm. Among thoracic malignancies, the majority happen to be carcinomas, and the proportion of STS among thoracic malignancies is estimated to be as low as 0.01% [1]. Synovial sarcomas are a rare variety of STS which combine features of both sarcomas and carcinomas. Synovial sarcomas usually are observed to occur in the extremities of young adults. Synovial sarcoma presenting in the mediastinum is exceedingly rare, with only a few reported cases in the world literature [2–7].

The current case report is possibly the first in the world of a patient with SVC obstruction due to a mediastinal synovial sarcoma who responded successfully to treatment with a combined modality approach utilizing neoadjuvant chemotherapy, surgery, postoperative chemotherapy, and radiotherapy. The patient has been rendered free of disease, currently at one-year follow-up after treatment completion.

2. Case Report

A 35-year-old nonsmoker male patient presented to the outpatient department with symptoms of rapidly progressive dyspnoea, facial puffiness, and voice-hoarseness developing over a span of 15 days prior to presentation. There was no history of any haemoptysis, abnormal swelling, breathing difficulty, headache, dizziness, tinnitus, epistaxis, or tuberculosis in the past. His overall past medical and surgical history was uneventful.

On examination, the patient was tachypneic with stable vitals. There was a characteristic plethoric face with periorbital and upper body edema with dilated veins over the anterior wall of the chest and neck. There was no pallor, clubbing, lymphadenopathy, ptosis, or any signs of Horner's syndrome. On thoracic auscultation, there were decreased breath sounds in the third and fourth intercostal spaces in the right parasternal area and infraclavicular areas. The rest of the systemic examination was within normal limits.

His blood investigations at presentation revealed hemoglobin level of 11.5 gm/dL, total leukocyte counts of 8500 cells/mm^3, and platelet counts of 3,20,000/mm^3. His serum electrolytes, renal function tests, and liver function tests were within normal range. Germ cell tumor markers like lactate-dehydrogenase (LDH), alpha-fetoprotein (AFP), and β-human chorionic gonadotropin (β-HCG) levels were within normal limits. Bone marrow examination did not show any malignant marrow infiltration. Serology was negative for human immunodeficiency virus (HIV), viral hepatitis B and C.

Contrast-enhanced computed tomography (CT) of the thorax showed an enhancing well-defined soft tissue density lesion of size 10.3 × 9.3 cm involving superior mediastinum, with compression of trachea, SVC, right upper lobe bronchus, and its branches (Figure 1(a)). The mass was also seen encasing the right brachiocephalic trunk, right subclavian artery, and right common carotid artery.

Histopathological examination of the biopsy specimen was characterized by a monotonous proliferation of tumor cells with oval to spindle, vesicular nuclei surrounded by an indistinct rim of amphophilic to lightly eosinophilic cytoplasm (Figure 1(b)). Immunohistochemistry of the biopsied sample showed positive reactivity to vimentin (Figure 1(c)) and S-100 (Figure 1(d)), epithelial membrane antigen, cytokeratin AE1/AE3, bcl-2, and E-cadherin. Negativity was established for CD34. Cytogenetic analysis by fluorescent in situ hybridization (FISH) sample showed the t(X:18) translocation abnormality. So by combining the histopathological features, IHC, and cytogenetic analysis, diagnosis of monophasic synovial sarcoma was confirmed.

Patient was initially managed symptomatically with diuretics, dexamethasone, oxygen inhalation, and propped up position for symptomatic superior vena cava syndrome. Palliative radiotherapy was omitted owing to the radioresistance of sarcomas. Three cycles of neoadjuvant chemotherapy (ifosfamide 2400 mg/m^2 on days 1–5 and doxorubicin 37.5 mg/m^2 on days 1 and 2) were given. Patient tolerated chemotherapy well, and there was partial response to the above mentioned chemotherapeutic drugs according to the RECIST criteria. Surgical excision of the mediastinal mass was carried out via a median sternotomy incision. Postoperative recovery was uneventful.

On cut section, the tumor was composed of gray-white to tan homogeneous soft tissue with focal areas of gelatinous consistency, as well as areas of hemorrhage and necrosis. Histopathological appearance was characterized by a monotonous proliferation of tumor cells with oval to spindle, vesicular nuclei surrounded by an indistinct rim of amphophilic to lightly eosinophilic cytoplasm. Thus the diagnosis of monophasic type of synovial sarcoma of the mediastinum was reconfirmed. The resected surgical margins were free of tumor (R0 resection). Patient was managed postoperatively with adjuvant postoperative radiotherapy (50 Gray in 25 fractions over 5 weeks), followed by three more cycles of chemotherapy. After completion of treatment, the patient is under regular surveillance and for the past one year remains free of recurrence.

3. Discussion

The term synovial sarcoma was earlier coined for the tumors arising near the joints. "Synovial sarcoma" owes the name to its resemblance to developing synovial tissue when seen under light microscopy. It however does not arise from the synovial tissue but arises from the pluripotential mesenchymal cells near joint surfaces, tendons, tendon sheaths, juxta-articular membranes, and fascial aponeurosis. These tumors comprise up to 5–10% of all soft tissue sarcomas. The most common age group of occurrence is in the second to fourth decades of life. The most common site of occurrence of these tumors is near the joints and lower extremities. The other sites that may be involved may be the head, neck, trunk, esophagus, intestine, mediastinum, and retroperitoneum. Primary mediastinal synovial sarcoma is a rare malignancy with only a few cases reported so far [2–7].

The differential diagnoses for mediastinal synovial sarcomas would include other rare tumors such as malignant peripheral nerve sheath tumor (MPNST), thymoma, mesothelioma, pulmonary blastoma, and sarcomatoid carcinoma [8].

Since diagnosis based on histopathological appearance in itself is difficult, it is imperative that additional methods such as immunohistochemistry and fluorescent in situ hybridization are necessary. Synovial sarcomas are usually positive for vimentin, epithelial membrane antigen (EMA), bcl-2, CD99 (60–90%), and S-100 (30%). Negativity for myogenin and myoD1 expression is seen, and these markers differentiate synovial sarcomas from rhabdomyosarcomas. Further, the presence of the translocation t(X:18) on fluorescent in situ hybridization is also confirmatory of synovial sarcoma [9–11].

There are three subtypes of synovial sarcoma: the monophasic form (further subdivided into the monophasic spindle cell type, monophasic epithelial cell type, or the monophasic fibrous type), poorly differentiated form, and biphasic form. Monophasic type may be misdiagnosed as leiomyosarcoma, fibrosarcoma, hemangiopericytoma, and malignant peripheral nerve sheath tumor; thus the use of immunohistochemistry will be very much required to confirm a diagnosis. Poorly differentiated variant of synovial sarcoma can be diagnosed on the basis of expression of CD56 and CD59.

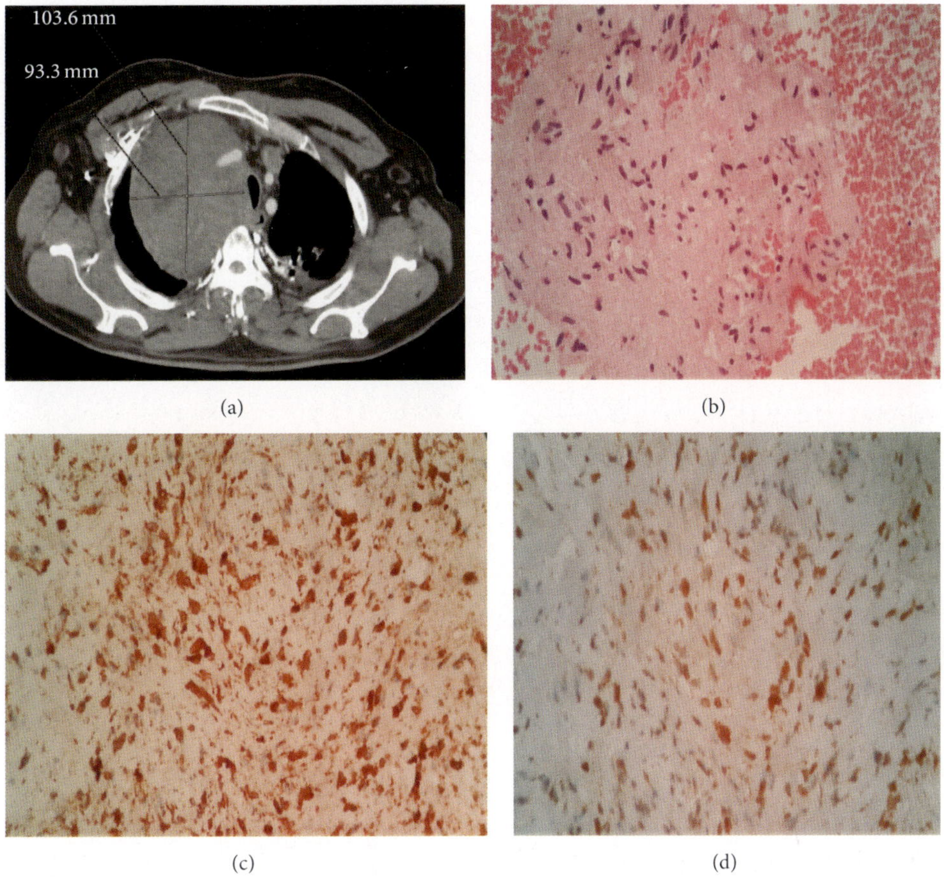

FIGURE 1: (a) Computed tomography (CT) of the thorax showed a well-defined enhancing soft tissue density lesion of size 10.3 × 9.3 cm involving superior mediastinum, with compression of trachea, SVC, right upper lobe bronchus, and its branches. (b) Histopathological examination of the biopsy specimen from the mediastinal mass was characterized by a monotonous proliferation of tumor cells with oval to spindle, vesicular nuclei surrounded by an indistinct rim of amphophilic to lightly eosinophilic cytoplasm. (c) Immunohistochemical image shows strong vimentin positivity. (d) Immunohistochemical image shows strong S-100 positivity.

Biphasic form is histologically composed of two sharply contrasted types of tissues: one of synovial element, the other of fibromatous element. Hence, the biphasic synovial sarcoma can be very easily identified based on characteristic histopathological findings alone [9, 12].

Thus, adequate tissue biopsy will be required for definitive diagnosis based on morphology, special staining, and chromosomal studies. Usually 90% of the synovial sarcomas demonstrate translocation involving fusion of two genes *SYT* located on chromosome 18q11 and *SSX 1*, *SSX2* or *SSX 4* located on Xp11 breakpoint [13].

Synovial sarcomas traditionally have been regarded as being highly aggressive. The most common site of metastasis is lung; however other sites that are less commonly involved include lymph nodes, bone, and bone marrow. Important factors of prognostic significance include the presence of distant metastasis, tumour size (>5 cm), resection margin status, and degree of histological differentiation. Achieving negative surgical margins is highly important, and in case of gross residual disease, reexcision should always be considered. Radiotherapy and adjuvant chemotherapy can enhance the likelihood of disease control.

When complete surgical resection is not possible due to factors such as proximity of tumor to critical structures, maximum possible resection followed by adjuvant radiotherapy is the favored treatment [5]. Synovial sarcoma is one of the few sarcoma subtypes that has a considerable sensitivity to chemotherapy with reported response rates of 30–55%. Two nonrandomized studies had suggested that high dose chemotherapy using agents such as ifosfamide, cisplatin, and doxorubicin may improve disease-free and overall survival rates [14–18].

Patients with unresectable localized disease can be managed with the aim of curing by the use of neoadjuvant chemotherapy and/or radiotherapy so as to obtain a regression which may allow subsequent surgical resection [19]. In our case the primary tumor mass was large enough, making it inoperable. After stabilizing the patients general condition, three cycles of doxorubicin-ifosfamide based chemotherapy were given, and there was partial response to the above mentioned chemotherapeutic drugs according to RECIST criteria. Surgical excision of the mediastinal mass was carried out with median sternotomy incision, and all the margins were free of tumor (R0 resection). Patient was managed postoperatively with radiotherapy (50 Gray in 25 fractions) and three more cycles of doxorubicin-ifosfamide chemotherapy. Patient is under regular surveillance at our clinic for any recurrence for one year without any signs and symptoms of recurrence. This case report makes an evidence of early diagnosis and treatment can make a venue available for resectable as well as for nonresectable tumours so as to achieve complete cure. This case report emphasizes the importance of prompt clinical suspicion, accurate histopathological diagnosis, and use of appropriate immunohistochemical markers and specific chromosomal translocations in the diagnosis of this unusual tumor in an unusual site. This case also illustrates the successful outlook with the use of a combined modality approach for a synovial sarcoma located in a location as difficult as the mediastinum.

References

[1] D. M. Salter, "Pulmonary and thoracic sarcomas," *Current Diagnostic Pathology*, vol. 12, no. 6, pp. 409–417, 2006.

[2] R. Jeganathan, R. Davis, L. Wilson, J. McGuigan, and P. Sidhu, "Primary mediastinal synovial sarcoma," *Ulster Medical Journal*, vol. 76, no. 2, pp. 109–111, 2007.

[3] M. A. Balieiro, A. J. Lopes, B. P. Costa et al., "The surprising outcome of a giant primary mediastinal synovial sarcoma treated with neoadjuvant chemotherapy," *Journal of Thoracic Disease*, vol. 5, no. 1, pp. 94–96, 2013.

[4] S. Salah, A. Al-Ibraheem, A. Daboor, and M. Al-Hussaini, "Synovial sarcoma presenting with huge mediastinal mass: a case report and review of literature," *BMC Research Notes*, vol. 6, article 240, 2013.

[5] B. Henninger, M. Freund, B. Zelger et al., "Primary mediastinal synovial sarcoma: a case report and review of the literature," *Cases Journal*, vol. 2, no. 8, article 6948, 2009.

[6] S. Suster and C. A. Moran, "Primary synovial sarcomas of the mediastinum: a clinicopathologic, immunohistochemical, and ultrastructural study of 15 cases," *The American Journal of Surgical Pathology*, vol. 29, no. 5, pp. 569–578, 2005.

[7] M. Pal, B. N. Ghosh, C. Roy, and A. K. Manna, "Posterior mediastinal biphasic synovial sarcoma in a 12 year-old boy: a case report and review of literature," *Journal of Cancer Research and Therapeutics*, vol. 6, no. 4, pp. 564–566, 2010.

[8] M.-C. Aubry, J. A. Bridge, R. Wickert, and H. D. Tazelaar, "Primary monophasic synovial sarcoma of the pleura: five cases confirmed by the presence of SYT-SSX fusion transcript," *American Journal of Surgical Pathology*, vol. 25, no. 6, pp. 776–781, 2001.

[9] A. Korula, A. Shah, M. A. Philip et al., "Primary mediastinal synovial sarcoma with transdiaphragmatic extension presenting as a pericardial effusion," *Singapore Medical Journal*, vol. 50, no. 1, pp. e26–e28, 2009.

[10] M. H. Cessna, H. Zhou, S. L. Perkins et al., "Are Myogenin and MyoD1 expression specific for rhabdomyosarcoma? A study of 150 cases, with emphasis on spindle cell mimics," *The American Journal of Surgical Pathology*, vol. 25, no. 9, pp. 1150–1157, 2001.

[11] M. Pelmus, L. Guillou, I. Hostein, G. Sierankowski, C. Lussan, and J.-M. Coindre, "Monophasic fibrous and poorly differentiated synovial sarcoma: immunohistochemical reassessment of 60 t(X;18)(SYT-SSX)-positive cases," *The American Journal of Surgical Pathology*, vol. 26, no. 11, pp. 1434–1440, 2002.

[12] S. Suster and C. A. Moran, "Primary synovial sarcomas of the mediastinum: a clinicopathologic, immunohistochemical, and ultrastructural study of 15 cases," *The American Journal of Surgical Pathology*, vol. 29, no. 5, pp. 569–578, 2005.

[13] O. Y. Kwon, S. K. Lee, M. K. Cho, and Y. J. Kim, "A case of biphasic synovial sarcoma of frontal bone in an elderly patient," *Journal of Korean Neurosurgical Society*, vol. 42, pp. 67–70, 2007.

[14] M. van Glabbeke, A. T. van Oosterom, J. W. Oosterhuis et al., "Prognostic factors for the outcome of chemotherapy in advanced soft tissue sarcoma: an analysis of 2,185 patients treated with anthracycline-containing first-line regimens—a European organization for research and treatment of cancer soft tissue and bone sarcoma group study," *Journal of Clinical Oncology*, vol. 17, no. 1, pp. 150–157, 1999.

[15] S. Singer, E. H. Baldini, G. D. Demetri, J. A. Fletcher, and J. M. Corson, "Synovial sarcoma: prognostic significance of tumor size, margin of resection, and mitotic activity for survival," *Journal of Clinical Oncology*, vol. 14, no. 4, pp. 1201–1208, 1996.

[16] C. E. Kampe, G. Rosen, F. Eilber et al., "Synovial sarcoma: a study of intensive chemotherapy in 14 patients with localized disease," *Cancer*, vol. 72, no. 7, pp. 2161–2169, 1993.

[17] G. Rosen, C. Forscher, S. Lowenbraun et al., "Synovial sarcoma. Uniform response of metastases to high dose ifosfamide," *Cancer*, vol. 73, no. 10, pp. 2506–2511, 1994.

[18] A. J. Spillane, R. A'Hern, I. R. Judson, C. Fisher, and M. J. M. Thomas, "Synovial sarcoma: a clinicopathologic, staging, and prognostic assessment," *Journal of Clinical Oncology*, vol. 18, no. 22, pp. 3794–3803, 2000.

[19] M. A. Balieiro, A. J. Lopes, B. P. Costa et al., "The surprising outcome of a giant primary mediastinal synovial sarcoma treated with neoadjuvant chemotherapy," *Journal of Thoracic Disease*, vol. 5, no. 1, pp. 94–96, 2013.

7

Prolonged Complete Response in a Patient with Metastatic Pancreatic Adenocarcinoma after FOLFIRINOX Chemotherapy and Maintenance with FOLFIRI

Christos Nikolaou,[1] Alexios Matikas,[1] Maria Papavasilopoulou,[2] Dimitris Mavroudis,[1] and Lampros Vamvakas[1]

[1] *Department of Medical Oncology, University Hospital of Heraklion, Voutes, P.O. Box 1352, Heraklion, 71110 Crete, Greece*
[2] *Olympion General Clinic, Volou & Meilichou, 26443 Patra, Greece*

Correspondence should be addressed to Lampros Vamvakas; vamvakasla@yahoo.gr

Academic Editor: Jose I. Mayordomo

Metastatic pancreatic adenocarcinoma confers a poor prognosis. Even with recent advances in the treatment of this disease with the introduction of two modestly effective chemotherapy regimens, complete responses are still very rare. Moreover, there are no published data on how to further manage the patients who achieve a sustained remission following treatment. Herein, we report the case of a patient with metastatic pancreatic adenocarcinoma who achieved a complete response lasting for more than three years after receiving induction chemotherapy with FOLFIRINOX followed by maintenance with FOLFIRI.

1. Introduction

Primary adenocarcinoma of the pancreas is the eighth most common cancer and fourth leading cause of cancer-related death in the United States; the vast majority of newly diagnosed patients will eventually die of the disease [1]. Even when amenable to "curative" surgery, most patients eventually relapse. Despite recent advances, metastatic pancreatic cancer remains a devastating disease and carries a grim prognosis, with less than 1% of patients surviving for more than 5 years [1].

Until 2011, monotherapy with gemcitabine was the standard of care leading to an overall survival (OS) of approximately 6 months and a one-year survival rate of less than 20%; objective radiographic responses were rare [2]. Gemcitabine has been combined with a variety of cytotoxic and targeted agents, such as oxaliplatin [3], capecitabine [4, 5], 5-fluorouracil [6], irinotecan [7], and erlotinib [8]. However, the improvement in OS has been either statistically or clinically insignificant. In 2011, the results of the ACCORD 11 trial were published, which showed that the combination of 5-fluorouracil, irinotecan, and oxaliplatin (FOLFIRINOX) produced superior response rate, progression-free survival (PFS), and OS compared to single agent gemcitabine [9]. More recently, the combination of gemcitabine plus nanoparticle albumin bound paclitaxel (nab-paclitaxel) was also shown to be superior in terms of OS compared to gemcitabine [10]. Despite the aforementioned advances, almost all patients with metastatic pancreatic cancer eventually die of progressive disease, underscoring the clearly unmet need of curative therapy and the lack of data on how to best sequence existing active regimens when treating these patients.

In this case report, we present the case of a 51-year-old man with lung metastases from pancreatic adenocarcinoma who achieved a complete response after initial chemotherapy with FOLFIRINOX followed by maintenance chemotherapy with irinotecan, leucovorin, and 5-fluorouracil (FOLFIRI) and who has not yet recurred after 3 years from the initial diagnosis of metastatic disease. We propose this approach for highly selected patients with sustained responses to chemotherapy.

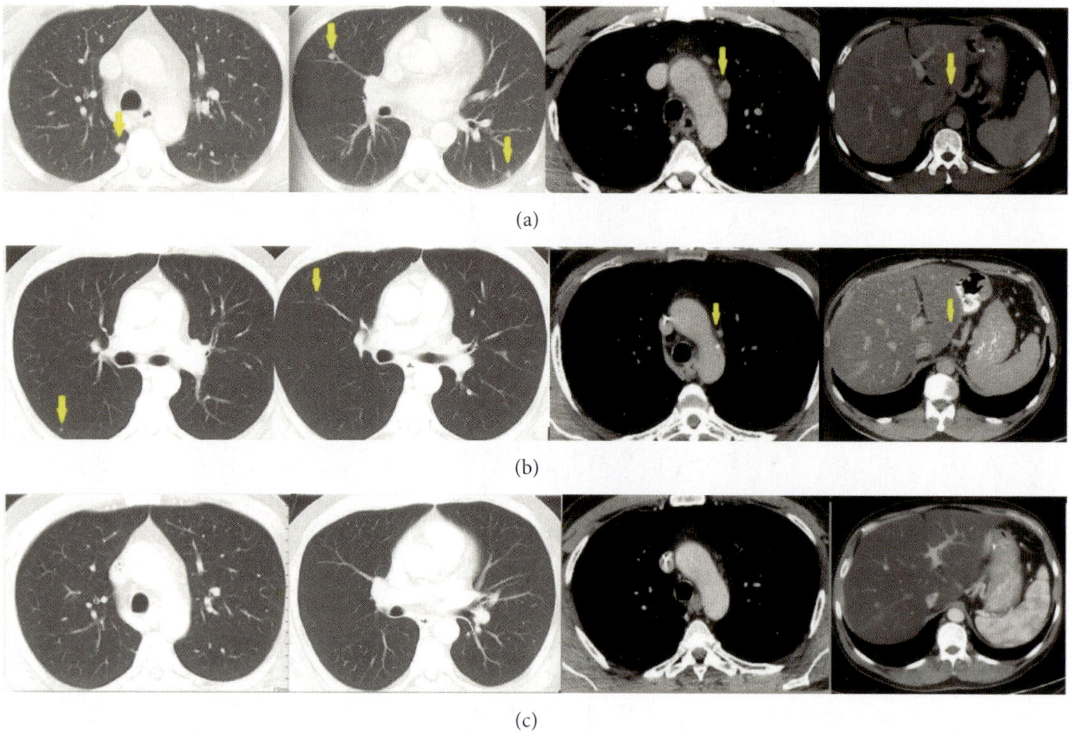

FIGURE 1: CT scan, axial images, at the same level, at the beginning of the therapy (a), after three cycles of chemotherapy (b) showing partial response (PR), and after the seventh cycle (c) in competence with complete response (CR). Yellow arrows indicate the pulmonary nodules (first two images) that are easily recognized at the first scan, are faintly differentiable at the following, and have disappeared at the final. In the remaining images, arrows indicate the pathologic mediastinal lymph node (third image) and the liver lesion.

2. Case Presentation

A 51-year-old male patient with a medical history of type II diabetes and a smoking history of over 30 pack-years presented with a 2-month history of worsening epigastric pain, jaundice, and weight loss of approximately 10 kg. Physical examination was otherwise unremarkable. An abdominal computed tomography (CT) scan revealed a mass at the head of the pancreas with a maximal diameter of 2.4 cm which caused dilatation of the pancreatic and biliary tract. Further testing revealed markedly elevated levels of CA 19-9 tumor marker exceeding 12000 U/mL (normal range: 0–37 U/mL). Subsequent staging with chest CT and abdominal magnetic resonance imaging (MRI) showed absence of metastases and the patient underwent a Whipple procedure. The pathology exam was diagnostic of a primary pancreatic adenocarcinoma with a maximal diameter of 3.2 cm, with perivascular and perineural invasion. Four out of seven excised peripancreatic lymph nodes were positive for metastatic disease and all surgical margins were negative. According to the American Joint Committee on Cancer (AJCC) staging system, pathologic stage was pT2N1M0, stage II.

The patient's recovery was uneventful. Postsurgery CT scans showed no evidence of metastatic or residual disease and CA 19-9 tumor marker levels were 1203 U/mL. Adjuvant chemotherapy with gemcitabine 1000 mg/m^2 on days 1, 8, and 15 on 28-day cycles was started 2.5 months after surgery, with a plan of administering 6 cycles. After completing 2 cycles, a gradual increase of CA 19-9 levels was noted and new imaging was performed. New multiple bilateral pulmonary nodules as well as para-aortic lymph nodes and one new liver lesion were shown, findings consistent with metastatic disease. On physical examination the patient remained asymptomatic, with an Eastern Cooperative Oncology Group (ECOG) performance status of 0. A palpable left supraclavicular lymph node approximately 1.5 cm in diameter was noted. CA 19-9 levels were increased to over 12000 U/mL.

First-line chemotherapy with the combination of oxaliplatin 85 mg/m^2, irinotecan 180 mg/m^2, leucovorin 400 mg/m^2, and fluorouracil 400 mg/m^2 given as a bolus followed by 2400 mg/m^2 given as a 46-hour continuous infusion, every 2 weeks (FOLFIRINOX), was initiated. After 4 administrations of chemotherapy a gradual decrease of CA 19-9 levels to 550 U/mL was evident, while the left supraclavicular lymph node was no longer palpable. Imaging revealed a partial response of the pulmonary nodes and a complete response of the para-aortic lymph nodes and liver lesion (Figure 1). After 4 more administrations (8 cycles in total) the patient attained a complete response which he maintained after seven months of FOLFIRINOX chemotherapy despite dose reductions due to hematologic toxicity. Because of worsening neurotoxicity caused by oxaliplatin which peaked at grade 3 and taking into account the absence of published data regarding the optimal management of this patient, maintenance chemotherapy with FOLFIRI was commenced. Due to sustained complete remission on reimaging studies, the patient completed a total of two years of chemotherapy and discontinued treatment due to steatohepatitis with grade 1 transaminitis probably caused by irinotecan. Eight months after treatment discontinuation he remained alive and in complete radiographic and biochemical remission.

3. Discussion

In spite of the use of more active combination regimens, complete responses are a rare occurrence in metastatic pancreatic cancer; in the ACCORD 11 trial, there was only one complete response among the 171 patients who received FOLFIRINOX (0.6%) [9]. Published case series propose total gross resection for locally advanced pancreatic cancer following dramatic responses from first-line chemotherapy [11, 12]. Complete radiological or pathologic complete responses after neoadjuvant FOLFIRINOX are rare but well documented in this setting [13–15]; these patients may have a better prognosis compared to those who experience lesser responses [16]. However, there is no published literature on how to best treat the rare patient with distant metastases who achieves a sustained partial or complete response, due to the rarity of such cases [17]. Current guidelines support the continuation of intensive chemotherapy until disease progression or unacceptable toxicities, as was the case with our patient [18]. Also, the role of Positron Emission Tomography (PET and PET/CT) scan in the initial staging of pancreatic cancer is controversial and there are no data to support its use in the metastatic setting [19].

Taking into account the absence of measurable disease after achieving a complete response and grade 3 neurotoxicity which affected our patient's activities of daily living and his unwillingness to stop treatment altogether, we proposed omitting oxaliplatin and continue with FOLFIRI. To our knowledge, this is the first published report of maintenance FOLFIRI after initial response to FOLFIRINOX in a patient with pancreatic cancer. How much benefit the patient actually derived from FOLFIRI cannot be determined, especially in light of the modest activity of irinotecan in metastatic pancreatic cancer [20].

In recent years, the traditional approach of distinct chemotherapy lines when treating metastatic solid tumors is being challenged in favor of a continuum of care paradigm where periods of intensive chemotherapy are followed by less toxic maintenance strategies. Whether such an approach can be successfully implemented in the treatment of metastatic pancreatic cancer remains to be seen in future trials. In addition, the optimal sequence of active regimens and whether surgical excision of metastatic sites in patients who exhibit significant response to systemic treatment has a role in the treatment strategy are questions that also remain unanswered, although the feasibility of the latter strategy has been demonstrated in case reports [21].

In conclusion, we present the case of a patient with prolonged complete response after initial chemotherapy with FOLFIRINOX and maintenance with FOLFIRI. Until data from prospective randomized trials are available and taking into account the absence of any relevant published literature, case reports and retrospective case series may offer a guide on how to treat the selected population of long-term (i.e., more than two years) survivors with metastatic pancreatic cancer.

Consent

Written informed consent was obtained from the patient for publication of this case report and any accompanying images.

References

[1] R. Siegel, J. Ma, Z. Zou, and A. Jemal, "Cancer statistics, 2014," *CA—Cancer Journal for Clinicians*, vol. 64, no. 1, pp. 9–29, 2014.

[2] H. A. Burris III, M. J. Moore, J. Andersen et al., "Improvements in survival and clinical benefit with gemcitabine as first-line therapy for patients with advanced pancreas cancer: a randomized trial," *Journal of Clinical Oncology*, vol. 15, no. 6, pp. 2403–2413, 1997.

[3] C. Louvet, R. Labianca, P. Hammel et al., "Gemcitabine in combination with oxaliplatin compared with gemcitabine alone in locally advanced or metastatic pancreatic cancer: Results of a GERCOR and GISCAD phase III trial," *Journal of Clinical Oncology*, vol. 23, no. 15, pp. 3509–3516, 2005.

[4] D. Cunningham, I. Chau, D. D. Stocken et al., "Phase III randomized comparison of gemcitabine versus gemcitabine plus capecitabine in patients with advanced pancreatic cancer," *Journal of Clinical Oncology*, vol. 27, no. 33, pp. 5513–5518, 2009.

[5] R. Herrmann, G. Bodoky, T. Ruhstaller et al., "Gemcitabine plus capecitabine compared with gemcitabine alone in advanced pancreatic cancer: a randomized, multicenter, phase III trial of the Swiss Group for Clinical Cancer Research and the Central European Cooperative Oncology Group," *Journal of Clinical Oncology*, vol. 25, no. 16, pp. 2212–2217, 2007.

[6] J. D. Berlin, P. Catalano, J. P. Thomas, J. W. Kugler, D. G. Haller, and A. B. Benson III, "Phase III study of gemcitabine in combination with fluorouracil versus gemcitabine alone in patients with advanced pancreatic carcinoma: eastern Cooperative Oncology Group trial E2297," *Journal of Clinical Oncology*, vol. 20, no. 15, pp. 3270–3275, 2002.

[7] G. P. Stathopoulos, K. Syrigos, G. Aravantinos et al., "A multicenter phase III trial comparing irinotecan-gemcitabine (IG) with gemcitabine (G) monotherapy as first-line treatment in patients with locally advanced or metastatic pancreatic cancer," *British Journal of Cancer*, vol. 95, no. 5, pp. 587–592, 2006.

[8] M. J. Moore, D. Goldstein, J. Hamm et al., "Erlotinib plus gemcitabine compared with gemcitabine alone in patients with advanced pancreatic cancer: a phase III trial of the National Cancer Institute of Canada Clinical Trials Group," *Journal of Clinical Oncology*, vol. 25, no. 15, pp. 1960–1966, 2007.

[9] T. Conroy, F. Desseigne, M. Ychou et al., "FOLFIRINOX versus gemcitabine for metastatic pancreatic cancer," *The New England Journal of Medicine*, vol. 364, no. 19, pp. 1817–1825, 2011.

[10] D. D. von Hoff, T. Ervin, F. P. Arena et al., "Increased survival in pancreatic cancer with nab-paclitaxel plus gemcitabine," *The New England Journal of Medicine*, vol. 369, no. 18, pp. 1691–1703, 2013.

[11] P. J. Hosein, J. Macintyre, C. Kawamura et al., "A retrospective study of neoadjuvant FOLFIRINOX in unresectable or borderline-resectable locally advanced pancreatic adenocarcinoma," *BMC Cancer*, vol. 12, article 199, 2012.

[12] P. F. Peddi, S. Lubner, R. McWilliams et al., "Multi-institutional experience with FOLFIRINOX in pancreatic adenocarcinoma," *Journal of the Pancreas*, vol. 13, no. 5, pp. 497–501, 2012.

[13] S. Valeri, D. Borzomati, G. Nappo, G. Perrone, D. Santini, and R. Coppola, "Complete pathological response after FOLFIRINOX for locally advanced pancreatic cancer. The beginning of a new era? Case report and review of the literature," *Pancreatology*, vol. 14, no. 5, pp. 425–430, 2014.

[14] K. Turner, G. B. L. Sandri, E. Boucher et al., "Complete radiological response of an initially locally advanced unresectable pancreatic cancer to chemoradiotherapy using FOLFIRINOX regimen: report of a case," *Clinics and Research in Hepatology and Gastroenterology*, vol. 39, no. 2, pp. e29–e31, 2015.

[15] I. Hartlapp, J. Müller, W. Kenn et al., "Complete pathological remission of locally advanced, unresectable pancreatic cancer (LAPC) after intensified neoadjuvant chemotherapy," *Onkologie*, vol. 36, no. 3, pp. 123–125, 2013.

[16] H. Wang, Q. Zhao, A. Rashid et al., "Pathologic complete response to neoadjuvant therapy in patients with pancreatic ductal adenocarcinoma is associated with a better prognosis," *Annals of Diagnostic Pathology*, vol. 16, no. 1, pp. 29–37, 2012.

[17] A. R. Shakir, "A near-complete response to treatment with gemcitabine plus nab-paclitaxel in a patient with metastatic pancreatic cancer and poor performance status: a case report," *Case Reports in Oncology*, vol. 7, no. 3, pp. 711–717, 2014.

[18] National Comprehensive Cancer Network (NCCN), Clinical Practice Guidelines in Oncology, Pancreatic Adenocarcinoma, Version 2.2014, 2014, http://www.nccn.org/professionals/physician_gls/pdf/pancreatic.pdf.

[19] K. Izuishi, Y. Yamamoto, T. Sano, R. Takebayashi, T. Masaki, and Y. Suzuki, "Impact of 18-fluorodeoxyglucose positron emission tomography on the management of pancreatic cancer," *Journal of Gastrointestinal Surgery*, vol. 14, no. 7, pp. 1151–1158, 2010.

[20] D. J. T. Wagener, H. E. R. Verdonk, L. Y. Dirix et al., "Phase II trial of CPT-11 in patients with advanced pancreatic cancer, an EORTC early clinical trials group study," *Annals of Oncology*, vol. 6, no. 2, pp. 129–132, 1995.

[21] T. Iida, Y. Nakabayashi, N. Okui, H. Shiba, M. Otsuka, and K. Yanaga, "Successful management of metachronous liver metastasis after pancreaticoduodectomy for pancreatic ductal carcinoma using hepatectomy and chemotherapy: a case report," *Anticancer Research*, vol. 34, no. 5, pp. 2417–2420, 2014.

8

Recurrence of Pelvic Chondrosarcoma through Fascial Defect into Abdominal Cavity

Kemal Gökkuş,[1,2] Tolgay Akin,[3] Ergin Sagtas,[4] Murat Saylik,[5] and Ahmet Turan Aydın[2]

[1] *Private Memorial Antalya Hospital, Zafer Mahallesi, Yildirim Beyazit Caddesi, No. 91, Kepez, 07020 Antalya, Turkey*
[2] *Orthopaedics and Trauma Department, Antalya Memorial Hospital, 07020 Antalya, Turkey*
[3] *General Surgery Department, Antalya Memorial Hospital, 07020 Antalya, Turkey*
[4] *Radiodiagnostic Department, Antalya Memorial Hospital, 07020 Antalya, Turkey*
[5] *Orthopaedics and Trauma Department, Ozel Bahar Hospital, 16100 Bursa, Turkey*

Correspondence should be addressed to Kemal Gökkuş; kgokkus@yahoo.com

Academic Editor: Constantine Gennatas

Our patient was a 76-year-old female who has been operated on 2 times in 8 years for pelvic chondrosarcoma. The patient came to our clinic with a large mass in left iliac region which extended into the paravertebral area. Physical examination and preoperative imagining studies revealed a mass at the left iliac area that infiltrated sciatic notch and extended from posterior iliac region towards the anterior side of iliac bone through the sciatic notch and an incisional hernia including descending colon. The mass was also penetrating the abdominal cavity through the hernia. Surgical intervention was planned. Since the tumor infiltrated the sciatic nerve, hemipelvectomy was indicated. Patient refused hemipelvectomy. Therefore, palliative debulking surgery was considered. We treated the case with marginal excision and abdominal wall reconstruction employing prolene and vicryl suture materials in order to prevent a postoperative visceral herniation and local invasion. At the latest follow-up appointment in 2 years, the patient still had no signs of tumor recurrence. This case showed us that an incisional hernia can serve as a pathway for the recurrence invasion of the chondrosarcoma.

1. Introduction

Chondrosarcomas constitute a heterogeneous group of neoplasms that have the production of cartilage matrix by tumor cells in common [1]. Chondrosarcoma is the third most common primary bone malignancy following myeloma and osteosarcoma, accounting for approximately 20% of bone sarcomas and mainly affecting the middle-aged population [2–4].

The pelvis is the most common site of occurrence with the ilium being the most frequently involved bone, followed by the pubis and ischium [5]. Although the majority of these tumors have a slow growth rate, rarely metastasize, and have a very good prognosis after surgery, local recurrence is a quite common occurrence, especially following inadequate excision. Since radiotherapy and chemotherapy were proven to be ineffective for the treatment of chondrosarcomas, wide en-bloc excision remains the treatment of choice [2, 6]. We hereby present a case of a second recurrent pelvic chondrosarcoma invading the pelvic region and locally extended into the abdominal cavity through the incisional hernia that caused by the abdominal wall defect which was a result of the previous operations. We treated the case with marginal excision and abdominal wall reconstruction employing prolene and vicryl suture materials in order to prevent a postoperative visceral herniation and local invasion.

2. Case

A 76-year-old woman came to our clinic with a large mass of the left iliac region.

According to the patient's history, she had a pelvic tumor removal surgery in 2006 and she was reoperated on for local recurrence in 2009. During admission to our oncosurgical clinic, an incisional hernia and a large mass of left iliac region were diagnosed. The patient was neurovascularly intact.

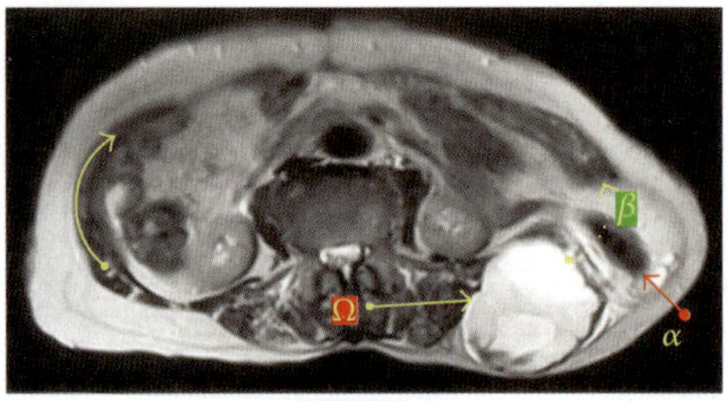

Figure 1: MRI imagining shows tumor (omega arrow), herniated descending colon (alpha arrow), and abdominal wall defect (dotted beta arrow).

Radiological studies showed a mass at the left iliac area that infiltrated sciatic notch and extended from posterior iliac region towards the anterior side of iliac bone through the sciatic notch and incisional hernia. The mass was also penetrating the abdominal cavity through the fascial defect and infiltrating the mesosigmoid that herniated through the fascial defect out of abdominal cavity (Figures 1 and 2). Surgical intervention was planned. Since the tumor infiltrated the sciatic nerve, hemipelvectomy was indicated. Patient refused hemipelvectomy. Therefore, palliative debulking surgery was considered.

The tumor was approached through the utilitarian pelvic incision that extended into the inner side of thigh and lateral border of the abdomen (the incision begins at the posterior inferior iliac spine and extends along the iliac crest to the anterior superior iliac spine. It is separated into two arms: one is carried along the inguinal ligament up to the symphysis pubis and the other turns distally over the anterior thigh for one-third the length of the thigh and then curves laterally just posterior to the shaft of the femur below the greater trochanter and follows the insertion of the gluteus maximus muscle).

The tumor in the pelvic and paravertebral area was marginally excised (Figure 3). Abdominal exploration was also performed using the same incision and tumors which infiltrated the omentum and mesosigmoid area were excised (Figure 4). Pelvic region and the abdominal cavity were separated using prolene and vicryl suture materials and hernia repair was done without using mesh. The operation lasted 8 hours. Recorded blood loss was 1500 mL and urine output was 1200 mL. The patient was transfused with 3 units of 500 mL erythrocyte suspension with sodium chloride-hydroxyethyl starch 120/0.4, 3000 mL Isolyte S, and 1 unit of fresh frozen plasma during the operation. In the post-op period, patient was held in Intensive Care Unit (ICU) for a day. During the ICU stay, 2 units of erythrocyte suspension and 1 unit of frozen plasma were used for transfusion. Two units of erythrocyte suspension were additionally transfused because of a drop in HB levels (8.2) on the 4th day of operation. Patient started mobilizing in bed on the 6th day and started to walk on the 9th day of the operation with assistance of a physiotherapist. Total hospital stay was 9 days. The patient was discharged without any complication. Patient had still no sign of tumor recurrence at the latest appointment of a 2-year follow-up period. Histological examination confirmed grade II chondrosarcoma diagnosis (Figure 5).

3. Discussion

Wide surgical tumor excision with adequate margins appears to be the procedure of choice in chondrosarcoma treatment, since this is the most effective way of reducing tumor recurrence rate [3–9]. Although local recurrence after inadequate surgical removal does not seem to significantly influence the overall survival, it must be kept in mind that each local recurrence bears the risk of the tumor evolving towards a higher-grade chondrosarcoma (up to 21.4%) [9].

The key point of our paper was to define an unusual way of local recurrence. To the best of our knowledge, no case of clearly defined pelvic chondrosarcoma developing local recurrence through the abdominal hernia into the abdomen was reported previously. Regarding the originality and rarity of our case, we performed a literature scan by employing PubMed database. The research criteria were as follows: (1) the research had to be in English, (2) papers examining pelvic chondrosarcoma related with colon and small intestines, (3) cases involving chondrosarcoma and abdominal wall repair, (4) cases involving bone resection that resulted abdominal hernia, and (5) cases involving chondrosarcoma, bone resection, and abdominal hernia altogether. Out of 252 articles, only 14 studies fulfilled the criteria described above. There was no case related with local recurrence and invasion into mesocolon area through the abdominal hernia. Considering this fact, we can say that our paper is unique in terms of focus on a local recurrence and invasion into mesocolon through the abdominal hernia.

Two articles (references [10, 11]) documented the involvement of small intestine and colon [10, 11].

Extraskeletal myxoid chondrosarcoma is differentiated by a biological structure that is distinct from the genetic heterogeneity observed in other forms of chondrosarcoma. Despite its high tendency to local recurrences and distant metastases, it has a relatively slow growth and a lazy clinical course [12, 13].

Bustinza-Linares et al. [10] presented a case of chest wall extraskeletal myxoid chondrosarcoma with small bowel metastasis (distant metastasis) which caused bowel obstruction. On the other hand, in our case the tumor locally invaded the omentum and sigmoid mesocolon through the abdominal wall defect and it might be described as local recurrence, as it is done in our case.

Hull [11] reported a case of chondrosarcoma originating from ribs (costochondral junction) that extended into colon. He performed a colon resection with wide resection of tumor together (resection of left 7th, 8th, 9th, 10th, 11th, and 12th ribs with a portion sternum with splenic flexura of the colon). He repaired the abdominal wall using tantalum mesh to prevent visceral hernia. No recurrence was reported during the 9-month follow-up period. This paper is important because of the emphasis on both colon involvement and abdominal wall repair (this article was similar to our case regarding abdominal involvement and abdominal wall repair. Even in this article, the link between the abdominal incisional hernia

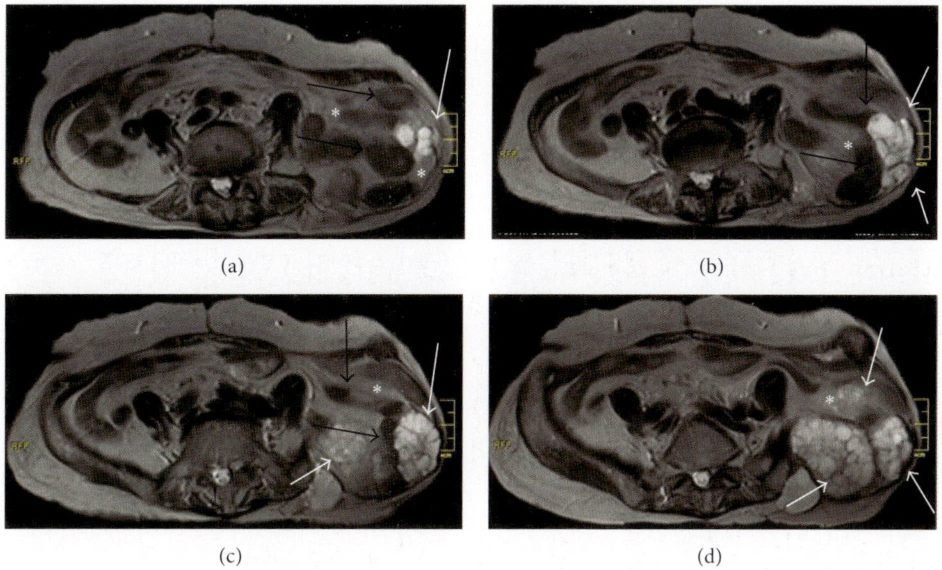

FIGURE 2: White arrows show tumoral mass (chondrosarcoma mass), black arrows show intestine or colon, and asterisk shows mesenteric fatty tissue.

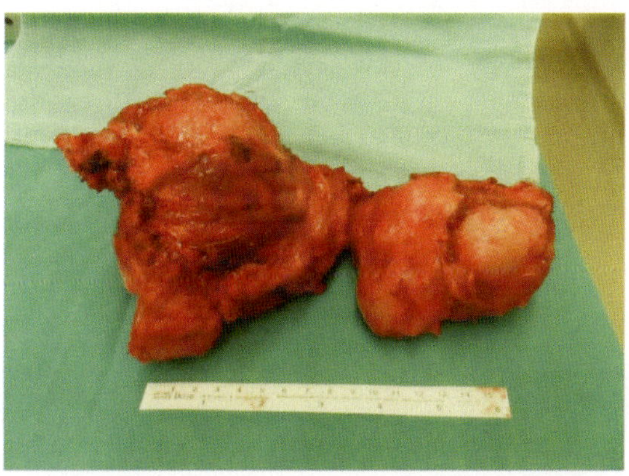

FIGURE 3: Excised tumor mass from the pelvic region.

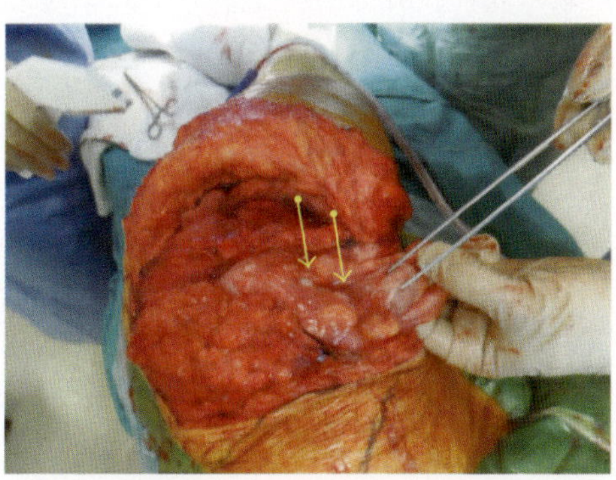

FIGURE 4: The intraoperative photograph, note the chondrosarcoma nodes in mesocolon (yellow arrows).

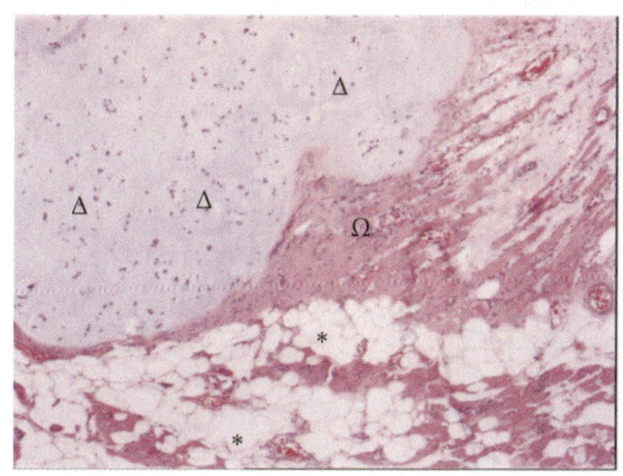

FIGURE 5: Hematoxylin-eosin stain with (x4) magnification. Asterisk: adipose tissue, omega: muscle tissue, and delta: atypical chondrocytes. Grade II chondrosarcoma.

and local recurrence or invasion of chondrosarcoma through hernia has not been shown)

We searched the literature for the link between bone resection (the resected bone was used for bone grafting) and abdominal hernia (cases involving bone resection that resulted with abdominal hernia) and 7 articles were found [14–20].

Petsatodis et al. performed radical excision of the tumor (chondrosarcoma) at symphysis pubis and used synthetic mesh in order to reduce the possibility of a postoperative visceral herniation [21]. They emphasized the importance of abdominal wall repair. No recurrence was reported during the 2-year follow-up period.

Juan-García et al. [22] reported abdominal hernia after resection of a chondrosarcoma of the pelvis. In contrast with our case, their case had no local recurrence invasion through the hernia. The link between the abdominal incisional hernia and local recurrence or invasion of chondrosarcoma through hernia was not discussed. We would like to stress the contribution to literature by presenting the evidence about this relationship.

In our case we repaired abdominal wall carefully with prolene and vicryl suture materials to prevent future herniation and local invasion of pelvic chondrosarcoma.

This case showed us that an incisional hernia can serve as a pathway for the recurrence invasion of the chondrosarcoma.

In conclusion, surgeons should separate compartments by materials like mesh or sutures to minimize the ratio of intercompartmental recurrence.

References

[1] World Health Organization, "Cartilage tumours," in *Pathology and Genetics of Tumours of Soft Tissue and Bone*, C. D. M. Fletcher, K. K. Unni, and F. Mertens, Eds., IARC WHO Classification of Tumours, pp. 234–257, IARC Press, Lyon, France, 2002.

[2] H. Gelderblom, P. C. W. Hogendoorn, S. D. Dijkstra et al., "The clinical approach towards chondrosarcoma," *Oncologist*, vol. 13, no. 3, pp. 320–329, 2008.

[3] T. Ozaki, A. Hillmann, N. Lindner, S. Blasius, and W. Winkelmann, "Chondrosarcoma of the pelvis," *Clinical Orthopaedics and Related Research*, no. 337, pp. 226–239, 1997.

[4] R. J. Wirbel, M. Schulte, B. Maier, M. Koschnik, and W. E. Mutschler, "Chondrosarcoma of the pelvis: oncologic and functional outcome," *Sarcoma*, vol. 4, no. 4, pp. 161–168, 2000.

[5] D. Donati, A. El Ghoneimy, F. Bertoni, C. Di Bella, and M. Mercuri, "Surgical treatment and outcome of conventional pelvic chondrosarcoma," *Journal of Bone and Joint Surgery—Series B*, vol. 87, no. 11, pp. 1527–1530, 2005.

[6] M. E. Pring, K. L. Weber, K. K. Unni, and F. H. Sim, "Chondrosarcoma of the pelvis: a review of sixty-four cases," *Journal of Bone and Joint Surgery—Series A*, vol. 83, no. 11, article 1630, 2001.

[7] A. Kawai, J. H. Healey, P. J. Boland, P. P. Lin, A. G. Huvos, and P. A. Meyers, "Prognostic factors for patients with sarcomas of the pelvic bones," *Cancer*, vol. 82, no. 5, pp. 851–859, 1998.

[8] J. S. Spratt and J. S. Meyer, "Biological considerations with pelvic neoplasms," *Journal of Surgical Oncology*, vol. 71, no. 3, pp. 198–205, 1999.

[9] A. Streitbürger, H. Ahrens, M. Balke et al., "Grade i chondrosarcoma of bone: the Münster experience," *Journal of Cancer Research and Clinical Oncology*, vol. 135, no. 4, pp. 543–550, 2009.

[10] E. Bustinza-Linares, F. Socola, V. Ernani, S. A. Miller, and J. C. Trent, "Extraskeletal myxoid chondrosarcoma with small bowel metastasis causing bowel obstruction," *Case Reports in Oncological Medicine*, vol. 2012, Article ID 621025, 4 pages, 2012.

[11] D. Hull, "Massive chondrosarcoma of the rib with extension into the colon: repair with tantalum mesh," *Annals of Surgery*, vol. 140, no. 6, pp. 886–891, 1954.

[12] S. Kawaguchi, T. Wada, S. Nagoya et al., "Extraskeletal myxoid chondrosarcoma: a multi-institutional study of 42 cases in Japan," *Cancer*, vol. 97, no. 5, pp. 1285–1292, 2003.

[13] M. R. D'Aprile, A. Stasolla, R. Guerrisi et al., "Extraskeletal myxoid chondrosarcoma of the thoracic wall," *Journal of Experimental & Clinical Cancer Research*, vol. 22, no. 2, pp. 333–335, 2003.

[14] S. P. Cowley and L. D. Anderson, "Hernias through donor sites for iliac-bone grafts," *Journal of Bone and Joint Surgery A*, vol. 65, no. 7, pp. 1023–1025, 1983.

[15] A. I. Froimson and A. G. Cummings Jr., "Iliac hernia following hip arthrodesis," *Clinical Orthopaedics and Related Research*, vol. 80, pp. 89–91, 1971.

[16] M. Lotem, P. Maor, H. Haimoff, and Y. Woloch, "Lumbar hernia at an iliac bone graft donor site. A case report.," *Clinical Orthopaedics and Related Research*, vol. 80, pp. 130–132, 1971.

[17] M. C. Oldfield, "Iliac hernia after bone grafting," *The Lancet*, vol. 1, pp. 810–812, 1945.

[18] L. J. Pyrtek and C. C. Kelly, "Management of herniation through large iliac bone defects," *Annals of Surgery*, vol. 152, pp. 998–1003, 1960.

[19] R. L. Reid, "Hernia through an iliac bone-graft donor site," *Journal of Bone and Joint Surgery A*, vol. 50, no. 4, pp. 757–760, 1968.

[20] P. Verheugen, R. Goffin, and L. Musin, "Iliac hernia after bone removal: subobstruction," *Acta Chirurgica Belgica*, vol. 64, no. 8, pp. 1051–1056, 1965.

[21] G. Petsatodis, S. I. Stavridis, D. Karataglis, and A. Christodoulou, "Surgical treatment of a twice recurrent chondrosarcoma of the pubic symphysis: a case report and review of the literature," *Cases Journal*, vol. 2, no. 6, article 6769, 2009.

[22] E. Juan-García, V. Canales, A. Peguero, A. Herrera, and A. Martínez, "Abdominal hernia through a defect in the iliac bone after resection of a chondrosarcoma of the pelvis," *Acta Orthopaedica Belgica*, vol. 68, no. 1, pp. 79–82, 2002.

9

A Rare Initial Presentation of Gastric Cancer with Multiple Osteolytic Lesions

Asad Jehangir,[1] Kim Aderhold,[1] Priya Rajagopalan,[1] Oluwaseun Shogbesan,[1] Sharon Swierczynski,[2] Anam Qureshi,[3] Qasim Jehangir,[4] and Christian Espana Schmidt[5]

[1] *Department of Internal Medicine, Reading Health System, Spruce Street/6th Avenue, West Reading, PA 19610, USA*
[2] *Department of Pathology, Reading Health System, Spruce Street/6th Avenue, West Reading, PA 19610, USA*
[3] *King Edward Medical University, Mayo Hospital Road, Nelagumbad, Anarkali, Lahore 54000, Pakistan*
[4] *Rawalpindi Medical College, Tipu Road, Rawalpindi 46000, Pakistan*
[5] *Reading Health System, Spruce Street/6th Avenue, West Reading, PA 19610, USA*

Correspondence should be addressed to Asad Jehangir; asadjehangir@gmail.com

Academic Editor: Se-Hoon Lee

Gastric cancer is the 12th leading cause of cancer-related deaths in the United States and commonly metastasizes to the bones. However, the presentation of gastric cancer as bony metastases without preceding gastrointestinal symptoms is rare which has been infrequently reported in the literature. Moreover, leptomeningeal carcinomatosis is an unusual complication of gastric cancer accounting for less than 1 percent of these patients. We present a unique case of a middle aged male who presented to the emergency department with worsening backache which started one month priorly. The only abnormal laboratory test was an elevated alkaline phosphatase of 154 IU/L. The imaging of his spine showed osteolytic lesions which on biopsy revealed signet ring cells. A small 2 cm ulcerated mass was found on esophagogastroduodenoscopy at the gastric cardia which on biopsy revealed signet ring gastric carcinoma. The patient received chemotherapy with capecitabine and oxaliplatin as well as radiation and showed a good response initially. A few months later, he presented with persistent worsening headaches and on brain imaging was found to have leptomeningeal carcinomatosis. Ten months after the diagnosis of gastric carcinoma, he passed away.

1. Introduction

Fifty percent of gastric adenocarcinomas can initially present with distant metastasis. Disseminated bony metastases as the first clinical manifestation are seen in exceptional cases and generally present in the later stages of an established disease. Furthermore, leptomeningeal carcinomatosis (LMC) is a rare complication of gastric cancer seen in only about 0.16 to 0.69% of cases [1]. We describe an unusual presentation of gastric cancer with multiple osteolytic metastases complicated by LMC few months after the diagnosis despite chemotherapy.

2. Case

A 48-year-old male with history of mild gastroesophageal reflux disease presented to the emergency with a one-month history of worsening low back pain without a preceding trauma. The pain had gradually increased to 10/10 in severity and impaired his ambulation over the previous 2 days. He denied any lower extremity pain, weakness, numbness or tingling, or fecal or urinary incontinence. He also reported right chest discomfort that began with a "painful crack" while he was bowling about a week before. His backache and chest pain did not improve with a brief course of NSAIDs. He denied nausea, vomiting, hematochezia, melena, or weight loss. His family history was negative for any malignancies.

On examination the patient did not have any spinal tenderness or signs of spinal cord compression and had normal strength, sensation, and reflexes in the lower extremities. The only significant abnormality on the laboratory tests was an elevated alkaline phosphatase of 154 IU/L (reference range 38–110 IU/L). Other laboratory values including calcium (9.9 MG/DL), creatinine (0.94 MG/DL),

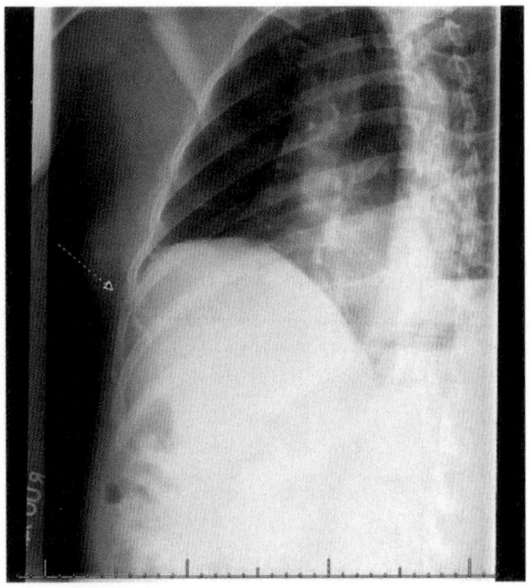

FIGURE 1: X-ray of the right sided ribs revealing a fracture involving the lateral aspect of the 7th rib.

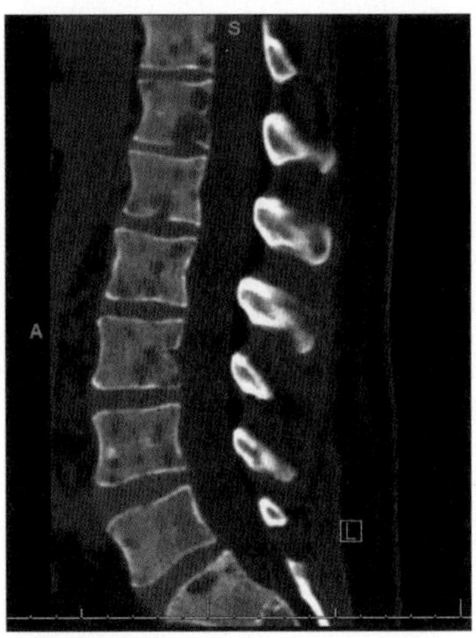

FIGURE 2: CT lumbar spine without contrast showing innumerable lytic lesions seen throughout the lumbar spine.

hemoglobin (15.6 G/DL), platelet count (320 CMM), and PSA (0.45 NG/ML) were all normal. An X-ray of the chest showed a fracture of the lateral aspect of the right 7th rib (Figure 1). Computerized tomography (CT) of the spine revealed several lytic lesions throughout most of his spine (Figure 2) which initially raised suspicion for multiple myeloma; however the findings of normal calcium, creatinine, and protein levels prompted evaluation for an alternative diagnosis. A CT chest did not reveal any lung or thyroid masses. A left transpedicular core biopsy of the L3 vertebra was performed which surprisingly was consistent with adenocarcinoma with signet cell features (Figures 3(a) and 3(b)). A CT of the abdomen and pelvis showed multiple prominent retroperitoneal lymph nodes which were not pathologically enlarged; however, their abnormal number was suspicious for early metastatic disease. Esophagogastroduodenoscopy revealed a small 2 cm ulcerated mass at the gastric cardia which was not visualized on the CT scan. A biopsy indicated invasive poorly differentiated gastric adenocarcinoma with signet ring cells (Figures 4(a) and 4(b)). An immunohistochemical stain for human epidermal growth factor receptor 2 (HER2) was\ equivocal (Figure 4(c)). HER2 fluorescence in situ hybridization analysis was performed which did not reveal any evidence of HER2 gene amplification.

The patient underwent chemotherapy with capecitabine and oxaliplatin along with radiation with good initial response; however, after a few months he reported persistent headaches. Head imaging demonstrated leptomeningeal carcinomatosis. Ten months after the initial diagnosis of metastatic gastric cancer, he was brought to the emergency department after multiple episodes of loss of consciousness. A brain MRI revealed acute infarcts in multiple vascular territories (Figure 5), presumably caused by a hypercoagulable state secondary to malignancy. The patient's condition continued to deteriorate, and he expired approximately two weeks later.

3. Discussion

Gastric cancer is the 12th leading cause of cancer-related death in the United States and accounted for approximately 11,000 deaths nationwide in 2014 [2]. There has been a progressive decline in the incidence of intestinal type gastric cancer; on the contrary, the diffuse type of gastric carcinoma is being diagnosed more frequently, particularly the signet ring cell type, which constitutes 3.4 to 29% of all cases of gastric carcinomas [3, 4]. The diffuse type often presents in an advanced stage and at a younger age [4]. Most cases (99%) of signet ring cell carcinoma originate in the stomach [4].

Bone metastases from gastric cancer, more commonly seen in signet ring cell type, portend a poor prognosis. The reported incidence of bones metastases varies widely from as low as 1% in clinical practice to as high as 45% in screening studies for bone metastases, implying that many cases are asymptomatic [5]. Bone metastases are usually detected after a diagnosis of gastric cancer has already been established. Gastric cancer presenting as bone metastases without any preceding gastrointestinal symptoms has been infrequently reported in the literature [6, 7]. Such rare cases are generally associated with significantly larger primary gastric lesions in contrast to the small 2 cm mass of the gastric cardia seen in our patient. The most likely route of spread from a primary gastric lesion to the bone is via lymphatic channels, although dissemination may also occur through portal and nonportal veins [8]. The most common sites of involvement reported in the literature include spine, ribs, scapula, and pelvis [9]. Patients with bone metastases may present with refractory pain or pathological fractures. Various laboratory abnormalities that suggest the possibility of bone metastases include elevated alkaline phosphatase (ALP), increased LDH, and anemia or thrombocytopenia. Of interest, the only deranged laboratory finding in our patient was elevated ALP [8, 10].

Our patient also developed leptomeningeal carcinomatosis which is usually seen as a complication of hematological malignancies and manifests less commonly in solid malignancies [11]. Melanoma and lung and breast cancer are the more common solid tumors associated with LMC [11]. LMC resulting from an underlying gastric malignancy has

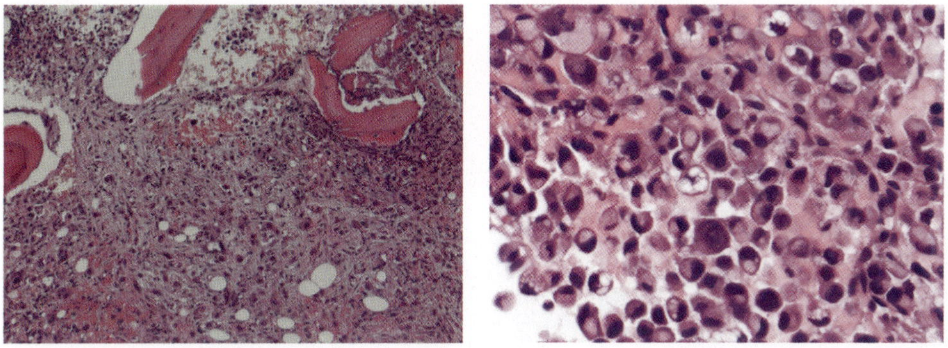

(a) (b)

Figure 3: (a) Metastasis to the lumbar spine. Histologic sections of a core biopsy of the L3 vertebral body demonstrate near complete marrow replacement by a proliferation of malignant cells with associated fibrosis ((a), 10x). (b) Metastasis to the lumbar spine. On high power (40x), the infiltrate is comprised of signet ring cells morphologically identical to the gastric cardia biopsy (see Figure 4(b)).

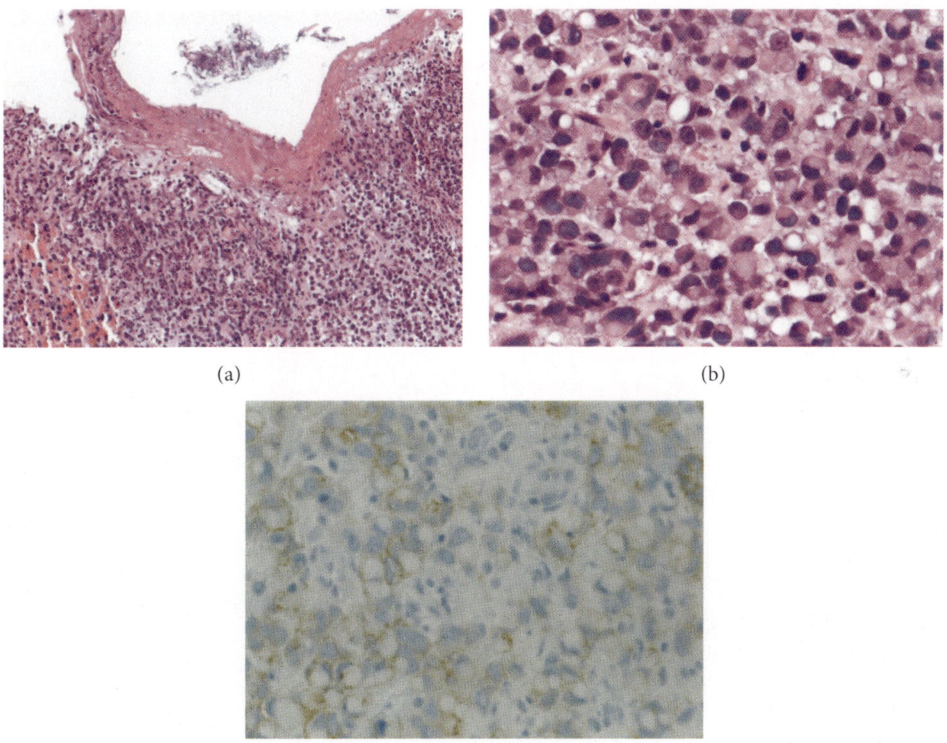

(a) (b)

(c)

Figure 4: (a) Poorly differentiated adenocarcinoma of the gastric cardia. Histologic sections demonstrate erosion of the surface epithelium with diffuse involvement of the lamina propria by an atypical infiltrate comprised predominantly of discohesive cells ((a), 10x). (b) Poorly differentiated adenocarcinoma of the gastric cardia. On high power (40x), the cells in the infiltrate demonstrate prominent signet ring cell morphology, diagnostic of poorly differentiated adenocarcinoma. (c) Poorly differentiated adenocarcinoma of the gastric cardia. An immunohistochemical stain for HER2 interpreted as being equivocal ((c), 40x).

been rarely reported in the literature and is associated with poor outcomes. It commonly manifests as headaches; other neurological manifestations may include weakness, dizziness, altered mental status, or seizures [12]. There is no single test sensitive enough to establish the diagnosis, although a combination of CSF cytology and MRI imaging can assist with a combined sensitivity of over 90% [13].

Chemotherapy for the treatment of advanced metastatic gastric carcinomas may be associated with better quality of life than symptomatic treatment alone. Intrathecal chemotherapy may be used in cases of LMC [11, 14]. Adjuvant trastuzumab may also be utilized for HER2 positive lesions [14]. However, chemotherapy is not advised for patients with Eastern Cooperative Oncology Group score of 3 or higher

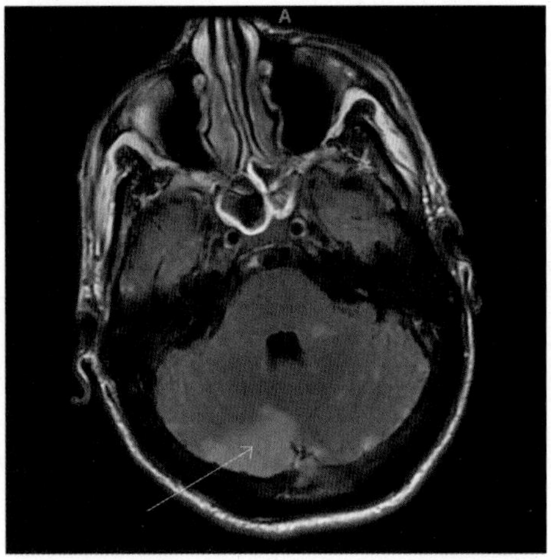

Figure 5: MRI brain with and without contrast revealing multiple foci of predominantly cortical signal change with the largest area involving the medial right cerebellar hemisphere (white arrow). The appearance is most compatible with subacute infarcts, presumably from an embolic source. There are no enhancing masses to suggest metastatic disease.

and must be carefully utilized in a selective group of patients after extensive counseling. Those patients not responding should be recognized early [9]. Advanced signet ring cell carcinoma carries a poor prognosis compared to other types of gastric cancer [4]. Other factors associated with poor outcomes include microinvasion of vessels and tumor location; tumors involving the whole stomach understandably have a worse prognosis compared to lesions localized in the antrum and the body [4]. Mean survival time is 4-5 months with bone metastases from gastric cancer and even less about 3 months with LMC [10, 15, 16].

4. Conclusion

Multiple rounded osteolytic lesions and pathologic fractures are often presumed to be multiple myeloma. Also included in the differential are metastases from solid organs like prostate, breast, lung, thyroid, or kidney. However, it is prudent to consider gastric cancer as the possible primary site of disease even in the absence of overt gastrointestinal symptoms. Leptomeningeal carcinomatosis is a rare but invariably fatal complication of gastric cancer that frequently manifests as headaches; however, other neurological complaints may also be present.

References

[1] M. Kim, "Intracranial involvement by metastatic advanced gastric carcinoma," *Journal of Neuro-Oncology*, vol. 43, no. 1, pp. 59–62, 1999.

[2] R. Siegel, J. Ma, Z. Zou, and A. Jemal, "Cancer statistics, 2014," *CA Cancer Journal for Clinicians*, vol. 64, no. 1, pp. 9–29, 2014.

[3] D. E. Henson, C. Dittus, M. Younes, H. Nguyen, and J. Albores-Saavedra, "Differential trends in the intestinal diffuse types of gastric carcinoma in the United States, 1973–2000: increase in the signet ring cell type," *Archives of Pathology and Laboratory Medicine*, vol. 128, no. 7, pp. 765–770, 2004.

[4] T. Yokota, Y. Kunii, S. Teshima et al., "Signet ring cell carcinoma of the stomach: a clinicopathological comparison with the other histological types," *Tohoku Journal of Experimental Medicine*, vol. 186, no. 2, pp. 121–130, 1998.

[5] F. P. Turkoz, M. Solak, S. Kilickap et al., "Bone metastasis from gastric cancer: the incidence, clinicopathological features, and influence on survival," *Journal of Gastric Cancer*, vol. 14, no. 3, pp. 164–172, 2014.

[6] C. Dittus, H. Mathew, A. Malek, and A. Negroiu, "Bone marrow infiltration as the initial presentation of gastric signet ring cell adenocarcinoma," *Journal of Gastrointestinal Oncology*, vol. 5, no. 6, pp. E113–E116, 2014.

[7] M. Nottebaert, G. U. Exner, A. R. von Hochstetter, and A. Schreiber, "Metastatic bone disease from occult carcinoma: a profile," *International Orthopaedics*, vol. 13, no. 2, pp. 119–123, 1989.

[8] A. Basheer, J. Daniel, and S. Padhi, "Compressive myeloradiculopathy from bony metastasis as the initial presentation of poorly differentiated adenocarcinoma stomach—a case report," *Australasian Medical Journal*, vol. 6, no. 10, pp. 515–519, 2013.

[9] J. B. Ahn, T. K. Ha, and S. J. Kwon, "Bone metastasis in gastric cancer patients," *Journal of Gastric Cancer*, vol. 11, no. 1, pp. 38–45, 2011.

[10] H. S. Kim, S. Y. Yi, H. J. Jun et al., "Clinical outcome of gastric cancer patients with bone marrow metastases," *Oncology*, vol. 73, no. 3-4, pp. 192–197, 2007.

[11] N. Saad, A. Alsibai, and T. H. Hadid, "Carcinomatous meningitis due to gastric adenocarcinoma: a rare presentation of relapse," *World Journal of Gastrointestinal Oncology*, vol. 6, no. 12, pp. 450–453, 2014.

[12] S. Y. Oh, S.-J. Lee, J. Lee et al., "Gastric leptomeningeal carcinomatosis: multi-center retrospective analysis of 54 cases," *World Journal of Gastroenterology*, vol. 15, no. 40, pp. 5086–5090, 2009.

[13] S. J. Kim, J. T. Kwon, S. K. Mun, and Y. H. Hong, "Leptomeningeal carcinomatosis of gastric cancer misdiagnosed as vestibular schwannoma," *Journal of Korean Neurosurgical Society*, vol. 56, no. 1, pp. 51–54, 2014.

[14] N. Ahmed, X. Li, and J. Rathmann, "Bone marrow metastasis as first recurrence of gastric cancer: a case report," *Connecticut Medicine*, vol. 75, no. 10, pp. 599–602, 2011.

[15] N.-H. Kim, J.-H. Kim, H.-M. Chin, and K.-H. Jun, "Leptomeningeal carcinomatosis from gastric cancer: single institute retrospective analysis of 9 cases," *Annals of Surgical Treatment and Research*, vol. 86, no. 1, pp. 16–21, 2014.

[16] S. Hussain and S. Chui, "Gastric carcinoma presenting with extensive bone metastases and marrow infiltration causing extradural spinal haemorrhage," *British Journal of Radiology*, vol. 79, no. 939, pp. 261–263, 2006.

10

Late Onset Ipilimumab-Induced Pericarditis and Pericardial Effusion: A Rare but Life Threatening Complication

Seongseok Yun,[1] Nicole D. Vincelette,[2] Iyad Mansour,[1] Dana Hariri,[3] and Sara Motamed[4]

[1]*Department of Medicine, University of Arizona, Tucson, AZ 85721, USA*
[2]*Molecular Pharmacology and Experimental Therapeutics, Mayo Clinic, Rochester, MN 55905, USA*
[3]*Department of Pathology, University of Arizona, Tucson, AZ 85721, USA*
[4]*Midwestern University, Arizona College of Osteopathic Medicine, Glendale, AZ 85308, USA*

Correspondence should be addressed to Seongseok Yun; namaska97@gmail.com

Academic Editor: Francesco A. Mauri

Metastatic cutaneous melanoma has poor prognosis with 2-year survival rate of 10–20%. Melanoma cells express various antigens including gp100, melanoma antigen recognized by T cells 1 (MART-1), and tyrosinase, which can induce immune-mediated anticancer response via T cell activation. Cytotoxic T-lymphocyte associated antigen-4 (CTLA-4) is an immune check point molecule that negatively regulates T cell activation and proliferation. Accordingly, recent phase III clinical trials demonstrated significant survival benefit with ipilimumab, a human monoclonal antibody (IgG1) that blocks the interaction of CTLA-4 with its ligands. Since the efficacy of ipilimumab depends on T cell activation, it is associated with substantial risk of immune mediated adverse reactions such as colitis, hepatitis, thyroiditis, and hypophysitis. We report the first case of late onset pericarditis and cardiac tamponade associated with ipilimumab treatment in patient with metastatic cutaneous melanoma.

1. Case Presentation

A 59-year-old male patient with no significant history of autoimmune disease presented to clinic with bleeding from a mole in the right forearm. Biopsy and mutation testing identified melanoma with $BRAF^{V600E}$ mutation. PET/CT showed four FDG avid soft tissue nodules in the subcutaneous tissues of chest and back, abdominal mesentery, and right retroperitoneum. Excisional biopsy from right axillary lymph node was positive for melanin A staining and showed extracapsular invasion, confirming the diagnosis of stage M1c metastatic melanoma. Therefore, patient received 4 cycles of ipilimumab (3 mg/kg) treatment every 3 weeks without significant adverse reaction except skin rash on the infusion site.

Twelve weeks after the last cycle of ipilimumab treatment, the patient presented to ED with acute onset chest pain and shortness of breath which started 1 day prior to the presentation. Vital sign showed BP 97/55 mmHg, HR 106 beats/min, RR 20 breaths/min, and O_2 saturation 99% while breathing room air and temperature 36.9°C. Physical examination revealed distant heart sound and 5 cm of jugular venous distension. Electrocardiogram showed low QRS voltage and T wave inversion on V_1–V_4 leads, and troponin I was negative. CT angiogram showed negative for pulmonary embolism; however, it demonstrated pericardial thickening and moderate sized pericardial effusion which are new compared to the prior study (Figures 1(a) and 1(b)). Subsequent echocardiogram showed septal bouncing and respiratory septal shift, suggesting ventricular interdependence and constrictive effusive physiology. Total 3 L of fluid was given for low blood pressure. Bedsides pericardiocentesis drained 130 mL of serosanguinous fluid and subxiphoid pericardial window was performed the next day. Biochemical study from pericardial fluid showed LDH 794 IU/L, protein 4.3 g/dL, amylase 29 IU/L, and glucose 99 mg/dL. Fluid cytology, Gram stain, and culture were negative for neoplasm or microorganism, and adenosine deaminase PCR was also negative. WBC count was 19,600/μL with 90% of lymphocyte consistent with marked acute inflammation. Pathology from pericardial tissue demonstrated acute fibrinous pericarditis without any evidence of malignancy or microorganism (Figure 2). Additional examinations for autoimmune disease including

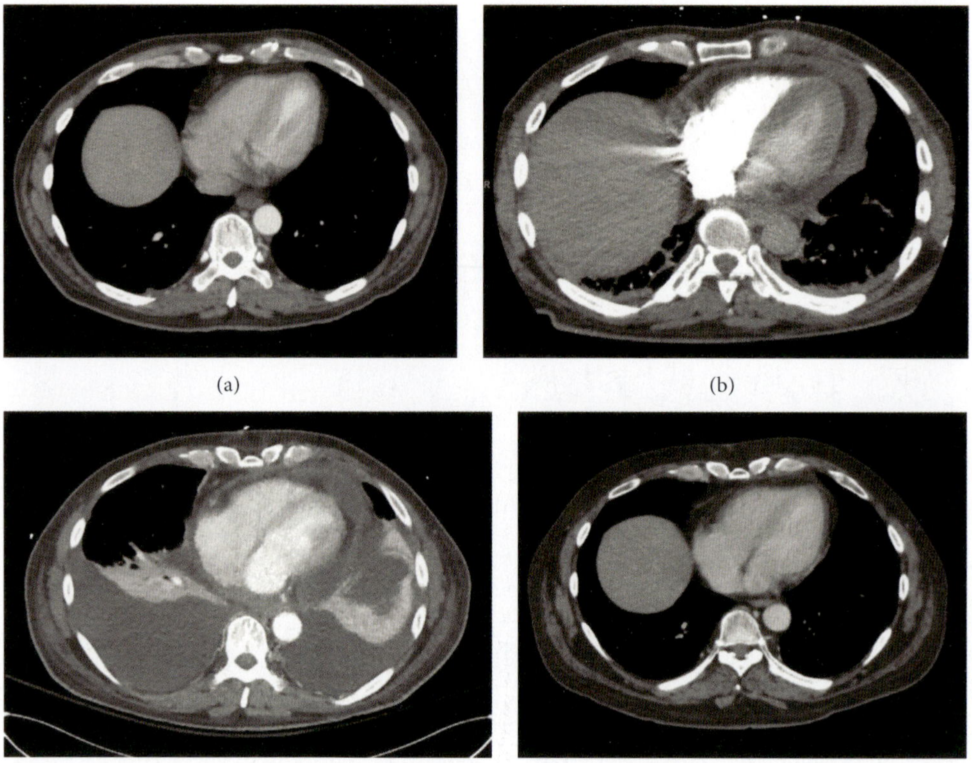

(a) (b)

(c) (d)

Figure 1: CT chest on admission showed pericardial thickening, moderate-sized pericardial effusion, and adjacent inflammatory changes within the epicardial fat and mediastinum (b), which were new compared to the prior study (a). New large bilateral pleural effusion with associated compressive atelectasis in the lower lungs and stable pericardial effusion is observed on day 10 (c), which resolved after systemic steroid treatment (d).

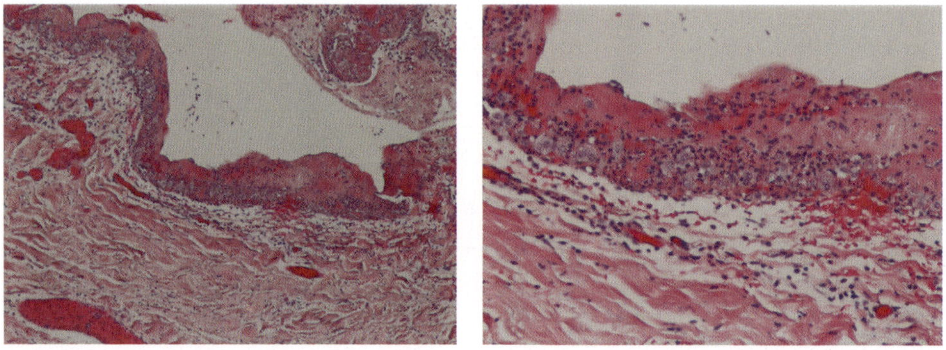

(a) (b)

Figure 2: Biopsy specimen from pericardium, sections through the pericardium show acute fibrinous pericarditis, characterized by mixed inflammatory infiltrates in the pericardial wall, accompanied by abundant surface fibrin. No microorganisms were identified on hematoxylin-eosin-stained sections.

rheumatoid factor, anti-nuclear antibodies (ANA), double strand DNA (dsDNA), anti-neutrophil cytoplasmic antibodies (ANCA), proteinase 3, and myeloperoxidase antibodies were all negative. Further infectious work-up including blood culture, sputum culture, and respiratory viral panel were all negative as well.

Indomethacin (50 mg three times a day) was started for the treatment of acute pericarditis; however, patient developed worsening shortness of breath, generalized weakness, somnolence, and diarrhea. Blood pressure dropped down to 64/42 for which levophed and aggressive fluid resuscitation was initiated. Repeat CT scan demonstrated persistent pericardial effusion and large bilateral pleural effusion with compressive atelectasis in the lower lobes (Figure 1(c)). Thoracentesis was performed to drain 1.4 L of pleural fluid and biochemistry revealed borderline exudates with LDH ratio 0.27, protein ratio 0.51, and WBC 667/μL with lymphocyte dominance (57%) but no evidence of malignancy or infection.

Table 1: Lab values during the hospitalization, baseline TSH, free T4, and cortisol levels were within normal range; however, patient presented with elevated TSH, low free T4, and decreased cortisol levels, suggesting immune-mediated hypothyroidism and adrenal insufficiency.

Labs (reference range)	Baseline	Admission	Day 7 after steroid Tx	Day 21 after steroid Tx	Day 35 after steroid Tx
TSH (0.35–4.00 μIU/mL)	3.26	6.78	8.10	5.85	2.85
Free T4 (0.7–1.5 ng/dL)	0.8	0.4	0.4	1.2	1.0
ACTH (7–69 pg/mL)	NR	NR	<5	<5	<5
Cortisol at 8 AM (4.2–38.4 μg/dL)	10.6	<1.0	<1.0	<1.0	1.5
AST (5–34 IU/L)	28	30	24	18	21
ALT (0–55 IU/L)	13	14	28	33	19
Total bilirubin (0.2–1.2 mg/dL)	1.1	1.9	0.8	0.6	0.6
Troponin I (0.00–0.02 ng/mL)	NR	<0.02	0.07	<0.02	NR

Brain MRI showed no pathologic changes. TSH, free T4, and morning random cortisol levels after the last cycle of ipilimumab treatment were 3.26 μIU/mL, 0.8 ng/dL, and 10.6 μg/dL, respectively, and rechecked levels on admission showed 6.78 μIU/mL, 0.4 ng/dL, and 1.0 μg/dL, indicating hypothyroidism and adrenal insufficiency (Table 1). Screening colonoscopy prior to ipilimumab treatment had shown normal finding and infectious work-up for the new onset diarrhea including *C. diff* toxin PCR, stool Gram stain, culture, and parasites was all negative. Collectively, these results suggested ipilimumab induced immune-mediated pericarditis, hypothyroidism, adrenal insufficiency, and diarrhea for which high dose intravenous methylprednisolone (125 mg daily) was started. Patient achieved remarkable clinical improvement over the 48 hours, and methylprednisolone was switched to prednisone (40 mg daily) and budesonide (9 mg daily) on the third day, and they were tapered down over a month. Repeat chest X-ray and CT scan showed resolved pleural and pericardial effusion (Figure 1(d)), and diarrhea improved gradually over the month. Rechecked TSH and random cortisol levels also showed normal range of 2.85 μIU/mL (without thyroid hormone replacement) and 1.5 μg/dL, respectively (Table 1).

2. Discussion

Over the past decades, the incidence of cutaneous melanoma has increased by more than 60%, and 10–15% of patients present at stage III or IV [1]. Unresectable disease is used to be treated with best supportive care, radiation, or systemic treatments such as dacarbazine and temozolomide; however, the prognosis of metastatic disease is dismal with median survival of less than 12 months [2, 3]. Immune system plays a pivotal role to eradicate cancer cells, making immune modulation a novel therapeutic target. Recognition of various tumor antigens by antigen presenting cells induces cytotoxic T cell activation via interaction of T cell receptor with major histocompatibility complex 1 molecule. For the full T cell activation, additional engagement of costimulatory pathway is required and this is antagonized by CTLA-4, an immune check point molecule. CTLA-4 competes with CD28 to bind CD80 (B7-1) and CD86 (B7-2) and negatively regulates T cell activation and proliferation [4, 5]. Accordingly, CTLA-4 knockout mice were shown to develop lymphoproliferative disorder with excessive accumulation of activated T cells and preclinical study with antibodies against CTLA-4 demonstrated tumor cells suppression [6, 7].

Ipilimumab is a human monoclonal antibody (IgG1) that blocks the interaction of CTLA-4 with its ligands and recent phase III clinical trials in patients with unresectable metastatic melanoma showed overall survival benefit with ipilimumab treatment compared to gp100 vaccination or dacarbazine monotherapy [8, 9]. Because antagonizing CTLA-4 stimulates T cell proliferation, ipilimumab treatment is associated with substantial risk of immune mediated adverse reactions and current guideline recommends ipilimumab treatment with careful monitor for these side effects [10]. Previous phase II and III clinical trials showed that grade 3-4 immune related adverse events including enterocolitis, hepatitis, dermatitis, and endocrinopathy can occur in 10–40% of patients [5, 8, 9, 11–13] and rare complications such as pericarditis, nephritis, pneumonitis, meningitis, uveitis, and hemolytic anemia in less than 1% of patients who were treated with ipilimumab (Table 2) [14].

The halflife of ipilimumab clearance is 14.7 days [14]; however, immune cell activation and proliferation are slow process [15]. Accordingly, the effect of ipilimumab treatment evolves over months and delayed responses and adverse events (18–20 weeks after treatment) are well known as in this case [15]. Our patient completed the last cycle of ipilimumab treatment 12 weeks prior to admission and he presented with pericarditis and pericardial effusion. Infectious work-up including bacterial and viral etiologies was negative. There was no significant history of autoimmune disease and additional examinations for autoimmune disease were all negative. Moreover, pericardial and pleural fluids cytology showed lymphocytes dominance with no evidence of malignancy or infection and pericardial tissue biopsy demonstrated acute inflammation, suggesting ipilimumab induced immune mediated pericarditis and pericardial effusion, most likely.

TABLE 2: Ipilimumab induced immune related adverse events in Phases II and III trials.

Study	Pathology	Stage	Range of median Age	Pt. No.	Treatments	Overall survival rate Ipilimumab (1)	Overall survival rate Ipilimumab (2)	Overall survival rate Ctrl	Grade 3/4 immune related adverse events rate Ipilimumab (1)	Grade 3/4 immune related adverse events rate Ipilimumab (2)	Grade 3/4 immune related adverse events rate Ctrl
Robert et al., 2011 [9]	Cutaneous melanoma	III IV	56.4–57.5	502	Ipilimumab (10 mg/kg) + dacarbazine (1) versus placebo + dacarbazine	47.3% (1 yr) 28.5% (2 yr) 20.8% (3 yr)		36.3% (1 yr) 17.9% (2 yr) 12.2% (3 yr)	†Any events: 41.7% dermatologic: 3.2% GI: 5.6% hepatic: 30%		Any events: 6.0% dermatologic: 0% GI: 0% hepatic: 1.2%
Hodi et al., 2010 [8]	LHA-A*0201 (+) cutaneous melanoma	III IV	55.6–57.4	676	Ipilimumab (3 mg/kg) + gp100 (1) versus ipilimumab (3 mg/kg) (2) versus gp100	43.6% (1 yr) 21.6% (2 yr)	45.6% (1 yr) 23.5% (2 yr)	25.3% (1 yr) 13.7% (2 yr)	‡¶Any events: 10.2% dermatologic: 2.4% GI: 5.8% hepatic: 3.2% endocrine: 1.1% others: 1.3%	Any events: 14.5% dermatologic: 1.5% GI: 7.6% hepatic: 0% endocrine: 3.8% others: 2.3%	Any events: 3.0% dermatologic: 0% GI: 0.8% hepatic: 2.3% endocrine: 0% others: 3.1%
Wolchok et al., 2010 [11]	Cutaneous melanoma	III IV	56–59	217	Ipilimumab (10 mg/kg) (1) versus ipilimumab (3 mg/kg) (2)	48.6% (1 yr) 29.8% (2 yr)	39.6% (1 yr) 24.2% (2 yr)		¶Any events: 25.4% dermatologic: 4.2% GI: 15.5% hepatic: 3.0% endocrine: 1.4% δothers: 2.8%	Any events: 7.0% dermatologic: 1.4% GI: 2.8% hepatic: 0% endocrine: 2.8% others: 0%	
Hersh et al., 2011 [13]	Cutaneous melanoma	III IV	60–66	76	Ipilimumab (3 mg/kg) + dacarbazine (1) versus ipilimumab (3 mg/kg) (2)	62.0% (1 yr) 24.0% (2 yr) 20.0% (3 yr)	45.0% (1 yr) 21.0% (2 yr) 9.0% (3 yr)		ΦAny events: 17.1% dermatologic: 42.9% GI: 28.6%	Any events: 7.1% dermatologic: 48.7% GI: 20.5%	
Weber et al., 2009 [12]	Cutaneous melanoma	III IV	58–61	115	Ipilimumab (10 mg/kg) + placebo (1) versus ipilimumab (10 mg/kg) + budesonide (2)	62.4% (1 yr) 41.7% (2 yr)	55.9% (1 yr) 40.5% (2 yr)		¶Any events: 38.0% dermatologic: 0% GI: 23.0% hepatic: 12.0% endocrine: 5.0% others: 2.0%	Any events: 41.0% dermatologic: 5.0% GI: 24.0% hepatic: 9.0% endocrine: 5.0% others: 2.0%	

†The immune-related adverse events were prospectively defined (medical dictionary for regulatory activities, version 13.0).
‡The immune-related adverse events were defined as an adverse event that was associated with exposure to the study drug and that was consistent with an immune phenomenon.
¶The adverse events were graded by the National Cancer Institute's common terminology criteria for adverse events version 3.0.
δOther immune related adverse events included scleritis ($n = 1$) and pneumonitis ($n = 1$).
ΦImmune related adverse events were coded according to the Medical Dictionary for Regulatory Affairs, and severities were graded using Common Toxicity Criteria version 2.0. Dermatologic and GI adverse events included grade ≥1 in this study.

This is supported by associated hypothyroidism, adrenal insufficiency, and diarrhea, all of which showed remarkable improvement with systemic steroid treatment and without hormone replacement.

As shown in phase II and III clinical trials, most of the ipilimumab induced immune related adverse effects are reversible with early recognition and appropriate management. For the severe immune reactions, early administration of high dose systemic corticosteroid is critical and adverse reactions resolve within a median of 2-3 weeks as in our case [5, 8, 9, 11]. Collectively, ipilimumab treatment is associated with significant survival benefit and, however, also with life threatening immune mediated adverse effects that require close monitor, early diagnosis, and appropriate management.

3. Conclusion

To the best of our knowledge, this is the first case of late onset pericarditis and pericardial effusion associated with ipilimumab treatment in patient with metastatic cutaneous melanoma. Ipilimumab induced immune mediated adverse events could be life threatening as shown in our case, and early diagnosis and intervention with systemic corticosteroid are critical for the better clinical outcome.

Authors' Contribution

Seongseok Yun, Nicole D. Vincelette, Dana Hariri, and Iyad Mansour contributed to acquisition, analysis, and interpretation of data. Seongseok Yun, Iyad Mansour, and Dana Hariri were responsible for patient care. Seongseok Yun, Nicole D. Vincelette, Iyad Mansour, and Sara Motamed contributed to drafting the paper.

References

[1] R. Siegel, J. Ma, Z. Zou, and A. Jemal, "Cancer statistics, 2014," *CA: A Cancer Journal for Clinicians*, vol. 64, no. 1, pp. 9–29, 2014.

[2] H. Tsao, M. B. Atkins, and A. J. Sober, "Management of cutaneous melanoma," *The New England Journal of Medicine*, vol. 351, no. 10, pp. 998–1042, 2004.

[3] S. S. Agarwala, "Current systemic therapy for metastatic melanoma," *Expert Review of Anticancer Therapy*, vol. 9, no. 5, pp. 587–595, 2009.

[4] I. Melero, S. Hervas-Stubbs, M. Glennie, D. M. Pardoll, and L. Chen, "Immunostimulatory monoclonal antibodies for cancer therapy," *Nature Reviews Cancer*, vol. 7, no. 2, pp. 95–106, 2007.

[5] S. J. O'Day, O. Hamid, and W. J. Urba, "Targeting cytotoxic T-lymphocyte antigen-4 (CTLA-4): a novel strategy for the treatment of melanoma and other malignancies," *Cancer*, vol. 110, no. 12, pp. 2614–2627, 2007.

[6] P. Waterhouse, J. M. Penninger, E. Timms et al., "Lymphoproliferative disorders with early lethality in mice deficient in Ctla-4," *Science*, vol. 270, no. 5238, pp. 985–988, 1995.

[7] D. R. Leach, M. F. Krummel, and J. P. Allison, "Enhancement of antitumor immunity by CTLA-4 blockade," *Science*, vol. 271, no. 5256, pp. 1734–1736, 1996.

[8] F. S. Hodi, S. J. O'Day, D. F. McDermott et al., "Improved survival with ipilimumab in patients with metastatic melanoma," *The New England Journal of Medicine*, vol. 363, no. 8, pp. 711–723, 2010.

[9] C. Robert, L. Thomas, I. Bondarenko et al., "Ipilimumab plus dacarbazine for previously untreated metastatic melanoma," *The New England Journal of Medicine*, vol. 364, no. 26, pp. 2517–2526, 2011.

[10] NCCN, *NCCN Guideline, Melanoma, Version 2*, NCCN, 2015.

[11] J. D. Wolchok, B. Neyns, G. Linette et al., "Ipilimumab monotherapy in patients with pretreated advanced melanoma: a randomised, double-blind, multicentre, phase 2, dose-ranging study," *The Lancet Oncology*, vol. 11, no. 2, pp. 155–164, 2010.

[12] J. Weber, J. A. Thompson, O. Hamid et al., "A randomized, double-blind, placebo-controlled, phase II study comparing the tolerability and efficacy of ipilimumab administered with or without prophylactic budesonide in patients with unresectable stage III or IV melanoma," *Clinical Cancer Research*, vol. 15, no. 17, pp. 5591–5598, 2009.

[13] E. M. Hersh, S. J. O'Day, J. Powderly et al., "A phase II multicenter study of ipilimumab with or without dacarbazine in chemotherapy-naïve patients with advanced melanoma," *Investigational New Drugs*, vol. 29, no. 3, pp. 489–498, 2011.

[14] C. Fellne, "Ipilimumab (yervoy) prolongs survival in advanced melanoma: serious side effects and a hefty price tag may limit its use," *P & T*, vol. 37, no. 9, pp. 503–530, 2012.

[15] G. K. Pennock, W. Waterfield, and J. D. Wolchok, "Patient responses to ipilimumab, a novel immunopotentiator for metastatic melanoma: how different are these from conventional treatment responses?" *American Journal of Clinical Oncology*, vol. 35, no. 6, pp. 606–611, 2012.

11

Progression of an Invasive ACTH Pituitary Macroadenoma with Cushing's Disease to Pituitary Carcinoma

Clarissa Groberio Borba,[1] Rafael Loch Batista,[1] Nina Rosa de Castro Musolino,[1] Vanielle Carvalho Machado,[1] Ana Elisa Evangelista Alcantara,[1] Gilberto Ochman da Silva,[2] Valter Angelo Sperling Cescato,[2] and Malebranche Berardo Carneiro da Cunha Neto[1]

[1] *Neuroendocrinology Unit, Functional Neurosurgery Division, Hospital das Clinicas, Faculdade de Medicina, Universidade de São Paulo, Brazil*

[2] *Pituitary Neurosurgery Unit, Functional Neurosurgery Division, Hospital das Clinicas, Faculdade de Medicina, Universidade de São Paulo, Brazil*

Correspondence should be addressed to Rafael Loch Batista; rafael.loch@hc.fm.usp.br

Academic Editor: Cesar V. Reyes

Pituitary carcinomas are very rare tumors that in most cases produce prolactin and adrenocorticotropic hormone (ACTH). It is a challenge to diagnosis of a pituitary carcinoma before disclosed symptomatic metastasis. We report the case of a female patient with Cushing's disease who underwent three transsphenoidal surgeries, with pathological findings of common ACTH pituitary adenoma including Ki-67 expression <3%. She achieved hypocortisolism after the 3rd surgery although ACTH levels remained slightly elevated. The patient returned some time later with fast worsening of hypercortisolism. Magnetic resonance imaging showed clivus invasion, which led to a fourth surgery and radiation. This time, immunohistochemistry revealed strong Ki-67 (10% to 15%) and p53 expression. Liver and lumbar spine metastases were found on workup. The patient died after few months due to lung infection. Pituitary carcinomas are rare, and the transformation of an ACTH-secreting pituitary adenoma into a carcinoma is exceptional. The difficulty of defining markers for the diagnosis of carcinoma, before metastasis diagnosis, in order to change the management of the disease, is a challenge.

1. Introduction

Pituitary adenomas are a common type of intracranial tumor. The more effective approach is transsphenoidal surgery. Nonfunctioning pituitary adenomas and prolactinomas are more prevalent pituitary adenomas [1]. Pituitary adenomas can be classified according to pathological, radiological, or clinical behavior as typical or atypical, invasive or noninvasive, and aggressive or nonaggressive. The World Health Organization (WHO) classification categorizes pituitary adenomas as typical and atypical and the pathological features of atypical adenoma are defined as a Ki-67 index greater than 3% and/or extensive p53 immunoreactivity [1]. Pituitary carcinomas are very rare (0.1%-0.2% of pituitary tumors) [2], with diagnosis requiring evidence of metastasis and they, frequently, show a higher index of Ki-67 and p53 protein than aggressive adenomas. Most of these tumors secrete prolactin and/or ACTH and they are usually resistant to radiotheraphy [1, 3, 4].

2. Case Description

A 55-year-old female patient diagnosed with Cushing's disease (CD) due to a macroadenoma ($2,39 \times 2,54 \times 3,36$ cm) underwent two transsphenoidal surgeries (TS) at another medical center (2008 and 2009, and we do not have data about the anatomopathological exam of these surgeries because these procedures were done in another region of country), without clinical improvement. She presented to our hospital by the end of 2009 with persistent CD symptoms. The patient did not use any medication when she came to our hospital. Laboratory tests revealed hypokalemia ($K = 2.4$ mEq/L, normal range 3.5–5 mEq/L) and very high serum ACTH and

TABLE 1: Clinical course.

Data	Condition	24 h urinary cortisol*	Late salivary cortisol**	Serum morning cortisol***	ACTH****
Dec 2009	Before 3rd surgery	>1,100	6.45	51.8	793
Dec 2009	**3rd TS surgery**				
Jan 2010	Postoperative (no GC replacement)			4.4	46
Feb 2010	No GC replacement	54.6	0.11	5.7	62
Jun 2010	GC dependency replacement	20	<0.1	2.3	60
Dec 2010	GC dependency replacement	25.2	0.04	3.2	45
Mar 2011	GC dependency replacement	25	0.08	2.8	59
Apr 2012	Clinical recurrence of CS	170	0.12	16.5	270
May 2012	No drug	435	0.21	25.3	336
Jul 2012	On 1,200 mg/d of ketoconazole	821	0.52	23.5	670
Jul 2012	**4th surgery**				
Sep 2012	Postoperative (no drug)	4,998	2.44	47.7	582
Nov 2012	**Radiotherapy**				
Feb 2013	Postradiotherapy	2,348	13.5	70.8	4,087

*24h urinary cortisol (NR: 30–310 μg/24 h).
**Late salivary cortisol (NR < 0.13 μg/dL).
***Serum morning cortisol (NR: 5–25 μg/dL).
****ACTH (NR: <46 pg/mL).
GC: glucocorticoid, CS: Cushing's syndrome.

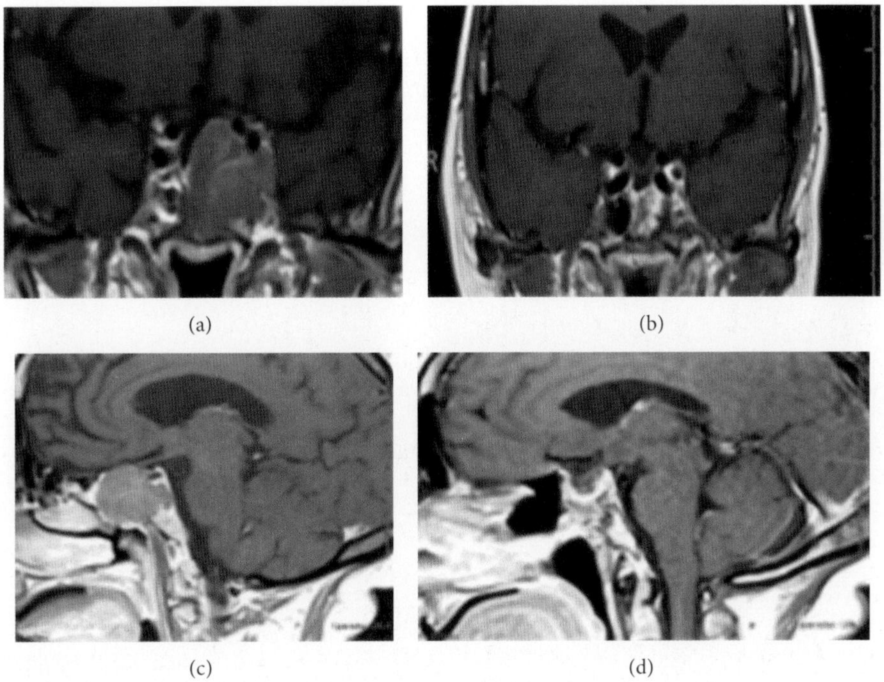

FIGURE 1: (a) Coronal image before the third surgery. (b) Sagittal image before the third surgery. (c) Coronal image after the third surgery. (d) Sagittal image after the third surgery.

cortisol levels (Table 1). Magnetic resonance imaging (MRI) showed an invasive sellar mass (Figures 1(a) and 1(b)). The patient exhibited symptoms of pituitary apoplexy confirmed after a third TS with radical tumor resection (Figures 1(c) and 1(d)). Histopathology confirmed a pituitary adenoma positive for ACTH (standard diffuse > 50%) and Ki-67 (<5%) and negative for p53 by immunohistochemistry (IHC) (Table 2). The patient achieved complete clinical and laboratory remission of hypercortisolism. In fact, she developed clinical and laboratory adrenal insufficiency requiring glucocorticoid replacement for two years. No tumor growth was detected, although ACTH levels remained slightly elevated (Table 1). In 2012, the patient returned with rapidly progressive recurrence of clinical and laboratory hypercortisolism (Table 1). Sellar

Table 2: Tumor markers comparison between third and fourth surgeries.

	Ki-67 (%)	p53	ACTH (IHQ)
2009 (after 3rd surgery)	<5%	No evidence	>50%
2012 (after 4th surgery)	10–15%	25%	>50%

Considerations: The Ki-67 and p53 immunohistochemical exams were made with primary monoclonal antibody performed with 1 : 50 dilution, according to the manufacturer's protocol.

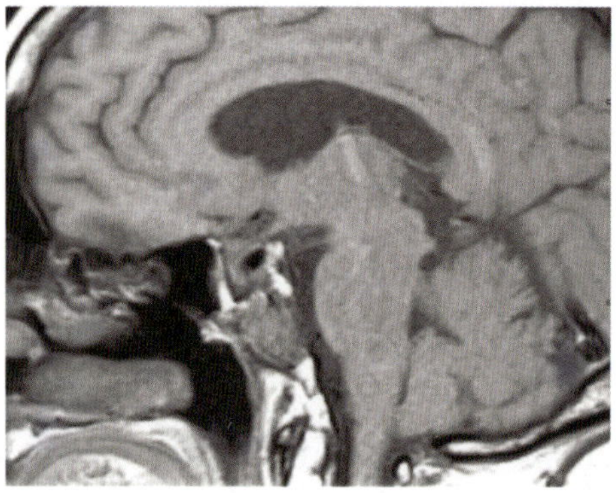

Figure 2: Sagittal image on clinical recurrence showing tumor invasion of the clivus.

MRI showed tumor extension into the clivus (Figure 2). The patient was started on ketoconazole (1200 mg/day) and underwent radiotherapy (5040 cGy in 28 sessions) after another subtotal TS resection. Immunohistochemical analysis after this fourth surgery showed a pituitary adenoma with ACTH expression (>50%) and diffuse immunoreactivity to Ki-67 (10%–15%) and to p53. The patient returned 3 months later, showing accelerated clinical deterioration: hyperpigmentation, severe myopathy and low back pain, dyspnea, generalized edema, severe hypertension, and diabetes mellitus. Laboratory tests showed hypokalemia (2 mEq/L) and very high ACTH and cortisol levels (Table 1). Positron emission tomography (PET/CT) was performed using 10.4 fluoro-2-deoxyglucose mCi labeled with fluorine-18, which showed multiple hypodense nodules in the liver parenchyma, measuring up to 3.3 cm in segment VIII (Figure 3). Liver biopsy showed a neuroendocrine pattern with immunopositive ACTH (>50%) and Ki-67 (5%–10%), Table 1. MRI also showed metastasis in the lumbar spine (Figure 4). The patient was reassigned the oncology team for discussion of the possibility of using temozolomide and adrenalectomy was considered at time. But the patient developed important lung infection, probably due to hypercortisolism, and she died one month later.

3. Discussion

Pituitary carcinomas are rare tumors, accounting for an average of 0.2% of pituitary neoplasms. They are defined by the presence of craniospinal and/or systemic metastases and are associated with high mortality rates. Most are invasive sellar tumors, characterized by their expansion beyond the limits of the sella turcica. They show endocrine activity and consist of PRL- and/or ACTH-secreting tumors in most cases. However, these tumors can also be nonfunctioning and produce symptoms only when adjacent structures are compressed [3]. Primary pituitary carcinoma metastases are of difficult diagnosis because they are not always present at the time of initial diagnosis [2, 3]. According to Pernicone et al., the latency period between the diagnosis of a primary carcinoma and the manifestation of metastases ranges between 3 months and 18 years (mean, 6.6 years). This time interval is longer for ACTH-secreting carcinomas than prolactinomas (9.5 versus 4.7 years) [4]. The protein Ki-67 is a cell proliferation marker detected by the monoclonal antibody MIB-1 and is expressed as a percentage of immunopositive nuclei in the form of a Ki-67 proliferation index [5]. According to Thapar et al. Ki-67 over 3% is a criterion to distinguish invasive from noninvasive adenomas with 97% specificity and 73% sensitivity [5, 6]. In this case, after 3 years, the adenoma progressed to a carcinoma, as evidenced by p53 expression and diffuse Ki-67 staining. Typically, pituitary carcinomas develop craniospinal, lung, liver, and ovary metastases. Immunohistochemical staining of these metastases reveals elevated rates of oncoproteins

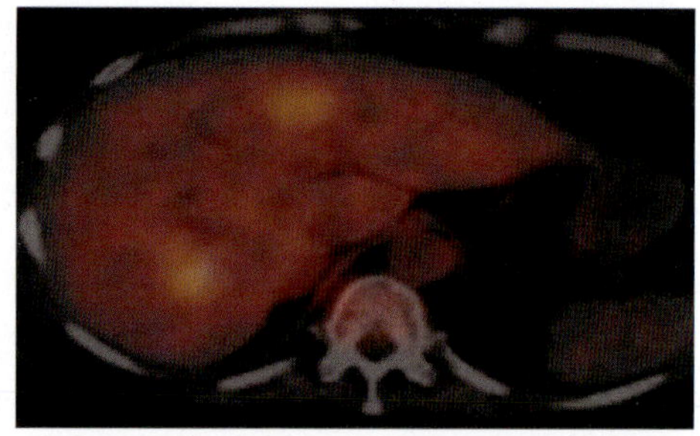

Figure 3: Liver metastasis (PET/CT).

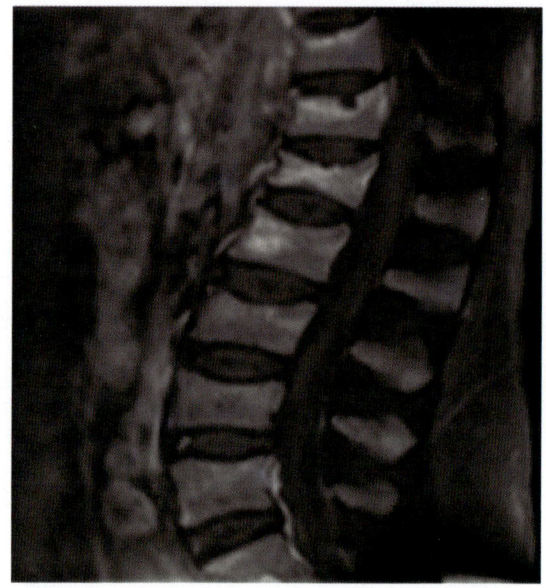

Figure 4: Lumbar spine metastasis on MRI.

such as p53 and cell proliferation marker (Ki-67), which is helpful for diagnosis and prognostic relevance in these cases [4, 6]. It is worth noting that the levels of those markers are typically higher in metastases than in the primary tumor [6]. The most interesting and unusual aspect in the reported case was that the patient had a diagnosis of an adenoma with low oncoprotein expression and later progressed to a carcinoma with increased oncoprotein expression in the primary tumor and in the liver metastasis, with rapid and severe clinical deterioration—thus demonstrating the malignancy and high mortality of pituitary carcinomas. The treatment options for these tumors are surgery, radiotherapy, and, more recently, chemotherapy with drugs such as temozolomide [7]. The response to these treatment modalities is poor, as 66% of the patients die within 1 year, which illustrates the inexorable course of this serious disease [4].

4. Conclusion

Pituitary carcinomas are rare, and the progression of an ACTH-secreting pituitary adenoma to a carcinoma is exceptional. The difficulty of defining before metastasis markers for the diagnosis of carcinoma is a challenge that can be solved by changing the approach to this disease.

References

[1] A. Sav, F. Rotondo, L. V. Syro, A. Di Ieva, M. D. Cusimano, and K. Kovacs, "Invasive, atypical and aggressive pituitary adenomas and carcinomas," *Endocrinology and Metabolism Clinics of North America*, vol. 44, no. 1, pp. 99–104, 2014.

[2] M. B. S. Lopes, B. W. Scheithauer, and D. Schiff, "Pituitary carcinoma: diagnosis and treatment," *Endocrine*, vol. 28, no. 1, pp. 115–121, 2005.

[3] B. T. Ragel and W. T. Couldwell, "Pituitary carcinoma: a review of the literature," *Neurosurgical focus*, vol. 16, no. 4, p. E7, 2004.

[4] P. J. Pernicone, B. W. Scheithauer, T. J. Sebo et al., "Pituitary carcinoma: a clinicopathologic study of 15 cases," *Cancer*, vol. 79, no. 4, pp. 804–812, 1997.

[5] K. Thapar, K. Kovacs, B. W. Scheithauer et al., "Proliferative activity and invasiveness among pituitary adenomas and carcinomas: an analysis using the MIB-1 antibody," *Neurosurgery*, vol. 38, no. 1, pp. 99–107, 1996.

[6] P. Marques, M. Mafra, C. Calado, A. Martins, J. Monteiro, and V. Leite, "Aggressive pituitary lesion with a remarkably high Ki-67," *Arquivos Brasileiros de Endocrinologia e Metabologia*, vol. 58, no. 6, pp. 656–660, 2014.

[7] B. W. Scheithauer, Ö. Kurtkaya-Yapicier, K. T. Kovacs, W. F. Young Jr., and R. V. Lloyd, "Pituitary carcinoma: a clinicopathological review," *Neurosurgery*, vol. 56, no. 5, pp. 1066–1074, 2005.

12

A Case of Biphasic Pulmonary Blastoma Treated with Carboplatin and Paclitaxel plus Bevacizumab

Shinya Sakata, Sho Saeki, Sayuri Hirooka, Susumu Hirosako, Hidenori Ichiyasu, and Hirotsugu Kohrogi

Department of Respiratory Medicine, Kumamoto University Hospital, 1-1-1 Honjo, Chuo-ku, Kumamoto 860-8556, Japan

Correspondence should be addressed to Hirotsugu Kohrogi; kohrogi@kumamoto-u.ac.jp

Academic Editor: Cesar V. Reyes

Background. Pulmonary blastoma is a rare lung tumor similar to fetal lung tissues. Surgical resection at early stage is more curative than other treatments, but there is no standard treatment in unresectable cases. We show a case treated with carboplatin and paclitaxel plus bevacizumab. *Case.* A 68-year-old man received surgical resection and was diagnosed with biphasic pulmonary blastoma (pT3N0M0 stage IIB). Metastasis to the spleen was detected six weeks after the surgery. Carboplatin, paclitaxel, and bevacizumab were administered and showed an effect on the metastasis. Four courses of the chemotherapy were completed, but a metastasis was found and the metastatic tumor in the spleen was enlarged. After that, chemotherapy was not effective afterward and he died of the progression of biphasic pulmonary blastoma on the 292nd day of illness. *Conclusion.* In this case, chemotherapy with carboplatin and paclitaxel plus bevacizumab was temporarily efficacious for biphasic pulmonary blastoma.

1. Introduction

Pulmonary blastoma is a rare lung tumor similar to fetal lung tissues and is considered to be 0.25–0.5% of the primary pulmonary malignant tumor [1]. Surgical resection at early stage of pulmonary blastoma is more curative than other treatments, but its 5-year survival rate is 25% in stage I. At present, in unresectable cases chemotherapy and radiotherapy do not statistically reach the establishment of the standard treatment. Biphasic pulmonary blastoma, a subgroup of pulmonary blastoma, is characterized by histopathological heterogeneity intermixing of epithelial and mesenchymal malignant cells [2]. We show a case of biphasic pulmonary blastoma effectively treated with carboplatin and paclitaxel plus bevacizumab.

2. Case Report

A 68-year-old man was admitted to our hospital because of a mass lesion (55 × 45 mm) in the left upper lobe of the lung on chest radiograph and computed tomography (CT) scan (Figure 1(a)).

Physical examinations were normal, and laboratory tests showed an elevated level of serum carcinoembryonic antigen (CEA) level (4.7 ng/mL). Ultrasound-guided biopsy of the tumor was performed. Pathology of the tissue stained with hematoxylin and eosin (H&E) staining showed malignant cells which were suspected large cell neuroendocrine carcinoma of the lung. Fluorodeoxyglucose-positron-emission tomography (FDG-PET) and brain magnetic resonance imaging (MRI) showed no apparent metastasis, and the clinical stage was cT3N0M0 stage IIB. Then, left upper lobectomy and lymph node dissection were performed.

The pathology of the surgically resected tumor with H&E staining demonstrated mixed epithelial and mesenchymal malignancies, biphasic pulmonary blastoma showing slit-formed duct formation of carcinoma, and immature mesenchymal cells (Figure 1(b)). Immunohistochemical staining for epithelial markers, CAM5.2 and TTF-1, was positive in epithelial areas (Figure 1(d)). The mesenchymal markers, vimentin and desmin, were positive in the mesenchymal areas (Figure 1(c)). These findings confirmed the diagnosis of biphasic pulmonary blastoma.

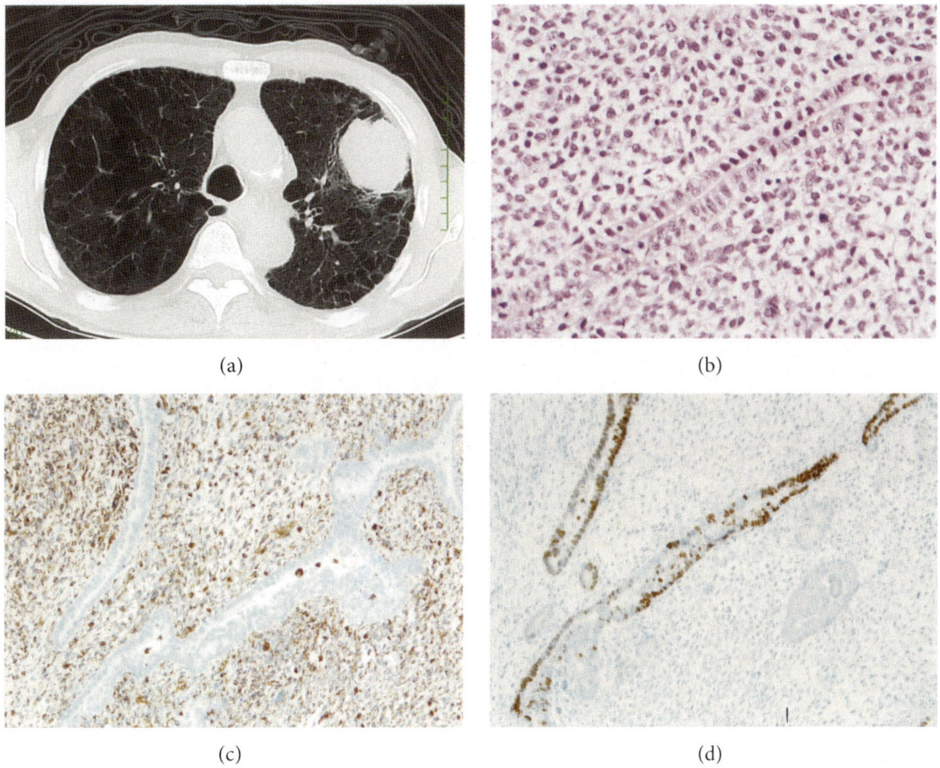

FIGURE 1: (a) Chest CT showing the mass opacity of the diameter 55 × 45 mm in size in the left upper lobe. Severe emphysema is visible in the background. (b) Pathology (hematoxylin and eosin staining, 400x) shows a part of carcinoma with slit-formed duct formation of carcinoma and immature mesenchymal cells. (c) Vimentin (100x) is diffusely positive for the mesenchymal cells. (d) TTF-1 (100x) is positive in parts of carcinoma with the slit-formed duct formation.

When he was admitted to our hospital to receive adjuvant chemotherapy six weeks after the surgery, abdominal CT showed a metastasis to the spleen (Figures 2(a) and 2(b)). Carboplatin area under the curve 6 and paclitaxel 200 mg/m^2 plus bevacizumab 15 mg/kg on day 1 every 3 weeks were administered and the effect measurement in CT after two courses of the chemotherapy showed reduction of the metastatic lesion and its inhomogeneous opacity changed to homogeneous opacity (Figure 2(c)), and levels of tumor markers were decreased (Figure 3). After two courses of the chemotherapy, serum levels of AFP decreased from 1120.0 to 441.2 ng/mL, those of NSE decreased from 15.2 to 9.6 ng/mL, and those of CEA decreased from 4.7 to 3.1 ng/mL. Four courses of the chemotherapy were completed, but a new liver metastasis was found and the metastatic tumor in the spleen was enlarged (Figure 2(d)). On the 292nd day of illness he died of the progression of pulmonary blastoma without showing a response to pemetrexed 500 mg/m^2 on day 1 every 3 weeks, docetaxel 60 mg/m^2 on day 1 every 3 weeks, and S-1 80 mg/m^2/day on days 1 to 14 plus bevacizumab 15 mg/kg on day 1 every 3 weeks as the latter treatment (Figure 3). Autopsy showed multiple metastases to the spleen, liver, pleura, rib, stomach, duodenum, heart, and cervical lymph nodes. The cut surface of metastatic tumors showed significant necrosis and hemorrhage.

3. Discussion

Pulmonary blastoma is classified into three subgroups: (1) biphasic pulmonary blastoma, characterized by histopathological heterogeneity intermixing of epithelial and mesenchymal malignant cells, (2) well-differentiated fetus adenocarcinoma, characterized by a monophasic epithelial tumor, and (3) pleuropulmonary blastoma, characterized by a monophasic mesenchymal tumor. However, according to World Health Organization (WHO) classification of lung tumors published in 1999, well-differentiated fetus adenocarcinoma is classified into a histological variant of adenocarcinoma, and pleuropulmonary blastoma is classified into soft tissue tumors [2].

Pulmonary blastoma is a rare lung tumor similar to fetal lung tissues and is considered to be 0.25–0.5% of the primary pulmonary malignant tumor [1]. The mean tumor diameter is known to be 101 mm (20–270 mm) [3]. In the present case, tumor developed in peripheral area, and the diameter 55 mm at the initial diagnosis showed a rapid growth to 80 mm in three weeks at the surgical resection. Serum levels of tumor markers, AFP, NSE, and CEA, were increased as shown in the previous reports [4]. In particular, AFP positive tumor cells are seen in many pulmonary blastoma cases [5]. Therefore, an elevated level of AFP in a patient with lung tumor is one of suggestions to suspect pulmonary

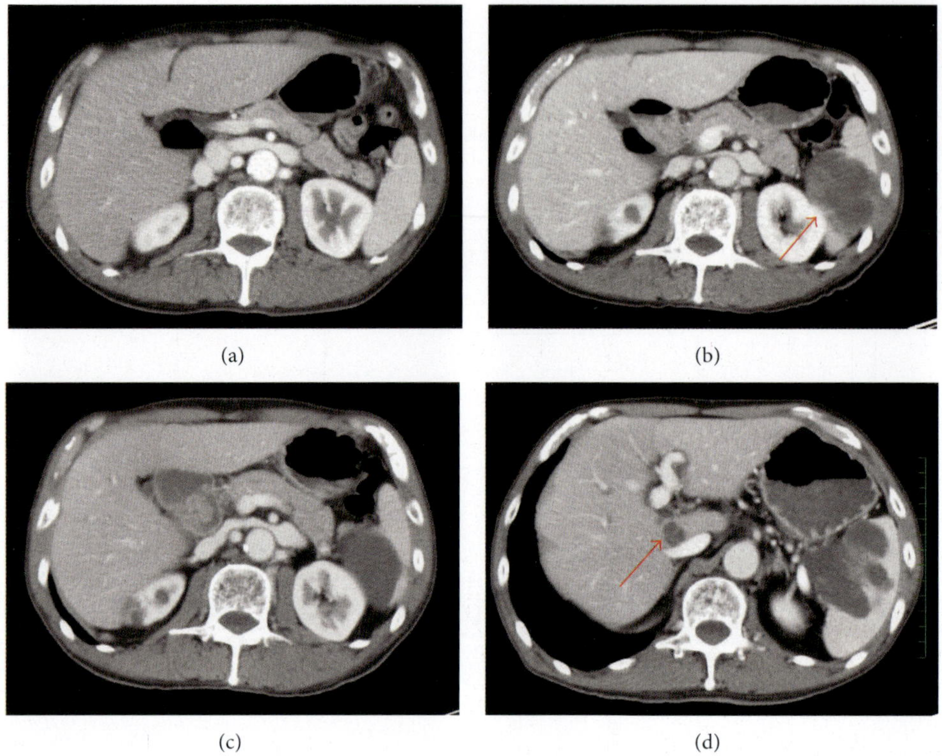

FIGURE 2: (a) There are no abnormal findings in abdominal CT scan before surgery. (b) Abdominal CT scan with contrast 6 weeks after surgery shows a mass with inhomogeneous opacity in the spleen (arrow). (c) Abdominal CT scan with contrast after the 3 courses of chemotherapy by carboplatin and paclitaxel plus bevacizumab. The tumor size is reduced and its inhomogeneous opacity changed to homogeneous opacity. (d) Abdominal CT scan with contrast after the 4 courses of chemotherapy shows a new metastasis to the liver and enlarged metastatic tumor in the spleen (arrow).

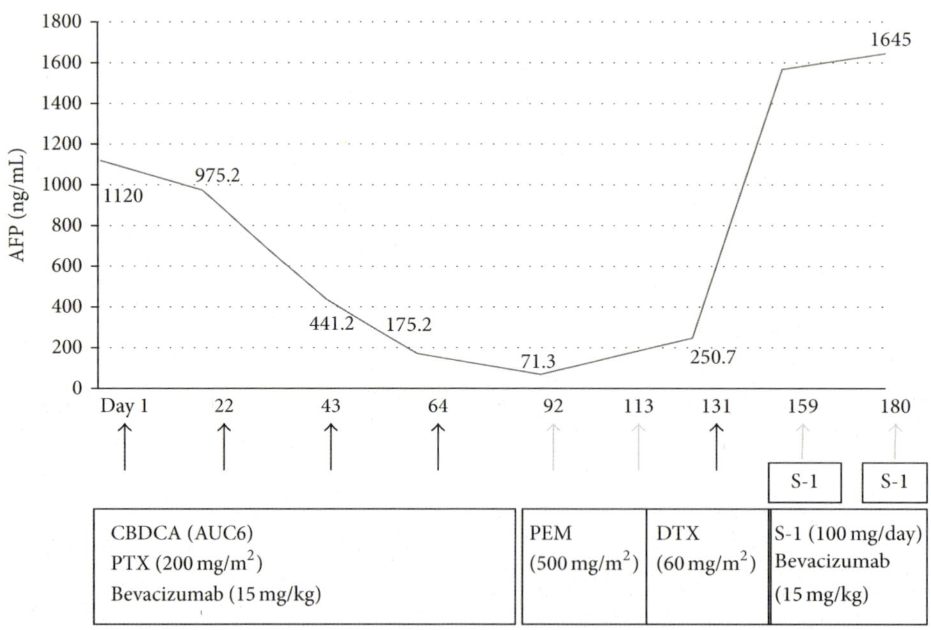

FIGURE 3: Clinical course showing decreased levels of AFP after the serial courses of chemotherapy with carboplatin and paclitaxel plus bevacizumab. After the recurrence, levels of AFP rapidly increased regardless of latter treatment with pemetrexed (PEM), docetaxel (DTX), and S-1 plus bevacizumab.

blastoma. Because it is difficult to obtain tissues containing both epithelial and mesenchymal tumor by transbronchial biopsy, its pathological diagnosis is done by tissues obtained by surgical resection in most cases of pulmonary blastoma. In fact, the present case was preoperatively diagnosed as large cell neuroendocrine carcinoma by percutaneous needle biopsy.

The prognosis of biphasic pulmonary blastoma is extremely poor. The size of more than 50 mm is a significant predictor of a poor prognosis [3]. In the present case, the tumor was 80 mm in diameter at the surgical resection. Although surgical resection at early stage of pulmonary blastoma is more curative than any other treatment [3], its 5-year survival rate is 25% in stage I. At present, in unresectable cases, chemotherapy and radiotherapy do not statistically reach the establishment of the standard treatment.

One case showed partial response to ifosfamide plus doxorubicin with radiotherapy for a postoperative recurrence [6]. In another case, cisplatin plus etoposide with radiotherapy made surgical resection possible for postoperative recurrence. Also, a case of pulmonary blastoma responding to sorafenib was reported [7].

The present case showed recurrence with the distant metastasis six weeks after the surgery. Because pulmonary blastoma was nonsquamous cell carcinoma, we selected the regimen carboplatin and paclitaxel plus bevacizumab as one of the standard treatments. Bevacizumab is the IgG1 hominization monoclonal antibody targeting the vascular endothelial growth factor (VEGF), and it inhibits neovascularization by binding to blood VEGF inhibiting the bond with the VEGF receptor of vascular endothelial cells and shows antitumor effect [8].

In the present case, the treatment after the 3 courses showed decreased levels of AFP and decreased tumor size of the metastasis, suggesting that this regimen is effective on biphasic pulmonary blastoma. Further accumulation of knowledge and experience is needed to establish effective treatment (including chemotherapy) of biphasic pulmonary blastoma.

4. Conclusion

To our knowledge, there is no report of responders to bevacizumab combination regimen for the biphasic pulmonary blastoma so far. The present case is valuable to establish future chemotherapy for biphasic pulmonary blastoma. Accumulation of the future cases is expected.

Acknowledgment

The authors thank all of the staffs in this paper.

References

[1] D. Francis and M. Jacobsen, "Pulmonary blastoma," *Current Topics in Pathology*, vol. 73, pp. 265–294, 1983.

[2] E. Brambilla, W. D. Travis, T. V. Colby, B. Corrin, and Y. Shimosato, "The new World Health Organization classification of lung tumours," *European Respiratory Journal*, vol. 18, no. 6, pp. 1059–1068, 2001.

[3] M. N. Koss, L. Hochholzer, and T. O'Leary, "Pulmonary blastomas," *Cancer*, vol. 67, no. 9, pp. 2368–2381, 1991.

[4] T. Iwata, N. Nishiyama, K. Inoue et al., "Biphasic pulmonary blastoma: report of a case," *Annals of Thoracic and Cardiovascular Surgery*, vol. 13, no. 1, pp. 40–43, 2007.

[5] Y. Nakatani, H. Kitamura, Y. Inayama et al., "Pulmonary adenocarcinomas of the fetal lung type: a clinicopathologic study indicating differences in histology, epidemiology, and natural history of low-grade and high-grade forms," *American Journal of Surgical Pathology*, vol. 22, no. 4, pp. 399–411, 1998.

[6] C. Lindet, M. Vanhuyse, E. Thebaud, Y.-M. Robin, and N. Penel, "Pulmonary blastoma in adult: dramatic but transient response to doxorubicin plus ifosfamide," *Acta Oncologica*, vol. 50, no. 1, pp. 156–157, 2011.

[7] K. Mulamalla, A. M. Truskinovsky, and A. Z. Dudek, "Pulmonary blastoma with renal metastasis responds to sorafenib," *Journal of Thoracic Oncology*, vol. 2, no. 4, pp. 344–347, 2007.

[8] H.-P. Gerber and N. Ferrara, "Pharmacology and pharmacodynamics of bevacizumab as monotherapy or in combination with cytotoxic therapy in preclinical studies," *Cancer Research*, vol. 65, no. 3, pp. 671–680, 2005.

13

A Case of Primary Breast Diffuse Large B-Cell Lymphoma Treated with Chemotherapy Followed by Elective Field Radiation Therapy: A Brief Treatment Pattern Review from a Radiation Oncologist's Point of View

Kyu Chan Lee,[1] Seung Heon Lee,[1] KiHoon Sung,[1] So Hyun Ahn,[1] Jinho Choi,[1] Seok Ho Lee,[1] Jae Hoon Lee,[2] Junshik Hong,[2] and Sang Hui Park[3]

[1] *Department of Radiation Oncology, Gil Medical Center, School of Medicine, Gachon University, Incheon 405-760, Republic of Korea*
[2] *Department of Internal Medicine, Gil Medical Center, School of Medicine, Gachon University, Incheon 405-760, Republic of Korea*
[3] *Department of Pathology, Ewha Womans University School of Medicine, Seoul 158-710, Republic of Korea*

Correspondence should be addressed to Seok Ho Lee; souko@gilhospital.com

Academic Editor: Katsuhiro Tanaka

We here report a case of primary breast lymphoma (PBL). A 44-year-old woman presented with a painless mass in the right breast. Fine needle aspiration cytology and excisional biopsy were performed. Excisional biopsy revealed low grade lymphoma, which was subsequently confirmed with histopathology and diagnosed as diffuse large B-cell lymphoma (DLBCL). A chest computed tomography scan revealed a 3.5 cm sized breast mass with skin thickening and a small sized lymphadenopathy in the ipsilateral axilla. Radiation therapy including the right whole breast and ipsilateral axilla and supraclavicular lymph node was performed after the patient received four courses of R-CHOP (cyclophosphamide, doxorubicin, vincristine, and prednisolone plus rituximab) chemotherapy. At the follow-up period of 42 months, the patient is surviving with no evidence of disease. No morbidities occurred in this patient during the follow-up period. We also briefly review the current practice pattern in PBL patients with DLBCL.

1. Introduction

Primary breast lymphoma (PBL) is a rare tumor that originates from lymph tissues. The reported incidence is 0.04–0.5% of malignant breast tumors [1]. The incidence of PBL in all non-Hodgkin's lymphoma (NHL) cases is less than 1%. And the most common histology in PBL was diffuse large B-cell lymphoma (DLBCL) [2]. Although PBL may behave in a similar clinical and radiological presentation as breast carcinoma, treatment modalities and outcomes differ. Because of its rarity, the treatment approach varies greatly. Although the use of radiation therapy (RT) and/or chemotherapy (CTx) differs in the literature, combined therapy with surgery, CTx, and involved field radiation therapy (IFRT) or elective field radiation therapy (EFRT) is currently considered to be the standard treatment approach for PBL patients with DLBCL [2, 3].

However, confidential data regarding appropriate treatment strategy including RT techniques such as RT field, RT dose, and RT fraction size of DLBCL in PBL are still lacking. Here, we present a case of PBL treated with chemotherapy followed by EFRT and also performed a brief literature review of the current practice pattern of PBL patients with DLBCL.

2. Case Report

A 44-year-old woman was admitted to our hospital with a mass in the right breast. A physical examination revealed a hard mass in the upper outer quadrant (UOQ) of the right breast, located approximately 2 cm from the nipple. The exam also revealed a nontender mass that was about 3 cm in size. The contralateral breast was normal. The patient had no previous history of liver cirrhosis, hepatitis B infection, and

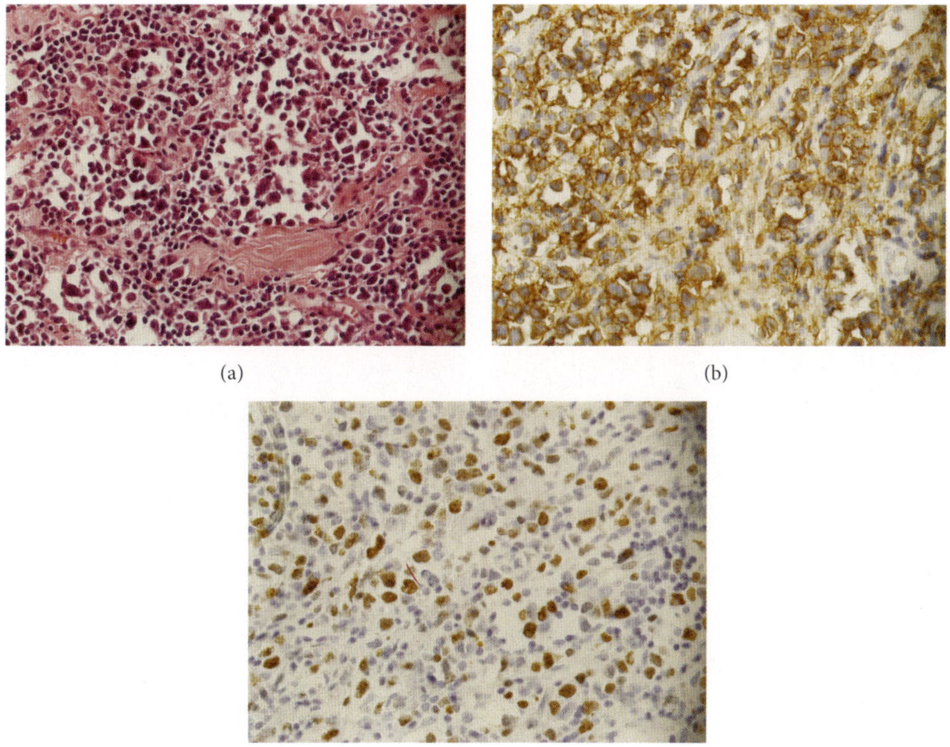

(a) (b) (c)

Figure 1: Histopathological examination shows diffuse dense infiltration of small and large lymphoid cells (a, ×400), composed of predominantly CD20 positive cells (b, ×400). Excisional biopsy revealed low grade lymphoma subsequently confirmed by histopathology and diagnosed as diffuse large B-cell lymphoma. CD 20+/CD 30−/CD 3−/cyclin D1- and index of proliferation Ki-67 positive for tumor cells (c).

diabetes mellitus. The ethnicity of patient was East Asian. A physical examination of the neck and axilla was negative for enlarged lymph nodes. Beta2-microglobulin level was 890.4 ng/mL and the lactate dehydrogenase (LDH) level was 390 IU/L. The patient had no B symptoms (fever, weight loss, or night sweats).

Fine needle aspiration cytology (FNAC) and excisional biopsy were performed. FNAC showed small lymphocytic infiltration with some large atypical cells and recommended additional ancillary test such as immunochemistry or excisional biopsy for confirmative diagnosis. Therefore, an excisional biopsy was performed and showed atypical lymphocytic infiltration suspicious for lymphoid malignancy. Additional immunohistochemical stains were performed for a confirmative diagnosis. CD20 and Ki-67 expression were positive by immunochemistry (Figure 1). Finally, excisional biopsy revealed low grade lymphoma, which was subsequently confirmed by histopathology and diagnosed as DLBCL.

Chest and abdominal computed tomography (CT) and positive emission tomography (PET) scans were evaluated for the staging workup. A bone-marrow (BM) biopsy was also performed. The chest CT revealed a 3.5 cm sized breast mass with skin thickening and a small (7 mm) sized lymphadenopathy in the ipsilateral axilla. A PET scan showed hypermetabolic uptake in the UOQ of the right breast with mild hypermetabolic uptake in the ipsilateral axilla (Figure 2). The patient was diagnosed with DLBCL. The BM biopsy showed a negative result for lymphomatous infiltration. The patient was diagnosed with stage IEA primary breast lymphoma according to the Ann Arbor staging system.

The patient received four courses of R-CHOP (cyclophosphamide, doxorubicin, vincristine, and prednisolone plus rituximab) CTx. After two courses of R-CHOP CTx, the follow-up chest CT showed decreased size of the right breast mass (3.5 cm → 2 cm) and right axillary lymph node (7 mm → 3 mm). After four courses of R-CHOP CTx, the follow-up chest CT showed no visible mass in the breast or axilla. The EFRT including the right whole breast, ipsilateral axilla, and supraclavicular lymph node (SCLN) was performed. An RT dose of 36 Gy in 1.8 Gy daily fractions was given to the whole right breast, ipsilateral axilla, and SCLN. After whole breast RT, a boost to the primary tumor bed was performed with a direct 12 MeV electron beam at a dose of 14.4 Gy. The primary tumor bed was irradiated with a total dose of 50.4 Gy in 28 fractions (Figure 3).

Follow-up chest CT and breast ultrasonography (USG), performed 32 months after RT, were normal. At a follow-up period of 42 months, the patient is surviving with no evidence of disease. No morbidities (such as radiation pneumonitis or arm edema) occurred in this patient during the follow-up period.

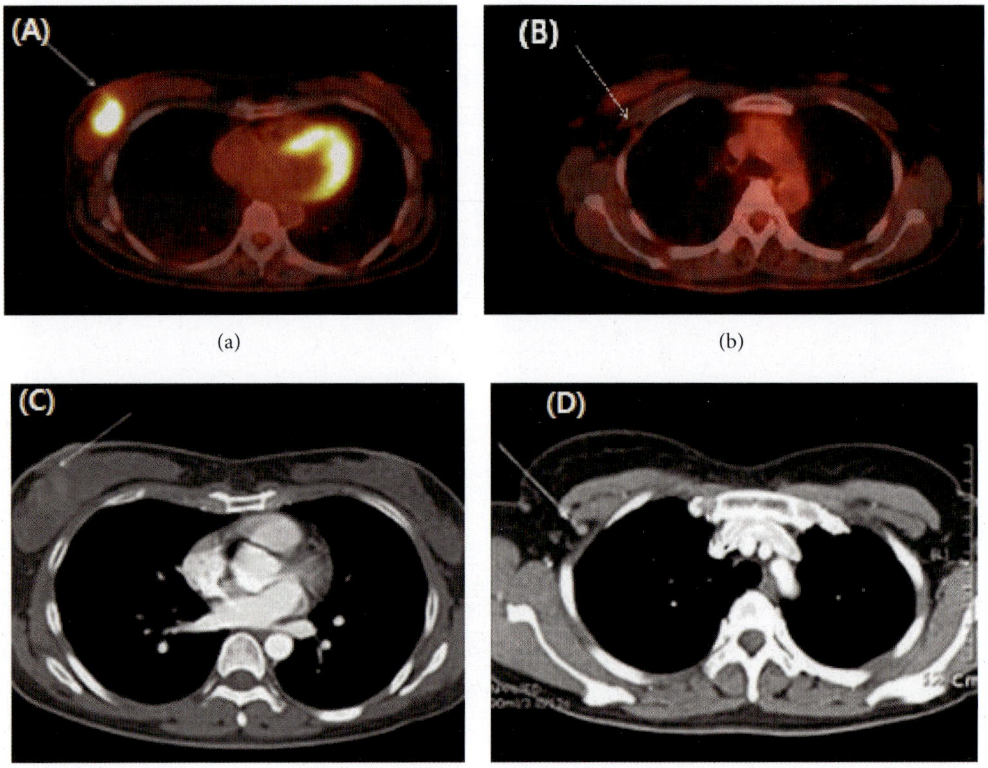

(a) (b) (c) (d)

FIGURE 2: F-18 fluorodeoxyglucose positron emission tomography/computed tomography (CT) reveals a hypermetabolic lesion (arrows) in the right breast (a) with mild hypermetabolic uptake in the ipsilateral axilla (b) and about a 3.5 cm sized right breast mass (c) with skin thickening. A small (7 mm) sized lymphadenopathy is observed in the ipsilateral axilla (d) on a plain contrast CT scan of the chest.

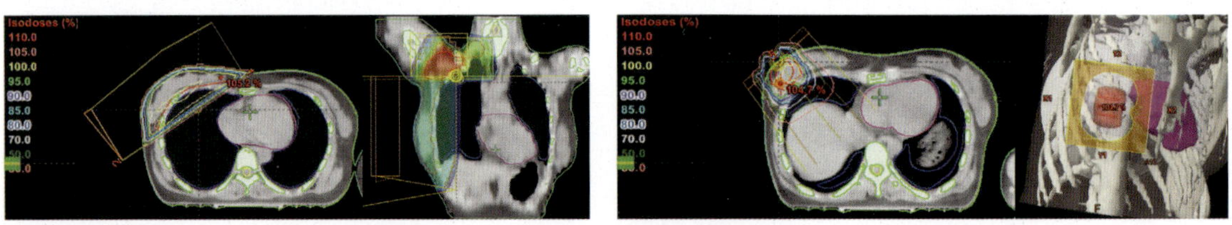

(a) (b)

FIGURE 3: The patient received elective field radiation therapy including the whole right breast, ipsilateral axilla, and supraclavicular lymph node (a) with dose prescription of 3,600 cGy in 20 fractions over 4 weeks plus a local boost (b) of 1,440 cGy to the primary site in 8 fractions over 1 week.

3. Discussion

The rarity of this cancer is because the breast contains less lymphoid tissue than other organs, such as the intestines and lungs, where primary lymphomas are more common [4]. PBL was traditionally defined as localized lymphoma to one or both breasts with or without regional lymph nodes such as ipsilateral axillary and/or SCLNs [5]. The most common pathological diagnosis in PBL is DLBCL. The following should also be included in the differential diagnosis of PBL: primary breast cancer, inflammatory breast cancer, fibroadenoma, phyllodes tumor, pseudolymphoma, metastatic disease, and benign breast neoplasm [6–8]. DLBCL is the most common histopathological type of PBL. The other frequent histological types are follicular lymphoma (15%), mucosa associated lymphoid tissue lymphoma (12.2%), Burkitt's lymphoma, and Burkitt-like lymphoma (10.3%) [9].

Although the present case was diagnosed with PBL in the fifth decade, the peak age for PBL is usually the sixth decade. The peak age of PBL is different between ethnicities. The median age in Western countries is over sixty years (62–64 years), whereas the median age in East Asian countries (45–53 years) is lower [10]. The right breast was involved in our case. PBL occurs more frequently in the right breast, with a 3 : 2 ratio [3, 11]. Breast USG was not performed in our case after biopsy results were obtained. Instead, chest CT and PET scans were conducted. The CT features in our study were circumscribed or ill-defined masses with homogenous, heterogeneous, or rim enhancement. Because none of these imaging features of PBL are pathognomonic, a biopsy was performed. Not only a histopathological examination but also immunophenotyping is an effective way to confirm aspiration cytology findings. In this report, we performed not only aspiration cytology but also excisional biopsy, and the histopathological examination showed diffuse infiltration of the small and large lymphoid cells, which were composed predominantly of CD20 positive cells.

No consensus exists on the best way to treat PBL, but the current treatment modality is considered as combined therapy consisting of CTx and RT. It has been previously reported that CTx with CHOP regimens and RT can significantly increase the overall survival and progression-free survival compared to CTx alone in localized intermediate- and high-grade NHL. Miller et al. concluded that CTx with three cycles of CHOP regimen followed by IFRT is superior to CTx with eight cycles alone [12]. Nowadays, the most common chemotherapeutic regimen for treating PBL is the R-CHOP regimen. In particular, rituximab, a monoclonal antibody targeting the CD20 antigen, is reported to have high efficacy for DLBCL [13]. The use of rituximab for CHOP CTx has been reported to reduce the overall CNS relapse risk in PBL patients with DLBCL [14].

We briefly reviewed the role of surgery, CTx, and RT in PBL patients with DLBCL as follows. Initially, most patients received surgery ranging from lumpectomy to mastectomy [9]; however, most studies have been inconclusive regarding the effects of surgery on PBL. The study reported by Ryan et al. [3] showed that surgeries including mastectomy were associated with increased risk of mortality. And this study of 204 patients with PBL showed that there was no benefit from mastectomy, as opposed to biopsy or lumpectomy. Even axillary node dissection did not show survival benefits [11]. They reported that the combination of limited surgery, anthracycline-based CTx, and IFRT produced the best outcome in the pre-rituximab era and concluded that combined therapy was the best method for treating patients with PBL [3]. They also suggested prophylactic therapy for avoiding central nervous system (CNS) involvement. It is now well established that limited surgery should be performed for diagnostic purposes for PBL and should not be considered a treatment modality. The CTx, especially with an anthracycline-based regimen which showed positive effects on overall survival, is a main treatment component of PBL patients with DLBCL [3]. The addition of rituximab to the CHOP regimen was also evaluated by several studies [13–15]. Avilés et al. [15] reported that there were no CNS relapses in patients treated with rituximab, whereas a relapse rate of 11% occurred in patients treated without rituximab. The ultimate goal of RT is to consolidate the primary lesions after CTx. The CTx followed by RT has shown a significantly improved survival benefit compared to CTx or RT alone [3, 9, 15]. However, the appropriate RT volume in PBL with DLBCL has not yet been settled. Although initial RT techniques encompassed the ipsilateral breast with or without regional nodes and even contralateral breast in some patients, the current RT approach is to minimize the RT volume into the involved site [16]. The involved site RT technique (IFRT) encompasses the pre-CTx tumor volume with enough margins to include the subclinical disease, setup margin, and so forth. In our case, the EFRT including prophylactic RT to SCLN was performed, which is somewhat different from the IFRT technique. In EFRT, the prophylactic RT to uninvolved nodes is used. We summarized the recent literatures published after the year 2005 on treatment modalities for the PBL patients with DLBCL in Table 1. Avilés et al. reported that a complete response (CR) in patients treated with RT, CTx, and RT and CTx arm was 66.7% (20/30), 59.4% (19/32), and 88.2% (30/34), respectively ($P < 0.01$). They also reported that the most common site of recurrence was the CNS (11.4% (11/96)) and that the acute toxicity was mild [17]. To improve the treatment outcome, the combination CTx that includes a high dose of methotrexate and/or Ara C for CNS prophylaxis should be considered for patients with aggressive forms of PBL, even in the early stage [18].

In the present study, the patient received the R-CHOP regimen followed by RT. Although the CR of the breast tumor after treatment of a four-cycle R-CHOP had been achieved, we then hypothesized that the ipsilateral whole breast, axilla, and SCLN may have the potential risk of subclinical disease. Therefore, we planned to treat the patient with EFRT including not only the whole right breast and ipsilateral axilla, but also SCLN. Because an axillary lymph node biopsy could not be performed for a pathological confirmation due to the deep-seated location, the initial stage before starting CTx was IEA according to the Ann Arbor staging system. However, we considered this patient could be staged as IIEA (limited to the breast and ipsilateral axilla) because axillary metastasis was strongly suspected considering the axillary response to CTx. One report indicates that the EFRT policy for PBL should include the breast, ipsilateral axilla, and supraclavicular region in RT fields [2]. Modern RT technology such as intensity modulated radiation therapy and respiratory gating techniques will further decrease the RT dose to normal tissues and the risk of RT related toxicities.

Although there are controversies regarding the prognostic factors in patients with PBL, a favorable international prognostic index (IPI) score, use of anthracycline-containing CTx, and RT have been reported as significant prognostic factors for longer overall survival (OS) [3]. The patient in our report had an initial IPI score of 0-1 and received anthracycline-containing CTx followed by RT. Thus, more favorable survival results may have been expected in our patient.

4. Conclusion

Here, we report a case of PBL with a review of the literature. The PBL was confirmed by histopathology and immunohistochemistry and treated with EFRT after CTx. We suggest that RT is an effective and safe option and combined CTx and EFRT can give a longer survival in PBL cases with axillary lymph node involvement.

Table 1: Brief review of treatment modalities and results in PBL patients with DLBCL.

Author [Ref]	N	Age (median)	Surgery (%)	Treatment modality					Results			
				CTx			RT (%)				Survival (%)	
				CHOP (%)	Rituximab (%)	N (%)	Field	RT dose (Gy/Fx)	CR (%)	CNS relapse (%)	5 Y-OS	PFS
Avilés et al. [17]	96	58	0	66 (69)	0	64 (67)	IFRT	45/20	69 (72)	11 (11.5)	76 (10 Y)	83 (10 Y)
Yoshida et al. [19]	15	68	11 (73)	12 (80)	0	NA	NA-	NA	NA	0	NA	NA
Avilés et al. [15]	32	46	NA	32 (100)	32 (100)	32 (100)	IFRT	45/20	28 (87)	0	63 (3 Y)	75 (3 Y)
Salzberg et al. [20]	75	62	NA	68 (91)	52 (69)	51 (68)	NA	NA	NA	10 (13.3)	75	65
Mouna et al. [21]	7	50	4 (57)	6 (86)	2 (29)	2 (29)	EFRT	36–50	7 (71.4)	0	NA	NA
Seker et al. [22]	9	49	0	8 (89)	7 (78)	5 (56)	IFRT, EFRT	NA	7 (77.7)	0	76.2	NA
Yhim et al. [5]	68	48	23 (34)	66 (97)	42 (62)	21 (31)	NA	NA	54 (83.1)	0	60.7	50.3
Niitsu et al. [23]	30	57	NA	30 (100)	11 (37)	18 (60)	IFRT	NA	29 (96.7)	2 (6.7)	87	77
Zhao et al. [24]	1	39	1 (100)	1 (100)	1 (100)	1 (100)	IFRT	40/NA	100	0	NA	NA
Validire et al. [25]	38	62	NA	36 (95)	4 (10)	27 (71)	IFRT, CNS PRT	40/20 18/10	34 (89)	3 (6.7)	61	54
Present study	1	44	no	1 (100)	1 (100)	1 (100)	EFRT	50.4/28	100	0	NA	NA

Ref: references; N: total number of patients; NA: not applicable; Gy: Gray; Fx: fractionation; CTx: chemotherapy; RT: radiation therapy; 5 Y-OS: 5-year overall survival; PFS: progression-free survival; CR: complete response; IFRT: involved field radiation therapy; EFRT: elective field radiation therapy; CNS PRT: central nervous system prophylactic radiation therapy.

Consent

Verbal consent was obtained from the patient for publication of this case report and any accompanying images.

Authors' Contribution

All the authors contributed equally to this paper.

References

[1] N. Avenia, A. Sanguinetti, R. Cirocchi et al., "Primary breast lymphomas: a multicentric experience," *World Journal of Surgical Oncology*, vol. 8, article 53, 2010.

[2] J. A. Lyons, J. Myles, B. Pohlman, R. M. Macklis, J. Crowe, and R. L. Crownover, "Treatment and prognosis of primary breast lymphoma: a review of 13 cases," *American Journal of Clinical Oncology*, vol. 23, no. 4, pp. 334–336, 2000.

[3] G. Ryan, G. Martinelli, M. Kuper-Hommel et al., "Primary diffuse large B-cell lymphoma of the breast: prognostic factors and outcomes of a study by the international extranodal lymphoma study group," *Annals of Oncology*, vol. 19, no. 2, pp. 233–241, 2008.

[4] D. J. P. Ferguson, "Intraepithelial lymphocytes and macrophages in the normal breast," *Virchows Archiv A*, vol. 407, no. 4, pp. 369–378, 1985.

[5] H.-Y. Yhim, H. J. Kang, Y. H. Choi et al., "Clinical outcomes and prognostic factors in patients with breast diffuse large B cell lymphoma; Consortium for Improving Survival of Lymphoma (CISL) study," *BMC Cancer*, vol. 10, article 321, 2010.

[6] H. Yang, R.-G. Lang, F.-F. Liu et al., "Primary lymphoma of breast: a clinicopathologic and prognostic study of 40 cases," *Zhonghua Bing Li Xue Za Zhi*, vol. 40, no. 2, pp. 79–84, 2011.

[7] N. Anne and R. Pallapothu, "Lymphoma of the breast: a mimic of inflammatory breast cancer," *World Journal of Surgical Oncology*, vol. 9, article 125, 2011.

[8] J. R. Zack, S. G. Trevisan, and M. Gupta, "Primary breast lymphoma originating in a benign intramammary lymph node," *The American Journal of Roentgenology*, vol. 177, no. 1, pp. 177–178, 2001.

[9] W. C. Jennings, R. S. Baker, S. S. Murray et al., "Primary breast lymphoma: the role of mastectomy and the importance of lymph node status," *Annals of Surgery*, vol. 245, no. 5, pp. 784–789, 2007.

[10] C. Y. Cheah, B. A. Campbell, and J. F. Seymour, "Primary breast lymphoma," *Cancer Treatments Reviews*, vol. 40, no. 8, pp. 900–908, 2014.

[11] M. Uesato, Y. Miyazawa, Y. Gunji, and T. Ochiai, "Primary non-Hodgkin's lymphoma of the breast: report of a case with special reference to 380 cases in the Japanese literature," *Breast Cancer*, vol. 12, no. 2, pp. 154–158, 2005.

[12] T. P. Miller, S. Dahlberg, J. R. Cassady et al., "Chemotherapy alone compared with chemotherapy plus radiotherapy for localized intermediate- and high-grade non-Hodgkin's lymphoma," *The New England Journal of Medicine*, vol. 339, no. 1, pp. 21–26, 1998.

[13] B. Coiffier, "Rituximab therapy in malignant lymphoma," *Oncogene*, vol. 26, no. 25, pp. 3603–3613, 2007.

[14] D. Villa, J. M. Connors, T. N. Shenkier, R. D. Gascoyne, L. H. Sehn, and K. J. Savage, "Incidence and risk factors for central nervous system relapse in patients with diffuse large B-cell lymphoma: the impact of the addition of rituximab to CHOP chemotherapy," *Annals of Oncology*, vol. 21, no. 5, pp. 1046–1052, 2009.

[15] A. Avilés, C. Castañeda, N. Neri, S. Cleto, and M. J. Nambo, "Rituximab and dose dense chemotherapy in primary breast lymphoma," *Haematologica*, vol. 92, no. 8, pp. 1147–1148, 2007.

[16] B. A. Campbell, "The role of radiation therapy in the treatment of stage I-II diffuse large B-cell lymphoma," *Current Hematologic Malignancy Reports*, vol. 8, pp. 236–238, 2013.

[17] A. Avilés, S. Delgado, M. J. Nambo, N. Neri, E. Murillo, and S. Cleto, "Primary breast lymphoma: results of a controlled clinical trial," *Oncology*, vol. 69, no. 3, pp. 256–260, 2005.

[18] C. Haioun, C. Besson, E. Lepage et al., "Incidence and risk factors of central nervous system relapse in histologically aggressive non-Hodgkin's lymphoma uniformly treated and receiving intrathecal central nervous system prophylaxis: a GELA study on 974 patients," *Annals of Oncology*, vol. 11, no. 6, pp. 685–690, 2000.

[19] S. Yoshida, N. Nakamura, Y. Sasaki et al., "Primary breast diffuse large B-cell lymphoma shows a non-germinal center B-cell phenotype," *Modern Pathology*, vol. 18, no. 3, pp. 398–405, 2005.

[20] M. P. Salzberg, J. C. Maragulia, O. W. Press et al., "Primary breast diffuse large B cell lymphoma: a distinct clinical entity," in *Proceedings of the 54th Annual Meeting and Exposition of the American Society of Hematology (ASH '12)*, Atlanta, Ga, USA, December 2012.

[21] B. Mouna, B. Saber, E. H. Tijaniel, M. Hind, T. Amina, and E. Hassan, "Primary malignant non-Hodgkin's lymphoma of the breast: a study of seven cases and literature review," *World Journal of Surgical Oncology*, vol. 10, article 151, 2012.

[22] M. Seker, A. Bilici, B. O. Ustaalioglu et al., "Clinicopathologic features of the nine patients with primary diffuse large B cell lymphoma of the breast," *Archives of Gynecology and Obstetrics*, vol. 284, no. 2, pp. 405–409, 2011.

[23] N. Niitsu, M. Okamoto, H. Nakamine, and M. Hirano, "Clinicopathologic features and treatment outcome of primary breast diffuse large B-cell lymphoma," *Leukemia Research*, vol. 32, no. 12, pp. 1837–1841, 2008.

[24] Y.-F. Zhao, F. Jiao, H.-Q. Liang, Q.-C. Luo, and L.-W. Zhao, "Primary malignant non-Hodgkin's lymphoma of the breast: a case report," *Oncology Letters*, vol. 8, no. 6, pp. 2596–2600, 2014.

[25] P. Validire, M. Capovilla, B. Asselain et al., "Primary breast non-Hodgkin's lymphoma: a large single center study of initial characteristics, natural history, and prognostic factors," *The American Journal of Hematology*, vol. 84, no. 3, pp. 133–139, 2009.

14

Foreign Body Granulomas Induced by Intramuscular Leuprorelin Acetate Injection for Prostate Cancer: Clinical Mimics of Soft Tissue Sarcoma

Khin Thway, Dirk C. Strauss, Myles J. Smith, and Cyril Fisher

Sarcoma Unit, Royal Marsden Hospital, London SW3 6JJ, UK

Correspondence should be addressed to Khin Thway; khin.thway@rmh.nhs.uk

Academic Editor: Annekathryn Goodman

We describe two cases of florid, foreign body granulomatous reaction occurring in the upper arms of males in their eighth decade, who were undergoing treatment with depot injection of leuprorelin acetate for prostatic carcinoma. These patients presented with rapidly enlarging extremity soft tissue masses and were referred to a tertiary sarcoma center with clinical suspicion of a primary soft tissue neoplasm. The occurrence of injection site granulomas secondary to leuprorelin acetate administration is rarely known outside the urological and dermatological communities, and their recognition is important due to the spectrum of clinical differential diagnoses and potential for diagnostic confusion with metastatic prostatic cancer and primary sarcoma and in order to avoid unnecessary stress and clinical intervention for patients.

1. Introduction

Leuprorelin acetate is a synthetic analogue of gonadotropin-releasing hormone (GnRH)/luteinizing hormone-releasing hormone (LHRH), which is indicated in the treatment of prostatic cancer, and is injectable as a depot formulation for long term, controlled drug release. It can cause florid granulomatous inflammation at the site of subcutaneous or intramuscular injection, which can present clinically as a rapidly enlarging soft tissue mass. We describe two cases, occurring either subcutaneously or deeply within the skeletal muscle of the upper arms of males in their eighth decades, who were undergoing androgen deprivation therapy for prostatic carcinoma with depot injection of leuprorelin acetate and who were referred to a tertiary sarcoma center with the suspicion of a soft tissue neoplasm. The occurrence of injection site granulomas secondary to leuprorelin acetate is little known outside the urological and dermatological communities. As these lesions can occur deeply and their clinical and radiological features can be concerning for malignancy, we highlight the importance of recognizing this phenomenon and of clinical correlation in diagnosis.

2. Case Report

The patients were 73- and 75-year-old males. Case 1 presented with an 11-week history of sudden onset, painful swelling of the right upper arm. He was referred to our sarcoma unit with the clinical and radiological suspicion of sarcoma. He had been diagnosed with T3bN0M0 Gleason score 4 + 5 prostatic adenocarcinoma 6 months prior to this, for which he had elected for systemic treatment. LHRH injections were commenced 3 months prior to presentation to sarcoma unit, and he was currently treated with leuprorelin acetate injection (brand name Prostap) at a dose of 11.25 mg once every 3 months. He had no other past medical history and no known history of travel or infection. On examination, there was an approximately 5 cm hard mass in the distal right biceps, just above the tendon. Clinically, the differential diagnoses were of organized hematoma, previous biceps muscle tear with healing by fibrosis, and myositis ossificans. Magnetic resonance imaging (MRI) showed a maximally 5.4 cm, ill-defined heterogeneous mass arising within the distal right biceps muscle, just proximal to the tendon, with peripheral enhancement and slightly increased T2/T1 signal relative

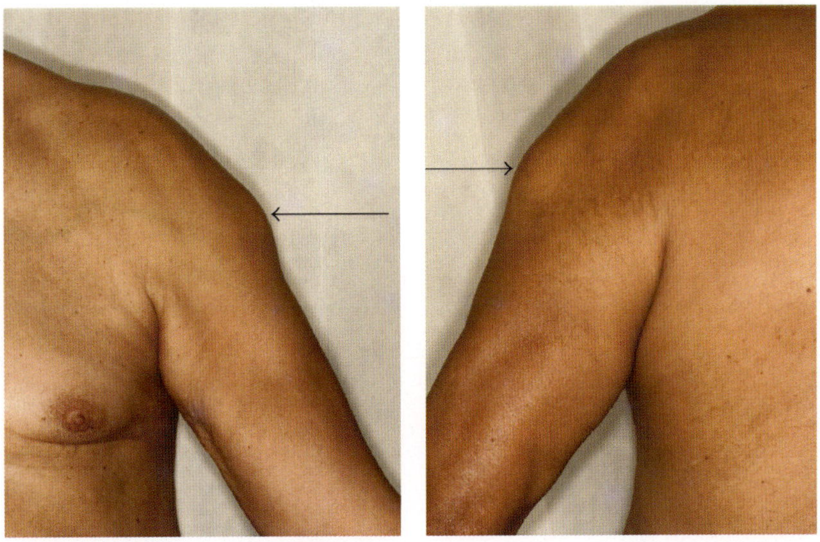

(a) (b)

Figure 1: Clinically, the lesion was a relatively well defined, firm approximately 7 cm mass over the left biceps muscle, fixed to the underlying structures. No erythema of the overlying skin is seen in this example (case 2).

to skeletal muscle, which was radiologically concerning for sarcoma. No evidence of disease was present elsewhere. Two needle core biopsies (initial and repeat) were performed. Six weeks after the initial biopsy and following the histological result for both biopsies, the patient was well and his right arm lesion was seen to be resolving. At this appointment, he was also noted to have a severe inflammatory reaction involving the skin and subcutis following a subsequent injection on the contralateral (left) upper arm. It was unknown whether the leuprorelin injections had been intramuscular or subcutaneous, but it was considered that he had intramuscular injection at the time of the first biopsy (with the reaction involving the biceps muscle) and then subcutaneous injections at the time of the second, which caused reaction in the superficial tissues. He was discharged from the sarcoma clinic; treatment with leuprorelin was stopped and he underwent surgical castration with subcapsular orchidectomy. Four months after initial diagnosis, he has subsequently developed skeletal metastases and is being treated with radiotherapy to the spine. Case 2 presented with an 8-week history of a rapidly enlarging, maximally 7 cm diameter left deltoid mass. He had a history of T3bN0Mx Gleason score 3 + 4 prostatic adenocarcinoma, had been previously treated with prostate radiotherapy, and was currently being treated with neoadjuvant and adjuvant hormone therapy including leuprorelin acetate. 13 weeks before presentation, he had been administered the first of a 3-year course of 3-monthly injections of subcutaneous leuprorelin acetate, prior to which he had been receiving monthly injection, and his symptoms appeared 2 months after changing from monthly to 3-monthly formulations of the leuprorelin preparation. There was no other past medical history or known history of travel or infection. Serum testosterone at presentation was <0.35 nmol/L (normal range 6.1–27 nmol/L). On examination, there was an approximately 7 cm firm

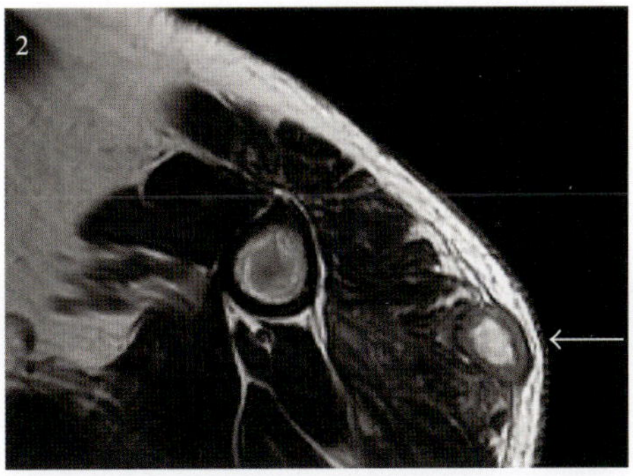

Figure 2: Magnetic resonance imaging (MRI) shows a complex, infiltrative maximally 9 cm mass in the left deltoid, extending from subcutaneous to deep tissues to abut the humerus, with underlying normal marrow. The lesion is composed of interlinked foci of abnormal tissue with intense central enhancement, suggesting necrosis.

mass over the left biceps muscle, fixed to the underlying structures (Figures 1(a) and 1(b)). Clinically it was of indeterminate nature but was thought to represent a primary soft tissue neoplasm. MRI showed a complex, infiltrative maximally 9 cm lesion in the left deltoid, which extended from subcutaneous to deep tissues to abut the humerus, with underlying normal marrow (Figure 2). This was composed of interlinked foci of abnormal tissue with intense central enhancement, possibly representing necrosis and suggestive of an aggressive inflammatory lesion or sarcoma. The lesion was biopsied.

3. Pathology

Histologically, the core biopsies of both cases showed similar features of fibrous tissue and skeletal muscle with extensive,

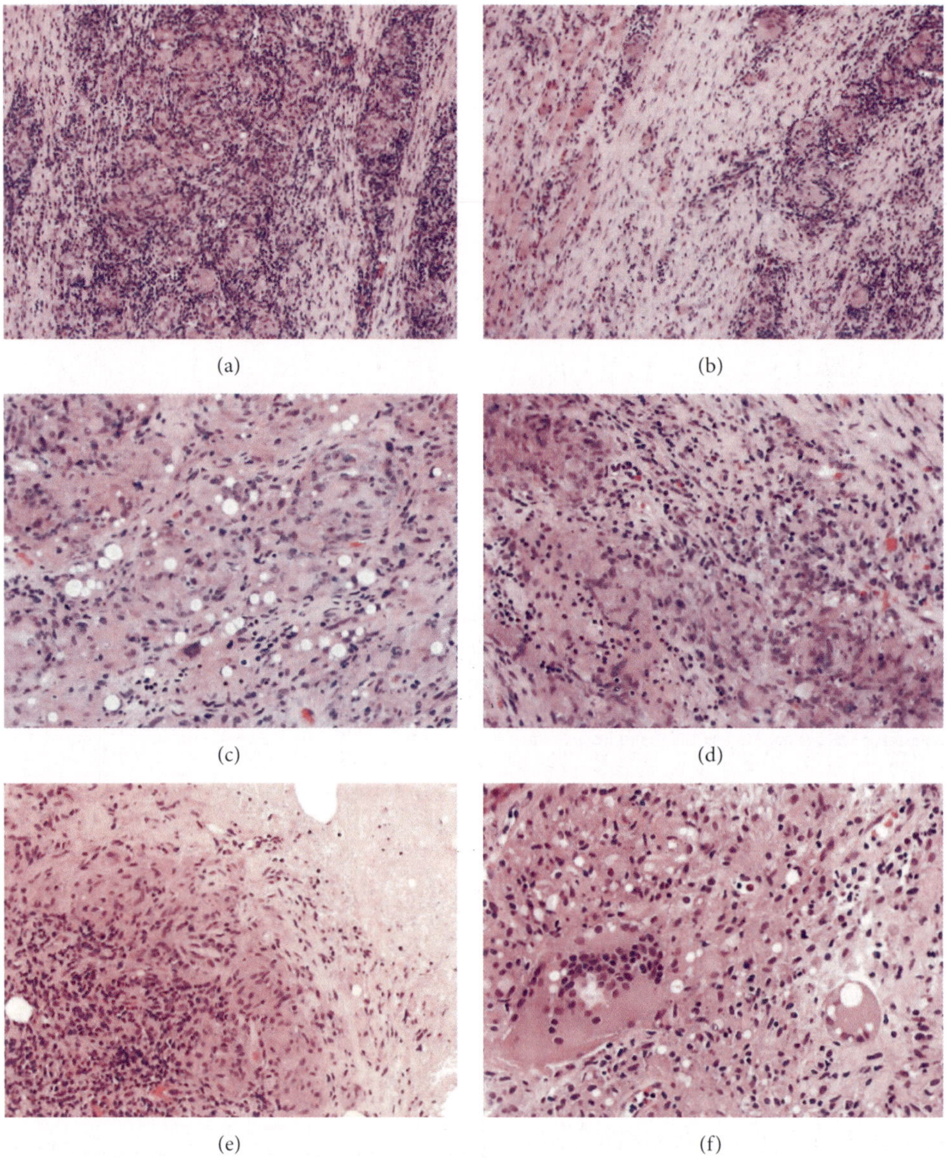

Figure 3: (a) These are relatively ill-defined granulomas comprising sheets of epithelioid histiocytes and giant cells and are surrounded by prominent mixed inflammation rich in small lymphocytes. (b) This example occurred deeply within the biceps muscle. There is atrophy of skeletal muscle fibers, with surrounding fibrosis and chronic inflammation. (c) In areas, there are rounded clear intracytoplasmic vacuoles within the histiocytic population. This is thought to represent foreign body reaction to polylactic acid. Luteinising hormone-releasing hormone (LHRH) has been shown to have lipolytic activity *in vitro*, and the degenerate lipid granules may induce foreign body granulomas. (d) The chronic inflammatory infiltrate comprises largely histiocytes and small lymphocytes, but there are smaller numbers of plasma cells and eosinophils. (e) This example shows areas of necrosis. (f) The giant cells can contain twenty or thirty nuclei. Engulfment of vacuoles corresponding to degenerate elements of leuprorelin acetate is apparent.

florid and destructive granulomatous inflammation, composed of relatively ill-defined granulomas containing sheets of epithelioid histiocytes and giant cells, including those of foreign body type (Figures 3(a)–3(f)). The histiocytes had plump, ovoid vesicular nuclei without atypia (Figures 3(a)–3(d)). Case 1 showed no caseation or necrosis, but case 2 showed focal areas of necrosis (Figure 3(e)). No foreign material was identified, but there were prominent rounded clear fatty vacuoles within the histiocytes (Figures 3(c) and 3(f)). There was marked surrounding chronic inflammation, largely composed of small lymphocytes, along with plasma cells and small numbers of eosinophils (Figure 3(d)). The granulomatous inflammation caused prominent skeletal muscle fiber atrophy in case 1 (Figure 3(b)). No neoplasm was identified with desmin, smooth muscle actin (SMA), S100 protein, AE1/AE3, CD117, or CD34. No microorganisms were identified with Ziehl-Neelsen, periodic acid-Schiff or Grocott's stains. In view of the continued clinical suspicion of neoplastic disease, patient 1 had a repeat biopsy, which showed similar findings.

4. Discussion

These are rare examples of florid, foreign body granulomas occurring within the subcutis and skeletal muscle of two males in their eighth decades, who were undergoing treatment for prostatic cancer with the luteinizing hormone-releasing hormone analogue leuprorelin acetate. LHRH analogues are widely used in the treatment of diseases that are responsive to the sex hormones, including advanced prostatic carcinoma, breast cancer, endometriosis, and central precocious puberty. When administered continuously, leuprorelin acetate is a potent inhibitor of gonadotropin secretion. After initial gonadotropin stimulation, chronic stimulation with leuprorelin acetate causes downregulation or suppression of these hormones, with subsequent suppression of testicular or ovarian steroidogenesis [1]. LHRH analogues are the mainstay of treatment for advanced prostatic carcinoma, either as primary therapy for metastatic disease or as salvage therapy following surgery or radiation therapy for clinically localized disease [2, 3]. Chemical castration using androgen deprivation therapy with LHRH analogues has been considered equivalent to bilateral orchidectomy in terms of reported testosterone suppression [4]. A sustained-action depot injection system is used to deliver long term controlled chemical castration [5], and to achieve this leuprorelin acetate is coupled to spherical microcapsules made of synthetic biodegradable lactic acid polymers or lactic acid and glycolic acid copolymers [6]. The interior of the polymer matrix contains many fine drug cores containing leuprorelin acetate [6, 7]. This long acting suspension of leuprorelin acetate is injected intramuscularly or subcutaneously and can be given as a monthly injection (3.75 mg) or longer acting 3-monthly preparation (11.25 mg).

There are several known side effects of leuprorelin acetate, including hot flushes, fatigue, nausea and vomiting, loss of libido, and osteoporosis. However, granulomatous nodules occurring at the site of injection are infrequently recognized. While leuprorelin acetate injection site granulomas have been occasionally reported in the urology and dermatology literature [8–13], they are not widely recognized outside these communities. This phenomenon warrants highlighting because of the wide clinical and radiological differential diagnosis, which includes both benign and malignant neoplastic disease and hence the significant potential patient and clinical impact, particularly when lesions are deeply sited (as they have greater propensity to mimic primary or metastatic cancer), which may cause unnecessary patient stress, clinical investigations, or possibly unnecessary surgical intervention [14, 15].

Injection granulomas of leuprorelin acetate are thought to arise from foreign body reaction to polylactic acid [16]. LHRH has been shown to have lipolytic activity *in vitro* [17, 18] and the degenerate lipid granules may induce foreign body granulomas [6]. Granuloma formation may also be dependent on the amount of leuprorelin acetate injected, as most of the reported cases were after injection of the larger 11.25 mg product [5, 6, 19]. Local reactions to depot leuprorelin acetate were first reported in 1992, in the treatment of patients with central precocious puberty [20]. While histology was not described in these cases, "apparent sterile abscess formation" was noted in one patient [20]. Rarely, leuprorelin acetate-induced granulomas have been documented in the arm after subcutaneous injection in the treatment of endometriosis [21], but the overwhelming majority of cases are in men being treated for prostate cancer. While these are still considered to be rare phenomena, many of the reported occurrences are from Japan, where, in a large study of 118 patients who were administered LHRH analogues, there was an incidence of injection site granulomas of 4.2% [19]. Many fewer cases have been reported in Europe and the USA, and authors have hypothesized that the administration of leuprorelin acetate intramuscularly in these areas, but subcutaneously in Japan, might account for the variable geographic incidence of leuprorelin granulomas [19]. The cases we report here occurred within 4 months of each other at our tertiary sarcoma center, but it is difficult to gauge whether this might truly represent an increasing finding in the UK. The reason for the much greater incidence of leuprorelin acetate granulomas occurring in patients with prostate cancer is unclear, although Watanabe et al. postulated that this might be due to the quantitative or qualitative differences in responsiveness of leuprorelin acetate to the LHRH receptor of adipose tissue between men and women [6].

Clinically leuprorelin acetate injection site granulomas tend to manifest as firm, often multiple erythematous nodules measuring approximately 2–6 cm [1, 21], often with a suppurative appearance [22], in the subcutis or sometimes skeletal muscle. The duration from time of first injection to onset of clinical findings varies from 35 to 350 days (mean 150 days), and it has been reported that most granulomas occurred after the first or second administration of the 11.25 mg quantity [19]. Development of granulomas is also noted to occur after the depot type was changed from a 1-monthly to 3-monthly formulation [1]. The clinical differential diagnosis is wide, ranging from inflammatory or reparative lesions such as traumatic panniculitis or hematoma or infective nodules from bacterial, mycobacterial, or fungal infection [21] to benign and malignant neoplasms. Because of their rapid enlargement, they can be mistaken for metastatic deposits [9, 14] or soft tissue sarcoma, such as epithelioid sarcoma, which can present similarly as numerous erythematous nodules at an extremity site. Alternatively, leuprorelin acetate granulomas can be mistaken for primary benign soft tissue neoplasms associated with rapid growth, such as nodular fasciitis or myositis ossificans.

Histologically, there are prominent granulomas usually centered within the subcutis but sometimes seen within the dermis or skeletal muscle and composed of sheets and nodules of epithelioid histiocytes with foreign body giant cells [6]. The histiocytes typically contain numerous translucent intracytoplasmic vacuoles of varying sizes, as well as variable degeneration of the adipose tissue. Sometimes the granulomas have a palisading appearance with eosinophils, and occasionally there may be central necrosis and abscess formation [6]. It is important not to miss a necrotic neoplasm, however, so immunohistochemistry with a basic panel of markers (AE1/AE3, desmin, SMA, CD34, S100 protein, and CD45/CD20/CD3) is likely to be contributory to excluding this. Ultrastructurally, within the cells of the granulomas, there are electron-lucent spherical bodies conforming to microcapsules of leuprorelin acetate products, as well as needle-shaped crystalloid structures in lipid droplets (degenerated lipid droplets) within both the granuloma cells and adipose tissue [6].

The phenomenon of leuprorelin acetate-induced injection site granulomas is still relatively little known outside the fields of urology and dermatology, and, with the increasing subspecialization of medicine, lesional biopsy may be performed at a tertiary sarcoma or orthopedic center, rather than the patient's local hospital, without access to or knowledge of the patient's medical history. This highlights the importance of clinical correlation and diagnostic recognition, in order to avoid misdiagnosis of these generally self-limiting lesions as malignant neoplasms.

Acknowledgments

The authors acknowledge support from the NIHR Royal Marsden/ICR Biomedical Research Centre.

References

[1] K. Yasukawa, D. Sawamura, H. Sugawara, and N. Kato, "Leuprorelin acetate granulomas: case reports and review of the literature," *British Journal of Dermatology*, vol. 152, no. 5, pp. 1045–1047, 2005.

[2] N. Sharifi, J. L. Gulley, and W. L. Dahut, "Androgen deprivation therapy for prostate cancer," *The Journal of the American Medical Association*, vol. 294, no. 2, pp. 238–244, 2005.

[3] M. R. Smith, "Obesity and sex steroids during gonadotropin-releasing hormone agonist treatment for prostate cancer," *Clinical Cancer Research*, vol. 13, no. 1, pp. 241–245, 2007.

[4] J. W. Moul, "Utility of LHRH antagonists for advanced prostate cancer," *The Canadian Journal of Urology*, vol. 21, no. 2, supplement 1, pp. 22–27, 2014.

[5] T. Ouchi, T. Koyama, N. Miyata, and M. Sugiura, "Granuloma caused by subcutaneous injection of leuprorelin acetate product: case report and histopathological findings," *Journal of Dermatology*, vol. 33, no. 10, pp. 719–721, 2006.

[6] T. Watanabe, N. Yamada, Y. Yoshida, and O. Yamamoto, "A morphological study of granulomas induced by subcutaneous injection of leuprorelin acetate," *Journal of Cutaneous Pathology*, vol. 36, no. 12, pp. 1299–1302, 2009.

[7] H. Okada, Y. Doken, and Y. Ogawa, "Persistent suppression of the pituitary-gonadal system in female rats by three-month depot injectable microspheres of leuprorelin acetate," *Journal of Pharmaceutical Sciences*, vol. 85, no. 10, pp. 1044–1048, 1996.

[8] I. S. Whitaker, M. Z. Fazel, H. B. Joshi, R. P. Moseley, and W. H. Turner, "Leuprorelin acetate granulomas: recurrent subcutaneous nodules mimicking metastatic deposits at injection sites," *BJU International*, vol. 90, no. 3, p. 350, 2002.

[9] M. Saxby, "Leuprorelin acetate granulomas: recurrent subcutaneous nodules mimicking metastatic deposits at injections sites," *BJU International*, vol. 91, no. 1, p. 125, 2003.

[10] R. Sakamoto, Y. Higashi, K. Mera, T. Kanekura, and T. Kanzaki, "Granulomas induced by subcutaneous injection of leuprorelin acetate," *The Journal of Dermatology*, vol. 33, no. 1, pp. 43–45, 2006.

[11] T. Oida, Y. Shichiri, N. Takao, T. Kanno, and H. Kanamaru, "Surgical management of inflammatory granuloma which developed following subcutaneous injection of leuprorelin acetate: a case report," *Acta Urologica Japonica*, vol. 51, no. 7, pp. 487–489, 2005.

[12] M. Tachibana, Z. Yamano, Y. Kusuda, S. Hara, H. Shimogaki, and G. Hamami, "Cutaneous epithelioid granulomas caused by subcutaneous infusion of leuprorelin acetate: a case report," *Acta Urologica Japonica*, vol. 50, no. 3, pp. 199–202, 2004.

[13] P. Dangle, V. Palit, S. K. Sundaram, and P. Weston, "Noninfective cutaneous granuloma with leuprorelin acetate—reality or myth," *Urology*, vol. 69, no. 4, pp. 779.e5–779.e6, 2007.

[14] M. Shiota, N. Tokuda, T. Kanou, and H. Yamasaki, "Injection-site granulomas due to the administration of leuprorelin acetate for the treatment of prostatic cancer," *Fukuoka Igaku Zasshi*, vol. 98, no. 7, pp. 301–304, 2007.

[15] R. Kitazawa, F. Yamamichi, T. Hidaka et al., "Bilateral injection-site granuloma by subcutaneous administration of luteinizing hormone-releasing hormone analogue: a case report," *Cases Journal*, vol. 2, article 8326, 2009.

[16] C. Vieu, J.-P. Arnault, N. Petitpain et al., "Granuloma at the injection site of leuprorelin acetate: foreign body reaction to polylactic acid," *Annales de Dermatologie et de Venereologie*, vol. 134, part 1, no. 10, pp. 771–773, 2007.

[17] G. G. Murthy and R. R. Modesto, "Effects of luteinizing hormone releasing hormone and thyrotrophin releasing hormone on rabbit adipose tissue," *Journal of Endocrinology*, vol. 62, no. 3, pp. 639–643, 1974.

[18] A. J. Kastin, T. W. Redding, R. Hall, G. M. Besser, and A. V. Schally, "Lipid mobilizing hormones of the hypothalamus and pituitary," *Pharmacology Biochemistry and Behavior*, vol. 3, no. 1, supplement, pp. 121–126, 1975.

[19] M. Shiota, N. Tokuda, T. Kanou, and H. Yamasaki, "Incidence rate of injection-site granulomas resulting from the administration of Luteinizing hormone-releasing hormone analogues for the treatment of prostatic cancer," *Yonsei Medical Journal*, vol. 48, no. 3, pp. 421–424, 2007.

[20] E. K. Neely, R. L. Hintz, B. Parker et al., "Two-year results of treatment with depot leuprolide acetate for central precocious puberty," *The Journal of Pediatrics*, vol. 121, no. 4, pp. 634–640, 1992.

[21] B. I. Lee, J. Y. Lee, H. O. Kim, and Y. M. Park, "Foreign body granuloma secondary to leuprorelin acetate," *Annals of Dermatology*, vol. 26, no. 2, pp. 254–255, 2014.

[22] M. Ferran, A. Giménez-Arnau, A. Toll et al., "Depot leuprorelin acetate-induced granulomas manifested as persistent suppurative nodules," *Acta Dermato-Venereologica*, vol. 86, no. 5, pp. 453–455, 2006.

15

Male Pelvic Squamous Cell Carcinoma of Unknown Primary Origin

Lauren Chiec,[1] Sadhna Verma,[2] Ady Kendler,[3] and Nagla Abdel Karim[4]

[1] *University of Cincinnati College of Medicine, Cincinnati, OH 45267, USA*
[2] *Division of Radiology, University of Cincinnati College of Medicine, Cincinnati, OH 45267, USA*
[3] *Division of Pathology, University of Cincinnati College of Medicine, Cincinnati, OH 45267, USA*
[4] *The Vontz Center for Molecular Studies, 3125 Eden Avenue, RM 1312, ML 0562, Cincinnati, OH 45267, USA*

Correspondence should be addressed to Nagla Abdel Karim; nagla.karim@uc.edu

Academic Editor: Constantine Gennatas

Pelvic squamous cell carcinoma of unknown primary origin has been described in several case reports of female patients. However, there have been no published reports describing male patients with pelvic squamous cell cancer of unknown primary origin. Our case describes a 52-year-old man who presented with right buttock pain, rectal urgency, and constipation. His physical examination demonstrated tenderness to palpation around his gluteal folds. Computed tomography scan of his abdomen and pelvis demonstrated a large mass in his retroperitoneum. The mass was determined to be squamous cell carcinoma of unknown primary origin. Additionally, the patient had small nodules in his right lower lung lobe and right hepatic lobe. The patient was treated with concomitant chemoradiation, including cisplatin and intensity-modulated radiation therapy, followed by carboplatin and paclitaxel. The patient achieved partial remission, in which he remained one year after his presentation. Our case is consistent with the literature which suggests that squamous cell carcinoma of unknown primary origin occurring outside of the head and neck region may have a more favorable prognosis than other carcinomas of unknown primary origin. Further studies are necessary to determine the most appropriate work-up, diagnosis, and optimal treatment strategies.

1. Introduction

Carcinomas of unknown primary (CUP) origin account for 3–5% of all malignancies and can be defined as "a heterogeneous group of metastatic tumors for which a standardized diagnostic work-up fails to identify the site of origin at the time of diagnosis" [1]. Among CUPs, squamous cell carcinoma accounts for 5–10%, often presenting in the cervical, supraclavicular, and inguinal lymph nodes [2]. Metastatic squamous cell CUP occurring in the pelvic cavity is extremely rare, with several case reports described involving female patients. These cases include a patient presenting with iliac lymph node metastases and a patient with an incidental pelvic mass found upon work-up for dysfunctional uterine bleeding [3, 4]. There have been no published reports describing male patients with pelvic squamous cell CUP. We herein describe a case of metastatic squamous cell CUP occurring in the pelvic cavity of a 52-year-old male patient.

2. Case Presentation

A 52-year-old Caucasian male presented to the emergency department after several weeks of right buttock pain, rectal urgency, and constipation. He denied systemic symptoms and had a normal physical examination, including digital rectal examination. The patient was given polyethylene glycol and discharged. Upon follow-up with his primary care physician, he continued to complain of buttock pain (now bilateral and tender to palpation around his gluteal folds), along with alternating diarrhea and constipation, and new urinary frequency. His physical examination was again normal and it was recommended for him to obtain a computed tomography (CT) scan of his abdomen and pelvis to evaluate for any neoplasm.

Of note, the patient's past medical history was significant for excision of a penile lesion 14 months prior to his presentation. The lesion was a granular cell tumor with overlying

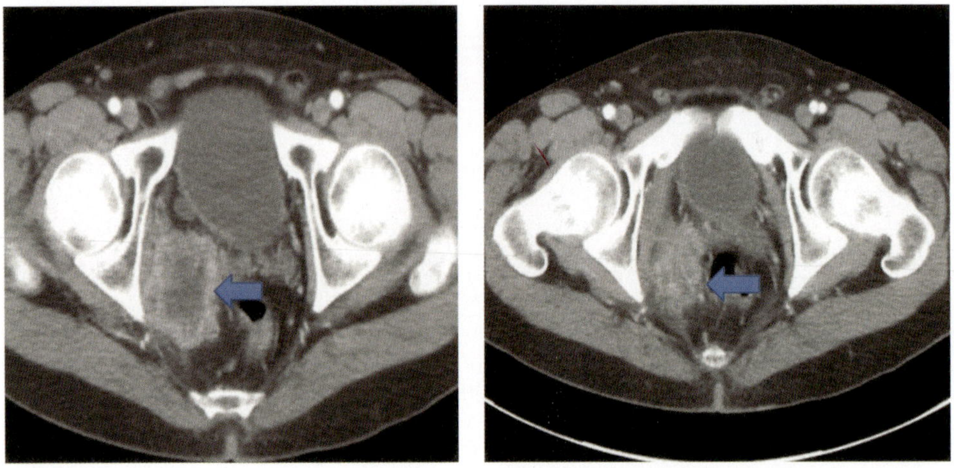

(a) (b)

FIGURE 1: Contrast-enhanced CT scan of the pelvis demonstrates a 6.5 × 5.1 cm mass within the right pelvis (arrows), bordered by the right obturator internus, right seminal vesicles, and bladder diverticulum. The epicenter of the mass is centered at the internal iliac neurovascular bundle.

pseudo epitheliomatous hyperplasia with no evidence of malignancy.

The CT scan was delayed for three months due to insurance issues. Subsequently when performed, it showed a large mass in his retroperitoneum. CT showed a 7 × 5 cm mass within the right pelvis, bordered by the right obturator internus, right seminal vesicles, and bladder diverticulum (Figures 1(a) and 1(b)). The epicenter of the mass was centered at the internal iliac neurovascular bundle. In addition to his pelvic mass, 5 and 3 mm nodules were discovered in his right lower lung lobe and right hepatic lobe, respectively.

CT guided percutaneous biopsy showed a perirectal, invasive, moderately differentiated, keratinizing, squamous cell carcinoma (Figures 2(a), 2(b), and 2(c)). Immunostain was strongly positive for pankeratin and positive for CK5, CK6, and P16 (Figures 3(a) and 3(b)). It was negative for CK7 and PSA.

The patient began to have systemic symptoms of chills, diaphoresis, weight loss, decreased appetite, and fatigue, as well as increased hip, groin and abdominal pain, dysuria and frequency, and dizziness. Although anoscopy, cystoscopy, and CT chest were recommended for further work-up, these were not obtained given the patient's financial situation. Chemoradiation was started with 2 cycles of cisplatin (targeting penile, anal, lung, and bladder carcinoma) and intensity-modulated radiation therapy with 6000 centigray in 30 fractions. This was tolerated well.

Follow-up CT chest, abdomen, and pelvis after 2 cycles of cisplatin and concurrent radiation showed a decrease in the size of the right pelvic mass to 4.2 × 2 cm (35% decrease). At that time, the lesion was a well-defined fluid collection with no substantial soft-tissue component. The liver lesion was stable, and several pulmonary nodules were discovered. Several of the pulmonary nodules were stable from prior CT. No evidence of brain metastases were seen on brain MRI. The patient was incidentally found to have bilateral acute on chronic pulmonary emboli on CT chest and was admitted to the hospital and begun on low molecular weight heparin therapy. Systemic chemotherapy with weekly carboplatin and paclitaxel was begun soon after and the patient received two cycles of carboplatin and paclitaxel. This was tolerated well except for neutropenia which led to the delay of one cycle of his systemic therapy and continued grade 1 peripheral neuropathy.

Cystoscopy with biopsy was performed and showed urothelial mucosa with mild chronic inflammation, reactive epithelial changes, and focal squamous metaplasia. There was no evidence of malignancy.

Follow-up CT chest, abdomen, and pelvis at 12 months after diagnosis (8 months after beginning treatment) showed a continued interval decrease in size of the pelvic lesion to 3.4 × 1.7 cm (Figures 4(a) and 4(b)). The patient has thus achieved a partial remission per RECIST 1.1 criteria [5], with an overall 47% decrease in the size of the lesion. In addition, the total response may be underestimated given that the residual mass had a linear and elongated shape and consisted of mainly necrotic tissue. Liver and lung lesions remain stable.

3. Discussion

In our report, we describe a 52-year-old male with pelvic squamous cell carcinoma of unknown primary origin, who achieved partial remission after platinum-based therapy in addition to paclitaxel. The uniqueness of this case is supported by the lack of published case reports describing male patients with this malignancy. Of the published literature regarding squamous cell CUP in the pelvic region, the patients described were all female, with gynecologic malignancies considered as possible etiologies.

One report describes a 47-year-old female with an incidental pelvic mass found during a work-up for dysfunctional

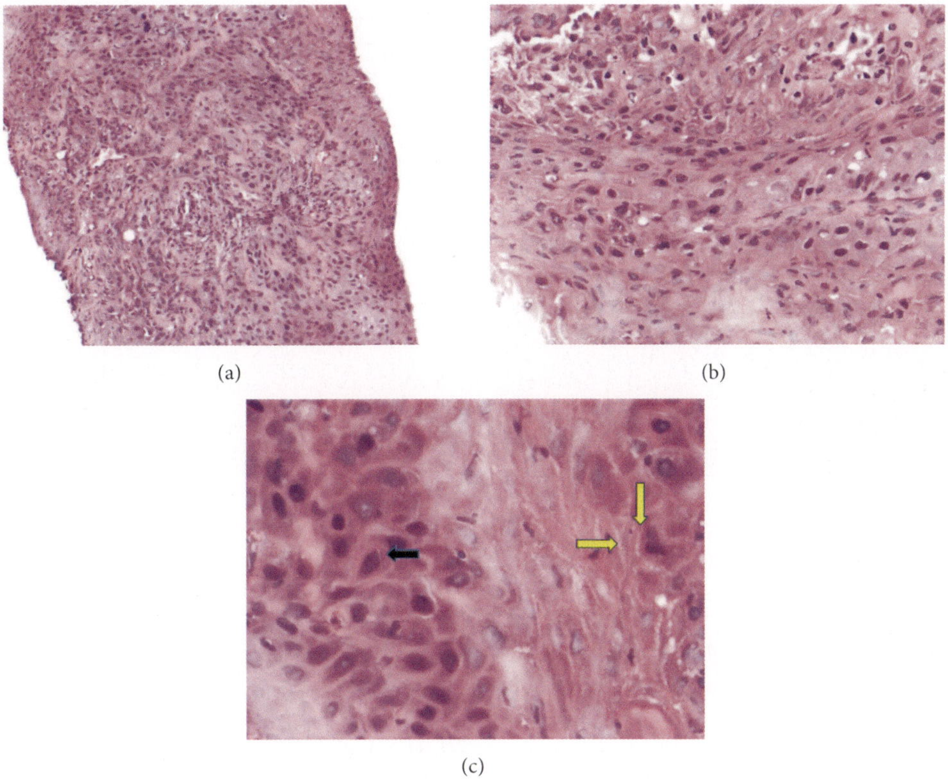

FIGURE 2: Hematoxylin and eosin (H&E) stain at 100x, 200x, and 400x power, respectively, demonstrates metastatic squamous cell carcinoma. At 400x power (c), intracellular bridges (yellow arrows) and eosinophilic, intracytoplasmic keratin (black arrow) are seen, indicating squamous differentiation.

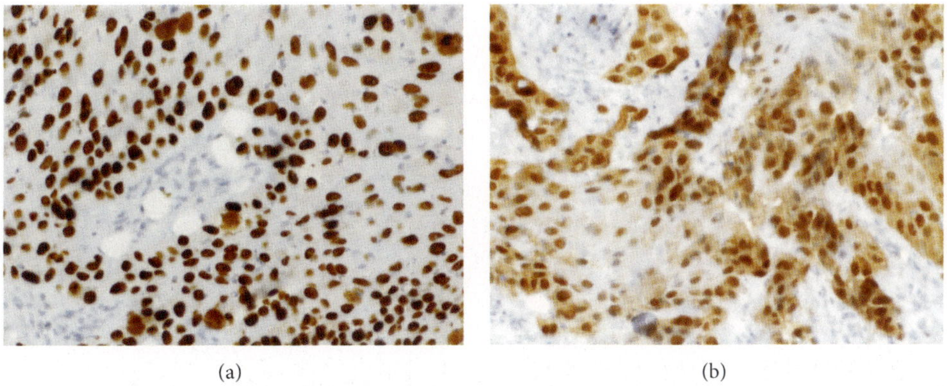

FIGURE 3: P63 immunostain shows positive nuclear staining in tumor cells ((a), (b)), as well as cytoplasmic staining (b), supporting the diagnosis of squamous cell carcinoma.

uterine bleeding. It was classified as squamous cell CUP and the patient showed a complete response after radiotherapy and intensive long-term chemotherapy (six cycles of 5-FU, cisplatin and leucovorin; four cycles of etoposide, doxorubicin, and cisplatin; five cycles of ifosfamide, mesna, cisplatin, and etoposide). Although she had recurrence of her pelvic mass five years after completing treatment, her initial response was promising in demonstrating the effect of systemic chemotherapy on squamous cell CUP presenting in the pelvic cavity. The patient remained alive more than eight years after her diagnosis, suggesting the prognosis for this metastatic malignancy is more favorable than others [4].

Another report describes a 70-year-old female with persistent right leg edema, found to have squamous cell CUP metastatic to the iliac lymph nodes. She underwent surgical resection and radiation therapy and continued to show no recurrence after 17 months of follow-up. Her tumor was controlled with locoregional management; the role of systemic chemotherapy has not been evaluated in patients with CUP of the inguinal and or iliac lymph nodes [3].

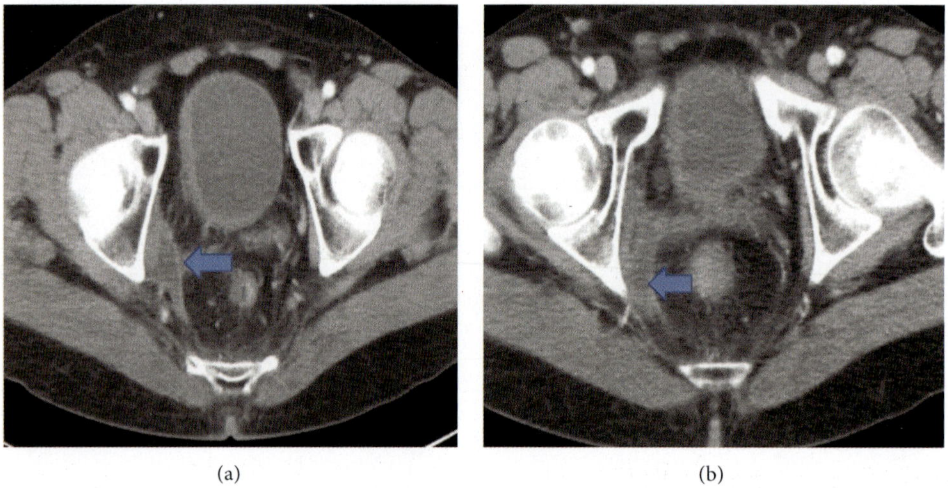

FIGURE 4: Contrast-enhanced CT scan of the pelvis demonstrates a 3.4 × 1.7 cm pelvic lesion (arrows) with no substantial soft-tissue component. The lesion is linear and elongated and appears to be comprised mainly of necrotic tissue, consistent with postradiation changes.

In general, CUP has a poor prognosis, with a median survival time of less than six months and only about 15% of patients surviving after 1 year in population-based studies [6]. However, it appears that squamous cell carcinomas with limited anatomic distribution in nodal regions outside the head and neck region may be a prognostically favorable subset of CUP, with a median survival time of almost 2 years [7]. Our patient's clinical course is consistent with the literature in that he remains in partial remission one year after presentation. Given the rarity of squamous cell CUP, especially in the pelvic region, further studies are needed to fully evaluate the prognosis of this malignancy.

In our case, we were able to rule out many common primary malignancies, including prostate (immunostain PSA negative), urinary bladder (no evidence of malignancy on cystoscopy), and lung (immunostain p16 positive and CK7 negative). Immunostaining is not generally helpful in differentiating metastatic squamous cell CUP, aside from in favoring an extrapulmonary neoplasm if results are p16 positive [8]. P16 positivity is also seen in other primary malignancies associated with human papillomavirus infection, including squamous cell carcinomas of the oropharynx, cervix, and anus. Studies have shown that in some cases, a clone of cells in an otherwise benign epithelium may be determined as a source for metastases through microsatellite analysis before histopathology can identify definite dysplasia or malignancy [9]. In our patient, a primary anal neoplasm was unlikely as no anal lesions were noted on digital rectal examination. It is possible that targeted biopsies of common primary sites may be helpful in determining the origin of the metastases, although the rarity of this presentation makes the diagnostic approach challenging, and there are several obvious risks and financial limitations of further biopsies. Although there has been a case report of a patient presenting with pelvic squamous cell CUP which was later discovered to be primary esophageal carcinoma, this is rare and our patient has not shown any sign of esophageal neoplasm on CT chest studies [10].

Although our patient's clinical course and diagnostic work-up were consistent with a CUP, it is important to note that his initial staging investigations were incomplete, as the patient had significant financial constraints which limited his ability to undergo complete testing. He chose not to undergo anoscopy or sigmoidoscopy, and CT chest and cystoscopy were both performed after the patient had begun receiving systemic treatment. Had these investigations been performed at the time of diagnosis, the likelihood of discovering a primary site would have been much higher. Performing these investigations after treatment was begun could mean that the primary was no longer visible and therefore missed. In addition, although routine serum tumor markers are often considered in the initial diagnostic evaluation, these were not performed in our case. Routine tumor markers have been shown to be nonspecifically elevated in more than 50% of patients with CUP and have not been proven to have any diagnostic or prognostic significance at this time [11].

Based on the limited data from reported cases, it appears that squamous cell CUP, especially outside of the head and neck region, has a more favorable prognosis compared to other CUPs. It also appears that these malignancies may respond well to a combination of surgical resection, when feasible, local radiotherapy, and platinum-based systemic chemotherapy. Given the rare nature of pelvic squamous cell CUP, further reports and studies on these cases are necessary to better determine the ideal work-up for diagnosing primary tumors, optimal treatment strategies, and accurate prognostic data.

4. Conclusion

Squamous cell carcinoma of unknown primary origin is a rare malignancy, and reports of this neoplasm occurring in the pelvic cavity are extremely limited. Further studies are needed to determine ideal strategies for diagnosis, treatment, and prognostication.

References

[1] K. Fizazi, F. A. Greco, N. Pavlidis, and G. Pentheroudakis, "Cancers of unknown primary site: ESMO clinical practice guidelines for diagnosis, treatment and follow-up," *Annals of Oncology*, vol. 22, no. 6, pp. vi64–vi68, 2011.

[2] K. A. Oien, "Pathologic evaluation of unknown primary cancer," *Seminars in Oncology*, vol. 36, no. 1, pp. 8–37, 2009.

[3] S. Matsuyama, Y. Nakafusa, M. Tanaka, Y. Yoda, D. Mori, and K. Miyazaki, "Iliac lymph node metastasis of an unknown primary tumor: report of a case," *Surgery Today*, vol. 36, no. 7, pp. 655–658, 2006.

[4] H. J. Lee, H. J. Yun, D. Y. Jo, K. S. Suh, and S. Kim, "Metastatic squamous cell carcinoma of unknown primary site occurring in pelvic cavity," *European Journal of Obstetrics Gynecology and Reproductive Biology*, vol. 138, no. 2, pp. 239–240, 2008.

[5] E. A. Eisenhauer, P. Therasse, J. Bogaerts et al., "New response evaluation criteria in solid tumours: revised RECIST guideline (version 1.1)," *European Journal of Cancer*, vol. 45, no. 2, pp. 228–247, 2009.

[6] A. J. Van de Wouw, M. L. G. Janssen-Heijnen, J. W. W. Coebergh, and H. F. P. Hillen, "Epidemiology of unknown primary tumours; incidence and population-based survival of 1285 patients in Southeast Netherlands, 1984-1992," *European Journal of Cancer*, vol. 38, no. 3, pp. 409–413, 2002.

[7] M. Randén, M. Helde-Frankling, S. Runesdotter, and P. Gunvén, "Unfavorable cancers of unknown primaries: presentation and prognostic factors. A population-based 8-year experience," *Medical Oncology*, vol. 30, no. 4, article 706, 2013.

[8] T. C. Pereira, S. M. Share, A. V. Magalhães, and J. F. Silverman, "Can we tell the site of origin of metastatic squamous cell carcinoma? An immunohistochemical tissue microarray study of 194 cases," *Applied Immunohistochemistry and Molecular Morphology*, vol. 19, no. 1, pp. 10–14, 2011.

[9] J. Califano, W. H. Westra, W. Koch et al., "Unknown primary head and neck squamous cell carcinoma: molecular identification of the site of origin," *Journal of the National Cancer Institute*, vol. 91, no. 7, pp. 599–604, 1999.

[10] L. Yu, X. Ge, S. Huang et al., "Primary squamous cell carcinoma of the esophagus initially presenting as a large retroperitoneal mass: a case diagnosed as cancer of unknown primary site," *Molecular Clinical Oncology*, vol. 1, pp. 503–506, 2013.

[11] M. Milovic, I. Popov, and S. Jelic, "Tumor markers in metastatic disease from cancer of unknown primary origin," *Medical Science Monitor*, vol. 8, no. 2, pp. MT25–MT30, 2002.

16

Nontargeted Effect after Radiotherapy in a Patient with Non-Small Cell Lung Cancer and Bullous Pemphigoid

Carsten Nieder,[1,2] Khalid Al-Shibli,[3] and Terje Tollåli[4]

[1] *Department of Oncology and Palliative Medicine, Nordland Hospital, 8092 Bodø, Norway*
[2] *Department of Clinical Medicine, Faculty of Health Sciences, University of Tromsø, 9038 Tromsø, Norway*
[3] *Department of Pathology, Nordland Hospital, 8092 Bodø, Norway*
[4] *Department of Pulmonology, Nordland Hospital, 8092 Bodø, Norway*

Correspondence should be addressed to Carsten Nieder; carsten.nieder@nlsh.no

Academic Editor: Jose I. Mayordomo

Purpose. To describe tumor shrinkage of nonirradiated lung metastases in a patient with non-small cell lung cancer. *Case Report.* The patient had a concurrent autoimmune condition, bullous pemphigoid, which was clinically exacerbated during radiotherapy of mediastinal and axillary lymph node metastases. He also developed a series of infections during and after irradiation, and we hypothesize that the immunological events during this phase might have influenced the size of the nonirradiated metastases. *Conclusion.* Ionizing radiation generates inflammatory signals and, in principle, could provide both tumor-specific antigens from dying cells and maturation stimuli that are necessary for dendritic cells' activation of tumor-specific T cells. Even if the detailed mechanisms causing nontargeted immune modulatory effects in individual patients are poorly understood, clinical development of radioimmunotherapy is underway.

1. Introduction

It has been long realized that ionizing radiation is able to influence cells and tissues that are not directly located in the radiation fields [1–3]. Several case reports, experimental studies, and reviews have addressed such phenomena, which typically are termed bystander, nontargeted immune modulatory, or abscopal effect. In clinical practice, few patients experience tumor response in metastatic sites that are distant from the radiation fields. Here we describe the clinical course of a patient with nonsmall cell lung cancer (NSCLC) and bullous pemphigoid, an autoimmune skin disease that typically manifests in older people and with male preponderance, without clear association to malignant diseases [4], who developed response of nonirradiated lung metastases, possibly related to immune activation by infection.

2. Case Report

A 67-year-old Caucasian male patient was treated for NSCLC of the left upper lobe in February 2013 (lobectomy). He had a history of heavy smoking, chronic kidney failure, and myocardial infarction. Furthermore, he had been treated with radical prostatectomy (2009) and salvage radiotherapy to the prostate bed (2010, stage pT4 N0 R1, Gleason score 4 + 4). Because of new biochemical relapse, he had started antiandrogen treatment with bicalutamide in November 2011. His prostate-specific antigen (PSA) value was <0.2 ng/mL after endocrine therapy. Cystectomy had been performed in March 2012 after diagnosis of WHO grade 3 urothelial cell bladder cancer (stage pT1). Medical treatment also included simvastatin 40 mg daily, acetylsalicylic acid 75 mg daily, cetirizine 5 mg daily, hydrochlorothiazide 25 mg daily, and valsartan 320 mg daily. Histology after lobectomy showed two foci of adenosquamous carcinoma (22 and 23 mm, resp.) invading the visceral pleura (stage pT3 pN1). Immunohistochemistry of the two tumors showed positive staining for p53 in only one of them. Adjuvant chemotherapy started in April 2013. Because of impaired renal function, carboplatin AUC6 and vinorelbine 30 mg/m^2 were prescribed. After three of four planned cycles, the patient developed local relapse in the thoracic wall and skin changes, mainly at the

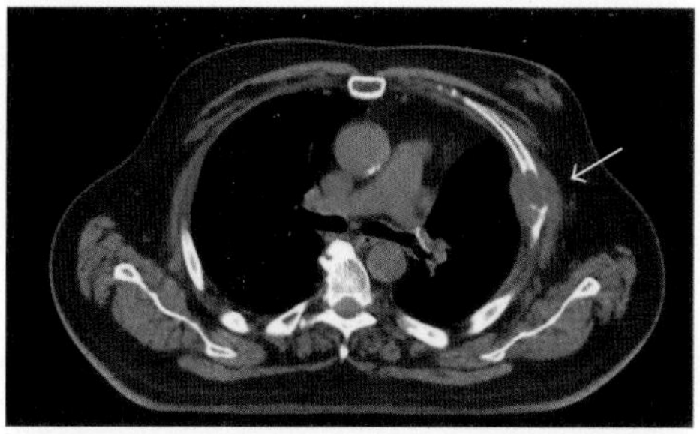

FIGURE 1: Computed tomography scan of the thorax showing left-sided local relapse in the pleura and thoracic wall after lobectomy. Status before palliative radiotherapy.

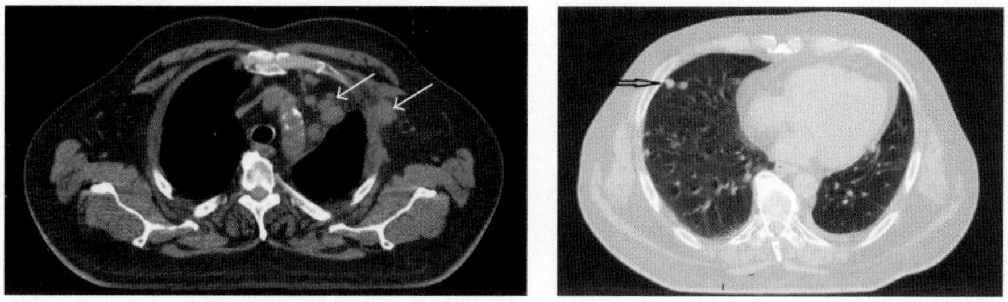

(a) (b)

FIGURE 2: (a) Computed tomography scan of the thorax showing left-sided axillary nodal metastasis and mediastinal lymph node metastases. Status before palliative radiotherapy. (b) Computed tomography scan of the thorax showing right-sided pulmonary metastases (example of the patient's bilateral metastases). During radiotherapy, this region received a cumulative dose of <1 Gy.

upper part of the body and arms, which were diagnosed as bullous pemphigoid. White blood cell count and differential were within the normal range. Treatment included prednisolone and topical desoxymethasone. In July 2013, 3D conformal palliative radiotherapy was administered to the region of pleural/thoracic wall recurrence (13 fractions of 3 Gy), Figure 1. In November 2013, systemic progression was detected, with new bilateral pulmonary metastases and mediastinal and left-sided axillary lymph node metastases, Figures 2(a) and 2(b). A new course of 3D conformal palliative radiotherapy was given (10 fractions of 3 Gy to all lymph node metastases). During radiotherapy, the bullous pemphigoid was exacerbated and secondary infection occurred (status at simulation shown in Figure 3). Serum C-reactive protein was elevated to 50 mg/L and leukocyte count was slightly elevated to 11.1×10^9/L (Figure 4). The daily dose of prednisolone during radiotherapy was 20 mg. The patient received antibiotic treatment with cefuroxime. Two weeks after the last fraction of radiotherapy, the patient was hospitalized and treated for pneumonia. Chest X-rays showed a pneumonic infiltrate in the left lower lobe. Microbiological tests did not reveal the cause of infection. Three weeks after discharge, he was hospitalized again, this time because of sepsis caused by *E. coli*. Computed tomography (CT) showed partial response of the irradiated and nonirradiated lesions (Figure 5, January 2014). The total radiation dose in the region of these lung metastases was <1 Gy, compared to the prescription dose of 30 Gy. Two weeks after discharge, he was treated for another infection, now caused by influenza A virus. In April 2014, CT showed progression of all pulmonary metastases (Figure 6). Further systemic therapy was not given because of reduced performance status, impaired kidney function, and frequent infections. The patient received analgetics and supportive treatment under guidance of the hospital's multidisciplinary palliative team. The bullous pemphigoid never disappeared completely. He died from pulmonary failure in July 2014, seventeen months after surgical resection of the primary tumor.

3. Discussion

NSCLC is often characterized by rapid development of distant metastases, even in patients receiving radical treatment upfront [5]. Palliative radiotherapy is an established and effective option in this setting [6, 7]. The patient described here experienced lasting local control of all irradiated tumors. Surprisingly, his unirradiated lung metastases also responded rapidly, followed by progression later on. This so-called nontargeted immune modulatory effect is a rare event. Previous case reports often related distant responses outside of the radiation fields to administration of immune modulating agents [8]. Immunogenic forms of tumor cell death induced by X-rays might include immune modulating danger signals like heat shock protein 70, adenosine triphosphate, and high-mobility group box 1 protein [9]. Moreover, antitumor effects exerted by cells of the innate (natural killer cells) as well

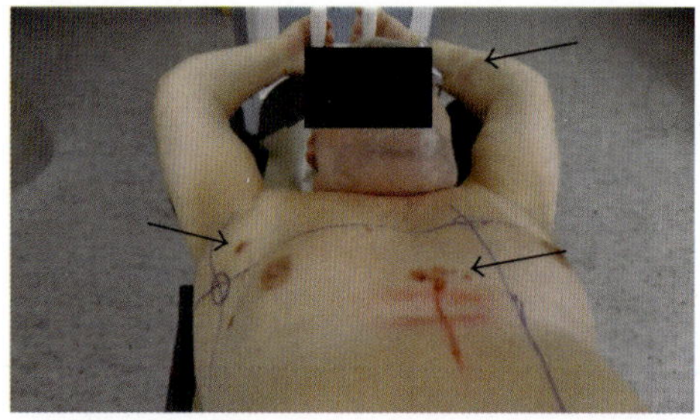

Figure 3: Skin lesions at the time of simulation before palliative radiotherapy to the mediastinum and left axilla. Bullous pemphigoid mainly involving trunk and arms.

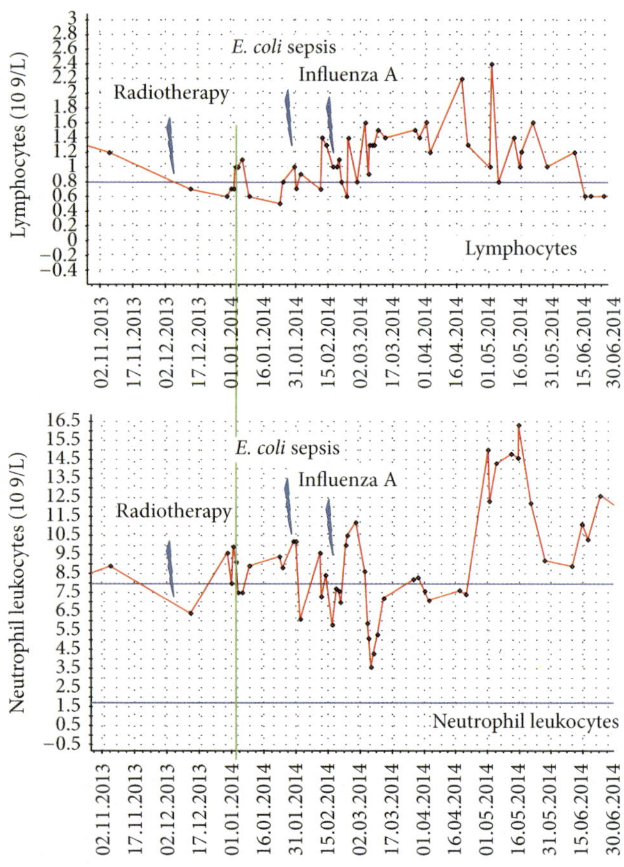

Figure 4: Time course of neutrophil leukocyte and lymphocyte counts during follow-up. The green line corresponds to the date of the computed tomography scan showing the nontargeted effect. At this time, the patient had recovered from presumably radiation-related lymphopenia. Abnormally high lymphocyte counts were never detected. In contrast, several episodes of leukocytosis occurred.

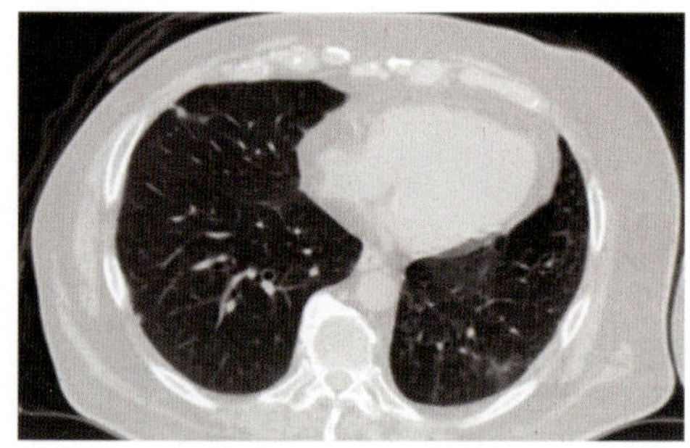

Figure 5: Computed tomography scan of the thorax showing right-sided pulmonary metastases approximately 3 weeks after radiotherapy to other targets. Marked reduction in size.

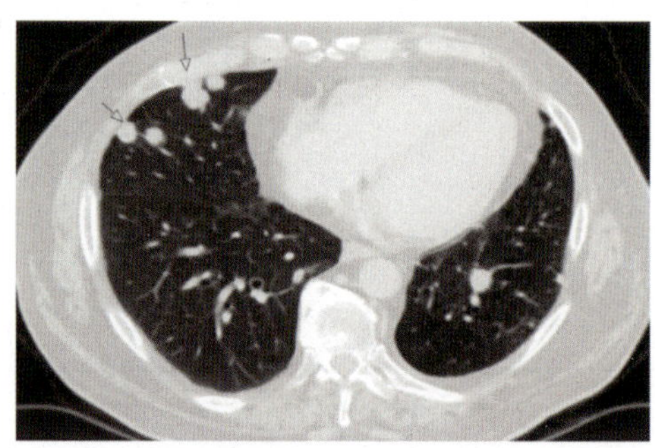

Figure 6: Computed tomography scan of the thorax showing progression of the right-sided pulmonary metastases approximately 3 months after radiotherapy to other targets. Temporary nontargeted effect.

as adaptive immune system (T cells activated by dendritic cells) might play a role. Ionizing radiation generates inflammatory signals and, in principle, could provide both tumor-specific antigens from dying cells and maturation stimuli that are necessary for dendritic cells' activation of tumor-specific T cells. Experimental data provided support for these mechanisms [1]. The patient described in our report had a concurrent autoimmune condition, bullous pemphigoid, which was clinically exacerbated during radiotherapy. He also developed a series of infections during and after irradiation, and we hypothesize that the complex immunological events during this phase might have influenced the shrinkage of the nonirradiated metastases. Unfortunately, his immunological status was not analyzed in detail. Future studies should include longitudinal analyses of different immune cell populations, ideally also tumor-infiltrating lymphocytes. Current research efforts aim at development of clinically applicable protocols of combined radio- and immunotherapy [10].

Consent

Consent to publish has been obtained from the participant to report individual patient data.

Authors' Contribution

All the authors participated in evaluation and treatment of this patient and drafted the paper together. All the authors read and approved the final paper.

References

[1] S. Demaria, B. Ng, M. L. Devitt et al., "Ionizing radiation inhibition of distant untreated tumors (abscopal effect) is immune mediated," *International Journal of Radiation Oncology, Biology, Physics*, vol. 58, no. 3, pp. 862–870, 2004.

[2] K. Shiraishi, Y. Ishiwata, K. Nakagawa et al., "Enhancement of antitumor radiation efficacy and consistent induction of the abscopal effect in mice by ECI301, an active variant of macrophage inflammatory protein-1α," *Clinical Cancer Research*, vol. 14, no. 4, pp. 1159–1166, 2008.

[3] F. Rödel, B. Frey, G. Multhoff, and U. Gaipl, "Contribution of the immune system to bystander and non-targeted effects of ionizing radiation," *Cancer Letters*, vol. 356, no. 1, pp. 105–113, 2015.

[4] E. Ong, R. Goldacre, U. Hoang, R. Sinclair, and M. Goldacre, "Associations between bullous pemphigoid and primary malignant cancers: an English national record linkage study, 1999–2011," *Archives of Dermatological Research*, vol. 306, no. 1, pp. 75–80, 2014.

[5] S. Kunisawa, K. Yamashita, H. Ikai, T. Otsubo, and Y. Imanaka, "Survival analyses of postoperative lung cancer patients: an investigation using Japanese administrative data," *SpringerPlus*, vol. 3, article 217, 2014.

[6] B. van Oorschot, B. Assenbrunner, M. Schuler, G. Beckmann, and M. Flentje, "Survival and prognostic factors after moderately hypofractionated palliative thoracic radiotherapy for non-small cell lung cancer," *Strahlentherapie und Onkologie*, vol. 190, no. 3, pp. 270–275, 2014.

[7] C. Schröder, M. Ivo, and A. Buchali, "Does high-dose radiotherapy benefit palliative lung cancer patients?: an intradepartmental comparison of two dose regimens," *Strahlentherapie und Onkologie*, vol. 189, no. 9, pp. 771–776, 2013.

[8] E. B. Golden, S. Demaria, P. B. Schiff, A. Chachoua, and S. C. Formenti, "An abscopal response to radiation and ipilimumab in a patient with metastatic non-small cell lung cancer," *Cancer Immunology Research*, vol. 1, no. 6, pp. 365–372, 2013.

[9] U. S. Gaipl, G. Multhoff, H. Scheithauer et al., "Kill and spread the word: stimulation of antitumor immune responses in the context of radiotherapy," *Immunotherapy*, vol. 6, no. 5, pp. 597–610, 2014.

[10] E. Sharon, M.-Y. Polley, M. B. Bernstein, and M. Ahmed, "Immunotherapy and radiation therapy: considerations for successfully combining radiation into the paradigm of immuno-oncology drug development," *Radiation Research*, vol. 182, no. 2, pp. 252–257, 2014.

17

Metastatic Prostate Cancer Manifesting as Cholestatic Jaundice: A Case Report

Deepak Ravindranathan,[1] Emilie Elise Hitron,[2] Greta Anne Russler,[2] Yue Xue,[3] and Mehmet Asim Bilen[2]

[1]*Department of Medicine, Emory University School of Medicine, Atlanta, GA, USA*
[2]*Department of Hematology and Medical Oncology, Winship Cancer Institute of Emory University, Atlanta, GA, USA*
[3]*Department of Pathology, Emory University School of Medicine, Atlanta, GA, USA*

Correspondence should be addressed to Mehmet Asim Bilen; mbilen@emory.edu

Academic Editor: Peter F. Lenehan

A paraneoplastic syndrome can often present as the first manifestation of an underlying malignancy. We report a patient who presented with cholestatic jaundice as a paraneoplastic syndrome from his newly diagnosed metastatic prostate cancer. He received initial treatment with androgen deprivation therapy followed by six cycles of docetaxel resulting in resolution of his cholestatic process, normalization of liver enzyme levels, and excellent biochemical and radiographic response. To the best of our knowledge, this is the first reported case of metastatic prostate cancer with cholestatic jaundice as a paraneoplastic phenomenon to be safely treated with androgen deprivation therapy and upfront docetaxel, reflecting the latest shift in the treatment of metastatic prostate cancer.

1. Introduction

Paraneoplastic syndrome refers to signs and symptoms that are found in the presence of a malignancy but are not attributable to direct compression or invasion of the tumor. Several of these syndromes have been found in genitourinary malignancies. Stauffer's syndrome, first described in 1961, is a paraneoplastic syndrome found in renal cell cancer that results in hepatic dysfunction [1]. Following renal cell cancer, prostate cancer ranks as the second most common genitourinary malignancy to be associated with paraneoplastic syndromes; however, finding a paraneoplastic syndrome associated with prostate cancer is still very uncommon. In the medical literature, there are about a hundred cases of paraneoplastic syndromes found in prostate cancer manifesting as endocrinological, neurological, or dermatological conditions [2].

Cholestasis in patients suffering from malignancies can typically result from a bile duct obstruction either by the primary tumor itself, metastasis to the liver, or enlarged lymph nodes [3]. In fact, the paraneoplastic syndrome of cholestatic jaundice in patients with metastatic prostate cancer without any evidence of biliary duct obstruction or hepatic infiltration has been described in the medical literature [4]. Androgen deprivation therapy (ADT) has resulted in improvement of the cholestatic process as demonstrated by decline in bilirubin, liver enzymes, and prostate-specific antigen (PSA) levels [5–7]. However, none of those patients were treated with early chemotherapy in combination with ADT as per the latest guidelines in the treatment of metastatic prostate cancer [8].

Here, we describe the first case, to the best of our knowledge, of a patient with metastatic prostate cancer who presented with cholestatic jaundice as a paraneoplastic syndrome and was safely treated with both ADT and chemotherapy, consisting of six cycles of docetaxel, resulting in excellent response.

2. Case Presentation

A 47-year-old African American male presented at Emory University Hospital with jaundice and dark urine. He had no previous history of liver or biliary disease, blood transfusions,

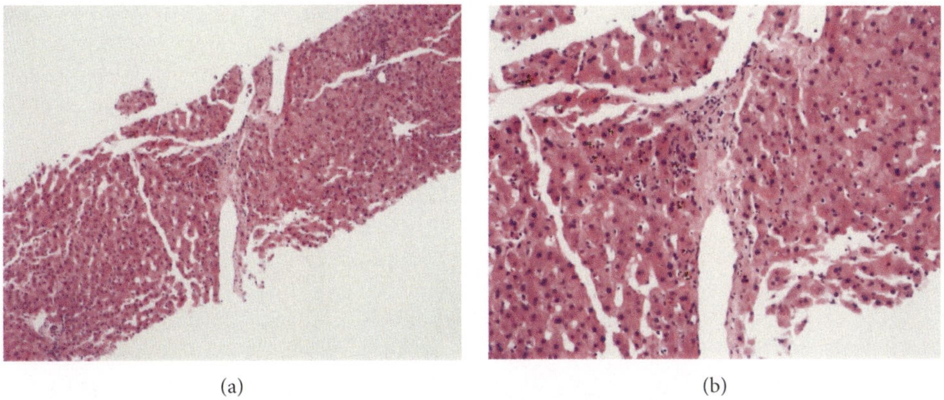

FIGURE 1: Hematoxylin-eosin staining of the liver biopsy showing canalicular cholestasis predominantly in the centrizonal areas with no obvious hepatocyte injury. (a) Magnification ×10. (b) Magnification ×20.

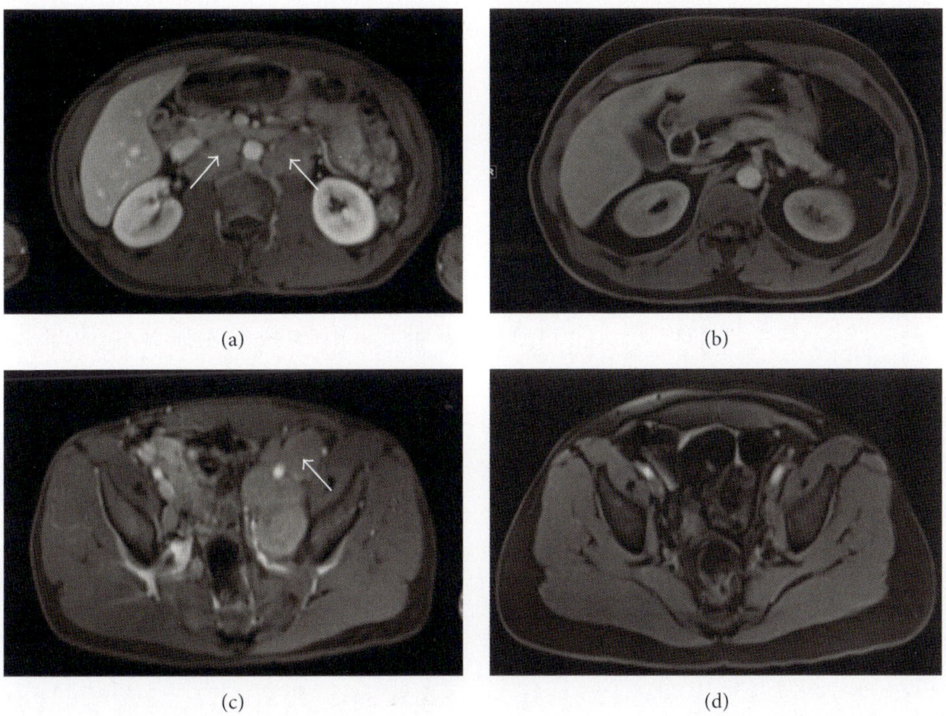

FIGURE 2: MRI of the patient's abdomen and pelvis showing resolution of paraaortic and iliac lymphadenopathy after ADT and docetaxel treatment. (a) Paraaortic lymphadenopathy (shown by white arrows) before treatment. (b) Resolution of paraaortic lymphadenopathy after treatment. (c) Left iliac lymphadenopathy (shown by white arrow) before treatment. (d) Resolution of left iliac lymphadenopathy after treatment.

or recent travel. He denied fevers, night sweats, chills, nausea, vomiting, abdominal pain, distention, diarrhea, or pale stools. Initial liver function test results were as follows: AST of 425 U/L (normal range: 7–52 U/L), ALT of 601 U/L (normal range: 13–39 U/L), alkaline phosphatase of 524 U/L (normal range: 34–104 U/L), gamma-glutamyltransferase of 1389 U/L (normal range: 9–64 U/L), and total bilirubin of 15.3 mg/dL (normal range: 0.3–1 mg/dL), with direct component of 9.24 mg/dL (normal range: $\leq$0.18). Urinalysis showed the presence of bilirubin and urobilinogen. Viral hepatitis panel was negative. Computed tomography (CT) of the patient's abdomen and pelvis with contrast showed retroperitoneal lymphadenopathy extending into bilateral iliac chains with mottled appearance of bone, concerning metastatic malignancy. Ultrasound of the abdomen showed no evidence of cirrhosis or cholelithiasis. On endoscopic retrograde cholangiopancreatography, the cholangiogram was normal ruling out extrahepatic cholestatic disorders. Biopsy of the patient's liver showed cholestasis, mild portal chronic, and minimal lobular inflammation (Figures 1(a) and 1(b)). Magnetic resonance imaging (MRI) of the patient's abdomen revealed bulky, diffuse lymphadenopathy and secondary lymphomatous involvement of the prostate gland (Figures 2(a) and 2(b)). CT-guided lymph node biopsy revealed malignant cells, consistent

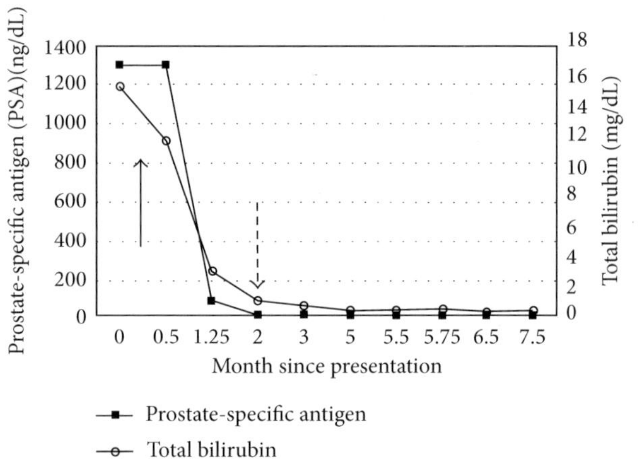

FIGURE 3: Trend in PSA and total bilirubin levels after diagnosis. Solid arrow represents the time of initiation of androgen deprivation therapy, and dotted arrow represents the time of initiation of docetaxel.

with prostate cancer based on staining markers. The patient's PSA level was greater than 1300 ng/mL (normal range: ≤4 ng/mL), and his jaundice was presumed secondary to paraneoplastic syndrome from underlying metastatic prostate cancer.

The patient was started on ADT initially with degarelix (240 mg subcutaneously) and a month later with leuprolide (22.5 mg intramuscularly every 3 months). Within 2 months of initiating ADT, his PSA level declined to 6.5 ng/mL (Figure 3). His liver enzyme levels reached normal ranges within two months, and subsequently, the first cycle of docetaxel was initiated. Patient tolerated six cycles of docetaxel without any adverse event, including no elevation in liver enzymes. The patient's most recent staging imaging after completion of chemotherapy revealed excellent response with resolution of retroperitoneal and pelvic lymphadenopathy with decreased enhancement of multiple bone lesions (Figures 2(c) and 2(d)). Notably, his most recent bilirubin was 0.3 mg/dL, and PSA was 0.84 ng/dL. At the time of writing, the patient was alive and clinically doing well.

3. Discussion

Timely and accurate diagnosis and treatment of paraneoplastic syndromes can greatly affect patient's clinical outcomes. Paraneoplastic syndromes may present before a cancer diagnosis; recognition of such syndrome may lead to the diagnosis of a possibly occult tumor at an early and treatable stage. The fact that this patient's jaundice was not associated with hepatocellular and cholestatic conditions and that the patient's symptoms resolved completely and shortly after initiation of antiandrogen treatment for prostate cancer suggest that the intrahepatic cholestasis in this patient was likely a paraneoplastic manifestation of prostate cancer.

The pathophysiology of this interesting paraneoplastic phenomenon is still not well delineated. Blay et al. reported that the cytokine, interleukin-6 (IL-6), is involved in the pathophysiology of paraneoplastic cholestasis in renal cell cancer. Treatment with anti-IL-6 monoclonal antibody was found to reverse most of the biochemical abnormalities in such patients. The general mechanism through which this occurs is still unknown, but this has also been thought to play a role in prostate cancer [9, 10].

There are case reports describing cholestasis as a paraneoplastic syndrome associated with several different malignancies, including Hodgkin's disease, thyroid cancer, T-cell lymphoma, chronic lymphocytic leukemia, and lung cancer [2, 11–14]. Karakolios reported a prostate cancer case that was metastatic only to the bone at the time of diagnosis and was treated with ADT, which had been the standard of care for men with metastatic prostate cancer [15]. Unfortunately, over time, patients develop castration resistance to such therapy.

Recently, there has been shift towards using upfront chemotherapy with ADT in castration-naive metastatic prostate cancer. In the CHAARTED trial, Sweeney et al. demonstrated in patients with metastatic prostate cancer that the administration of six cycles of docetaxel at the beginning of ADT treatment resulted in significantly longer survival of more than a year compared to ADT alone [16]. The STAMPEDE trial also showed survival benefit in patients with advanced prostate cancer treated with this combination [17]. Our case is the first report of a patient with metastatic prostate cancer presenting with cholestasis as a paraneoplastic syndrome to be safely treated with ADT and docetaxel. Fortunately, this treatment approach resulted in excellent response, reflecting the potential effectiveness of early chemotherapy in conjunction with ADT for advanced prostate cancer.

4. Conclusion

Paraneoplastic cholestasis resulting from prostate cancer should be considered in cases of jaundice in the absence of biliary or hepatic involvement or infectious etiology. We have reported such a case that was safely treated with the combination of ADT and docetaxel resulting in excellent response.

Acknowledgments

The authors thank Anthea Hammond for editing this manuscript.

References

[1] M. H. Stauffer, "Nephrogenic hepatosplenomegaly," *Gastroenterology*, vol. 40, p. 694, 1961.

[2] M. K. Hong, J. Kong, B. Namdarian et al., "Paraneoplastic syndromes in prostate carcinoma," *Nature Reviews Urology*, vol. 7, no. 12, pp. 681–692, 2010.

[3] M. Trauner, P. Fickert, and R. E. Stauber, "Inflammation-induced cholestasis," *Journal of Gastroenterology and Hepatology*, vol. 14, no. 10, pp. 946–959, 1999.

[4] A. C. Viera, M. J. Alvarenga, J. C. Santos, and M. A. Silva, "Paraneoplastic jaundice and prostate carcinoma," *BMJ Case Reports*, 2017.

[5] T. Kuramoto, H. Senzaki, H. Koike et al., "Cholestatic jaundice as a paraneoplastic manifestation of prostate carcinoma," *Case Reports in Urology*, vol. 2013, Article ID 303727, 3 pages, 2013.

[6] M. Koruk, M. Büyükberber, C. Savas, and A. Kdayifci, "Paraneoplastic cholestasis associated with prostate carcinoma," *Turkish Journal of Gastroenterology*, vol. 15, no. 1, pp. 53–55, 2004.

[7] J. Y. Blay, J. F. Rossi, J. Wijdenes et al., "Role of interleukin-6 in the paraneoplastic inflammatory syndrome associated with renal-cell carcinoma," *International Journal of Cancer*, vol. 72, no. 3, pp. 424–430, 1997.

[8] National Comprehensive Cancer Network, *Prostate Cancer, NCCN Clinical Practice Guidelines in Oncology, Version 2.2017*, 2017, https://www.nccn.org/professionals/physician_gls/pdf/prostate.pdf.

[9] A. Cole, D. Mendlnlatt, J. Aguayo et al., "Metastatic prostate carcinoma (with prostate-specific antigen of 9996) presenting as obstructive jaundice," *American Journal of the Medical Sciences*, vol. 319, no. 2, pp. 118–122, 2000.

[10] S. P. Dourakis, C. Sinani, M. Deutsch, E. Dimitriadou, and S. J. Hadziyannis, "Cholestatic jaundice as a paraneoplastic manifestation of renal cell carcinoma," *European Journal of Gastroenterology and Hepatology*, vol. 9, no. 3, pp. 311–314, 1997.

[11] J. Watterson and J. R. Priest, "Jaundice as a paraneoplastic phenomenon in a T-cell lymphoma," *Gastroenterology*, vol. 97, no. 5, pp. 1319–1322, 1989.

[12] J. Pandey and K. T. Bhowmik, "Chronic lymphocytic leukemia presenting as jaundice," *Indian Journal of Gastroenterology*, vol. 17, no. 1, p. 28, 1998.

[13] P. Saintigny, J. P. Spano, F. Tcherakian, M. C. Pailler, and J. L. Breau, "Non-metastatic intrahepatic cholestasis associated with bronchial adenocarcinoma," *Annales de Médecine Interne*, vol. 154, no. 3, pp. 171–175, 2003.

[14] S. Yalcin, A. Kars, C. Sokmensuer, and L. Atahan, "Extrahepatic Hodgkin's disease with intrahepatic cholestasis: report of two cases," *Oncology*, vol. 57, no. 1, pp. 83–85, 1999.

[15] A. Karakolios, C. Kasapis, T. Kallinikidis, P. Kalpidis, and N. Grigoriadis, "Cholestatic jaundice as a paraneoplastic manifestation of prostate adenocarcinoma," *Clinical Gastroenterology and Hepatology*, vol. 1, no. 6, pp. 480–483, 2003.

[16] C. J. Sweeney, Y. H. Chen, M. Carducci et al., "Chemohormonal therapy in metastatic hormone-sensitive prostate carcinoma," *New England Journal of Medicine*, vol. 373, no. 8, pp. 737–746, 2015.

[17] N. D. James, M. R. Sydes, N. W. Clarke et al., "Addition of docetaxel, zoledronic acid, or both to first-line long-term hormone therapy in prostate cancer (STAMPEDE): survival results from an adaptive, multiarm, multistage, platform randomized controlled trial," *The Lancet*, vol. 397, no. 10024, pp. 1163–1177, 2016.

18

External Beam Radiation and Brachytherapy for Prostate Cancer: Is It a Possible Trigger of Large Cell Neuroendocrine Carcinoma of the Urinary Bladder?

Ali Zakaria,[1] Bayan Al Share,[1] Sri Kollepara,[2] and Cynthia Vakhariya[2]

[1]*Department of Internal Medicine, Providence-Providence Park Hospital, Michigan State University College of Human Medicine, Southfield, MI, USA*
[2]*Division of Hematology & Oncology, Providence-Providence Park Hospital, Michigan State University College of Human Medicine, Southfield, MI, USA*

Correspondence should be addressed to Ali Zakaria; alizakaria86@hotmail.com

Academic Editor: Gerassimos P. Vandoros

Neuroendocrine tumors commonly involve the respiratory and gastrointestinal systems. Primary genitourinary neuroendocrine tumors are rare, accounting for less than 1% of all bladder carcinomas. Four histopathologic subtypes have been described. Among those, large cell neuroendocrine carcinoma (LCNEC) is the least common, is more aggressive, and generally presents in an advanced stage with poor prognosis compared to transitional cell bladder carcinoma. There is no standardized treatment regimen because of the rarity of the disease. Herein, we present a case of 72-year-old male patient with previously treated prostate cancer, who received external beam radiation therapy and high dose brachytherapy, presenting with intermittent hematuria. Cystoscopy and transurethral resection of bladder tumor (TURBT) were performed. The histopathology and immunohistochemistry were consistent with large cell neuroendocrine carcinoma (LCNEC). Further studies are required to proof the higher risk of neuroendocrine carcinoma of the bladder in patients treated with external beam radiation therapy and brachytherapy for prostate cancer.

1. Introduction

Neuroendocrine carcinomas of the urinary bladder are rare. They account for less than 1% of all bladder carcinomas. Four histopathologic subtypes have been described. Among those, large cell neuroendocrine carcinoma (LCNEC) is the least common, is more aggressive, and generally presents in an advanced stage with poor prognosis compared to transitional cell bladder carcinoma. We are reporting this case to demonstrate that further studies are required to explore the association between neuroendocrine carcinoma of the bladder in patients treated with external beam radiation therapy and brachytherapy for prostate cancer.

2. Case Report

A 72-year-old male presented to the emergency department complaining of 6-week history of intermittent hematuria. He was diagnosed with prostate cancer thirteen years prior to this presentation and was treated with external beam radiation therapy. His cancer recurred six years later and he was treated with high dose brachytherapy. Five-year posttreatment follow-up with computed tomography (CT) scans and prostate specific antigen (PSA) levels (range 0.63–0.8 ng/mL) revealed no evidence of disease. He had a past medical history of coronary artery disease status after percutaneous intervention with drug-eluting stent to the right coronary artery, diabetes mellitus type 2, hypertension, obstructive sleep apnea, and complicated necrotizing pancreatitis with walled-off necrosis. He had a past surgical history of cardiac catheterization, distal pancreatectomy, and brachytherapy seeds implantation. He denied any previous history of smoking and alcohol or illicit drug use. He has a family history of diabetes and hypertension, but no history of malignancy. His home medications included aspirin, clopidogrel, atenolol, lisinopril, simvastatin, insulin, and as needed acetaminophen-oxycodone for pain. He has no known allergies. On physical examination he was alert, oriented, and not in acute distress. His vital signs were as follows: temp 36.4°C; blood pressure 134/75 mmHg; respiratory rate 16 bpm; pulse 116 bpm; and oxygen saturation 97% on room air. Abdominal examination revealed normal active bowel sounds, which was soft and nontender to palpation, no evidence of organomegaly, left-side nephrostomy tube with clear urine, and an indwelling urinary catheter with gross hematuria. Digital rectal exam revealed normal sphincter tone, with the prostate being smooth, symmetric, and measuring 4 × 5 cm. Fecal occult blood test (FOBT) was negative.

The patient presented to another hospital with same complaint of hematuria two months prior to this admission. At that time workup revealed left sided hydronephrosis due to obstructive ureteric stones. Urgent cystoscopy with ureteric stent placement was performed which failed to relieve the obstruction. So, an emergent nephrostomy tube was inserted and he was discharged with indwelling urinary catheter and follow-up plans for revision and placement of another anterograde ureteric stent.

Upon admission to our hospital, the urinary catheter was replaced with a three-way urinary catheter and bladder irrigation was initiated. Computed tomography (CT) scan of abdomen and pelvis revealed no evidence of obstructive uropathy, diffuse thickening of the wall of the urinary bladder, and brachytherapy radiation seeds in the prostate (Figure 1). Cystoscopy revealed edematous mass over the left wall of the bladder. Transurethral resection of bladder tumor (TURBT) was performed and histopathology revealed invasive poorly differentiated carcinoma infiltrating lamina propria and muscularis propria, with foci suspicious for angiolymphatic invasion. Immunohistochemical stains were positive for Ber EP4, pankeratin, AE1/AE3, chromogranin, and TTF-1 and negative for CK-7, CK-20, PSA, and PAP (Figure 2). This carcinoma was histologically distinct from the previous prostate adenocarcinoma and consistent with large cell neuroendocrine carcinoma (LCNEC).

Further workup for staging of the disease was performed. Computed tomography (CT) scan of the chest revealed multiple bilateral pulmonary and pleural-based nodules suggestive of metastasis (Figure 3). Magnetic resonance imaging (MRI) of the brain and bone scan were both negative for metastatic disease.

Considering the rarity of the disease and unclear treatment guidelines a multidisciplinary team discussed the best treatment approach. The consensus was treatment with neoadjuvant chemotherapy using carboplatin and etoposide for five cycles followed by radical cystectomy. After completion of his fifth cycle of chemotherapy, a follow-up CT scan of the chest/abdomen/pelvis revealed interval increase in the size and number of bilateral pulmonary nodules and development of new liver lesions consistent with metastasis. He was started on anti-PD-1 immunotherapy with *pembrolizumab* "as an off-label prescription." Nevertheless, he was readmitted to the hospital due to intractable shoulder and back pain. Palliative care team met with the patient and his family. He stated his wishes to be transferred to hospice with comfort care due to his significant declining performance status and quality of life.

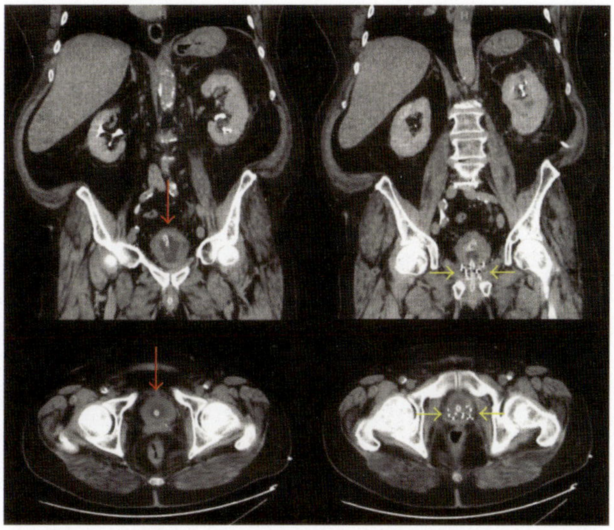

FIGURE 1: Computed tomography (CT) scan of the abdomen and pelvis revealed diffuse thickening of the wall of the urinary bladder with intravesical catheter *(red arrows)* and brachytherapy radiation seeds in the prostate *(yellow arrows)*.

3. Discussion

Neuroendocrine tumors commonly involve the respiratory and gastrointestinal systems. Primary genitourinary neuroendocrine tumors are rare, accounting for less than 1% of all bladder carcinomas [1, 2]. Four histopathologic subtypes have been described: small cell neuroendocrine carcinoma (SSNEC), large cell neuroendocrine carcinoma (LCNEC), carcinoid, and mixed histology. Literature review revealed the large cell subtype as the least common, with 25 cases reported as of 2013 [3]. It predominantly affects Caucasian men in seventh or eighth decade of life, with higher prevalence in patients with medical comorbidities, smoking history, and prior personal or family history of cancers [4–6]. However, the role of familial and genetic predisposition is still unknown. The etiology of bladder neuroendocrine tumor has not been clarified yet, with tumor development from stem cells or multipotent stem cells in urothelium being the widely accepted theory [7, 8]. In our case post-prostate-cancer external beam radiation therapy and high dose brachytherapy might be the trigger for this tumor.

The clinical presentation of LCNEC of the bladder may include abdominal pain, dysuria, obstructive voiding symptom, ureteral obstruction, or recurrent urinary tract infections (UTIs), yet painless hematuria is the most common presenting symptom [9, 10]. Given the rare incidence of the disease, treating physician should exclude other possible diagnoses such as metastasis of a pulmonary or gastrointestinal LCNEC, local invasion of the bladder by a poorly differentiated prostatic carcinoma, and poorly differentiated

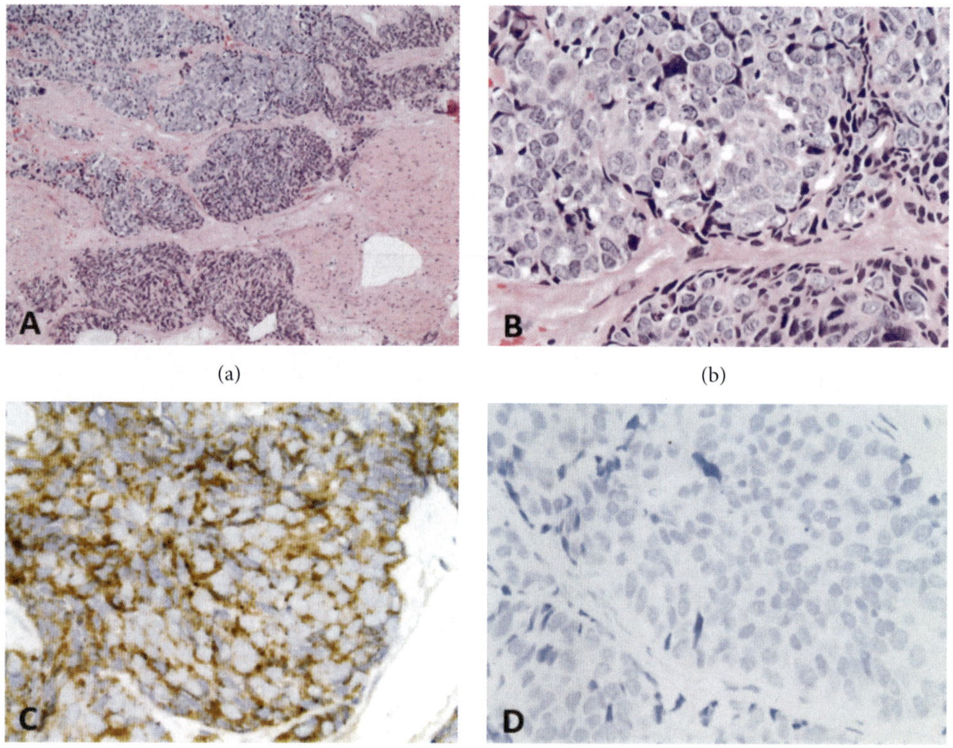

(a) (b) (c) (d)

Figure 2: Histopathology of the resected bladder lesion. (a) Low-power field H&E stain reveals invasive poorly differentiated carcinoma infiltrates lamina propria and muscularis propria. (b) High-power field H&E stain reveals large polygonal-shape cells with low nuclear to cytoplasmic ratio, coarse chromatin structure, multiple nucleoli, and high rate of mitosis. (c) Immunohistochemical stain positive for chromogranin and (d) negative for PSA.

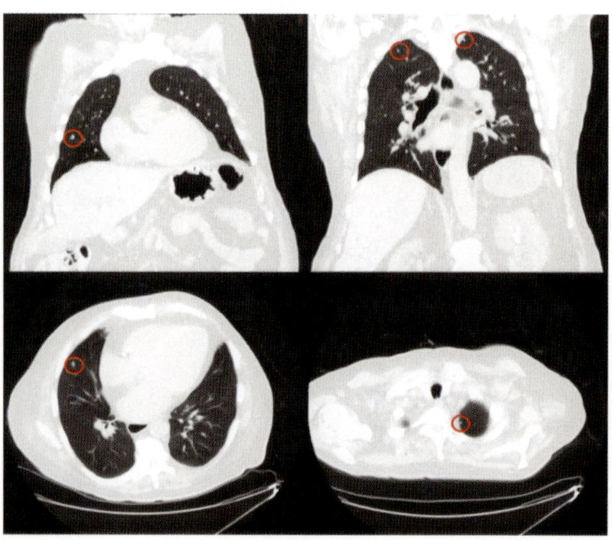

Figure 3: Computed tomography (CT) scan of the chest revealed multiple bilateral pulmonary and pleural-based nodules *(red circles)* suggestive of metastasis.

transitional cell carcinoma [8, 11, 12]. Tissue biopsy with characteristic histopathology and positive immunohistochemical markers demonstrating neuroendocrine differentiation (chromogranin, synaptophysin, neuron-specific enolase, and thyroid transcription factor-1) are required to establish and confirm the diagnosis of LCNEC [13–15].

Lung and liver have been reported as the most common sites for distant metastasis (and rarely the brain) in patients with LCNEC of the bladder either at time of diagnosis or later in the disease course [16]. Multiple imaging modalities have been suggested for staging of the disease, with computed tomography (CT) scan and/or magnetic resonance imaging (MRI) being most commonly used. In addition, positron emission tomography (PET) scan and octreoscan are other suggested modalities [17].

There is no standardized treatment regimen existing due to the rarity of the disease. Quek et al. reported that patients who received platinum based neoadjuvant chemotherapy using etoposide and cisplatin (or carboplatin) plus aggressive surgical approach with cystectomy and bilateral lymphadenectomy had significant better overall and recurrence-free survival than those treated with cystectomy alone [12]. Based on its rare incidence, prediction of overall survival and prognostic factors of LCNEC of the bladder is still difficult. However, overall survival in the reported cases ranged from <1 year for advanced disease to >2 years for early disease [8, 15, 17, 18]. Our patient had metastatic disease and his survival was 11 months after the initial diagnosis.

4. Conclusion

Large cell neuroendocrine carcinoma of the bladder is a very rare disease. Postradiation therapy for prostate cancer might be a risk factor for this disease as illustrated by our case. Unfortunately, there is no standardized treatment regimen so far, and the overall survival is poor.

Acknowledgments

Authors would like to express their deepest appreciation to Dr. Alan Braunstein for his valuable expertise in providing and reading the histopathology slides.

References

[1] J. R. Mackey, H.-J. Au, J. Hugh, and P. Venner, "Genitourinary small cell carcinoma: determination of clinical and therapeutic factors associated with survival," *Journal of Urology*, vol. 159, no. 5, pp. 1624–1629, 1998.

[2] N. W. W. Choong, J. F. Quevedo, and J. S. Kaur, "Small cell carcinoma of the urinary bladder: The mayo clinic experience," *Cancer*, vol. 103, no. 6, pp. 1172–1178, 2005.

[3] H. M. P. Coelho, B. A. G. J. Pereira, and P. A. S. T. Caetano, "Large cell neuroendocrine carcinoma of the urinary bladder: case report and review," *Current Urology*, vol. 7, no. 3, pp. 155–159, 2014.

[4] S. Thota, G. Kistangari, H. Daw, and T. Spiro, "A clinical review of small-cell carcinoma of the urinary bladder," *Clinical Genitourinary Cancer*, vol. 11, no. 2, pp. 73–77, 2013.

[5] E. J. Koay, B. S. Teh, A. C. Paulino, and E. B. Butler, "A Surveillance, Epidemiology, and End Results analysis of small cell carcinoma of the bladder: Epidemiology, prognostic variables, and treatment trends," *Cancer*, vol. 117, no. 23, pp. 5325–5333, 2011.

[6] V. R. Bhatt, F. R. Loberiza Jr., P. Tandra, J. Krishnamurthy, R. Shrestha, and J. Wang, "Risk factors, therapy and survival outcomes of small cell and large cell neuroendocrine carcinoma of urinary bladder," *Rare Tumors*, vol. 6, no. 1, pp. 10–14, 2014.

[7] I. J. Martin, D. G. Vilar, and J. M. Aquado, "Large cell neuroendocrine carcinoma of the urinary bladder. Bibliographic review," *Españoles de Urología*, vol. 64, no. 2, pp. 105–113, 2011.

[8] A. J. Evans, J. Al-Maghrabi, J. Tsihlias, G. Lajoie, J. M. Sweet, and W. B. Chapman, "Primary large cell neuroendocrine carcinoma of the urinary bladder," *Archives of Pathology and Laboratory Medicine*, vol. 126, no. 10, pp. 1229–1232, 2002.

[9] D. N. Church and A. Bahl, "Clinical review—small cell carcinoma of the bladder," *Cancer Treatment Reviews*, vol. 32, no. 8, pp. 588–593, 2006.

[10] R. T. Naturale and G. T. MacLennan, "Small Cell Carcinoma of the Bladder," *Journal of Urology*, vol. 176, no. 2, p. 781, 2006.

[11] S. Hailemariam, A. Gaspert, P. Komminoth, P. Tamboli, and M. Amin, "Primary, pure, large-cell neuroendocrine carcinoma of the urinary bladder," *Modern Pathology*, vol. 11, no. 10, pp. 1016–1020, 1998.

[12] M. L. Quek, P. W. Nichols, J. Yamzon et al., "Radical cystectomy for primary neuroendocrine tumors of the bladder: the University of Southern California experience," *The Journal of Urology*, vol. 174, no. 1, pp. 93–96, 2005.

[13] S. Akamatsu, S. Kanamaru, M. Ishihara, T. Sano, A. Soeda, and K. Hashimoto, "Primary large cell neuroendocrine carcinoma of the urinary bladder: Case report," *International Journal of Urology*, vol. 15, no. 12, pp. 1080–1083, 2008.

[14] K. H. Lee, S. B. Ryu, M. C. Lee, C. S. Park, S. W. Juhng, and C. Choi, "Primary large cell neuroendocrine carcinoma of the urinary bladder," *Pathology International*, vol. 56, no. 11, pp. 688–693, 2006.

[15] F. A. Serrano, N. Sánchez-Mora, J. A. Arranz, C. Hernández, and E. Álvarez-Fernández, "Large cell and small cell neuroendocrine bladder carcinoma: Immunohistochemical and outcome study in a single institution," *American Journal of Clinical Pathology*, vol. 128, no. 5, pp. 733–739, 2007.

[16] A. Tsugu, M. Yoshiyama, and M. Matsumae, "Brain metastasis from large cell neuroendocrine carcinoma of the urinary bladder," *Surgical Neurology International*, vol. 2, no. 1, p. 84, 2011.

[17] A. Bertaccini, D. Marchiori, A. Cricca et al., "Neuroendocrine carcinoma of the urinary bladder: Case report and review of the literature," *Anticancer Research*, vol. 28, no. 2 B, pp. 1369–1372, 2008.

[18] C. Colarossi, P. Pino, D. Giuffrida et al., "Large cell neuroendocrine carcinoma (LCNEC) of the urinary bladder: A case report," *Diagnostic Pathology*, vol. 8, no. 1, article no. 19, 2013.

19

Severe Hypocalcemia and Hypomagnesemia with Denosumab in Advanced Chronic Kidney Disease: Case Report

Christina F. Marlow,[1] Shailendra Sharma,[2] Faizan Babar,[2] and Jianqing Lin[3]

[1]*Department of Internal Medicine, George Washington University School of Medicine, USA*
[2]*Division of Kidney Diseases and Hypertension, George Washington University School of Medicine, USA*
[3]*Division of Hematology and Oncology, George Washington University School of Medicine, USA*

Correspondence should be addressed to Christina F. Marlow; christinafmarlow@gmail.com

Academic Editor: Constantine Gennatas

Background. Denosumab has become the preferred agent over zolendronic acid to help prevent skeletal-related events in patients with metastatic bone disease and multiple myeloma because it is approved for use in those with kidney dysfunction. However, denosumab has been linked to cases of hypocalcemia, particularly in those with advanced kidney disease. *Case Presentation.* We present the case of a patient with metastatic prostate cancer and chronic kidney disease due to obstructive nephropathy who developed severe hypocalcemia and hypomagnesemia after denosumab injection, which required intensive care unit admission, aggressive calcium supplementation, and hemodialysis assistance. We reviewed the evidence behind the safety profile of denosumab in chronic kidney disease, and we also looked at additional factors that may precipitate severe hypocalcemia with denosumab in advanced kidney disease. *Conclusion.* We believe that denosumab should be avoided in advanced chronic kidney disease due to the potential life-threatening, severe hypocalcemia that has been observed.

1. Introduction

Skeletal-related events (SREs) are a significant source of morbidity in patients with metastatic bone disease due to solid tumor malignancies and multiple myeloma. SREs are typically defined as pathologic fracture, spinal cord compression, need for bone radiation, or surgical intervention to bone [1]. SREs are associated with a significant decrease in quality of life and performance status. Zoledronic acid and denosumab are typically used to reduce SREs. Zoledronic acid is a bisphosphonate and denosumab is a monoclonal antibody that inhibits osteoclast-mediated bone resorption by binding to receptor activator of nuclear factor-κB ligand (RANKL). In 2011, a randomized controlled trial conducted by Fizazi et al. showed that denosumab significantly delayed time to first SRE when compared to zoledronic acid (20.7 months versus 17.1 months, $p = 0.0002$) [2]. In terms of adverse side effects, bisphosphonates have been associated with renal toxicity and are contraindicated in patients with CrCl < 30 ml/min. Denosumab has emerged as an alternative agent in prevention of SREs in metastatic bone disease. However, denosumab is associated with a greater incidence of hypocalcemia [2]. There have been a number of cases reporting mild hypocalcemia associated with denosumab use [3, 4]. We present the case of a patient with metastatic prostate cancer who developed severe hypocalcemia in the setting of advanced chronic kidney disease (CKD) after receiving denosumab. We also searched the literature to evaluate the safety of denosumab use in chronic kidney disease.

2. Case

A 70-year-old African American gentleman with a history of CKD, pseudogout, and metastatic castration-resistant prostate cancer (to bone, nodes, and lung) was admitted to the hospital due to left knee swelling. He was incidentally found to be severely hypocalcemic to 2.7 mg/dl with EKG showing a prolonged QTC interval to 525 ms. Physical examination was negative for Chvostek and Trousseau's sign. Home medications included acetaminophen, amlodipine, bicalutamide, docusate-senna, lidocaine patches, ondansetron, and polyethylene glycol. Twenty-eight days prior, he had received his first dose of denosumab (together with leuprolide) when his calcium level was 8.8 mg/dl. He was prescribed vitamin D and calcium supplementation, but never took it. He finished a five-day course of prednisone 10 mg daily thirteen days prior for a pseudogout flare of the right foot. Other labs on admission were significant for phosphorus 5.5 mg/dl, total vitamin D3 31 IU, iPTH 93, and Mg 1.1 mg/dl. He was admitted to the intensive care unit for continuous, high-dose IV calcium gluconate and frequent electrolyte monitoring. During his ICU course, he received a total of 21 grams of IV calcium gluconate. He was also given 1 μg of oral calcitriol BID, 1000 mg of oral calcium carbonate TID, and aggressive magnesium supplementation. Unfortunately, the patient's creatinine worsened to 7.5 mg and he developed severe metabolic acidosis and hyponatremia in the setting of *Clostridium difficile* colitis. The decision was made to initiate hemodialysis given the poor recovery in kidney function from obstructive uropathy. For one week, he received intermittent hemodialysis with high calcium baths. Calcium, magnesium, and phosphate levels were monitored daily and supplemented as needed. Calcium levels improved to 8.5 mg/dl and magnesium levels improved to 2.0 mg/dl. He was discharged on 0.5 μg oral calcitriol daily, calcium carbonate 1000 mg BID, and continued intermittent hemodialysis.

The patient was originally diagnosed with de novo metastatic prostate cancer two years prior. He had not been on ADT or chemotherapy for approximately one year until he presented to our hospital two months prior with evidence of prostate cancer progression. His PSA was elevated to 1472 and he was found to have acute kidney injury with a Cr 12.8 mg/dl and a BUN of 131 mg/dl due to obstructive uropathy. CT of the abdomen/pelvis showed marked bilateral hydronephrosis due to a 6.3 cm pelvic mass and a 3.8 cm mass in the left ureteropelvic junction. Extensive pelvic and retroperitoneal lymphadenopathy was evident in addition to innumerable metastatic lytic skeletal lesions. Bilateral percutaneous nephrostomy tubes were placed by interventional radiology and the patient's creatinine improved to 7.3 mg/dl with a BUN of 120 mg/dl. Combined androgen deprivation was resumed and he was discharged with plans for close monitoring of renal functions with the ultimate plan to place ureteral stents depending upon renal recovery.

3. Discussion

Denosumab is a RANKL monoclonal antibody that blocks the RANKL receptor on the osteoclast, which results in reduced osteoclast activation and resultant bone resorption. Denosumab is more potent compared to bisphosphonates in preventing skeletal-related events in metastatic prostate cancer [2]. However, compared to bisphosphonates, the incidence of hypocalcemia is higher in patients treated with denosumab [2]. Although denosumab does not require renal dosing, the manufacturer recommends extreme caution with close monitoring of calcium levels in chronic kidney disease [5]. The risk of hypocalcemia with denosumab increases in patients with advanced stage kidney disease due to inherent defects in bone mineral metabolism and dependence on PTH-mediated bone resorption to maintain calcium levels.

Knowledge of the pharmacokinetics of denosumab is critical in understanding the risk of hypocalcemia. Denosumab exhibits a nonlinear dose-dependent response [6, 7]. The volume of distribution is proportional to the body weight and central volume of distribution is 2.6 l/66 kg body weight [6, 7]. Maximum drug level is reached in seven to twenty-one days. The drug elimination is not dependent on renal or hepatic clearance [6, 7]. Hence, no dose adjustment is recommended for patients with CKD. Like other monoclonal antibodies, clearance is mediated by the reticuloendothelial system and receptor-mediated endocytosis [6, 7]. Given the long half-life of the medication, side effects may persist for a prolonged period.

Denosumab is preferred over zoledronic acid in patients with both metastatic bone disease and chronic kidney disease because it is not cleared renally and is technically not nephrotoxic. However, there is a paucity of data regarding the safety of denosumab use in patients with advanced renal disease, that is, GFR < 30 ml/min or on hemodialysis, for the prevention of skeletal-related events in metastatic bone disease. An abstract of an open-label prospective study describes the effectiveness of denosumab at different stages of CKD in preventing SREs at the standard dose [8, 9]. However, severe hypocalcemia (i.e., <7 meq/dl) or symptomatic hypocalcemia was seen in the late stages of renal disease [10–12]. Similarly, in one observational study, 45 percent of the patients with baseline eGFR < 30 ml/min ($n = 22$) developed hypocalcemia during treatment with denosumab [13]. A dose-reduction strategy in CKD has been evaluated in only one case series study by Cicci et al. of refractory hypercalcemia due to MM and AKI [14]. They proposed the novel dosing strategy of 0.3 mg/kg of denosumab based on 4 case reports in patients with multiple myeloma over a fixed, reduced dose of 60 mg (from the standard 120 mg) in patients with renal dysfunction. Denosumab was used to treat refractory hypercalcemia associated with MM. Despite dose reduction, three out of four patients developed mild hypocalcemia with the effect lasting for 15–40 days [14]. Dose reduction might be an effective strategy to reduce the risk of severe hypocalcemia in CKD, but it requires further validation in large scale studies.

The higher risk of severe hypocalcemia in advanced kidney disease is due to the secondary hyperparathyroidism that is known to occur in end stage chronic kidney disease (Figure 1). Denosumab then further compounds the risk for hypocalcemia by blocking calcium release from the bone. In two trials evaluating the safety and efficacy of denosumab in patients with CKD stages 4 and 5, all patients received supplementation with calcium and vitamin D [5]. Despite these measures, patients developed hypocalcemia of variable degrees [13]. Hence, we believe that supplementing a vitamin D analogue prior to denosumab use in advanced CKD is unlikely to be an effective way of reducing hypocalcemia risk.

We also identified additional factors that may predispose advanced kidney disease patients to severe hypocalcemia

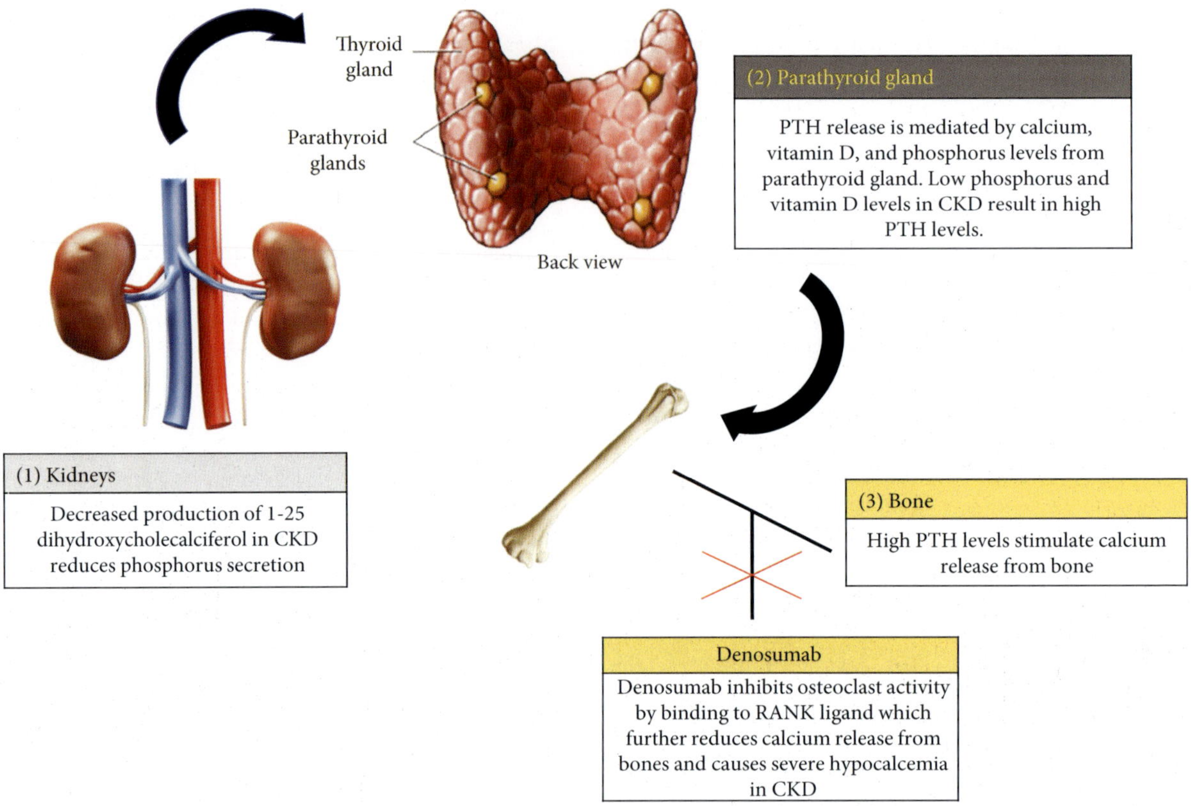

FIGURE 1: Calcium, phosphorus, and vitamin D metabolism in chronic kidney disease.

with denosumab use including high bone turnover markers, hypomagnesemia, and concomitant use of steroids or bisphosphonates. Bone turnover markers can be helpful in predicting patients at risk for hypocalcemia because high bone turnover is seen with both bone mineral disease and metastatic bone disease [15]. Several markers have been shown to correlate with bone activity in patients with CKD who were treated with denosumab for osteoporosis including bone specific alkaline phosphatase, CTX, total P1NP, and TRAP [15–17]. Further studies should explore the utility of checking these markers prior to administration of denosumab to those at greater risk of severe hypocalcemia.

Hypomagnesemia is another risk factor that can predispose to severe hypocalcemia with denosumab use in CKD which was evident in the case of this patient. Low magnesium is observed in chronic kidney disease patients with diabetes [18]. Magnesium acts as a cofactor to calcium-sensing receptors on the parathyroid gland to regulate PTH secretion [19]. Low Mg levels increase PTH release, which increases bone turnover. Hypomagnesemia is also associated with low calcitriol levels which can also increase the risk of hypocalcemia with denosumab use in CKD [20]. Additional risk factors for severe hypocalcemia with denosumab use include concomitant use of hypocalcemia agents such as steroids, bisphosphonates, and calcimimetics [13]. This was particularly evident in this case as the patient received five days of steroids for pseudogout prior to the first dose of denosumab.

4. Conclusion

Denosumab is an effective agent at reducing SREs in patients with metastatic bone disease and is technically approved for use in CKD patients without dose reduction. Inherent bone mineral disease in advanced kidney disease increases the risk of hypocalcemia with denosumab use. Prospective studies are needed to explore the safety profile of denosumab at a reduced dose in CKD patients. Further research is needed to determine the clinical utility of bone turnover markers; however, they may be helpful tools to physicians to help determine a patient's risk of hypocalcemia prior to starting denosumab. Until further evidence, we believe that denosumab should be avoided in advanced chronic kidney disease due to the potential life-threatening, severe hypocalcemia that has been observed.

References

[1] M. R. Smith, R. E. Coleman, L. Klotz et al., "Denosumab for the prevention of skeletal complications in metastatic castration-resistant prostate cancer: comparison of skeletal-related events and symptomatic skeletal events," *Annals of Oncology*, vol. 26, no. 2, pp. 368–374, 2015.

[2] K. Fizazi, M. Carducci, M. Smith et al., "Denosumab versus zoledronic acid for treatment of bone metastases in men with castration-resistant prostate cancer: a randomised, double-blind study," *The Lancet*, vol. 377, no. 9768, pp. 813–822, 2011.

[3] B. A. Gartrell, R. E. Coleman, K. Fizazi et al., "Toxicities following treatment with bisphosphonates and receptor activator of nuclear factor-κB ligand inhibitors in patients with advanced prostate cancer," *European Urology*, vol. 65, no. 2, pp. 278–286, 2014.

[4] M. I. Fokkema, L. J. de Heide, W. van Schelven, and N. A. Hamdy, "Severe hypocalcaemia associated with extensive osteoblastic metastases in a patient with prostate cancer," *The Netherlands Journal of Medicine*, vol. 63, no. 1, pp. 34–37, 2005.

[5] "Xegeva (denosumab) and renal function [Prescribing information]," Amgen Inc, Thousand Oaks, CA, USA, 2010.

[6] S. K. Tat, M. Padrines, S. Theoleyre et al., "OPG/membranous–RANKL complex is internalized via the clathrin pathway before a lysosomal and a proteasomal degradation," *Bone*, vol. 39, no. 4, pp. 706–715, 2006.

[7] R. J. Keizer, A. D. R. Huitema, J. H. M. Schellens, and J. H. Beijnen, "Clinical pharmacokinetics of therapeutic monoclonal antibodies," *Clinical Pharmacokinetics*, vol. 49, no. 8, pp. 493–507, 2010.

[8] G. Block, O. Egbuna, S. Zeig et al., "The evaluation of denosumab safety in patients with chronic kidney disease: an open-label study," *Journal of Clinical Oncology*, vol. 32, article e20649, Supplement 15, 2014.

[9] G. Block, O. Egbuna, S. Zeig et al., "Safety of denosumab (DMAB) in patients (pts) with stage 4 or stage 5D chronic kidney disease (CKD)," *Annals of Oncology*, vol. 25, article iv528, Supplement 4, 2014.

[10] A. L. H. Huynh, S. T. Baker, A. J. Stewardson, and D. F. Johnson, "Denosumab-associated hypocalcaemia: incidence, severity and patient characteristics in a tertiary hospital setting," *Pharmacoepidemiology and Drug Safety*, vol. 25, no. 11, pp. 1274–1278, 2016.

[11] J. J. Body, H. G. Bone, R. H. de Boer et al., "Hypocalcaemia in patients with metastatic bone disease treated with denosumab," *European Journal of Cancer*, vol. 51, no. 13, pp. 1812–1821, 2015.

[12] N. Okada, K. Kawazoe, K. Teraoka et al., "Identification of the risk factors associated with hypocalcemia induced by denosumab," *Biological and Pharmaceutical Bulletin*, vol. 36, no. 10, pp. 1622–1626, 2013.

[13] K. R. Watkins, J. E. Rogers, and B. Atkinson, "Tolerability of denosumab in metastatic solid tumor patients with renal insufficiency," *Support Care Cancer*, vol. 23, no. 6, pp. 1657–1662, 2015.

[14] J. D. Cicci, L. Buie, J. Bates, and H. van Deventer, "Denosumab for the management of hypercalcemia of malignancy in patients with multiple myeloma and renal dysfunction," *Clinical Lymphoma, Myeloma & Leukemia*, vol. 14, no. 6, pp. e207–e211, 2014.

[15] K. A. Autio, A. Farooki, I. G. Glezerman et al., "Severe hypocalcemia associated with denosumab in metastatic castration-resistant prostate cancer: risk factors and precautions for treating physicians," *Clinical Genitourinary Cancer*, vol. 13, no. 4, pp. e305–e309, 2015.

[16] M. Lein, K. Miller, M. Wirth et al., "Bone turnover markers as predictive tools for skeletal complications in men with metastatic prostate cancer treated with zoledronic acid," *The Prostate*, vol. 69, no. 6, pp. 624–632, 2009.

[17] K. Ishikawa, T. Nagai, K. Sakamoto et al., "High bone turnover elevates the risk of denosumab-induced hypocalcemia in women with postmenopausal osteoporosis," *Therapeutics and Clinical Risk Management*, vol. 12, pp. 1831–1840, 2016.

[18] A. Corsonello, R. Ientile, M. Buemi et al., "Serum ionized magnesium levels in type 2 diabetic patients with microalbuminuria or clinical proteinuria," *American Journal of Nephrology*, vol. 20, no. 3, pp. 187–192, 2000.

[19] Z. S. Agus, "Hypomagnesemia," *Journal of the American Society of Nephrology*, vol. 10, no. 7, pp. 1616–1622, 1999.

[20] R. K. Rude, J. S. Adams, E. Ryzen et al., "Low serum concentrations of 1,25-dihydroxyvitamin D in human magnesium deficiency," *The Journal of Clinical Endocrinology & Metabolism*, vol. 61, no. 5, pp. 933–940, 1985.

20

Successful Use of a Multidisciplinary Approach to Treat a Perforated Duodenal Malignant Lymphoma in an Elderly Patient

Tomoko Takagishi, Yuta Niimi, Goshi Matsuki, Shinta Nagano, Junsuke Hinami, Masaaki Kajiwara, Kiyoshi Kaneko, Yoshihiro Kubota, and Osamu Nakai

Department of Surgery, Uji Tokushukai Medical Center, Uji, Kyoto 611-0041, Japan

Correspondence should be addressed to Tomoko Takagishi; tomokobe0502@gmail.com

Academic Editor: Jose I. Mayordomo

Treatment of duodenal malignant lymphoma is difficult due to life-threatening complications such as intestinal obstruction, perforation, and pancreatitis. Thus, multidisciplinary procedures are required alongside surgical intervention. Contrast abdominal CT images of a 75-year-old female suffering from vomiting revealed thickening of the duodenal wall (from the second to third segment). Gastrojejunostomy and biopsy identified the tumor as diffuse large B-cell lymphoma. A diagnosis of stage II duodenal lymphoma was made. The lymphoma continued to grow, resulting in jaundice and intestinal perforation, which was first treated with two cycles of rituximab and antibiotics. Thereafter, less intensive chemotherapy (two cycles each of R-mini-CHP, CHP, and R-CHOP) was administered, which led to significant improvement upon assessment by PET-CT. Residual lymphoma was treated with consolidation radiotherapy (50 Gy in 25 fractions) over 5 weeks after chemotherapy. The patient attained a complete response and has been disease-free for more than 4 years. Thus, duodenal perforated lymphoma can be treated successfully using a multidisciplinary approach that combines surgery, immunochemotherapy, and radiation therapy.

1. Introduction

Primary gastrointestinal lymphoma accounts for 30–40% of all extranodal lymphomas but for only 1–8% of all gastrointestinal malignancies [1]. The majority of malignancies in the duodenum are adenocarcinoma; malignant lymphoma represents only 2% of cases [2]. Malignant gastrointestinal lymphomas increase the risk of stenosis and/or perforation, which is a serious life-threatening complication. Perforation can occur spontaneously due to enlargement of the tumor, or as a consequence of chemotherapy or irradiation [3]. Among the various types of gastrointestinal lymphoma, duodenal lymphoma is rare; however, it is highly morbid [4] and may develop as diffuse large B-cell lymphoma (DLBCL), mucosa-associated lymphoid tissue lymphoma, or Burkitt lymphoma [5, 6]. Duodenal lymphoma tends to be associated with life-threatening complications such as intestinal obstruction, jaundice, pancreatitis, and perforation [6–8]. Perforated gastrointestinal lymphoma increases the risk of peritoneal lymphomatous dissemination [9]. In terms of treatment, emergency surgical interventions are carried out to stall massive bleeding or performed electively to prevent intestinal obstruction or perforation [5]. In addition, recent progress in lymphoma immunochemotherapy means that patients may have a better outcome if treated using a multidisciplinary approach comprising a monoclonal antibody (rituximab, which is specific for CD20-positive B lymphoma cells), less intensive chemotherapy, radiotherapy, and surgical intervention (where needed) [10–13]. Here, we report successful use of a multidisciplinary approach to treat an elderly female patient with duodenal DLBCL complicated by obstruction and perforation.

2. Case Report

A 75-year-old female was referred to hospital due to a 5-day history of vomiting and reduced appetite. Over the previous 2 years, she had lost 10 kg. Her past medical history was

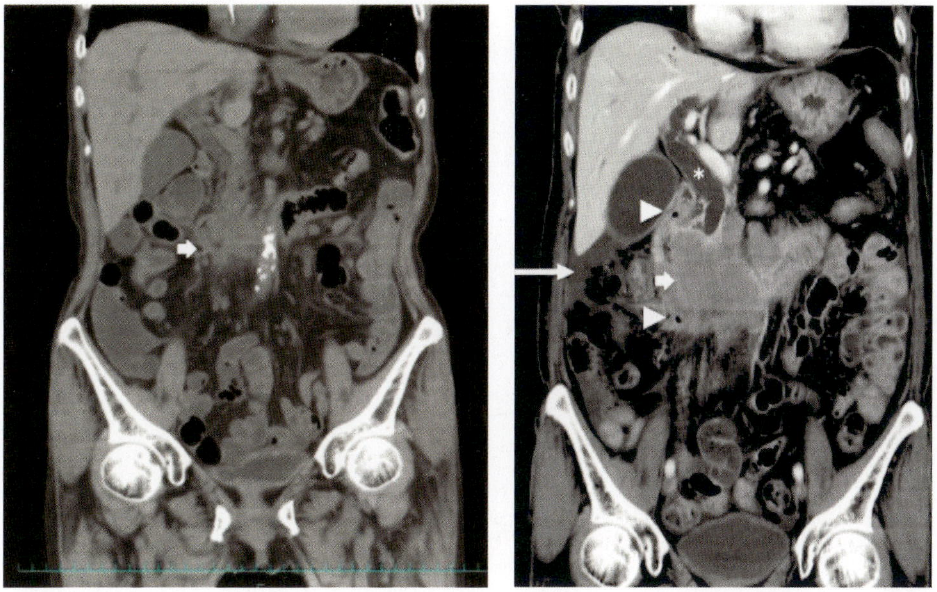

(a) (b)

Figure 1: Contrast abdominal CT (coronal) image upon admission. The scan shows (a) prominent thickening of the duodenal wall from the second to third portion (arrow), and (b) perforation 17 days after gastrojejunostomy revealing an enlarged duodenal mass (arrow), free air (arrow heads), ascites (long arrow), and expansion of the common bile duct/intrahepatic bile duct (*) due to tumor-related stenosis.

significant and included hypothyroidism and partial resection of the jejunum due to inflammatory (no malignancy) occlusion. On admission, the patient showed abdominal distention without pain, guarding, or rebound tenderness at the epigastric region. No superficial lymph nodes were palpable. Laboratory findings were as follows: white blood cell (WBC) count, 7,700/μL; hemoglobin (Hb), 10.7 g/dL; platelet count, 543 K/μL; serum lactate dehydrogenase (LDH), 703 U/L; total bilirubin (T-Bil), 1.52 mg/dL; and soluble interleukin-2 receptor (sIL-2R), 757 U/mL. Hepatic function and renal function were normal. Contrast abdominal computed tomography (CT) images showed a mass in the duodenum (Figure 1(a)). Esophagogastroduodenal endoscopy revealed marked thickening and bulging of the duodenal wall from the second to third portion (Figure 2). A diagnosis of duodenal obstruction led to performance of gastrojejunostomy. Histological examination of a biopsy from the duodenal lesion revealed DLBCL (phenotype: CD20+, CD79a+, Ki67+) (Figure 3). Eventually, the patient was diagnosed with stage II duodenal DLBCL.

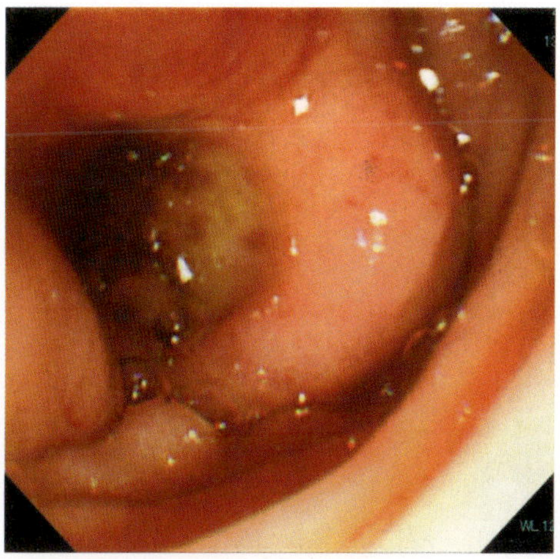

Figure 2: Endoscopic findings. Endoscopy revealed an ulcer and bulging of the thickened duodenal wall (second to third portion), where the perforation occurred.

Before starting chemotherapy, we planned to have positron emission tomography- (PET-) CT images to confirm the precise stage of lymphoma. Seventeen days after laparotomy during the time waiting for PET-CT, the duodenal mass had enlarged, resulting in obstructive jaundice and perforation of an ulcer in the second to third segment of the duodenum (Figure 1(b)), when the patient complained of severe abdominal pain, resulted in a state of shock with hypotension (76/42 mm Hg) and physical signs suggesting peritonitis. Serum LDH and sIL-2R increased rapidly (Figure 4). The patient was admitted to the intensive care unit and received a vasopressor and antibiotics (ABPC/SBT). In addition, the patient required a nasogastric tube for gastric decompression, along with percutaneous transhepatic biliary drainage to alleviate jaundice, but no need of percutaneous drainage for the periduodenal collection. We chose conservative therapy to manage this case of duodenal lymphoma with perforation. As shown in Figure 4, the patient received two cycles of rituximab, although because she was anti-HBs-Ab-negative and anti-HBc-Ab-positive, we were careful to monitor reactivation of HBV. The mass did not shrink significantly upon treatment with rituximab alone; however, CT revealed healed perforation of the duodenum, and symptoms associated with peritonitis and jaundice were relieved. Thereafter, we started immunochemotherapy by removing vincristine from the CHOP regimen due to concerns about adverse effects on the

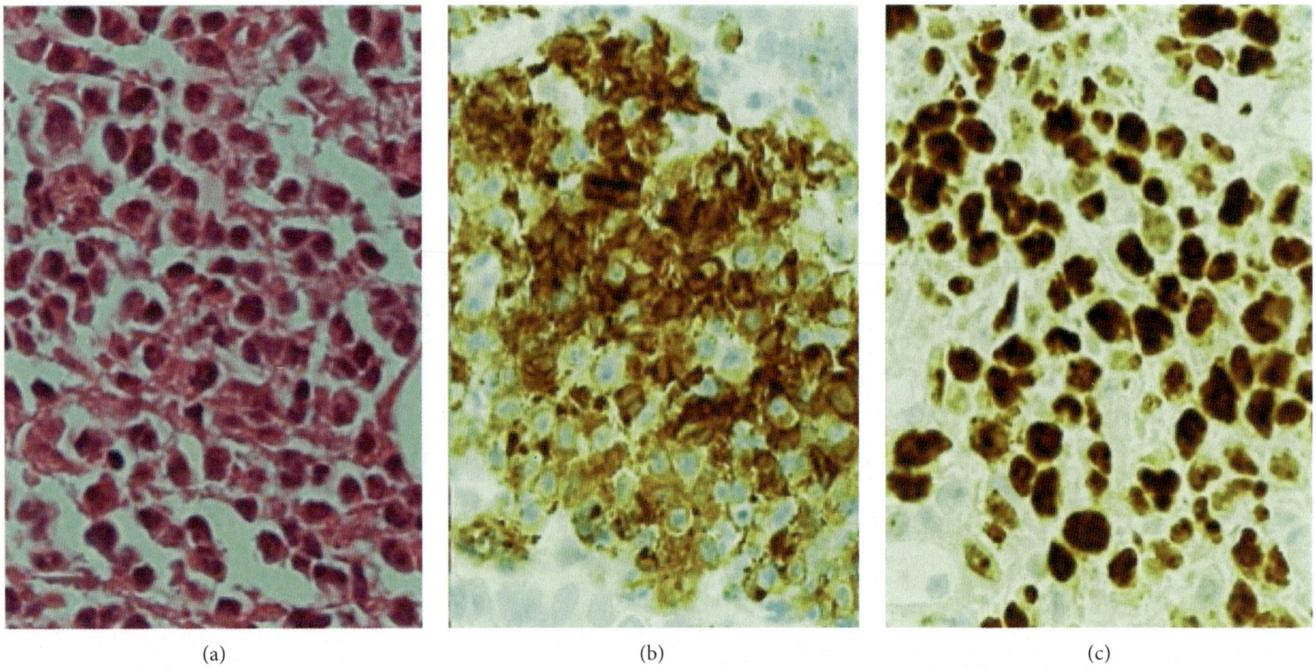

Figure 3: Histopathological findings. A biopsy led to a diagnosis of DLBCL. The tissue was diffusely infiltrated by lymphoblasts with nuclear atypia (a) (H&E stain; original magnification, ×400), which were diffusely stained with CD79a+ (b) and Ki67+ (c) (original magnification, ×400). CD20+ staining not shown.

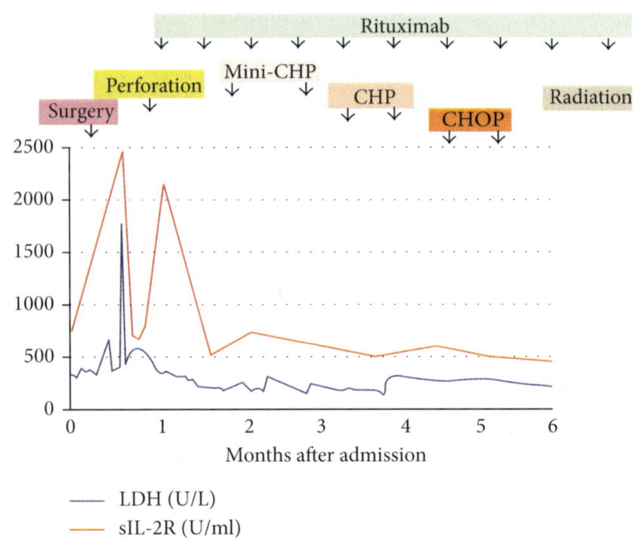

Figure 4: Time course of changes in laboratory data in response to treatment. Serum levels of lactate dehydrogenase (LDH) and sIL-2R in response to duodenal perforation and various therapeutic regimens. Details of treatment regimens are in the text.

gastrointestinal system (e.g., paralytic ileus), which might exacerbate perforation. First, the patient received two cycles of R-mini-CHP (rituximab (day 1; 375 mg/m^2), cyclophosphamide (day 1; 400 mg/m^2), doxorubicin (day 1; 25 mg/m^2), and prednisolone (days 1–5; 40 mg/m^2) in each cycle), with a 40–50% reduction in the dose of doxorubicin, cyclophosphamide, and prednisolone. This was followed by two cycles of R-CHP (rituximab (day 1; 375 mg/m^2), cyclophosphamide (day 1; 700 mg/m^2), doxorubicin (day 1; 50 mg/m^2), and prednisolone (days 1–5; 60 mg/m^2) in each cycle) with an interval of 21–28 days. Finally, the patient received two cycles of R-CHOP (rituximab (day 1; 375 mg/m^2), cyclophosphamide (day 1; 700 mg/m^2), doxorubicin (day 1; 50 mg/m^2), vincristine (day 1; 1.4 mg/m^2), and prednisolone (day 1–5; 60 mg/m^2) on days 1–5 of each cycle) because we thought vincristine could be given at this stage of the treatment. Thereafter, rituximab alone was given as maintenance therapy (total cumulative doses = 14).

In accordance with the Common Terminology Criteria for Adverse Events, grade 3 neutropenia (numbers of event/cycles) was noted during chemotherapy in rituximab alone (n = 0/14), R-mini CHP (n = 0/2), R-CHP (n = 2/2), or R-CHOP (n = 2/2); however, no peritoneal or bile duct infections were associated with grade 3 neutropenia.

After completing chemotherapy, the patient's condition improved markedly, although a residual high signal remained in the third segment of the duodenum and in the jejunum upon PET-CT (Figure 5). One month after finishing chemotherapy, the patient received radiotherapy (50 Gy; 25 fractions over 5 weeks) to treat residual lymphoma, after which the hot FDG uptake signal observed on PET-CT images disappeared (Figure 5). No grade 3 neutropenia (numbers of event/fractions) was noted during radiation therapy (n = 0/25). The patient has remained disease-free for more than 4 years.

3. Discussion

Because duodenal lymphoma is rare, there is little information about appropriate therapeutic regimens, especially for elderly patients. The duodenum is one of the most

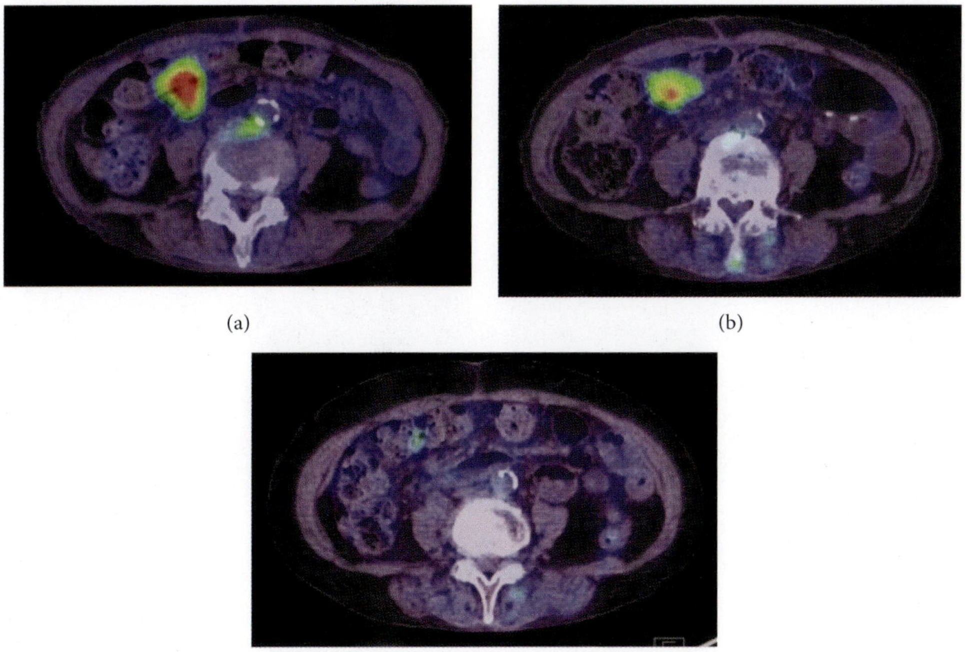

(a) (b) (c)

Figure 5: Time course of PET-CT findings regarding the duodenal mass in response to treatment, PET-CT shows (a) high FDG uptake (SUV max = 9.2) at the duodenum prior to immunochemotherapy, (b) reduced uptake (SUV max = 5.1) after radiation, and (c) barely detectable uptake (SUV max <1.0) after finishing treatment.

difficult anatomical sites with respect to surgical intervention; thus, radical resection of duodenal lymphoma is rarely performed. Considering the risk of perforation, intensive chemotherapy is not a good idea. Accordingly, a multidisciplinary approach using a combination of rituximab and less intensive chemotherapy followed by radiotherapy was chosen because we felt it would be both effective and safe. Here, we report successful treatment of duodenal lymphoma using this approach.

Sarkhosh et al. discuss surgical intervention for management of duodenal lymphoma [5]. They reviewed 23 cases: eight (35%) treated with surgery alone, eight (35%) with surgery plus chemotherapy, five (22%) with chemotherapy alone, and two (9%) with supportive care. Patients treated with surgery were mostly emergencies, that is, obstruction (58%), perforation (33%), and hemorrhage (8%). Here, we performed gastrojejunostomy prior to immunochemotherapy. The need for radiotherapy in the management of DLBCL in the rituximab era is controversial [13]. If radiotherapy is to be considered for DLBCL, patients with FDG uptake confined to a limited area after primary therapy with R-CHOP are likely to be the best candidates [14]. Indeed, in this case, we used radiotherapy to eradicate residual lymphoma after immunochemotherapy.

Thus, immunochemotherapy plays a key role in the treatment of duodenal lymphoma, which must be both safe and effective. Recently, rituximab has been used either alone or together with other chemotherapeutic agents [10]. Trials of less extensive regimens have also been conducted in frail elderly patients [11, 12]. The risk of paralytic ileus after treatment with vincristine must be borne in mind when treating gastrointestinal lymphomas [15, 16]. In addition, in gastrointestinal lymphomas, half of all perforations occur at the time of initial presentation; the other half occurs after chemotherapy [17–21]. Thus, our regimens were based on a cautious approach to chemotherapy-related paralytic ileus and ensuing perforation, a serious complication occurring in about 9% of gastrointestinal lymphomas along chemotherapy [3]. Here, spontaneous perforation was noted prior to, but not after, chemotherapy.

Gastrointestinal perforation due to lymphoma may extend into sepsis and/or peritoneal dissemination of disease, resulting in a poor outcome and a mortality rate of about 60% [3, 9]. A literature survey revealed reports of four cases of perforated duodenal lymphoma in Japan through 1980–2017 (written in Japanese without English abstracts [22–25]). The clinical characteristics of these four cases plus our own are summarized in Table 1. Of the five cases, three were DLBCL, and the remaining two were T-cell lymphomas. Three patients were alive at the time of reporting, one patient died, and the status of the remaining patient is unknown. In one case, complete resection of the tumor was performed, resulting in complete remission. In another case, minor leakage due to perforation was managed by argon plasma coagulation. Our case was the only one treated using a multidisciplinary approach.

In summary, when treating gastrointestinal lymphoma in the elderly, it is important not to attempt radical surgical resection or start intensive full-scale chemotherapy. We propose the following regimen: first, rituximab alone, followed by less intensive chemotherapy without vincristine. Once the mass size has reduced and the patient's condition

Table 1: Cases of perforated duodenal lymphoma reported in Japan.

Number	Reference	Age/sex	Sites of duodenum	Lymphoma type	Time of perforation	Surgery	Chemotherapy	Radiotherapy	Prognosis	Cause(s) of death
1	[22]	65/M	1st	DLBCL	At presentation	Pancreaticoduodenectomy	CHOP	–	Alive 9+ months	–
2	[23]	61/M	4th	T-cell lymphoma	After two cycles of SMILE	Argon plasma coagulation	Etoposide+ CHOP SMILE	–	Unknown	–
3	[24]	82/M	4th	T-cell lymphoma	After 6 cycles of CHOP	Partial resection	CHOP	–	12 months	Abdominal abscess
4	[25]	70/F	2nd	DLBCL	At presentation	Simple closure, peritoneal patch	R-CHOP	+	Alive 304 days	Sepsis
5	Our case	75/F	3rd	DLBCL	Day 21 after surgery, before chemotherapy	Gastrojejunostomy	R R-mini CHP R-CHP R-CHOP	+	Alive 4+ years	–

DLBCL = diffuse large B cell lymphoma; R-CHOP = rituximab (R), cyclophosphamide (C), doxorubicin (H), vincristine (O), prednisolone (P); CHP = cyclophosphamide (C), doxorubicin (H), prednisolone (P); SMILE = steroid (S), methotrexate (M), ifosfamide (I), L-asparaginase (L), etoposide (E).

has improved, full-scale chemotherapy can be given. If localized lymphoma persists, consolidation radiotherapy is effective at eradicating the residual mass. During treatment, assessment by PET-CT is essential for decision-making. We hope that further studies will confirm the effectiveness of this multidisciplinary approach.

Consent

Written informed consent was obtained from the patient for reporting her case.

Acknowledgments

The authors thank Dr. Shinsaku Imashuku for advice regarding patient care and critical reading of the manuscript.

References

[1] S. Nakamura and T. Matsumoto, "Gastrointestinal lymphoma: recent advances in diagnosis and treatment," *Digestion*, vol. 87, no. 3, pp. 182–188, 2013.

[2] T. Terada, "Pathologic observations of the duodenum in 615 consecutive duodenal specimens in a single Japanese hospital: II. malignant lesions," *International Journal of Clinical and Experimental Pathology*, vol. 5, no. 1, pp. 52–57, 2012.

[3] R. Vaidya, T. M. Habermann, J. H. Donohue et al., "Bowel perforation in intestinal lymphoma: incidence and clinical features," *Annals of Oncology*, vol. 24, no. 9, pp. 2439–2443, 2013.

[4] P. J. Chestovich, G. Schiller, S. Sasu, and J. R. Hiatt, "Duodenal lymphoma: a rare and morbid tumor," *Americal Surgeon*, vol. 73, no. 10, pp. 1057–1062, 2007.

[5] K. Sarkhosh, O. F. Bathe, D. A. Stewart, and L. A. Mack, "The role of surgical intervention in the management of duodenal lymphoma," *Journal of Surgical Oncology*, vol. 99, no. 7, pp. 428–432, 2009.

[6] S. Z. Usmani, L. Ding, A. H. Abu-Rashed, and H. A. Saleh, "Duodenal MALT lymphoma presenting with obstructive jaundice: report of a case and review of the literature," *Journal of Gastrointestinal Cancer*, vol. 38, no. 1, pp. 28–31, 2007.

[7] Z. Xiang, N. Onoda, M. Ohira et al., "Mucosa-associated lymphoid tissue lymphoma of the duodenum: report of a case resistant to *Helicobacter pylori* eradication," *Hepato-Gastroenterology*, vol. 51, no. 57, pp. 732–735, 2004.

[8] M. Corti, M. F. Villafañe, L. Souto, R. Schtirbu, M. Narbaitz, and M. de Dios Soler, "Burkitt's lymphoma of the duodenum in a patient with AIDS," *Revista da Sociedade Brasileira de Medicina*, vol. 40, no. 3, pp. 338–340, 2007.

[9] Y. Tanizawa, M. Terashima, M. Tokunaga et al., "Peritoneal disseminated recurrence after total gastrectomy for perforated gastric malignant lymphoma–a case report," *Gan To Kagaku Ryoho*, vol. 37, no. 11, pp. 2155–2160, 2010, in Japanese.

[10] D. G. Maloney, "Anti-CD20 antibody therapy for B-cell lymphomas," *New England Journal of Medicine*, vol. 366, no. 21, pp. 2008–2016, 2012.

[11] L. de Barros Pontes, J. Todaro, T. Karnakis et al., "Treatment of a frail older patient with diffuse large B-cell lymphoma on maintenance dialysis: attenuated immunochemotherapy and adapted care plan," *Case Reports in Oncology*, vol. 6, no. 1, pp. 197–203, 2013.

[12] Q. Huang, T. Yang, X. Jin, X. Ni, H. Qi, and Z. Yan, "Remission of late-onset post-heart transplantation lymphoproliferative disorder following treatment with rituximab and modified mini-CHOP chemotherapy: a case report," *Experimental and Therapeutic Medicine*, vol. 12, no. 1, pp. 262–266, 2016.

[13] P. Mondello, S. Cuzzocrea, V. Pitini, C. Aloisi, and M. Mian, "Is radiotherapy still necessary for diffuse large B-cell lymphoma therapy?," *Acta Oncologica*, vol. 54, no. 6, pp. 953–955, 2015.

[14] L. H. Sehn, R. Klasa, T. Shenkier et al., "Long-term experience with PET-guided consolidation radiation therapy (XRT) in patients with advanced stage diffuse large B-cell lymphoma (DLBCL) treated with R-CHOP," *Hematological Oncology*, vol. 31, pp. 96–150, 2013.

[15] P. J. Toghill and J. D. Burke, "Death from paralytic ileus following vincristine therapy," *Postgraduate Medical Journal*, vol. 46, no. 535, pp. 330-331, 1970.

[16] T. Yasu, N. Ohno, T. Kawamata, and Y. Kurokawa, "Vincristine-induced paralytic ileus during induction therapy of treatment protocols for acute lymphoblastic leukemia in adult patients," *International Journal of Clinical Pharmacology and Therapeutics*, vol. 54, no. 6, pp. 471–473, 2016.

[17] C. Ara, S. Coban, C. Kayaalp, S. Yilmaz, and V. Kirimlioglu, "Spontaneous intestinal perforation due to non-Hodgkin's lymphoma: evaluation of eight cases," *Digestive Diseases and Sciences*, vol. 52, no. 8, pp. 1752–1756, 2007.

[18] Y. Ohkura, S. Lee, D. Kaji et al., "Spontaneous perforation of primary gastric malignant lymphoma: a case report and review of the literature," *World Journal of Surgical Oncology*, vol. 13, no. 1, p. 35, 2015.

[19] M. Wada, M. Onda, A. Tokunaga et al., "Spontaneous gastrointestinal perforation in patients with lymphoma receiving chemotherapy and steroids. Report of three cases," *Nihon Ika Daigaku Zasshi*, vol. 66, no. 1, pp. 37–40, 1999.

[20] S. Yoshino, S. Nakamura, T. Matsumoto et al., "A case of primary gastric malignant lymphoma perforated immediately after administration of chemotherapy," *Nihon Shokakibyo Gakkai Zasshi*, vol. 103, no. 2, pp. 162–167, 2006, in Japanese.

[21] A. Sugimoto, M. Tada, T. Taji et al., "A case of malignant lymphoma of the jejunum that developed stenosis and perforation after a complete response to chemotherapy," *Gan To Kagaku Ryoho*, vol. 44, no. 4, pp. 341–343, 2017, in Japanese.

[22] T. Shoji, H. Konno, T. Tanaka et al., "Pancreaticoduodenectomy for perforated gastric malignant lymphoma: report of a case," *Surgery Today*, vol. 32, no. 5, pp. 468–471, 2002.

[23] W. Jyomen, H. Kuroda, T. Sakai et al., "Successful treatment of enteropathy-associated T cell lymphoma with SMILE therapy," *Medical Journal of Asahikawa Red Cross Hospital*, vol. 22, pp. 63–68, 2008.

[24] K. Fujiyoshi, S. Sueyoshi, T. Tsubuku et al., "Enteropathy-associated T-cell lymphoma in the ascending part of the duodenum," *Journal of Gastroenterological Surgery*, vol. 47, no. 10, pp. 580–587, 2014.

[25] Y. Shimoda, H. Sekikawa, T. Yamazaki et al., "A case of malignant lymphoma of the duodenum discovered by perforation," *Rinsho Zasshi Geka*, vol. 78, no. 4, pp. 422–425, 2016.

21

A Unique Case of Muscle-Invasive Metastatic Breast Cancer Mimicking Myositis

Janelle Gyorffy,[1] Samuel M. Philbrick,[1] Adrian R. Bersabe,[2] Richard J. Upton,[3] Derek A. Mathis,[3] Austin Peters,[4] and Alexander Brown[2]

[1]*Department of Internal Medicine, SAUSHEC, San Antonio, TX, USA*
[2]*Department of Hematology Oncology, SAUSHEC, San Antonio, TX, USA*
[3]*Department of Pathology, SAUSHEC, San Antonio, TX, USA*
[4]*Department of Radiology, SAUSHEC, San Antonio, TX, USA*

Correspondence should be addressed to Janelle Gyorffy; janelle.b.gyorffy.mil@mail.mil

Academic Editor: Jose I. Mayordomo

Breast cancer rarely metastasizes to the muscles, and it is even more unusual for this phenomenon to result in airway compromise. We present a unique case of an 84-year-old female who presented with neck swelling and upper airway obstruction due to metastatic breast cancer invading the sternocleidomastoid muscles. After establishing the diagnosis and discussing possible treatment options, the patient elected for antiestrogen therapy, palliative tracheostomy, radiation therapy, and hospice services.

1. Introduction

Breast cancer is the most commonly diagnosed cancer in women. The incidence of breast cancer increases with age, and a woman's lifetime risk is approximately 12.5%. While breast cancer is diagnosed at stage 1 in approximately half of non-Hispanic white women, diagnosis of metastatic disease as the initial presentation is seen in 6% of patients [1]. Breast cancer typically metastasizes to lung, liver, and bone [2]. Involvement of skeletal muscle is rare, but when it occurs, it usually presents with contiguous involvement of a soft tissue lesion and may appear clinically as a lump or mass. It may also occur in the setting of extensive bone involvement or in the presence of widely disseminated disease [3, 4]. Extranodal head and neck metastases are also uncommon with only a few case reports and case series documenting involvement of the thyroid, mandible, subcutaneous tissues, or pharynx [5–11]. Thus, metastases to muscles of the neck are almost unheard of, with only one such case documented in medical literature [12]. We report the exceedingly unusual case of an 84-year-old African-American female with neck swelling and airway obstruction due to metastatic breast cancer invading the musculature of the head and neck.

2. Case Report

An 84-year-old African-American female with no known history of malignancy initially presented at a local Emergency Department (ED) with complaint of dyspnea for several months. Patient was diagnosed with asthma and given an albuterol inhaler. Five months later, she presented to our ED with progressive neck swelling and dysphagia. Urgent evaluation with Otolaryngology (ENT) was arranged as she was noted to have difficulty controlling her secretions. During ENT evaluation, she acutely developed respiratory failure requiring emergent fiber-optic nasotracheal intubation and transfer to the medical intensive care unit (MICU).

A CT of the neck, chest, abdomen, and pelvis was remarkable for extensive inflammatory stranding of multiple muscular and fascial planes in the neck, mediastinum, and anterior chest. There was also moderate narrowing of the supraglottic airway (Figure 1). There was no evidence of other evidence of distant metastases. The CT did not reveal any bony lesions. A PET-CT and bone scan were unable to be performed given patient's unstable condition in the MICU.

Erythrocyte sedimentation rate (ESR) was within normal limits at 26 mm/hr, and C-reactive protein (CRP) was

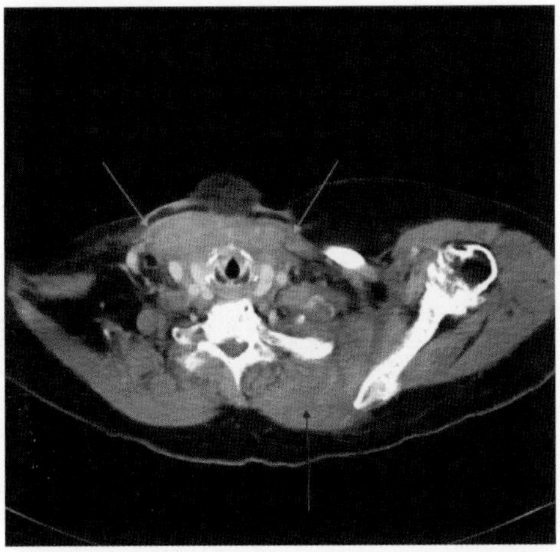

FIGURE 1: Significant thickening of the sternocleidomastoid muscles (blue arrows). Soft tissue density obliterating numerous fat planes extending into the mediastinum and completely encasing the major vessels and left paraspinal musculature including the left trapezius muscle (red arrow). The very few cases of breast cancer metastatic to the soft tissues predominantly describe focal or mass-like involvement. This diffuse, infiltrating appearance is highly unusual and most characteristic of severe infection/inflammation such as myositis or necrotizing fasciitis.

undetectable. Lactate dehydrogenase (LDH) was within the labs reference range at 155 U/L, and aspartate aminotransferase (AST) was normal at 26 U/L. Creatinine kinase (CK) was mildly elevated at 239 IU/L. Evaluation for an autoimmune etiology was negative, and the patient had no clinical improvement with high dose steroids.

A biopsy of the left sternocleidomastoid (SCM) was obtained which revealed infiltrating carcinoma. No associated inflammatory infiltrate or necrosis was identified. The tissue was strongly positive for estrogen receptor (ER), progesterone receptor (PR), pancytokeratin (Lu-5), high molecular weight cytokeratin (K903), GATA-3, and mammaglobin. Cells were mildly to moderately positive for GCDFP-15 and E-cadherin, and negative for HER-2/neu, S-100, TTF-1, CD34, CD30, and PAX-8 (Figure 2). Staining with mammaglobin showed strong positivity within malignant cells. These immunohistochemical findings were most consistent with a breast primary malignancy. Biopsies from vocal cord, arytenoid, epiglottis, and uvula biopsies demonstrated no malignant cells.

The patient had no palpable breast masses, and no axillary, supraclavicular, or cervical lymphadenopathy was clinically appreciable. A bilateral breast ultrasound showed a hypoechoic $1.7 \times 1.0 \times 1.5$ cm mass in the left breast with increased vascularity highly suggestive of malignancy (BI-RADS 5) and a $1.1 \times 1.1 \times 0.5$ cm mass in the right breast without increased vascularity also suspicious for malignancy (BI-RADS 4). There were no pathologic axillary lymph nodes appreciated on imaging. Serum tumor markers were remarkable for elevating CA 15-3 to 299 U/mL and CA 27.29 to 238 U/mL. CEA was elevated just above the reference range at 3.5 ng/L.

The diagnosis of metastatic breast cancer was discussed with the patient and her family. Given her critical illness and patient's desire for a less aggressive palliative approach, the patient elected for antiestrogen therapy with Fulvestrant over a trial of single-agent chemotherapy. She also agreed to palliative tracheostomy and radiotherapy (XRT) to expedite ventilator weaning. She underwent the four fractions of palliative XRT at 370 cGy for a total dose of 1480 cGY. She was successfully weaned off of ventilator support and transitioned to home hospice. The patient declined further treatment. She passed away approximately one month later after the definitive diagnosis of metastatic breast cancer was made.

3. Discussion

Breast cancer most frequently metastasizes to bone (70%), lung (66%), and liver (61%) but may involve other organs [2]. Malignant airway obstruction is more commonly found in patients with advanced local lung cancer but may rarely result from metastasis from cancers of the thyroid, breast, colon, melanoma, or kidneys [13]. This case demonstrates a rare instance of metastases to the SCM muscles along with the unusual presentation of airway obstruction due to local skeletal muscle invasion manifesting as myositis.

The patient's myositis caused by infiltrating carcinoma presented in a manner distinct from dermatomyositis (DM) and polymyositis (PM), idiopathic inflammatory myopathies that typically present with proximal muscle weakness and muscle inflammation. The differential diagnoses for DM and PM are broad and include sarcoidosis, amyloidosis, drug-induced myositis, and other infectious, familial, and autoimmune etiologies. Treatment is usually corticosteroids or immunosuppressive agents. Our patient did present with progressive dysphagia but had no other findings suggestive of proximal muscle weakness or cutaneous manifestations of DM. ESR, CRP, LDH, and AST, which are commonly elevated in DM and PM, were within normal limits, and CK levels were only mildly elevated. Furthermore, she was treated with steroids but did not demonstrate a significant clinical response. Diagnostic tissue biopsy did not reveal characteristic inflammatory cell infiltration, necrotic and regenerating muscle fibers, or atrophic muscle fibers that are characteristic of an inflammatory myositis. Although her CT scan was suspicious for myositis, her presentation and clinical course were not specifically suggestive of DM or PM.

The distinction between PM and the patient's myositis bears examination because PM is strongly associated with cancer, to such an extent that cancer surveillance and various imaging are warranted in new diagnoses [14]. Although less common, there are reported cases of paraneoplastic DM related to breast cancer [15, 16]. DM and PM are thought to manifest as paraneoplastic syndromes when cancer cells overexpress myositis-specific antigens (MSA) that cause autoimmune damage to both muscle and cancer mediated by T-cells [17]. However, in this case, myositis did not occur as a paraneoplastic syndrome mediated by T-cells; rather direct invasion of metastatic carcinoma cells caused the inflammatory changes seen on the patient's imaging and biopsy.

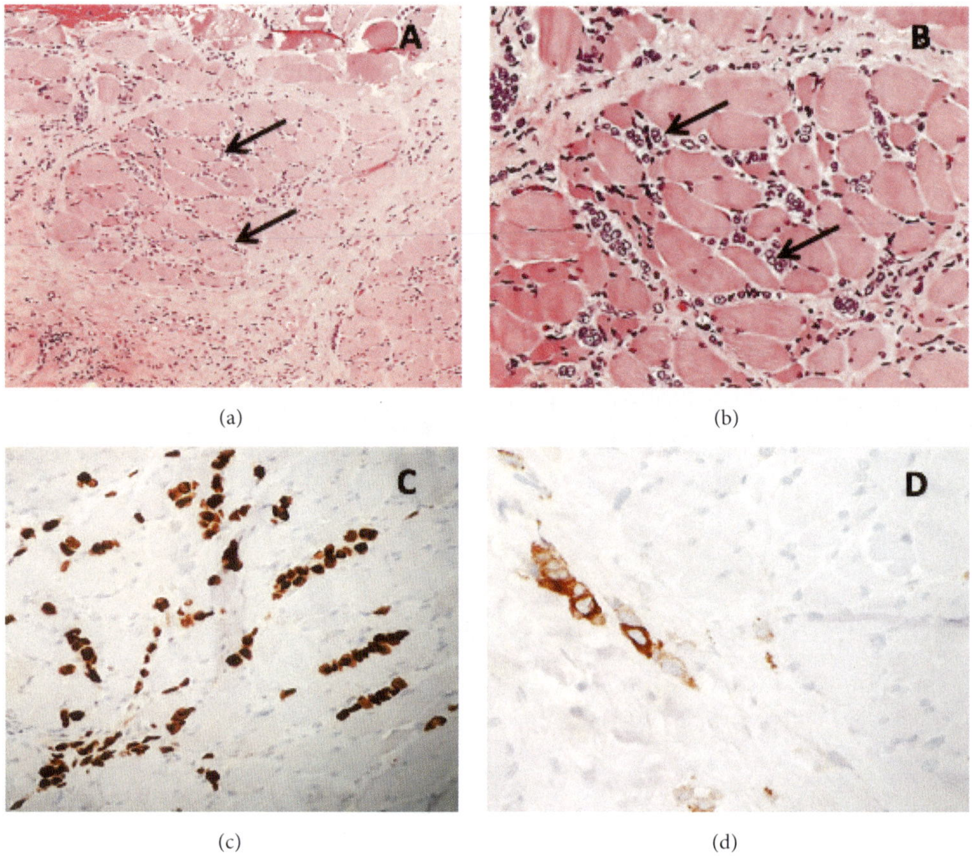

Figure 2: (a) Malignant cells (arrows) infiltrating through skeletal muscle and fibroconnective tissue (hematoxylin-eosin, original magnification ×100). (b) A higher power view shows malignant cells infiltrating singly or in small clusters through muscle and fibroconnective tissue. No tubule formation is identified, which is typical of invasive lobular breast carcinoma (hematoxylin-eosin, original magnification ×200). (c) Malignant cells alone and in single file strongly immunoreactive for GATA-3, a luminal marker for breast epithelium (original magnification ×200). (d) Malignant cells showing strong immunoreactivity for mammaglobin, another marker specific for breast carcinoma (original magnification ×400).

The nature of this breast cancer metastasis was also unusual. Skeletal muscle metastases are rare in and of themselves, likely due to a hostile microenvironment created by muscle's pH, ability to remove lactic acid associated with angiogenesis, the activation of lymphocytes and NK cells in skeletal muscles, and mechanical tumor destruction from motion. It is thought that for these reasons, skeletal muscle metastases from breast cancer are uncommon. However, this pattern of metastasis has been described and is usually seen with disseminated, multiorgan involvement [18]. When skeletal muscle metastases do develop, they often present as isolated, painful soft tissue masses in the involved areas [4, 18]. Typically, these metastases are challenging to evaluate with CT alone due to isodensity with surrounding muscle. They may be more appropriately identified with MRI or FDG PET-CT and are often found to have round or oval shapes with well-defined margins [19, 20]. However, in this case, the metastases manifested as diffuse infiltration of cervical musculature without a discrete lump or mass. Breast cancer presenting with direct muscle invasion in an infiltrative pattern mimicking myositis has only been reported in one other case [12]. Due to its relatively rare occurrence, there currently is no consensus on the standard treatment for skeletal muscle metastases, and further studies are needed to determine the prognosis and proper diagnostic and therapeutic treatment [18].

Given that imaging studies for this patient depicted what appeared to be impressive inflammatory stranding of the muscles of the neck, it is probable that subtler changes may have been detected earlier in the disease course prior to the development of respiratory failure. Earlier imaging in this case may have led to more timely intervention and prevention of this airway emergency. Various modalities to achieve airway patency are available. These options may include emergent tracheostomy, laser therapy, contact electrocautery, argon plasma coagulation, cryotherapy, photodynamic therapy, brachytherapy, and airway stenting [21].

4. Conclusion

This case illustrates a unique presentation of metastatic breast cancer presenting as a muscle infiltration mimicking myositis and resulted in airway compromise. Initial imaging showed distortion of tissue planes which appeared inflammatory in etiology thus confounding the differential diagnosis. This patient's initial subacute presentation of cough and dyspnea were nonspecific and would be unlikely to trigger a concern for breast cancer. However, close clinical follow-up and repeat imaging may have led to a more timely diagnosis thereby preventing the development of imminent respiratory failure. Earlier recognition may have allowed for the availability of wider array of palliative interventions to improve the patient's life expectancy and quality of life.

Unfortunately, this patient's clinical course was highly aggressive, and she ultimately required urgent intubation and subsequent tracheostomy. A high index of suspicion for neoplasm should be maintained when patients present with an indeterminate myositis. For patients with progressive dyspnea, dysphagia, and evidence of myositis by imaging, it is important to biopsy areas of involvement to evaluate for sarcoidosis, amyloidosis, drug-induced myositis, other infectious, and familial and autoimmune as well as neoplastic etiologies. A wide range of therapies are available to patients with airway compromise secondary to malignancy but should coincide with goals of care.

References

[1] J. Iqbal, O. Ginsburg, P. A. Rochon, P. Sun, and S. A. Narod, "Differences in breast cancer stage at diagnosis and cancer-specific survival by race and ethnicity in the United States," *Journal of the American Medical Association*, vol. 313, no. 2, pp. 165–173, 2015.

[2] S. P. L. Leong, B. Cady, D. M. Jablons et al., "Clinical patterns of metastasis," *Cancer and Metastasis Reviews*, vol. 25, no. 2, pp. 221–232, 2006.

[3] H. Kreisman, N. Wolkove, S. Finkelstein, C. Cohen, R. Margolese, and H. Frank, "Breast cancer and thoracic metastase: review of 119 patients," *Thorax*, vol. 38, no. 3, pp. 175–179, 1983.

[4] A. Ogiya, K. Takahashi, M. Sato et al., "Metastatic breast carcinoma of the abdominal wall muscle: a case report," *Breast Cancer*, vol. 22, no. 2, pp. 206–209, 2015.

[5] A. Surov, A. Machens, H.-J. Holzhausen, R. P. Spielmann, and H. Dralle, "Radiological features of metastases to the thyroid," *Acta Radiologica*, vol. 57, no. 4, pp. 444–450, 2016.

[6] K. Lacka, D. Breborowicz, A. Uliasz, and M. Teresiak, "Thyroid metastases from a breast cancer diagnosed by fine-needle aspiration biopsy. Case report and overview of the literature," *Experimental Oncology*, vol. 34, no. 2, pp. 129–133, 2012.

[7] M. Y. Rao and J. B. Wu, "Invasive ductal breast cancer with extensive subcutaneous metastases in trunk: a case report," *European Review for Medical and Pharmacological Sciences*, vol. 19, no. 21, pp. 4101–4104, 2015.

[8] S. Agrawal, K. Jayant, R. K. U. Agarwal, K. G. Dayama, and S. Arora, "An unusual case of metastatic male breast cancer to the nasopharynx-review of literature," *Annals of Palliative Medicine*, vol. 4, no. 4, pp. 233–238, 2015.

[9] V. Tiwari, S. C. H. Pande, K. Verma, and S. Goel, "Paranasal sinus and retro-orbital metastasis in a case of breast carcinoma: a clinicoradiological review," *BMJ Case Reports*, vol. 2014, 2014.

[10] S. Davey and S. Baer, "A rare case of breast cancer metastasising to the nasopharynx and paranasal sinuses," *International Journal of Surgery Case Reports*, vol. 3, no. 9, pp. 460–462, 2012.

[11] R. Bayon, S. K. Banas, and B. L. Wenig, "Case report: Metastatic breast cancer presenting as a hypopharyngeal mass," *Ear, Nose and Throat Journal*, vol. 92, no. 3, pp. E5–E6, 2013.

[12] S. Noda, S. Kashiwagi, H. Kawajiri, T. Takashima, N. Onoda, and K. Hirakawa, "A case of metastatic breast carcinoma of the cervical muscles," *Gan To Kagaku Ryoho*, vol. 40, no. 12, pp. 2405–2407, 2013.

[13] S. D. Murgu, K. Egressy, B. Laxmanan, G. Doblare, R. Ortiz-Comino, and D. K. Hogarth, "Central airway obstruction: benign strictures, tracheobronchomalacia, and malignancy-related obstruction," *Chest*, vol. 150, no. 2, pp. 426–441, 2016.

[14] Y.-F. Fang, Y.-J. J. Wu, C.-F. Kuo, S.-F. Luo, and K.-H. Yu, "Malignancy in dermatomyositis and polymyositis: analysis of 192 patients," *Clinical Rheumatology*, vol. 35, no. 8, pp. 1977–1984, 2016.

[15] T. Sakai, Y. Ogura, J. Narita et al., "Metachronous bilateral primary breast cancer associated with dermatomyositis," *The Breast Journal*, vol. 11, no. 3, pp. 225-226, 2005.

[16] N. Merali, M. Yousuff, V. Pronisceva, and A. Poddar, "Paraneoplastic polymyositis presenting as a clinically occult breast cancer," *The Annals of The Royal College of Surgeons of England*, vol. 99, no. 2, pp. e40–e43, 2017.

[17] S. M. Levine, "Cancer and myositis: new insights into an old association," *Current Opinion in Rheumatology*, vol. 18, no. 6, pp. 620–624, 2006.

[18] Y. W. Kim, K. J. Seo, S. L. Lee et al., "Skeletal muscle metastases from breast cancer: two case reports," *Journal of Breast Cancer*, vol. 16, no. 1, pp. 117–121, 2013.

[19] J. Emmering, W. V. Vogel, and M. P. M. Stokkel, "Intramuscular metastases on FDG PET-CT: a review of the literature," *Nuclear Medicine Communications*, vol. 33, no. 2, pp. 117–120, 2012.

[20] D. Bello-Roufai, D. G. Soares, K. Kerrou et al., "Long-term complete response in a breast cancer patient with skeletal muscle metastases diagnosed using 18F-FDG-PET," *Oxford Medical Case Reports*, vol. 2017, no. 2, pp. 12–14, 2017.

[21] A. Breitenbücher, P. N. Chhajed, M. H. Brutsche, C. Mordasini, D. Schilter, and M. Tamm, "Long-term follow-up and survival after Ultraflex stent insertion in the management of complex malignant airway stenoses," *Respiration*, vol. 75, no. 4, pp. 443–449, 2008.

22

Diffuse Bone Marrow Metastasis as the Initial Presentation of an Occult Breast Cancer

Frank S. Fan[1], **Chung-Fan Yang**[2], **and Yi-Fen Wang**[3]

[1]*Section of Hematology and Oncology, Department of Medicine, Changhua Hospital, Ministry of Health and Welfare, Chang-Hua County, Taiwan*
[2]*Department of Pathology, Changhua Hospital, Ministry of Health and Welfare, Chang-Hua County, Taiwan*
[3]*Department of Radiology, Changhua Hospital, Ministry of Health and Welfare, Chang-Hua County, Taiwan*

Correspondence should be addressed to Frank S. Fan; fantast.fan@msa.hinet.net

Academic Editor: Su Ming Tan

Introduction. Breast cancer is one of the malignancies which tend to involve the bone marrow, but initial presentation with diffuse bone marrow metastasis from an occult breast cancer is very rare. Prognosis is generally very poor for marrow metastasis from solid tumors except that breast cancer is a treatable disease even in such a dismal condition. *Case.* A 64-year-old woman's headache was found to result from diffuse adenocarcinoma metastasis in the bone marrow from an unknown primary site. Intensive immunohistochemistry study of bone marrow biopsy specimen confirmed the disease nature to be an estrogen receptor-positive/human epidermal growth factor receptor 2-negative breast cancer. Mammography and magnetic resonance imaging of breasts revealed a suspicious primary lesion in the right breast. Treatment with tamoxifen alone achieved a sustained response. *Discussion.* Mucin 1 (MUC1), also known as cancer antigen 15-3 (CA 15-3), facilitates motility and metastatic potential of breast cancer cells. Interleukin-1β (IL-1β) drives breast cancer cell growth and colonization in bone marrow adipose tissue niche. Receptor activator of nuclear factor kappa-B (RANK) and its ligand (RANKL) activate osteoclasts to make a favorable bone marrow microenvironment for tumor cells. Agents against MUC1, IL-1β, and RANKL might be of therapeutic effect for patients like ours.

1. Introduction

Bone marrow metastasis from nonhematological tumors is a well-known event. The most common origins identified are lung, breast, stomach, and prostate [1, 2]. But the primary sites of a large portion frequently still remain unknown with generally unfavorable prognosis [3, 4]. Nevertheless, symptomatic bone marrow metastasis from breast cancer seems to have a relatively longer median survival, probably due to its treatable characteristics [5]. We like to present a case of marrow carcinomatosis which was proven to originate from a hard-to-identify breast cancer by immunohistochemical staining and responded dramatically to tamoxifen alone. The possible underlying mechanisms of stealthy bone marrow metastasis from an occult breast cancer and recent progress in management of such a disastrous status will also be discussed.

2. Case Presentation

A 64-year-old woman was brought to the emergency unit with chief complaints of headache and fever for one week in September 2017. She felt pain over her whole calvarium without a specific trigger point. Her body temperature was 38.7 degrees Celsius. There was no nausea, vomiting, blurred vision, or nuchal stiffness. Cranial and peripheral neurologic function did not have any impairment. Superficial lymphadenopathy, breast nodules, and abdominal tumor mass were not detected on palpation. A Babinski sign was absent. She denied drug or alcohol abuse.

Laboratory examination disclosed a normocytic anemia with hemoglobin level of 7 g/dl, mean corpuscular volume of 89.3 fl, platelet count of 325000/μl, and white blood cell count of 12000/μl comprising neutrophils 61.7%, lymphocytes 26.7%, and monocytes 10.8%. A leucoerythroblastic

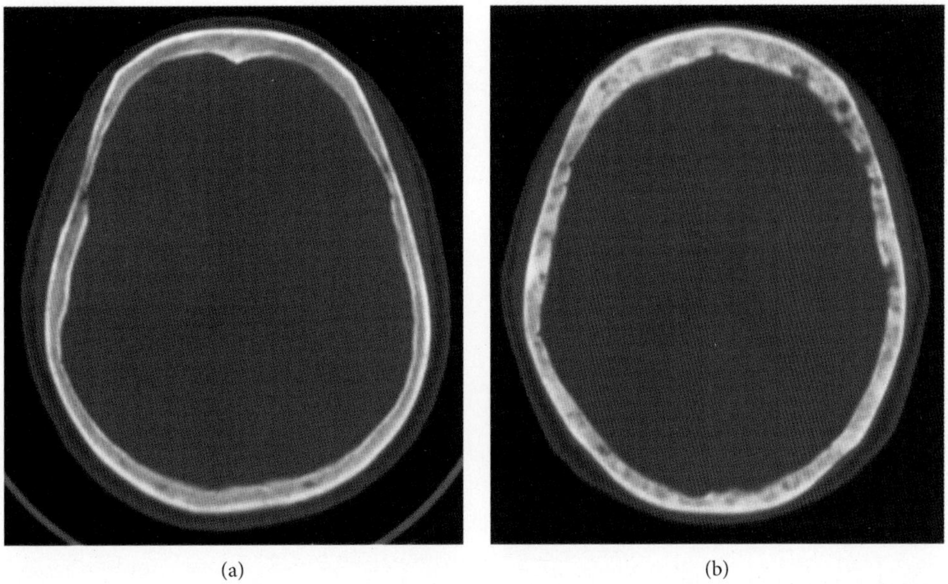

Figure 1: Axial head CT images on bone window. (a) The skull was intact on June 30, 2011. (b) Many osteolytic lesions were detected on September 13, 2017.

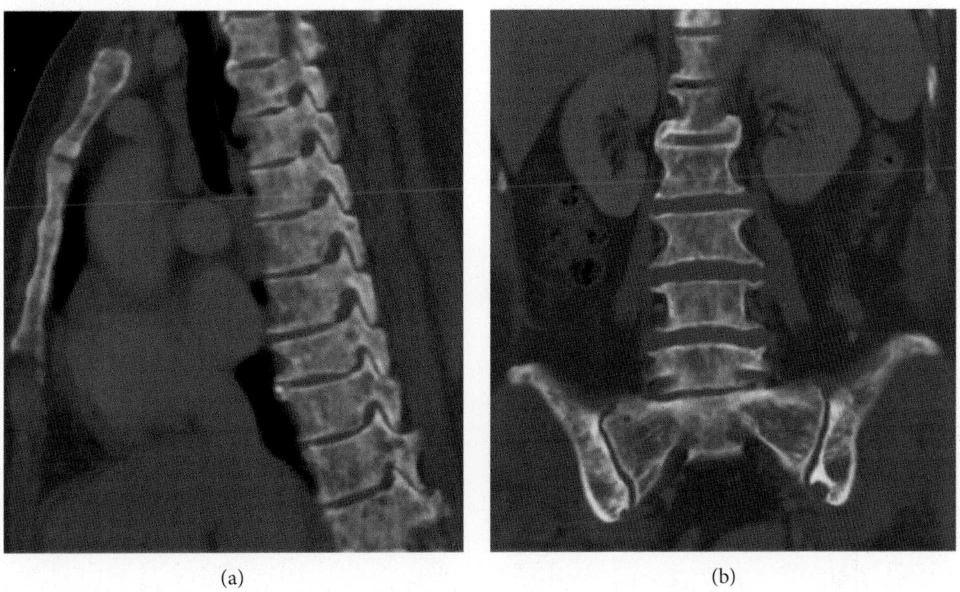

Figure 2: Chest and abdomen CT images on bone window, September 14, 2017. Multiple osteosclerotic and osteolytic lesions involved the sternum, vertebra, sacrum, and bilateral iliac bones.

picture was not present. Blood chemistry tests revealed abnormally elevated serum alkaline phosphatase of 158 iu/l (normal 32~91) and lactate dehydrogenase of 292 iu/l (normal 98~192). There was neither microhematuria nor stool occult blood. Both activated partial thromboplastin time and prothrombin time were normal in value but the D-dimer was extremely high: 6570 ng/ml (normal 0~500).

The chest X-ray routine film showed no active lung lesions. A computerized tomography (CT) scan of head was ordered to rule out intracranial abscess or other central nervous system problems. The brain turned out to be intact but, unexpectedly, multiple osteolytic lesions were detected in the skull, extraordinarily obvious upon comparison with previous films taken six years earlier for other reasons (Figure 1). She was then admitted to the ward under a suspicious impression of multiple myeloma.

Subsequent immunofixation electrophoresis analysis of serum, however, did not show any evidence of monoclonal gammopathy, and the levels of serum immunoglobulin G, A, and M were all within normal ranges. In contrast, serum tumor markers carcinoembryonic antigen (CEA) and cancer antigen 15-3 (CA 15-3) were meaningfully increased in concentration: CEA 8.1 ng/ml (normal 0~5) and CA 15-3 163.2 iu/ml (normal 0~31.3), respectively.

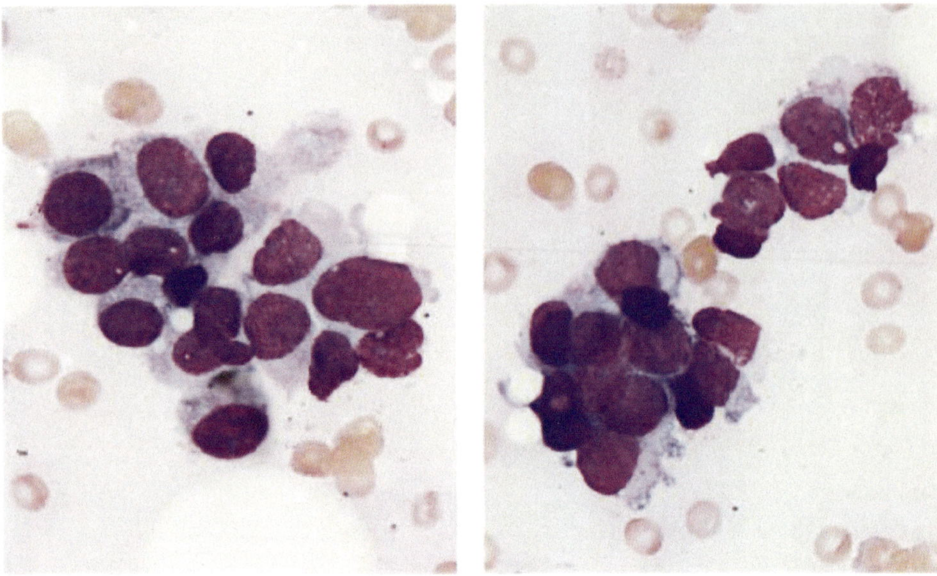

(a) (b)

FIGURE 3: Adenocarcinoma nests in bone marrow aspiration smears (Wright-Giemsa stain, 1000x).

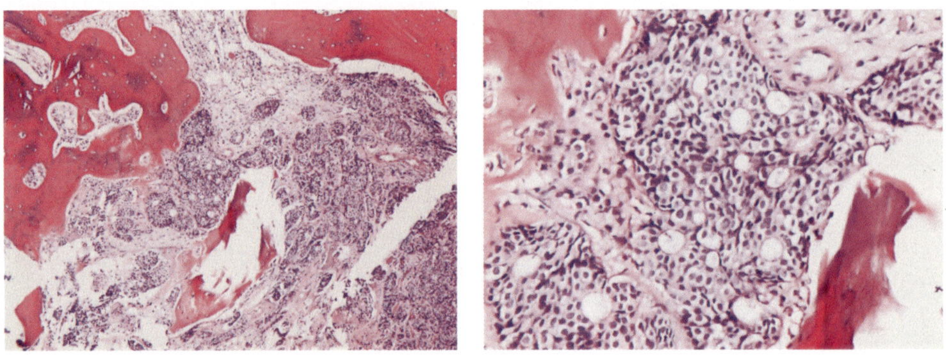

(a) (b)

FIGURE 4: Metastatic adenocarcinoma in bone marrow (Hematoxylin and eosin stain, (a) 100x; (b) 400x).

Levels of cancer antigen 19-9 (CA 19-9) and cancer antigen 125 (CA-125) were within normal limits. Afterwards, a CT scan of chest and abdomen revealed osteosclerotic and osteolytic lesions similar to that of skull involving almost the whole skeleton (Figure 2) but not a single clear-cut primary tumor site could be located.

Bone marrow aspiration and biopsy were performed on the right side posterior superior iliac crest. The aspiration smear demonstrated very scanty hematopoietic precursors scattered among crowded groups of oval neoplastic cells with large hyperchromatic nuclei, coarse chromatin, modest granular cytoplasm, and occasionally small nucleoli (Figure 3). Frequent rosette-like openings were seen in the tumor groups. A metastatic adenocarcinoma was considered as the most likely diagnosis.

Pathologic study of the biopsy specimen after decalcification displayed a picture of metastatic adenocarcinoma composed of round to oval tumor cells arranged in ovoid clusters, small rounded nests, cribriform nests, and focal microacinar pattern stuffed in bone marrow cavity (Figure 4). The immunohistochemical stains gave positive results for cytokeratin 7 (CK7), cytokeratin 8 (CK8), estrogen receptor (ER) (strong, 99%), progesterone receptor (PR) (strong, 99%) (Figure 5), Smad4 (DPC4), GATA binding protein 3 (GATA-3), gross cystic disease fluid protein 15 (GCDFP-15), and mammaglobin (Figure 6). While human epidermal growth factor receptor 2 (HER2/neu), cytokeratin 20 (CK20), thyroid transcription factor-1 (TTF-1), paired box gene 8 (PAX8), and synaptophysin were negative. The positive rate of Ki-67 in tumor cells was 20%. Diffuse bone marrow metastasis from breast carcinoma (invasive ductal carcinoma, not otherwise specified) thus should be considered firstly as the diagnosis based on aforementioned pathological findings and differential diagnosis markers recommended in the literature [6, 7].

Mammogram brought to light a suspect primary site in the right breast as compared with films taken five years earlier for cancer screening (Figure 7). The lesion was also

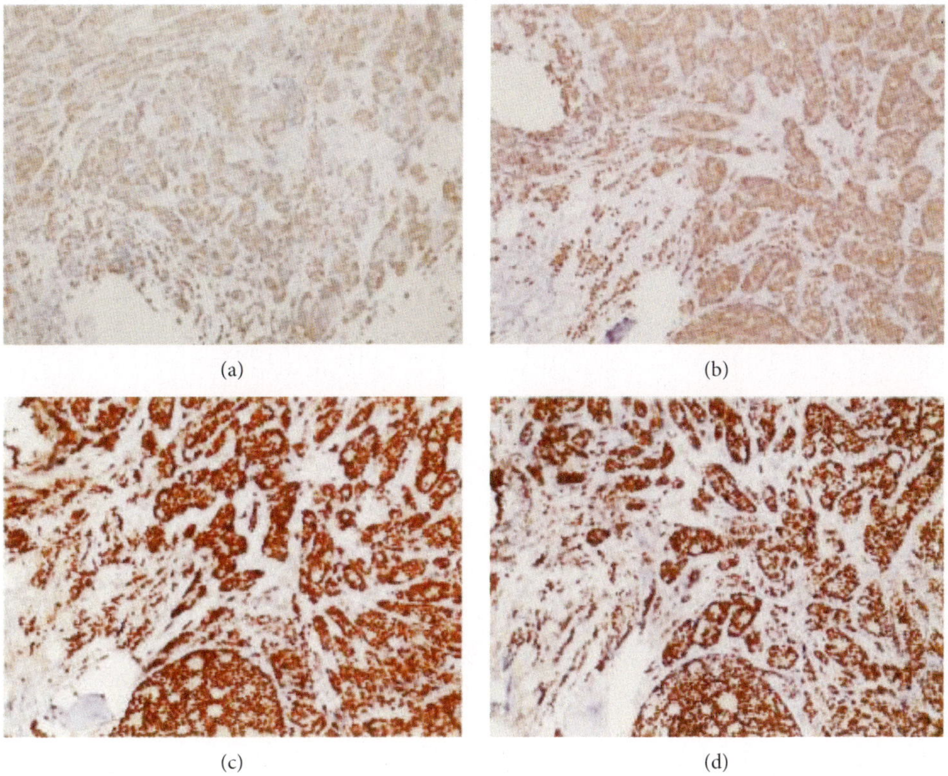

Figure 5: Immunohistochemical stain of adenocarcinoma in bone marrow. (a) CK7, (b) CK8, (c) ER, and (d) PR. All were positive.

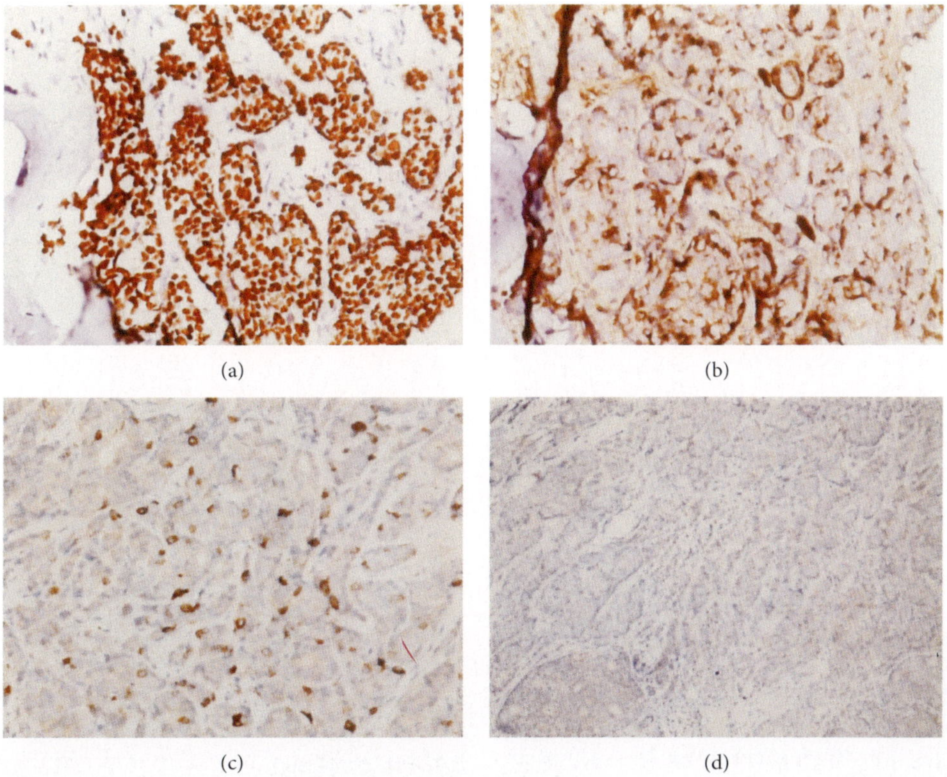

Figure 6: Immunohistochemical stain of adenocarcinoma in bone marrow. Positive for (a) GATA-3, (b) GCDFP-15 (patchy staining pattern), and (c) mammaglobin (scattered staining pattern). Negative for (d) HER2.

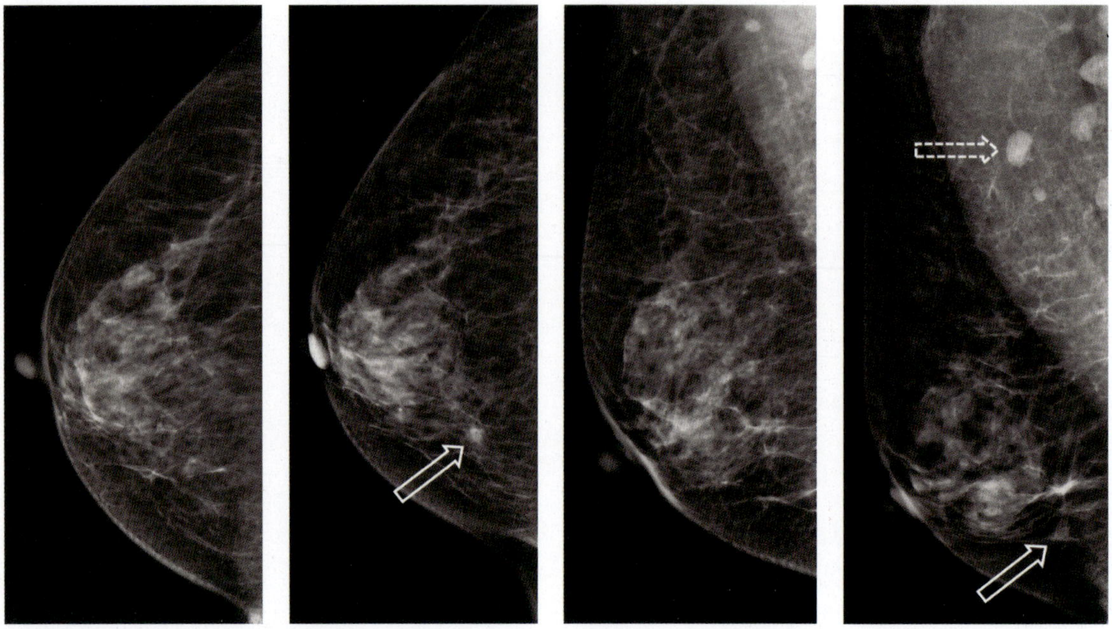

Figure 7: Mammography. (a and c) No suspicious lesions were detectable on June 25, 2012. (b and d) An about 7 to 8 mm focal asymmetry (solid arrows) at the posterior inner hemisphere of right breast and several enlarged lymph nodes at right axillary region (dashed arrow), diameter up to 12 mm, were noted on September 14, 2017.

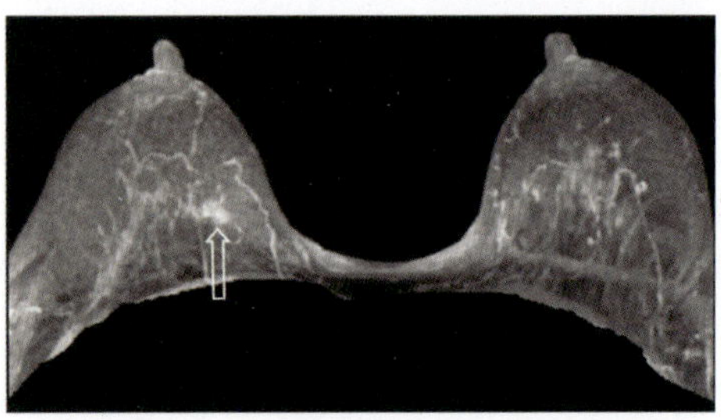

Figure 8: 3D maximum intensity projection (MIP) contrast subtraction study MRI of breast on September 15, 2017. There was an about 7 mm focal asymmetry at the posterior inner hemisphere of right breast (arrow).

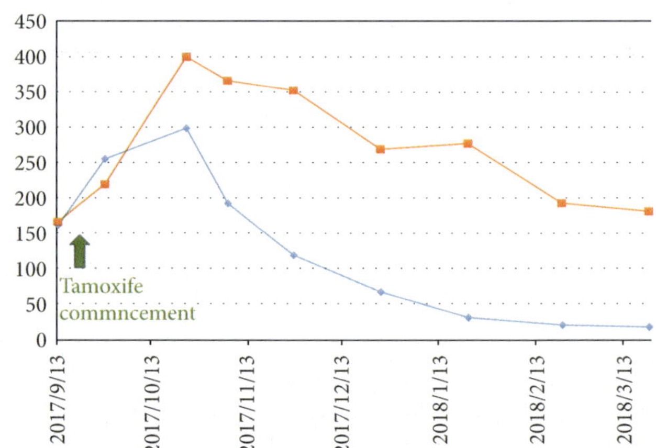

Figure 9: Change of serum CA 15-3 (blue diamond) and alkaline phosphatase (orange square) levels (iu/ml) along the clinical course. Green arrow: tamoxifen commencement date (September 21, 2017).

detectable in magnetic resonance imaging (MRI) (Figure 8). Nonetheless, no tumor was found by both physical examination and sonogram of breasts. Additionally, the patient's husband and sons did not want her to know the nature of the disease, so a breast biopsy was pitifully not done at last.

Due to our worry about the risk of fracture associated with aromatase inhibitors [8], the patient began to take tamoxifen, 20 mg twice daily, for treatment. The effect seemed very satisfactory. After a period of probable "tamoxifen flare" with elevation of serum CA 15-3 and alkaline phosphatase levels for six weeks [9], both of them dropped gradually within four months (Figure 9). Fortunately, there was no hypercalcemia noted during the whole clinical course. Serum CA15-3 was within normal limits at the last follow-up on March 21, 2018. Positron emission tomography/CT (PET/CT) scans during the treatment course confirmed an impressive improvement of the bone marrow uptake. The mild activity remained in the lumbar spine could be either residual metastasis or, more favored by us, compensatory hyperactive hematopoiesis in its recovery phase (Figure 10). The patient did not have headache or fever anymore and was enjoying a happy life up to the time of submitting this case report with a hemoglobin level of 12.2 g/dl.

3. Discussion

Occult micrometastasis to bone marrow in early stage breast cancer appeared in around 30% of the patients and was considered a poor prognostic factor [10]. Symptomatic diffuse

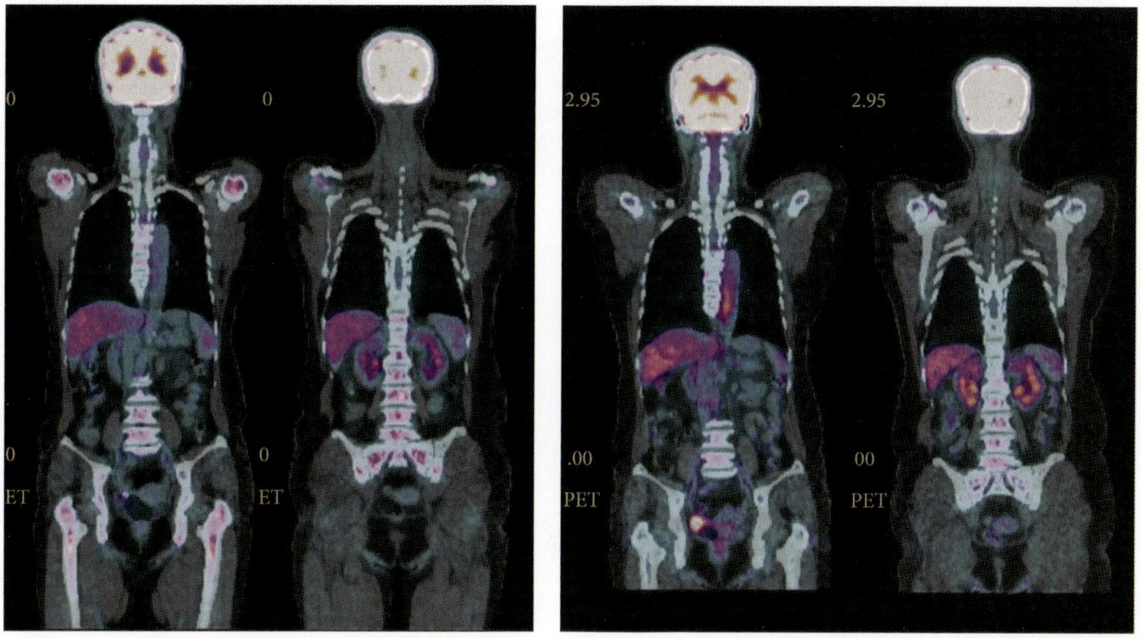

(a) (b)

Figure 10: PET/CT scans. (a) Profuse bone marrow uptake (SUVmax: liver 3.1, skeleton 4.2) 15 days after starting treatment with tamoxifen, October 16, 2017. (b) Obvious resolution of previous bone marrow uptake with some residual activity in the lumbar spine (SUVmax: liver 3.3, skeleton 3.2) while on continuous tamoxifen treatment, March 5, 2018.

bone marrow metastasis, on the contrary, is a relatively uncommon manifestation of breast cancer, estimated to happen in only 0.17% of the patients [5]. Most diffuse bone marrow metastasis took place in patients already diagnosed to have breast cancer. The median time from initial diagnosis of breast cancer to bone marrow involvement was reported to be from 36 to 46 months with anemia as the most frequent symptom at presentation [5, 11]. Our patient's presenting symptoms also included anemia, compatible with aforementioned reports, but her breast cancer remained almost as an unknown primary site. This scenario is indeed quite rare.

Despite that a bone marrow metastasis usually leads to an incurable stage of malignant disease, adequate treatment with endocrine agents, chemotherapy, and targeted therapy might still prolong survival in case the origin is the breast [12]. Our patient turned out to have a very successful treatment result with tamoxifen, which could be predicted from the absence of HER2 and the strong ER/PR expression in her tumor cells [13]. In the long run, when the disease becomes resistant to the present tamoxifen therapy, or even a prominent primary site lesion develops, a rebiopsy of metastatic lesions and total excision of the primary tumor are planned for investigation of possible characteristic changes of the tumor. At that time, if the cancer is still hormone receptor positive, aromatase inhibitors, selective estrogen receptor degradators, mechanistic target of rapamycin (mTOR) inhibitors, and cyclin-dependent kinase 4/6 inhibitors would accordingly be prescribed in sequence or in combination to benefit this postmenopausal patient most in regard of her quality of life [14].

Bone window of the patient's CT scan disclosed not only bone marrow involvement but also bony destruction by her metastatic cancer. It is believed that receptor activator of nuclear factor kappa-B (RANK) and its ligand (RANKL) play an important role in activating osteoclasts which constitute a vicious cycle with tumor cells to make a favorable bone marrow microenvironment facilitating bony destruction and tumor growth. Furthermore, recent studies pointed out that RANKL participates in progesterone-mediated breast cancer development [15]. Anti-RANKL monoclonal antibody, denosumab, which was more efficient than zoledronic acid in preventing skeletal events in patients with bony metastasis from breast cancer and might have direct antitumor effect against breast cancer [16], thus should be integrated into the treatment plan for patients like ours if it is reimbursed in the medical insurance system.

Cancer metastasis develops through a multistep process involving complex cell-cell interactions in microenvironments of both original and metastatic sites. Seeding into bone marrow and resulting in bony metastasis need not only RANK-RANKL pathway but also many other biologic targeting and stimulating molecules to establish an ample bone-specific tropism, fuel osteolysis, osteoblastogenesis, and T-cell differentiation [17]. Candidate genes promoting bone-specific metastasis from breast cancer have been deeply investigated. One of them was chemokine interleukin-1β (IL-1β) which drives breast cancer cell growth, colonization in the bone marrow adipose tissue compartment, and bony metastasis [18, 19]. Whether our patient's tumor produces more IL-1β than her normal breast tissue is currently unknown, but the possibility of treating bone marrow metastasis from breast cancer with interleukin-1 receptor antagonist (IL-1Ra), for example, anakinra, cannot be overlooked [20]. Estradiol increases IL-1β and decreased

IL-1Ra in normal breast tissue. On the contrary, tamoxifen increases IL-1Ra significantly [21] and might to some degree act through this mechanism to achieve its amazing treatment effect in this patient.

Mucin 1 (MUC1) is a transmembrane glycoprotein functioning as an adhesion molecule which, in its circulating form, is identified as the serum tumor marker CA 15-3. MUC1 is confined to the basolateral surface of normal epithelial cells. Loss of this polarity during carcinogenesis makes MUC1 overexpressed in a hypoglycosylated form all over the surface of cancer cells, closely associated with growth factor receptors [22]. Adhesion of MUC1 to E-selectin and intercellular adhesion molecule-1 (ICAM-1) on the surface of endothelium activates Src oncogene and thus facilitates motility and metastatic potential of breast cancer cells [23]. We can assume that MUC1 is overexpressed in our patient's tumor cells based on her highly elevated serum CA 15-3 levels. Various MUC1 targeted therapies have been under development as inhibitors of cancer metastasis [24]. Despite the absence of benefit upon adding an anti-MUC1 antibody to letrozole for hormone receptor-positive metastatic breast cancer when compared with letrozole alone in a phase II trial [25], we do hope other therapeutic modalities against MUC1 might turn out to be helpful for patients like ours in the future.

Consent

Written informed consent was obtained from the patient and her husband for publication of this case report and any accompanying images.

References

[1] L. Xiao, S. Luxi, T. Ying, L. Yizhi, W. Lingyun, and P. Quan, "Diagnosis of unknown nonhematological tumors by bone marrow biopsy: a retrospective analysis of 10,112 samples," *Journal of Cancer Research and Clinical Oncology*, vol. 135, no. 5, pp. 687–693, 2009.

[2] B. B. Kucukzeybek, A. O. Calli, Y. Kucukzeybek et al., "The prognostic significance of bone marrow metastases: evaluation of 58 cases," *Indian Journal of Pathology & Microbiology*, vol. 57, no. 3, pp. 396–399, 2014.

[3] Q. S. Ringenberg, D. C. Doll, J. W. Yarbro, and M. C. Perry, "Tumors of unknown origin in the bone marrow," *Archives of Internal Medicine*, vol. 146, no. 10, pp. 2027-2028, 1986.

[4] F. Ozkalemkas, R. Ali, V. Ozkocaman et al., "The bone marrow aspirate and biopsy in the diagnosis of unsuspected nonhematologic malignancy: a clinical study of 19 cases," *BMC Cancer*, vol. 5, no. 1, p. 144, 2005.

[5] H. G. Kopp, K. Krauss, T. Fehm et al., "Symptomatic bone marrow involvement in breast cancer – clinical presentation, treatment, and prognosis: a single institution review of 22 cases," *Anticancer Research*, vol. 31, no. 11, pp. 4025–4030, 2011.

[6] D. M. Abd El-Rehim, S. E. Pinder, C. E. Paish et al., "Expression of luminal and basal cytokeratins in human breast carcinoma," *The Journal of Pathology*, vol. 203, no. 2, pp. 661–671, 2004.

[7] A. M. Gown, R. S. Fulton, and P. L. Kandalaft, "Markers of metastatic carcinoma of breast origin," *Histopathology*, vol. 68, no. 1, pp. 86–95, 2016.

[8] O. L. Tseng, J. J. Spinelli, C. C. Gotay, W. Y. Ho, M. L. McBride, and M. G. Dawes, "Aromatase inhibitors are associated with a higher fracture risk than tamoxifen: a systematic review and meta-analysis," *Therapeutic Advances in Musculoskeletal Disease*, vol. 10, no. 4, pp. 71–90, 2018.

[9] D. Plotkin, J. J. Lechner, W. E. Jung, and P. J. Rosen, "Tamoxifen flare in advanced breast cancer," *JAMA*, vol. 240, no. 24, pp. 2644–2646, 1978.

[10] S. Braun, F. D. Vogl, B. Naume et al., "A pooled analysis of bone marrow micrometastasis in breast cancer," *The New England Journal of Medicine*, vol. 353, no. 8, pp. 793–802, 2005.

[11] L. Demir, M. Akyol, S. Bener et al., "Prognostic evaluation of breast cancer patients with evident bone marrow metastasis," *The Breast Journal*, vol. 20, no. 3, pp. 279–287, 2014.

[12] V. Bjelic-Radisic, H. Stöger, R. Winter, C. Beham-Schmid, and E. Petru, "Long-term control of bone marrow carcinosis and severe thrombocytopenia with standard-dose chemotherapy in a breast cancer patient: a case report," *Anticancer Research*, vol. 26, no. 2B, pp. 1627–1630, 2006.

[13] F. Rastelli and S. Crispino, "Factors predictive of response to hormone therapy in breast cancer," *Tumori*, vol. 94, no. 3, pp. 370–383, 2008.

[14] G. A. Başaran, C. Twelves, V. Diéras, J. Cortés, and A. Awada, "Ongoing unmet needs in treating estrogen receptor-positive/HER2-negative metastatic breast cancer," *Cancer Treatment Reviews*, vol. 63, pp. 144–155, 2018.

[15] H. Azim and H. A. Azim Jr., "Targeting RANKL in breast cancer: bone metastasis and beyond," *Expert Review of Anticancer Therapy*, vol. 13, no. 2, pp. 195–201, 2013.

[16] A. F. de Groot, N. M. Appelman-Dijkstra, S. H. van der Burg, and J. R. Kroep, "The anti-tumor effect of RANKL inhibition in malignant solid tumors – a systematic review," *Cancer Treatment Reviews*, vol. 62, pp. 18–28, 2018.

[17] L. R. Patel, D. F. Camacho, Y. Shiozawa, K. J. Pienta, and R. S. Taichman, "Mechanisms of cancer cell metastasis to the bone: a multistep process," *Future Oncology*, vol. 7, no. 11, pp. 1285–1297, 2011.

[18] Z. S. Templeton, W. R. Lie, W. Wang et al., "Breast cancer cell colonization of the human bone marrow adipose tissue niche," *Neoplasia*, vol. 17, no. 12, pp. 849–861, 2015.

[19] I. Holen, D. V. Lefley, S. E. Francis et al., "IL-1 drives breast cancer growth and bone metastasis in vivo," *Oncotarget*, vol. 7, no. 46, pp. 75571–75584, 2016.

[20] C. A. Dinarello, "Why not treat human cancer with interleukin-1 blockade?," *Cancer Metastasis Reviews*, vol. 29, no. 2, pp. 317–329, 2010.

[21] A. Abrahamsson, V. Morad, N. M. Saarinen, and C. Dabrosin, "Estradiol, tamoxifen, and flaxseed alter IL-1β and IL-1Ra levels in normal human breast tissue in vivo," *The Journal of Clinical Endocrinology & Metabolism*, vol. 97, no. 11, pp. E2044–E2054, 2012.

[22] S. Nath and P. Mukherjee, "MUC1: a multifaceted oncoprotein with a key role in cancer progression," *Trends in Molecular Medicine*, vol. 20, no. 6, pp. 332–342, 2014.

[23] L. Haddon and J. Hugh, "MUC1-mediated motility in breast cancer: a review highlighting the role of the MUC1/ICAM-1/Src signaling triad," *Clinical & Experimental Metastasis*, vol. 32, no. 4, pp. 393–403, 2015.

[24] T. M. Horm and J. A. Schroeder, "MUC1 and metastatic cancer: expression, function and therapeutic targeting," *Cell Adhesion & Migration*, vol. 7, no. 2, pp. 187–198, 2013.

[25] N. K. Ibrahim, K. O. Yariz, I. Bondarenko et al., "Randomized phase II trial of letrozole plus anti-MUC1 antibody AS1402 in hormone receptor–positive locally advanced or metastatic breast cancer," *Clinical Cancer Research*, vol. 17, no. 21, pp. 6822–6830, 2011.

23

Systemic Mastocytosis with Smoldering Multiple Myeloma: Report of a Case

Sassine Ghanem,[1] Gwenalyn Garcia,[2] Liu Ying,[3] Matthew Hurford,[3] and Marcel Odaimi[2]

[1]*Department of Medicine, Staten Island University Hospital, Northwell Health, 475 Seaview Avenue, Staten Island, NY 10305, USA*
[2]*Department of Hematology/Oncology, Staten Island University Hospital, Northwell Health, 475 Seaview Avenue, Staten Island, NY 10305, USA*
[3]*Department of Pathology, Staten Island University Hospital, Northwell Health, 475 Seaview Avenue, Staten Island, NY 10305, USA*

Correspondence should be addressed to Sassine Ghanem; sghanem@northwell.edu

Academic Editor: Junya Kuroda

Systemic mastocytosis (SM) is a disease characterized by a clonal infiltration of mast cells affecting various tissues of the body. It is grouped into six different subtypes according to the World Health Organization classification. It is called indolent systemic mastocytosis (ISM) when there is no evidence of end organ dysfunction, while the presence of end organ dysfunction defines aggressive systemic mastocytosis (ASM). When SM coexists with a clonal hematological disorder, it is classified as systemic mastocytosis with associated clonal hematological nonmast cell lineage disease (SM-AHNMD). Over 80% of SM-AHNMD cases involve disorders of the myeloid cell lines. To our knowledge, there are only 8 reported cases to date of SM associated with a plasma cell disorder. We report a patient with ISM who was found to have concomitant smoldering multiple myeloma. His disease later progressed to ASM. We discuss this rare association between SM and a plasma cell disorder, and potential common pathophysiologic mechanisms linking the two disorders will be reviewed. We also discuss prognostic factors in SM as well as the management options considered during the evolution of the patient's disease.

1. Introduction

Mastocytosis is a disease characterized by the abnormal infiltration of clonally derived mast cells in different tissues of the body. When the infiltration is limited to the skin, a diagnosis of cutaneous mastocytosis is made. Extracutaneous infiltration of clonal mast cells defines systemic mastocytosis (SM). It typically involves the bone marrow but can also affect any other organ [1].

The classification for systemic mastocytosis was established by Valent et al. [1] in a consensus proposal and later adopted in the World Health Organization 2008 classification [2]. It recognizes six different groups of SM: indolent systemic mastocytosis (ISM), systemic mastocytosis with associated clonal hematological nonmast cell lineage disease (SM-AHNMD), aggressive systemic mastocytosis (ASM), mast cell leukemia, mast cell sarcoma, and extracutaneous mastocytoma. The difference between indolent and aggressive SM depends on the presence of C findings, which indicate organ dysfunction secondary to excessive mast cell infiltration. C findings include gastrointestinal malabsorption, hypersplenism, hepatic dysfunction, cytopenias, and pathologic fractures [1, 2].

In a retrospective study of 66 patients with SM, Travis et al. found SM-AHNMD to be the second most common subtype (after ISM), with 22 patients affected. Over 80% of SM-AHNMD cases involved disorders of the myeloid cell lines [3].

To our knowledge, there are only 8 reported cases to date of SM associated with a plasma cell disorder (Table 1) [4–11]. We present a patient with ISM with concomitant smoldering multiple myeloma whose disease later progressed to ASM.

2. Case Presentation

A 59-year-old male with a known history of ISM incidentally found on pathologic review after surgery for osteoarthritis was referred to the hematology clinic for evaluation of

TABLE 1: Previously reported cases of SM with an associated plasma cell disorder.

Reference	Age/sex	Diagnosis
Sotlar et al. [4]	70/M	SM and multiple myeloma with secondary amyloidosis
Du et al. [5]	57/F	SM, chronic lymphocytic leukemia, and multiple myeloma
Jain et al. [6]	64/F	ASM and refractory multiple myeloma
Filanovsky et al. [7]	76/M	ISM and smoldering multiple myeloma
Motwani et al. [8]	71/M	SM and multiple myeloma
Stellmacher et al. [9]	51/M	SM and multiple myeloma
Hagen et al. [10]	48/F	SM and multiple myeloma
Pullarkat et al. [11]	84/M	SM and monoclonal gammopathy of undetermined significance

SM: systemic mastocytosis; ISM: indolent systemic mastocytosis; ASM: aggressive systemic mastocytosis.

TABLE 2: Laboratory test results upon initial presentation.

Lab test	Result	Unit
White blood cells	5.3	$\times 10^3/mm^3$
Hemoglobin	14.5	g/dL
Platelet	202	$\times 10^3/mm^3$
Blood urea nitrogen	26	mg/dL
Creatinine	1.31	mg/dL
Albumin	3.1	g/dL
Globulin	6.2	g/dL
Calcium	8.8	mg/dL
Serum protein electrophoresis (SPEP) and serum immunofixation	IgG kappa monoclonal protein	
M-spike	3.68	g/dL

suspected monoclonal gammopathy. His past medical history was significant for splenectomy. The exact indication for the procedure was unclear, but it was possibly done for involvement with lymphoma versus mastocytosis. He presented with suspected monoclonal gammopathy on previously done blood tests with the results shown in Table 2. His physical exam revealed no abnormalities.

Repeat serum protein electrophoresis and immunofixation again revealed an IgG kappa monoclonal protein. The M-spike was 3.8 g/dL. The serum IgG level was elevated at 4430 mg/dL, while IgA and IgM levels were within the normal range. Serum free kappa light chains were elevated at 203.1 mg/L with normal free lambda light chains of 9.4 mg/L and a free kappa/lambda ratio of 21.61. LDH was normal at 145 IU/L and beta-2 microglobulin was elevated at 3.8 mg/L. The tryptase level was elevated at 76 ng/mL.

Bone marrow aspiration and biopsy was performed, which showed an overall cellularity of 60–90%. Approximately 50% of the marrow was comprised of nodules of small mononuclear spindle cells (Figure 1(a)). Immunostains were positive for CD68, CD45, CD117, CD30, CD25, and M-tryptase but negative for CD56, consistent with a mast cell phenotype.

Plasma cells occupied at least 30% of the remaining marrow (Figure 1(b)). They were CD138 positive by immunohistochemistry (Figure 1(c)) and kappa restricted by *in situ* hybridization. Flow cytometry of the bone marrow aspirate detected a monoclonal IgG kappa plasma cell population comprising 4.7% of total cells in the sample. Cytogenetics testing revealed a normal male karyotype negative for mutations associated with multiple myeloma. Amyloid staining was negative.

Based on the above-mentioned morphology and immunohistochemical and molecular studies, in addition to the fact that the patient had no anemia, a normal calcium level, and no bone pain, a final diagnosis of ISM associated with smoldering multiple myeloma was established. The patient was followed up without specific treatment for either condition. An abdominal fat pad biopsy was done to rule out secondary amyloidosis as the cause of his chronic kidney disease, which came back negative.

Two years later, the patient presented to the emergency department with a 2-day history of generalized weakness, shortness of breath, and melena. A nasogastric lavage was done and showed bloody fluid. CBC on admission showed hemoglobin of 5.9 g/dL; WBC and platelet counts were within normal limits. The patient's coagulation parameters revealed a prolonged PT of >40 sec with an INR of >15 and a prolonged PTT of 65.6 sec. Of note, the patient was on anticoagulation with warfarin for atrial fibrillation. His transaminases and total bilirubin levels were within normal limits.

The patient received packed red cell and fresh frozen plasma transfusions. Emergent upper endoscopy showed grade IV gastroesophageal varices requiring band ligation. Severe hypertensive portal gastropathy was also found.

The patient had no known history of or obvious risk factors for liver cirrhosis; hence, workup was initiated for possible causes of portal hypertension. Ultrasound of the abdomen showed a normal sized liver with smooth contour and normal echogenicity. The portal and hepatic veins were both patent. There was small volume abdominal ascites. Screening for viral hepatitis was negative. Serum ceruloplasmin, alpha-1 antitrypsin, and ferritin levels were within normal limits. Testing for c-ANCA, p-ANCA, antimitochondrial, and antismooth muscle antibodies was negative.

Subsequently, liver biopsy was performed, which showed portal and periportal fibrosis with mild inflammation, compression of the portal veins, broad fibrous septa, and severe perisinusoidal fibrosis, confirmed by trichrome and reticulin stains. There was focal nodule formation. CD117 immunostaining demonstrated abundant mast cells in portal tracts. Rare cells were positive for CD25 and mast cell tryptase (Figure 2). Serum tryptase level was 104 ng/mL. These findings

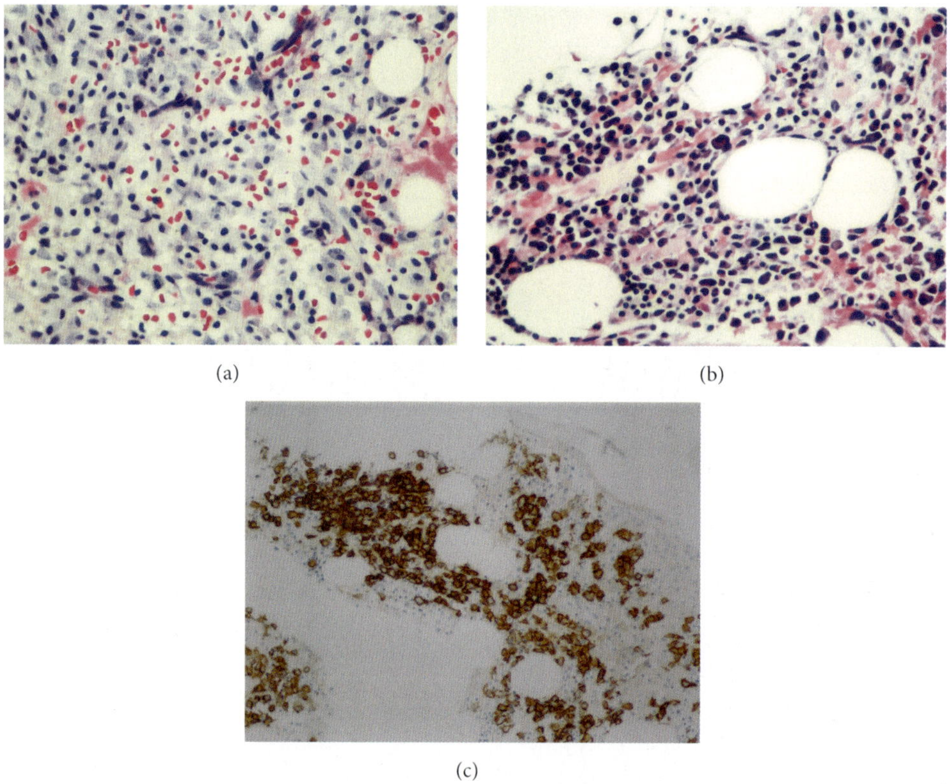

FIGURE 1: Bone marrow biopsy showing an infiltrate of spindle-shaped mast cells (a) comprising 50% of the marrow. Plasma cell infiltrate (b) occupying 30% of the remaining marrow, with an image showing CD138 staining (c).

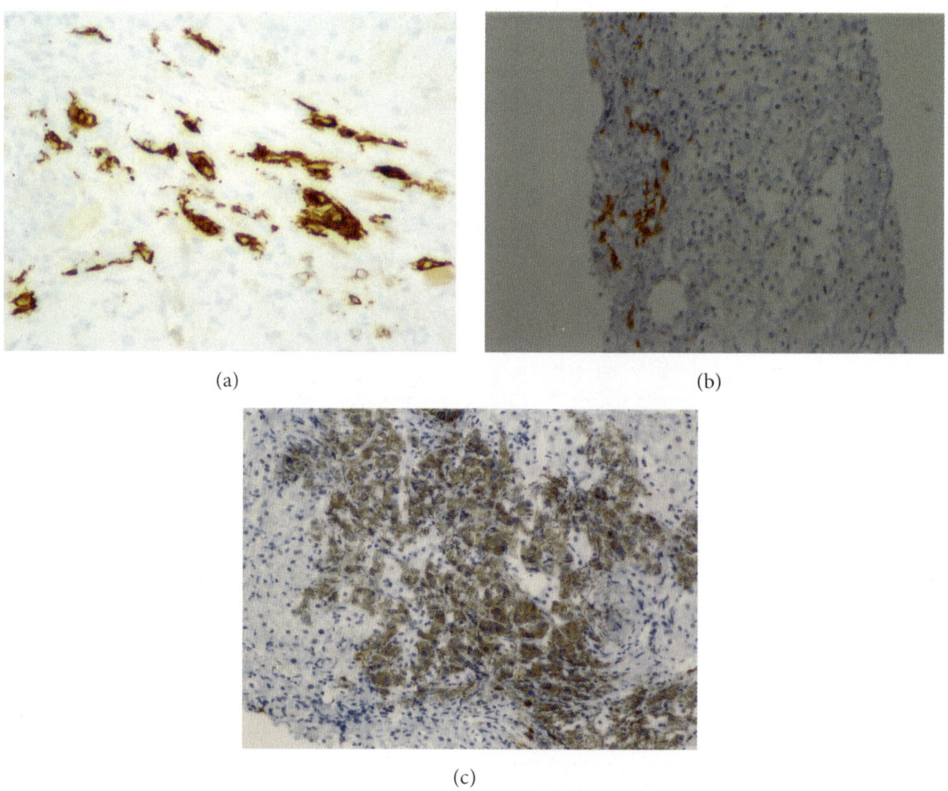

FIGURE 2: Liver biopsy immunohistochemical staining showing mast cells positive for CD117 (a), CD25 (b), and mast cell tryptase (c). Of note, (c) is zoomed in on the portion of the liver that is positive for mast cells.

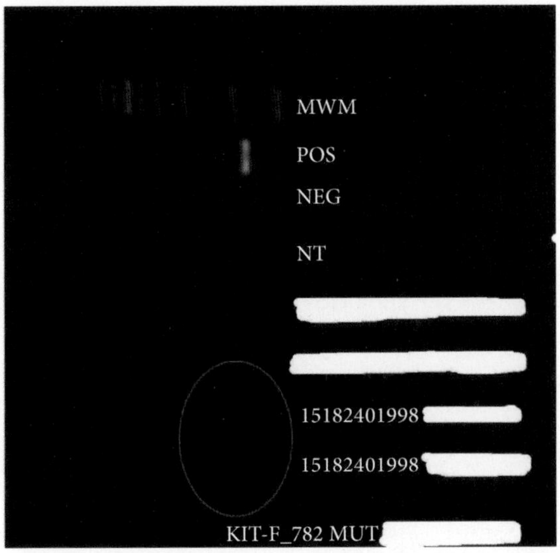

FIGURE 3: Sequence analysis of the KIT D816V mutation.

were consistent with mastocytosis involving the liver, resulting in extensive fibrosis. The patient's disease had progressed to ASM, and a course of treatment with cladribine as outpatient was recommended.

Subsequently, the patient followed up at a different institution where further evaluation showed a negative JAK 2 mutation and a positive KIT D816V mutation (Figure 3). A kidney biopsy was also performed to rule out secondary amyloidosis or multiple myeloma as the etiology of his chronic kidney disease; this showed interstitial fibrosis and tubular atrophy as well as features of thrombotic microangiopathy without any amyloid or immune-type deposits. The treating team however linked the chronic kidney disease to multiple myeloma and therefore started him on a treatment regimen of cyclophosphamide, bortezomib, and dexamethasone as well as hydroxyurea for the systemic mastocytosis. The patient tolerated therapy and only has complaints of fatigue in the days that follow the chemotherapy session.

3. Discussion

Criteria for the diagnosis of SM include 1 major criterion and 4 minor criteria. The major criterion is a multifocal dense infiltrate of mast cells (≥15 mast cells in aggregates) in sections from bone marrow and/or extracutaneous organs. The 4 minor criteria are as follows: (1) >25% of the mast cells in the infiltrate with spindle-shaped or atypical morphology or >25% of all mast cells in bone marrow aspirate smears characterized as immature or atypical, (2) presence of an activating point mutation at codon 816 of KIT, (3) expression of CD2 and/or CD25 in mast cells, and (4) total serum tryptase levels persistently exceeding 20 ng/mL. The first 3 minor criteria apply to samples obtained from blood, bone marrow, or other extracutaneous organs. The last criterion is not valid if there is an associated clonal myeloid disorder. The presence of the major criterion and 1 minor criterion or the presence of 3 minor criteria is required to establish the diagnosis of SM [2].

On evaluation in our clinic, the patient had a tryptase level of 76 ng/mL and a bone marrow biopsy showing CD25+ spindle-shaped mast cells occupying approximately 50% of the bone marrow, fulfilling the diagnostic criteria for SM. His bone marrow biopsy also showed CD138+ plasma cells occupying 30% of the remaining bone marrow. With this bone marrow finding along with a serum M-spike of 3.8 g/dL and the absence of end organ damage, the patient was diagnosed with concomitant smoldering multiple myeloma.

The coexistence of SM with multiple myeloma places our patient in the SM-AHNMD subtype. While associated myeloid/myelomonocytic neoplasia in SM-AHNMD accounts for 82%–89% of SM-AHNMD, associated lymphoproliferative disorders are rare [3, 4]. In their study of 138 cases of SM-AHNMD, Pardanani et al. found 7 patients (5.1%) with lymphoma, 5 patients (3.6%) with myeloma, and 2 patients (1.5%) with chronic lymphocytic leukemia (CLL) [12].

Since multiple myeloma occurring in an elderly patient is not uncommon, one could argue that the cooccurrence of SM with smoldering multiple myeloma was a coincidence. However, *in vitro* studies have shown the capacity of neoplastic mast cells to induce the growth of lymphocytic neoplasms. Tournilhac et al. demonstrated that the human mast cell line HMC-1 stimulated proliferation of the malignant lymphoplasmacytic cells of patients with Waldenstrom's macroglobulinemia through interactions between CD154 on the mast cells and CD40 on the lymphoplasmacytic cells [13]. *In vitro* studies also suggest a role of mast cells in the growth of Hodgkin lymphoma via their expression of CD30 ligand [14]. A similar relationship may exist between mast cells and plasma cells as well. Mast cells secrete multiple cytokines including IL-6 and stem cell factor, both of which have been shown to induce plasma cell proliferation [15–17].

Whether or not the neoplastic mast cells of SM and the associated hematologic malignancy are derived from the same clone has been examined. In 2 cases of SM associated with lymphoproliferative disorders, the D816V mutation was detected in the neoplastic mast cells but not in the malignant lymphocytes, suggesting that the SM and the coexisting lymphoid malignancy are clonally distinct [18, 19]. In contrast, in cases of acute myeloid leukemia, the leukemic translocation t(8;21) can be detected in the malignant myeloid cells as well as in the neoplastic mast cells. Therefore, they are presumed to have developed from the same clone [20, 21].

When confronted with cases of SM-AHNMD, the current strategy is to treat each entity on its own as if the other entity did not coexist in the patient [22–24]. With an M-spike greater than 3 g/dL but no myeloma-defining event such as anemia, hypercalcemia, bony disease, or renal insufficiency secondary to myeloma, our patient fit into the diagnosis of smoldering multiple myeloma, and management of his disease was close clinical monitoring for transformation to symptomatic multiple myeloma.

In SM, the difference between indolent and aggressive disease depends on the presence of C findings, which indicate organ dysfunction related to mast cell invasion. The patient's left hip replacement was performed for degenerative joint disease and no pathological fracture had occurred. Therefore, the finding of mast cells in the surgical specimen was incidental. In addition, the pathological finding of mast cells on the bone marrow biopsy was also an incidental finding during workup of the patient's hypergammaglobulinemia. Symptoms associated with mast cell degranulation, such as urticaria, flushing, or diarrhea, were also not present in the patient's history. The patient was therefore considered as having ISM.

The clinical presentation of patients with SM is highly variable. Thus, decisions regarding whether or not to initiate treatment are often complex. Patients with ISM rarely exhibit leukemic transformation and their life expectancy is not significantly different from the age- and sex-matched US population, as demonstrated in a retrospective study by Lim et al. on 342 patients with SM [25]. Thus, the treatment of ISM is mainly symptom-oriented [26]. Lim et al. also identified advanced age (defined as ≥65 years), weight loss, anemia, thrombocytopenia, hypoalbuminemia, and excess bone marrow blasts as independent adverse prognostic factors for survival [25]. Similarly, a retrospective study done by Butterfield and Weiler on 42 elderly patients with SM reported poor survival outcomes in patients with concomitant thrombocytopenia, leukemias, and myelodysplastic syndrome [27]. As our patient was asymptomatic with no poor prognostic factors, he was not treated for ISM on his initial presentation.

With the patient developing esophageal variceal bleed from portal hypertension due to a mast cell infiltrated liver, he was reclassified as having ASM, in which the primary goal of therapy is reducing the mast cell burden. Treatment options that have been studied in nonrandomized trials include hydroxyurea, interferon-alfa with or without prednisone, imatinib, and cladribine. A retrospective study by Lim et al. on 108 patients with SM favored interferon-alfa and cladribine as first line therapy, as hydroxyurea and imatinib were associated with lower overall response rates [28]. Imatinib is relatively ineffective in patients with SM who have a mutation of KIT D816V [29]. This patient therefore was a poor candidate for imatinib, and the lack of randomized controlled trials with evidence favoring one treatment over the others justified the use of hydroxyurea in this patient. A global phase II trial of the use of midostaurin, an oral multikinase inhibitor of both wild-type and D816-mutated KIT, is currently underway with primary results showing high overall response rates with reduction in mast cell burden, a favorable safety profile, as well as improvement in symptoms and quality of life [30]. Seeing this as the largest prospective trial in advanced systemic mastocytosis, midostaurin may become the future standard of care.

In summary, we report the case of a 59-year-old man who initially presented to our clinic with ISM associated with smoldering multiple myeloma. Using the 2008 WHO classification, he was diagnosed with SM-AHNMD. For both diseases, the clinical approach was close follow up until 2 years later when the patient progressed to ASM as evidenced by esophageal variceal bleed secondary to portal hypertension from mast cell infiltration of the liver. The patient was then offered cytoreductive therapy. The association of plasma cell disorders with systemic mastocytosis is rare and the neoplastic cells are believed to be derived from distinct clones. Some postulate that cytokines secreted by the neoplastic mast cells induce the proliferation of plasma cells. The treatment for each disease is planned as if the other did not coexist in the same patient.

Consent

A written and signed consent to publish the information was obtained from the patient prior to submission of the paper.

References

[1] P. Valent, H.-P. Horny, L. Escribano et al., "Diagnostic criteria and classification of mastocytosis: a consensus proposal," *Leukemia Research*, vol. 25, no. 7, pp. 603–625, 2001.

[2] H. P. Horny, J. M. Bennett, B. J. Bain et al., "Mastocytosis," in *WHO Classification of Tumours of Haematopoietic and Lymphoid Tissues*, S. H. Swerdlow, S. H. Camp, E. Harris et al., Eds., pp. 54–63, International Agency for Research on Cancer, Lyon, France, 4th edition, 2008.

[3] W. D. Travis, C.-Y. Li, L. T. Yam, E. J. Bergstralh, and R. G. Swee, "Significance of systemic mast cell disease with associated hematologic disorders," *Cancer*, vol. 62, no. 5, pp. 965–972, 1988.

[4] K. Sotlar, W. Saeger, F. Stellmacher et al., "'Occult' mastocytosis with activating c-kit point mutation evolving into systemic mastocytosis associated with plasma cell myeloma and secondary amyloidosis," *Journal of Clinical Pathology*, vol. 59, no. 8, pp. 875–878, 2006.

[5] S. Du, H. H. Rashidi, D. T. Le et al., "Systemic mastocytosis in association with chronic lymphocytic leukemia and plasma cell myeloma," *International Journal of Clinical and Experimental Pathology*, vol. 3, no. 4, pp. 448–457, 2010.

[6] P. Jain, S. Verstovsek, R. Z. Orlowski, E. Yap, and H. M. Amin, "An unusual case of aggressive systemic mastocytosis with associated refractory plasma cell myeloma," *Clinical Lymphoma, Myeloma and Leukemia*, vol. 12, no. 6, pp. 459–462, 2012.

[7] K. Filanovsky, S. Lev, M. Haran et al., "Systemic mastocytosis associated with smoldering multiple myeloma: an unexpected diagnosis in a patient with a rash," *Leukemia & Lymphoma*, vol. 51, no. 6, pp. 1152–1154, 2010.

[8] P. Motwani, M. Kocoglu, and R. B. Lorsbach, "Systemic mastocytosis in association with plasma cell dyscrasias: report of a case and review of the literature," *Leukemia Research*, vol. 33, no. 6, pp. 856–859, 2009.

[9] F. Stellmacher, K. Sotlar, L. Balleisen, P. Valent, and H.-P. Horny, "Bone marrow mastocytosis associated with IgM kappa plasma cell myeloma," *Leukemia and Lymphoma*, vol. 45, no. 4, pp. 801–805, 2004.

[10] W. Hagen, J. Schwarzmeier, S. Walchshofer et al., "A case of bone marrow mastocytosis associated with multiple myeloma," *Annals of Hematology*, vol. 76, no. 3-4, pp. 167–174, 1998.

[11] S. T. Pullarkat, F. Sedarat, R. Paquette, and J. Said, "Systemic mastocytosis with plasma cell dyscrasia: report of a case," *Leukemia Research*, vol. 32, no. 7, pp. 1160–1163, 2008.

[12] A. Pardanani, K.-H. Lim, T. L. Lasho et al., "Prognostically relevant breakdown of 123 patients with systemic mastocytosis associated with other myeloid malignancies," *Blood*, vol. 114, no. 18, pp. 3769–3772, 2009.

[13] O. Tournilhac, D. D. Santos, L. Xu et al., "Mast cells in Waldenstrom's macroglobulinemia support lymphoplasmacytic cell growth through CD154/CD40 signaling," *Annals of Oncology*, vol. 17, no. 8, pp. 1275–1282, 2006.

[14] D. Molin, M. Fischer, Z. Xiang et al., "Mast cells express functional CD30 ligand and are the predominant CD30L-positive cells in Hodgkin's disease," *British Journal of Haematology*, vol. 114, no. 3, pp. 616–623, 2001.

[15] R. Bataille, M. Jourdan, X.-G. Zhang, and B. Klein, "Serum levels of interleukin 6, a potent myeloma cell growth factor, as a reflect of disease severity in plasma cell dyscrasias," *Journal of Clinical Investigation*, vol. 84, no. 6, pp. 2008–2011, 1989.

[16] R. M. Lemoli, A. Fortuna, A. Grande et al., "Expression and functional role of c-kit ligand (SCF) in human multiple myeloma cells," *British Journal of Haematology*, vol. 88, no. 4, pp. 760–769, 1994.

[17] T. C. Theoharides, K.-D. Alysandratos, A. Angelidou et al., "Mast cells and inflammation," *Biochimica et Biophysica Acta (BBA)—Molecular Basis of Disease*, vol. 1822, no. 1, pp. 21–33, 2012.

[18] H.-P. Horny, K. Sotlar, F. Stellmacher, P. Valent, and J. Grabbe, "An unusual case of systemic mastocytosis associated with chronic lymphocytic leukaemia (SM-CLL)," *Journal of Clinical Pathology*, vol. 59, no. 3, pp. 264–268, 2006.

[19] Y. Kim, L. M. Weiss, Y.-Y. Chen, and V. Pullarkat, "Distinct clonal origins of systemic mastocytosis and associated B-cell lymphoma," *Leukemia Research*, vol. 31, no. 12, pp. 1749–1754, 2007.

[20] V. Pullarkat, V. Bedell, Y. Kim et al., "Neoplastic mast cells in systemic mastocytosis associated with t(8;21) acute myeloid leukemia are derived from the leukemic clone," *Leukemia Research*, vol. 31, no. 2, pp. 261–265, 2007.

[21] W. R. Sperr, J. Drach, A. W. Hauswirth et al., "Myelomastocytic leukemia: evidence for the origin of mast cells from the leukemic clone and eradication by allogeneic stem cell transplantation," *Clinical Cancer Research*, vol. 11, no. 19 I, pp. 6787–6792, 2005.

[22] P. Valent, C. Akin, W. R. Sperr et al., "Mastocytosis: pathology, genetics, and current options for therapy," *Leukemia and Lymphoma*, vol. 46, no. 1, pp. 35–48, 2005.

[23] W. R. Sperr and P. Valent, "Diagnosis, progression patterns and prognostication in mastocytosis," *Expert Review of Hematology*, vol. 5, no. 3, pp. 261–274, 2012.

[24] M. Arock and P. Valent, "Pathogenesis, classification and treatment of mastocytosis: state of the art in 2010 and future perspectives," *Expert Review of Hematology*, vol. 3, no. 4, pp. 497–516, 2010.

[25] K.-H. Lim, A. Tefferi, T. L. Lasho et al., "Systemic mastocytosis in 342 consecutive adults: survival studies and prognostic factors," *Blood*, vol. 113, no. 23, pp. 5727–5736, 2009.

[26] A. Pardanani, "How I treat patients with indolent and smoldering mastocytosis (rare conditions but difficult to manage)," *Blood*, vol. 121, no. 16, pp. 3085–3094, 2013.

[27] J. H. Butterfield and C. R. Weiler, "Systemic mastocytosis in the elderly," *American Journal of Hematology*, vol. 88, no. 5, pp. 406–408, 2013.

[28] K. H. Lim, A. Pardanani, J. H. Butterfield, C.-Y. Li, and A. Tefferi, "Cytoreductive therapy in 108 adults with systemic mastocytosis: outcome analysis and response prediction during treatment with interferon-alpha, hydroxyurea, imatinib mesylate or 2-chlorodeoxyadenosine," *American Journal of Hematology*, vol. 84, no. 12, pp. 790–794, 2009.

[29] A. Vega-Ruiz, J. E. Cortes, M. Sever et al., "Phase II study of imatinib mesylate as therapy for patients with systemic mastocytosis," *Leukemia Research*, vol. 33, no. 11, pp. 1481–1484, 2009.

[30] J. Gotlib, H. C. Kluin-Nelemans, T. I. George et al., "Demonstrates a high rate of durable responses in patients with advanced systemic mastocytosis: results from the fully accrued global phase 2 CPKC412D2201 trial," in *Proceedings of the 56th Annual Meeting of the American Society of Hematology*, vol. 124, no. 21, p. 636, San Francisco, Calif, USA, December 2014.

24

Misdiagnosis of a Giant Uterine Leiomyosarcoma: Clinic and Image Challenges

Jila Agah,[1] Sedighe Karimzadeh,[2] and Fateme Moharrer Ahmadi[2]

[1]*Department of Obstetrics and Gynecology, Faculty of Medicine, Sabzevar University of Medical Sciences, Sabzevar, Iran*
[2]*School of Medicine, Sabzevar University of Medical Sciences, Sabzevar, Iran*

Correspondence should be addressed to Jila Agah; jilaagah@yahoo.com

Academic Editor: Jeanine M. Buchanich

A 41-year-old woman ($G_3P_2L_2Ab_1$) was referred to gynecology clinic with chief complaints of abdominal distension and localized abdominal wall pruritus for three months. She was misdiagnosed with gastrointestinal disorder and ultimately had undergone imaging. Ultrasonography and computed tomography (CT) scan disclosed a huge solid-cystic mass originating from the ovary. On clinical examination the patient had no pain or tenderness and no gynecologic complaints. Laboratory tests showed normal tumor markers and hemoglobin at 8 g/dl. Laparotomy was carried out as diagnosis of ovarian serous cyst adenoma, but a huge tumor with attachment to uterus and ovaries and extension to pelvic floor, peripheral tissues of ureter, and upper abdomen was found. Hysterectomy with bilateral salpingooophorectomy was done. Pathology report demonstrated uterine leiomyosarcoma measuring 40 centimeters and weighing 10 kilograms. In conclusion, as pelvic masses even in a large size may present unspecific symptoms misdiagnosis may occur which lead to overgrowth, local invasion, or other complications. So, it is rather to suggest ultrasonography in patients with persistent abdominal or pelvic symptoms and if needed, more exact diagnostic modalities like magnetic resonance imaging (MRI) could be offered to avoid misdiagnosis and mismanagement.

1. Introduction

Pelvic masses are common findings in general gynecology [1]. Benign leiomyomas are the most uterine neoplastic mass which manifest clinically in about 30% of women older than 35 years [2]. Uterine sarcomas include 8% of all uterine malignancies with an incidence of about 0.4 per 100,000 women where leiomyosarcoma (LMS) consists 40% of them [3]. It occurs mostly in the 45–55 years of age. Leiomyosarcomas usually arise de novo from uterine smooth muscles; however rarely they may appear in a preexisting leiomyoma (0.2% of the cases) [4]. The gold standard of treatment for LMS is hysterectomy [5, 6]. Most leiomyosarcomas are accompanied with pain, sensation of pressure, and abnormal uterine bleeding or present only as a rapidly enlarging mass [7]. However, many imaging modalities are available and easy to accelerate the diagnosis; still some gigantic tumors are going to be neglected. Moreover, sometimes these tumors are erroneously reported as ovarian masses on imaging follow-up which can induce severe challenges for surgeon during operation. Herein we represent a huge uterine leiomyosarcoma mismanaged with incorrect diagnosis of dyspepsia for over two months and afterwards operated as misdiagnosis of ovarian mass reported in images.

2. Case Presentation

A 41-year-old woman ($G_3P_2L_2Ab_1$) was referred to gynecology clinic with chief complaints of abdominal distension and localized abdominal pruritus for three months. To rule out gastrointestinal disorders, she had visited a general physician given her symptoms. But she found no response to the drugs in spite of a long-term usage and was referred to our clinic after taking ultrasonography. Her past history showed menorrhagia but not menstrual irregularity and dysmenorrhea for several months. Laboratory tests including hemoglobin at 8 g/dl, hematocrit at 28,7%, ferritin at 6 ng/ml, and iron at 29 mcg/dl approved this claim but the patient had not expressed it initially as a complaint. Vital signs were in normal limits. In general appearance, the patient

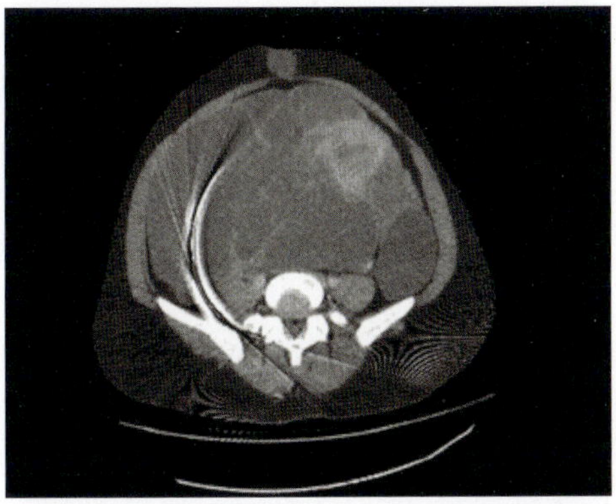

FIGURE 1: Intravenous contrast CT scan showing a large septated solid-cystic mass with report of serous cyst adenoma.

was not cachectic with full activity without vertigo, impairing appetite, constipation, nausea, vomiting, and urinary symptoms, but a distended abdomen that lacks rebound and tenderness. The origin of the mass was not detectable by vaginal examination. Ultrasonography had revealed a huge multicystic septated mass, 40 cm in diameter in abdominal cavity, probably a serous cystadenoma originating from ovary that was extended to epigastric area. Uterine and bladder were reported normal; however, these were impressed by extrinsic pressure of the mass. Uterine observation was not possible with vaginal sonography due to huge ovarian tumor. Tumor markers including cancer antigen-125, carcinoembryonic antigen, αFP, and CA19-9 were all within normal limits. Further assessment by computed tomography (CT) scan was done to show the nature of tumor which approved the diagnosis of ovarian serous cyst adenoma (Figure 1); other viscera like kidneys, spleen, and liver were all in normal status; no free fluid and no lymphadenopathy were observed in abdominal cavity. Chest X-ray also did not show any lesion. The patient was hospitalized and advised with operation. The surgery was performed under general anesthesia through a vertical incision. Laparotomy revealed a huge multilocular mass with firm consistency, originating from pelvic with extension to adjacent tissues like ureter and upward to diaphragm with adhesion to ovaries and uterine. Obviously, gentle adhesiolysis to avoid damage to ureter and intestine took a long time. The whole solid-multicystic tumor measuring 40 cm and weighing 10 kg and with attached uterine and ovaries was removed (Figure 2). Lymph nodes and other visceral organs were normal. Regarding previous chronic anemia of the patient, transfusion of two-packed cell-blood was done. Patient's weight was 82 kg before operation and 69 kg subsequently. Three days later, the patient was discharged in a good health status. Pathology report showed uterine leiomyosarcoma (Figure 3). The CT scan for patient's follow-up presents no metastatic mass and lymph node involvement. The patient is under observation and has no problem in one year.

3. Discussion

Leiomyosarcomas (LMS) are the most common sarcomatous malignancies of uterus that represent 1-2% of all uterine

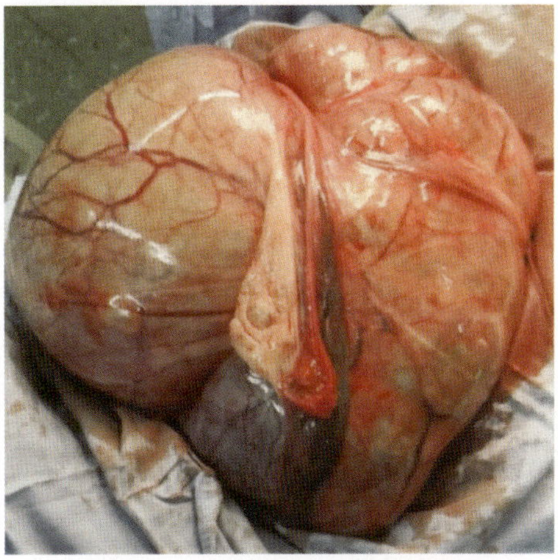

FIGURE 2: Gross appearance of tumor.

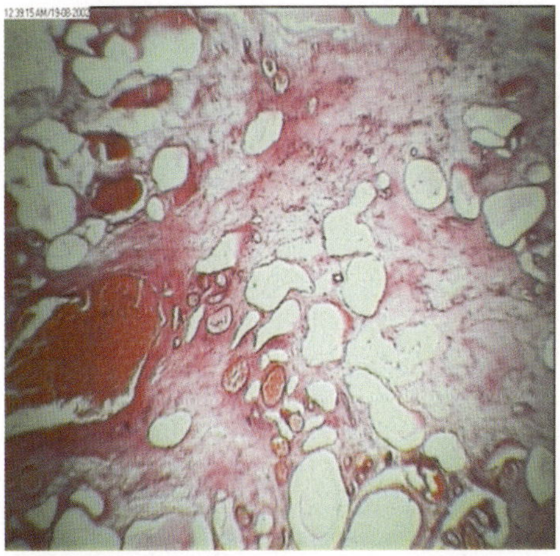

FIGURE 3: Microscopic appearance of tumor cells.

malignancies [8, 9]. Most patients with leiomyosarcoma have no recognizable risk factors. Patients who carry a germ line p53 gene mutation (Li-Fraumeni syndrome) have an increased risk of soft tissue cancers, including uterine LMS [10]. Some studies have suggested an increased risk for uterine sarcoma among women with obesity and also diabetes [11]. Our case had no identifiable risk factor except her BMI which was 27 kg/m^2.

The absolute diagnosis of uterine leiomyosarcoma is made by histologic confirmation. In most cases, the diagnosis of these tumors is made by specimen examination in hysterectomized patients who was managed as leiomyoma [5, 12].

The main treatment of LMS is surgical excision which consists of total abdominal hysterectomy and debulking of any tumor invading outside the uterus. It is considered appropriate to preserve ovaries in young women and routine dissection of pelvic and para-aortic lymph nodes, since lymph node involvement is seen in less than 3% of patients [13]. Its five-year survival rate varies from 18.8% to 68% and the risk of recurrence is reported from 45% to 73% [4]. As sarcomas are very aggressive tumors and have the propensity for early hematogenous spread, recurrence and relapse can occur even in completely resected tumors. So it is recommended to prescribe adjuvant chemotherapy in nonmetastatic cases by some authors. The utility of systemic lymph node dissection and adjuvant radiotherapy (RT) in the treatment of uterine LMS remains unclear. Although radiotherapy for reduction of local recurrence and/or chemotherapy for managing distant metastasis have been stated, the literature shows no efficacy concerning overall survival by these modalities actually. Anyway, attention to quality of life which may be influenced by the side effects and toxicity of adjuvant therapy is mandatory [8, 14]. Most cases include women over 40 years old, who are usually referred with abnormal vaginal bleeding (56%), palpable pelvic mass (54%), and pelvic pain (22%) [15]. Kaur et al. reported postmenopausal bleeding and lower abdominal pain in a 60-year-old female with uterine leiomyosarcoma while our patient had no gynecologic problem and no pain [8]. Senol et al. reported a very large leiomyosarcoma in a 62-year-old female presenting with abdominal mass, fatigue, and associated tenderness [16]. Vellanki et al. also reported a uterine leiomyosarcoma in a 40-year-old nulliparous woman presenting with abdominal pain and no menstrual irregularity and no vaginal bleeding [17]; our patient had no vaginal bleeding and no abdominal pain, just complains from 3 months' period of abdominal distension attributed to gastrointestinal diseases. However, abdominal distension is usually attributed to gastrointestinal diseases which leads to misdiagnosis, mismanagement, and overgrowth of tumor [18]. So, it would be reasonable to take an exact history to find out associated symptoms like menorrhagia seen in our case. Besides obtaining a complete history, physical examination, advising appropriate laboratory tests and imaging procedures, is very mandatory particularly in patients who do not respond to usual medications. In this case, severe anemia could be regarded as an alarm sign for her physician if detected. Ultrasonography is considered more appropriate as the first modality for detection of abdominopelvic mass, because it is harmless, available, inexpensive, and applicable by all radiologists and many gynecologists. It cannot reliably determine the origin of huge masses, the nature of malignancy point, and probable invasion of adjacent organs. The role of magnetic resonance imaging (MRI) is developing in the assessment of malignancies. leiomyosarcomas commonly manifest as large infiltrating myometrial mass on MRI with irregular and ill-defined margins and heterogeneous hypointensity on T1-weighted images and also hemorrhage, necrosis, and foci of calcifications may make heterogeneous features of enhancement which can be a hallmark for differentiating from benign leiomyomas [4, 19]. Researchers believe that the sensitivity of MRI for distinguishing the nature and origin of pelvic masses is more than CT scan [4, 20]. To verify, CT scan determined the abovementioned characteristics of the mass in our case but could not define its origin correctly. Subsequently, the patient was operated with diagnosis of ovarian serous cyst adenoma. However, the main advantage of CT scan is that it is cheaper than MRI and more tolerable for patients [4, 20].

In conclusion, pelvic masses even in a large size may be without any specific symptoms. Delay in diagnosis may lead to overgrowth, torsion, or hemorrhagic tear of tumors and invasion to surrounding visceral organs. So, it is considered more appropriate to suggest ultrasonography in patients with persistent abdominal pain or distension who do not respond to recommended drugs and in case of presence of a mass, MRI as a preferable imaging could be offered to avoid misdiagnosis.

Acknowledgments

The authors would like to thank the authorities and the staff of Mobini Hospital for their contribution and cooperation in performing the patient follow-up.

References

[1] B. Kamalimanesh, R. J. Esfehani, and J. Agah, "Papillary serous cystadenoma of ovary: a huge ovarian cyst complicating the pregnancy".

[2] N. Fasih, A. K. P. Shanbhogue, D. B. Macdonald et al., "Leiomyomas beyond the uterus: unusual locations, rare manifestations," *Radiographics*, vol. 28, no. 7, pp. 1931–1948, 2008.

[3] R. Koivisto-Korander, J. I. Martinsen, E. Weiderpass, A. Leminen, and E. Pukkala, "Incidence of uterine leiomyosarcoma and endometrial stromal sarcoma in Nordic countries: results from NORDCAN and NOCCA databases," *Maturitas*, vol. 72, no. 1, pp. 56–60, 2012.

[4] P. Santos and T. M. Cunha, "Uterine sarcomas: Clinical presentation and MRI features," *Diagnostic and Interventional Radiology*, vol. 21, no. 1, pp. 4–9, 2015.

[5] H. K. Sait, N. M. Anfinan, M. E. El Sayed et al., "Uterine sarcoma: Clinico-pathological characteristics and outcome," *Saudi Medical Journal*, vol. 35, no. 10, pp. 1215–1222, 2014.

[6] A. Gadducci, S. Cosio, A. Romanini, and A. R. Genazzani, "The management of patients with uterine sarcoma: a debated clinical challenge," *Critical Reviews in Oncology/Hematology*, vol. 65, no. 2, pp. 129–142, 2008.

[7] O. Zivanovic, M. M. Leitao, A. Iasonos et al., "Stage-specific outcomes of patients with uterine leiomyosarcoma: a comparison of the international Federation of gynecology and obstetrics and american joint committee on cancer staging systems," *Journal of Clinical Oncology*, vol. 27, no. 12, pp. 2066–2072, 2009.

[8] P. Kaur, A. Kaur, A. Singla, and K. Kaur, "Uterine leiomyosarcoma: A case report," *Journal of Mid-life Health*, vol. 5, no. 4, p. 200, 2014.

[9] S. E. Brooks, M. Zhan, T. Cote, and C. R. Baquet, "Surveillance, epidemiology, and end results analysis of 2677 cases of uterine sarcoma 1989–1999," *Gynecologic Oncology*, vol. 93, no. 1, pp. 204–208, 2004.

[10] K. D. Gonzalez, K. A. Noltner, C. H. Buzin et al., "Beyond li fraumeni syndrome: clinical characteristics of families with p53 germline mutations," *Journal of Clinical Oncology*, vol. 27, no. 8, pp. 1250–1256, 2009.

[11] A. S. Felix, L. S. Cook, M. M. Gaudet et al., "The etiology of uterine sarcomas: a pooled analysis of the epidemiology of endometrial cancer consortium," *British journal of cancer*, vol. 108, no. 3, pp. 727–734, 2013.

[12] S. Sagae, K. Yamashita, S. Ishioka et al., "Preoperative diagnosis and treatment results in 106 patients with uterine sarcoma in Hokkaido, Japan," *Oncology*, vol. 67, no. 1, pp. 33–39, 2004.

[13] P. Reichardt, "The treatment of uterine sarcomas," *Annals of Oncology*, vol. 23, supplement 10, pp. x151–x157, 2012.

[14] P. Eifel, D. Gershenson, and J. Kavanagh, *MD Anderson Cancer Care Series: Gynecologic Cancer*, Springer, New York, USA, 2006.

[15] E. D'Angelo and J. Prat, "Uterine sarcomas: a review," *Gynecologic Oncology*, vol. 116, no. 1, pp. 131–139, 2010.

[16] T. Senol, I. Kahramanoglu, B. Muezzinoglu, and I. Yucesoy, "Giant leiomyosarcoma: A case report," *International Journal of Surgery Case Reports*, vol. 19, pp. 109–111, 2016.

[17] V. Vellanki, M. Rao, C. Sunkavalli, R. Chinamotu, and S. Kaja, "A rare case of uterine leiomyosarcoma: A case report," *Journal of Medical Case Reports*, vol. 4, article no. 222, 2010.

[18] J. Agah, R. J. Esfehani, B. Kamalimanesh, M. F. Abdizadeh, and A. R. Jalilian, "Mismanagement of a Huge Ovarian Serous Cystadenoma in a Young Girl; a Case Report," *Journal of Midwifery and Reproductive Health*, vol. 3, no. 1, pp. 315–317, 2015.

[19] F. Zamani, S. Goodarzi, F. Hallaji et al., "Diagnostic value of pelvic MRI for assessment of the depth of myometrial invasion and cervical involvement in endometrial cancer: comparison of new versus old FIGO staging," *Iranian Journal of Radiology*, vol. 9, no. 4, pp. 202–208, 2012.

[20] C. J. Garvey and R. Hanlon, "Computed tomography in clinical practice," *British Medical Journal*, vol. 324, no. 7345, pp. 1077–1080, 2002.

25

Everolimus Implicated in Case of Severe Gastrointestinal Hemorrhage

Paul Gonzales,[1] Seth Klusewitz,[1] Johanna Marowske,[2] John Gancayco,[2] Michael B. Osswald,[3] and Robert Setlik[3]

[1] *Department of Internal Medicine, San Antonio Military Medical Center, Fort Sam Houston, San Antonio, TX 78234, USA*
[2] *Gastroenterology Service, San Antonio Military Medical Center, Fort Sam Houston, San Antonio, TX 78234, USA*
[3] *Hematology/Oncology Service, San Antonio Military Medical Center, Fort Sam Houston, San Antonio, TX 78234, USA*

Correspondence should be addressed to Paul Gonzales; paul.a.gonzales39.mil@mail.mil

Academic Editor: Gerassimos P. Vandoros

Breast cancer remains the leading cause of cancer and the third leading cause of cancer related deaths among our population with an estimated number of 246,660 new cases and 40,450 deaths in 2016. With treatment advancements, including targeted agents such as Everolimus, a mammalian target of rapamycin (mTOR) inhibitor, survivability and quality of life continue to improve. However, with the use of these agents come adverse effects, some of which are still being characterized. Our case demonstrates recurrent episodes of gastrointestinal bleeding in a 60-year-old woman being treated with Everolimus for progressive metastatic breast cancer. On endoscopy, bleeding was secondary to erosive gastritis. Previous case reports have described bleeding due to gastric antral vascular ectasia (GAVE), which was described in two prior reported cases. In our case, bleeding also occurred on a reduced dose of Everolimus compared to what is previously reported (5 mg versus 10 mg). As a result of her gastrointestinal bleeding, she required multiple endoscopic interventions including argon plasma coagulation and multipolar heater probe to achieve hemostasis. This is the first case reported of gastrointestinal bleeding not consistent with GAVE and occurring while being on a reduced dose of Everolimus. It is important to document our case so that the Gastroenterology and Hematology communities can be educated and made aware for their patient populations on Everolimus.

1. Introduction

Targeted agents, such as the mTOR inhibitor Everolimus, have increased the progression-free survival and quality of life of patients with numerous types of cancer. These targeted agents, while typically well-tolerated, have unique side effect profiles many of which are still being characterized. Given that patients treated with these agents are surviving longer, knowledge and mitigation of their side-effects are of paramount importance.

Since July 2012, the US Food and Drug Administration (FDA) has approved the use of Everolimus in combination with Exemestane for use in postmenopausal women with advanced hormone-receptor positive, HER2-negative breast cancer after failure of treatment with Letrozole or Anastrozole [1]. The FDA prescribing information addresses adverse reactions in a number of organ systems. Specifically, it lists the most common treatment-emergent, gastrointestinal adverse reactions as being stomatitis, diarrhea, abdominal pain, nausea, vomiting, constipation, and dry mouth. Notably, hemorrhage from all causes was only described in 3% of patients without specific mention of gastrointestinal bleeding [1].

Herein, we describe a patient with multiple episodes of life-threatening gastrointestinal bleeding while undergoing therapy with Everolimus with resolution following removal of therapy. As described by Fujihara et al. [2] and Assi and Abdel-Samad [3], there have been only 2 other reports of mTOR inhibitors and only 1 report of Everolimus implicated in life-threatening gastrointestinal bleeding. The case report describing Everolimus described gastrointestinal bleeding secondary to gastric antral vascular ectasia (GAVE); however we present a unique case in a patient with life-threatening

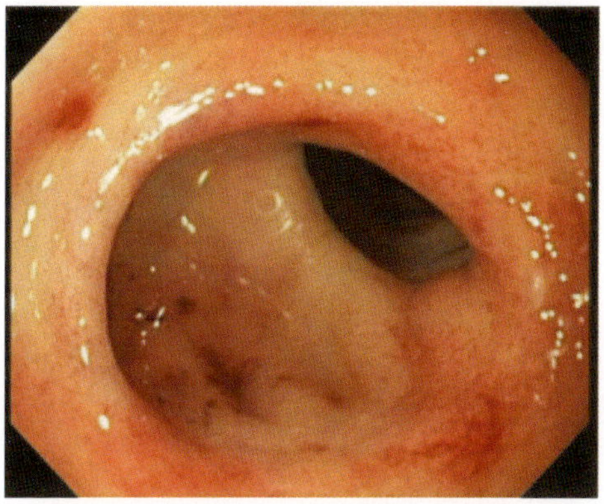

FIGURE 1: Antral stomach, several small punctate lesions observed.

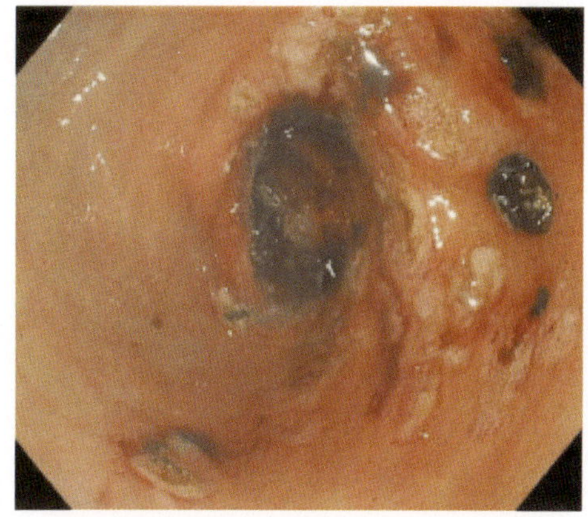

FIGURE 2: Following intraprocedural ERBE circumferential probe argon plasma coagulation, hemostasis was achieved.

gastrointestinal bleeding not consistent with GAVE. During the review of literature, this is the only case not consistent with GAVE and on reduced dose Everolimus and, given the potential life-threatening implications of this adverse reaction, awareness and vigilance are critical for any physician using this agent.

2. Case Description

Our patient is a 65-year-old Caucasian female with past medical history of estrogen receptor (ER) positive, progesterone receptor (PgR) negative, HER2 negative metastatic breast cancer treated with Everolimus and Fulvestrant after disease progression on first-line Anastrozole [4]. She initially started Fulvestrant as a single agent per the CONFIRM trial and then started Everolimus 5 mg daily one month later [5]. This treatment plan was devised in light of the patient's concerns over treatment-related side effects. Her initial gastrointestinal bleed began one month after starting Everolimus. On presentation, she had complaints of weakness, fatigue, and endorsed several episodes of melena. She was found to be anemic with hemoglobin of 6.1 g/dL, down from 11.7 g/dL (reference range 11.0–16.0 g/dL) just one week priorly. She was admitted for anemia secondary to suspected upper gastrointestinal bleed and after admission had further decrease of hemoglobin to 5.0 g/dL. She was transfused two units of packed red blood cells (pRBCs) with an appropriate rise in hemoglobin to 8.4 g/dL. Upper endoscopy performed by Gastroenterology revealed erosive gastritis. Multiple flat erosions with blood oozing were identified within the antral stomach (Figure 1). Hemostasis of these lesions was achieved with injections of epinephrine into the surrounding mucosa. One day following upper endoscopy, she required an additional transfusion of one unit of packed red blood cells for hemoglobin of 6.9 g/dL, again with appropriate response. She had no further melenic stools during her hospitalization and her hemoglobin stabilized at 9.2 g/dL. She was given prescription for Pantoprazole 20 mg twice daily and discharged home. Everolimus was held for two weeks, while continuing therapy with Fulvestrant.

Three weeks following discharge, the patient again developed index symptoms of fatigue, weakness, and melena after restarting Everolimus seven days priorly. The patient was admitted to an outside institution and transfused 8 units of pRBCs over the course of a two-week admission. During this time, she underwent both upper and lower endoscopy with upper endoscopy demonstrating friable mucosa, with no location of frank blood loss being identified. Lower endoscopy revealed normal mucosa with several nonbleeding diverticula and additional testing with radiologic mesenteric angiography was negative at that time. She was subsequently transferred to our hospital and hemoglobin on arrival was noted to be 6.5 g/dL. She was transfused two units of pRBCs with follow-up blood counts demonstrating adequate hemoglobin response to 8.9 g/dL. Gastroenterology was reconsulted and performed repeat upper endoscopy which demonstrated diffuse erosions with active oozing of blood in the gastric antrum. Hemostasis was achieved via intraprocedural ERBE circumferential probe argon plasma coagulation (Figure 2). Following her endoscopy, her hemoglobin level stabilized and melenic stools resolved. She was discharged home with hemoglobin of 9.2 g/dL, provided a prescription for Sucralfate 1 g twice daily, and increased dosing of her Pantoprazole to 40 mg twice daily. Everolimus treatment was permanently discontinued upon discharge.

Two weeks afterward, she was again admitted for symptomatic anemia with hemoglobin of 7.7 g/dL. Upper endoscopy was repeated which illustrated moderate clotted blood in the area of the gastric antrum with multiple 2-3 mm stellate, clean-based ulcers discovered following washing in the setting of friable mucosa. Definitive therapy was pursued with BICAP multipolar heater probe and epinephrine (Figure 3). The patient was subsequently discharged with stable hemoglobin and was seen in Hematology/Oncology Clinic one week later. Despite rising Cancer Ag 27–29 and increased tumor burden evidenced by CT-scan, it was decided that Everolimus therapy would not be restarted in light of the risk of continued gastrointestinal bleeding. The patient was started on palliative Capecitabine and has continued to have stable hemoglobin values since that time with no reoccurrences of gastrointestinal bleeding. She has not required further endoscopic evaluation since discharge.

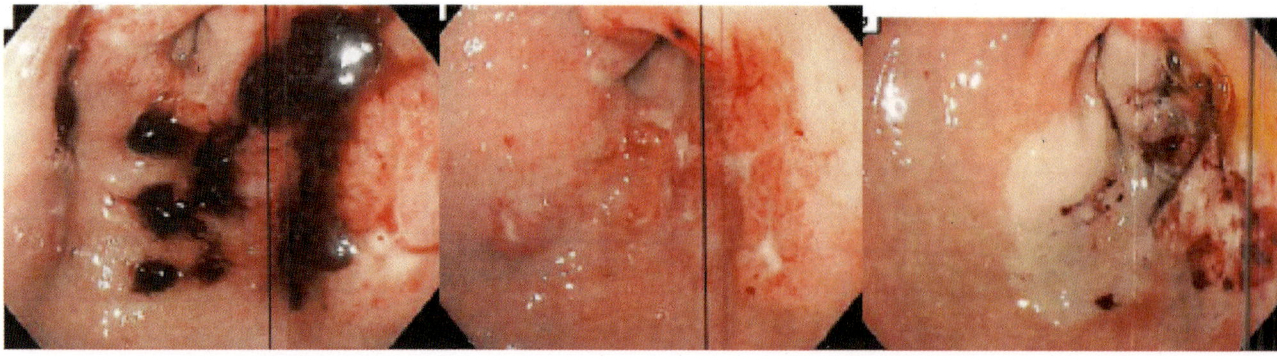

FIGURE 3: BICAP multipolar heater probe and epinephrine application following additional endoscopy.

3. Discussion

In two previous case reports, antineoplastic chemotherapy with an mTOR-based regimen was associated with gastric bleeding consistent with gastric antral vascular ectasia (GAVE). Despite our patient receiving a 50% Everolimus dose-reduction, she also developed gastric bleeding. However, our patient's endoscopic appearance is not consistent with typical findings in GAVE. In patients with GAVE, diagnosis is established with biopsy and visual evaluation on endoscopy demonstrating bleeding with appearance of red stripes radiating from the antrum of the stomach to the pylorus commonly described as watermelon stomach [6]. Our case is unique in that our patient had diffuse erosive gastritis with ulcerations likely secondary to the mTOR inhibitors which has not been demonstrated in the literature previously.

In our case, the patient required multiple modalities of endoscopic interventions to achieve hemostasis, ranging from mucosal injections of epinephrine to plasma argon coagulation and multipolar heater probes. While hemorrhage was adequately controlled in her case using more conventional methods, it is vital to have an understanding of all possible therapies available when treating life threatening hemorrhages, particularly associated with malignancy and their directed therapies. Of interest, the Ankahert blood stopper is a standardized mixture of plants, which acts as a topical hemostatic agent acting on the endothelium, blood cells, angiogenesis, cellular mediators and cellular proliferation and is becoming an effective alternative to conventional hemostatic measures [7]. In a literature review performed by Beyazit et al. [7], the Ankahert blood stopper was successfully used in the management of gastrointestinal hemorrhages from multiple etiologies including malignant and radiation associated bleeding. Additionally, in a case report by Ozdemir et al. [8], the blood stopper was successfully used in the management of bevacizumab-associated gastrointestinal hemorrhage.

In both prior instances of gastrointestinal bleeding associated with mTOR inhibitors described in case reports by Fujihara et al. [2] and Assi and Abdel-Samad [3], GAVE was identified as the likely etiology of bleeding. In our case, the patient's gastrointestinal bleeding was not only temporally associated with initiation of therapy but also resolved following its termination implicating Everolimus as the causative agent. As targeted drug therapy becomes more widely used in not only breast but many forms of cancer, knowledge of potentially life threatening adverse effects is of great importance to empower the caring physician to discontinue therapy when these events are recognized. This case further contributes to the literature that substantiates life-threatening gastrointestinal bleeding as a potential serious adverse outcome to Everolimus therapy.

Disclosure

The view(s) expressed herein are those of the authors and do not reflect the official policy or position of Brooke Army Medical Center, the US Army Medical Department, the US Army Office of the Surgeon General, the Department of the Army, the Department of the Air Force, and the Department of Defense or the US Government.

References

[1] "Food and Drug Administration," Afinitor® (Everolimus) Prescribing Information. June 2016. https://www.accessdata.fda.gov/drugsatfda_docs/label/2016/022334s036lbl.pdf, 01 Mar 2017.

[2] S. Fujihara, H. Mori, H. Kobara et al., "Life-threatening gastrointestinal bleeding during targeted therapy for advanced renal cell carcinoma: a case report," *BMC Nephrology*, vol. 14, no. 141, 2013.

[3] H. Assi and N. Abdel-Samad, "Severe gastrointestinal hemorrhage during targeted therapy for advanced breast carcinoma," *Current Oncology*, vol. 21, no. 5, pp. 732–735, 2014.

[4] S. Massarweh, E. Romond, E. P. Black et al., "Erratum to: A phase II study of combined Fulvestrant and Everolimus in patients with metastatic estrogen receptor (ER)-positive breast cancer after aromatase inhibitor (AI) failure," *Breast Cancer Research and Treatment*, vol. 143, pp. 325–332, 2014.

[5] M. Martin, J. Boyer, M. Stuart, and A. di Leo, "Final overall survival: fulvestrant 500 mg vs 250 mg in the randomized confirm trial," *JNCI: Journal of the National Cancer Institute*, vol. 106, djt337, no. 1, 2014.

[6] M. Jabbari, R. Cherry, J. O. Lough, D. S. Daly, D. G. Kinnear, and C. A. Goresky, "Gastric antral vascular ectasia: the watermelon stomach," *Gastroenterology*, vol. 87, pp. 1165–1170, 1984.

[7] Y. Beyazit, M. Kekilli, I. C. Haznedaroglu, E. Kayacetin, and M. Basaranoglu, "Ankaferd hemostat in the management of gastrointestinal hemorrhages," *World Journal of Gastroenterology*, vol. 17, no. 35, pp. 3962–3970, 2011.

[8] N. Ozdemir, S. Aksoy, T. Eren et al., "Successful management of bevacizumab-associated surgical bleeding with an Ankaferd blood stopper," *Asian Pacific Journal of Cancer Prevention*, vol. 12, no. 4, pp. 1103-1104, 2011.

A Rare Case of Metastasis to the Thyroid Gland from Renal Clear Cell Carcinoma 11 Years after Nephrectomy and Concurrent Primary Esophageal Carcinoma

Mohammad Saud Khan,[1] **Veena Balakrishnan Iyer,**[2,3] **and Neha Varshney**[4]

[1]*Department of Internal Medicine, University of Toledo Medical Center, Toledo, OH 43614, USA*
[2]*Department of Hematology and Oncology, Rhode Island Hospital, Providence, RI, USA*
[3]*Department of Oncology, University of Toledo Medical Center, Toledo, OH 43614, USA*
[4]*Department of Pathology, University of Toledo Medical Center, Toledo, OH 43614, USA*

Correspondence should be addressed to Mohammad Saud Khan; mohammad.khan2@utoledo.edu

Academic Editor: Katsuhiro Tanaka

Renal cell carcinoma is known to cause metastasis to unusual sites, which can be both synchronous or metachronous. Thyroid gland is a rare site for metastasis, but when it occurs, renal cell carcinoma is the most common primary neoplasm. We report the case of a 81-year-old female patient who had a significant medical history of right clear cell renal carcinoma with adrenal metastasis. She underwent right radical nephrectomy and adrenalectomy followed by radiofrequency ablation of left adrenal metastasis and systemic chemotherapy with sunitinib. Eleven years later, she presented with dysphagia and was found to have distal esophageal adenocarcinoma. On imaging, there was incidental detection of a left renal mass lesion and a right thyroid nodule, which on histopathology and immunohistochemistry were confirmed to be clear cell carcinoma of renal origin.

1. Introduction

Thyroid gland is a rare site for clinically detectable metastasis despite having rich blood supply [1]. Renal cell carcinoma (RCC) is the most common primary neoplasm that metastasizes to thyroid gland and accounts for more than 50% of clinically recognized cases [2]. Other neoplasm frequently identified with metastasis to thyroid gland includes breast, lung, skin, and colon cancers. Metastasis accounts for 2-3% of all thyroid malignancies detected clinically [3, 4]. However, the incidence of thyroid metastasis has been reported to be higher (ranging from 1.9 to 22.4%) on autopsy studies [5]. We report the case of a 81-year-old female patient who developed recurrence of RCC with thyroid metastasis after 11 years following nephrectomy of initial tumor.

2. Case Report

A eighty-one-year-old African American female patient presented to the hospital with the complaints of dysphagia and loss of appetite for past few weeks. She had a past medical history of right RCC, clear cell carcinoma subtype with bilateral adrenal metastasis (T3b, N0, and M1) diagnosed in May 2006. At that time, she was treated with right radical nephrectomy and right adrenalectomy followed by radiofrequency ablation of left adrenal metastasis and systemic chemotherapy with sunitinib. She tolerated the treatment well with adequate control of her malignant disease for 11 years. Recently, in June 2017, she presented with the complaints of dysphagia predominantly for solid food, loss of appetite, and generalized fatigability. Physical examination was unremarkable. Esophagogastroduodenoscopy with endoscopic ultrasound showed a distal esophagus mass causing high-grade stricture extending up to the adventitia with no mediastinal lymphadenopathy. Metallic esophageal stent was placed in, and biopsies were obtained which showed adenocarcinoma of esophagus (T3N0M0). Computed tomography (CT) of the chest and abdomen showed distal esophageal thickening along with incidental findings of solid mass lesion involving the inferior pole of the

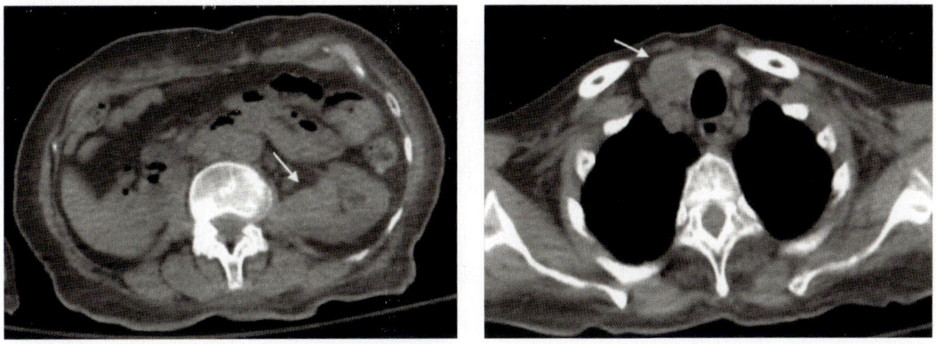

(a) (b)

FIGURE 1: (a) Axial CT scan of the abdomen showing a mass lesion involving the inferior pole of the left kidney (arrow), breaching the renal capsule and infiltrating into adjacent retroperitoneal space. (b) Axial CT scan of the chest at the level of thyroid showing a well-defined hypodense nodule in the right lobe of the thyroid gland (arrow).

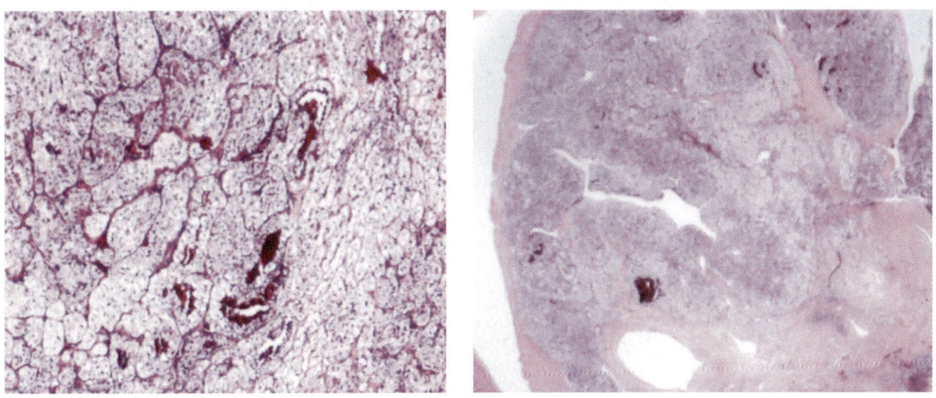

(a) (b)

FIGURE 2: (a) Clear cells with increased vasculature consistent clear cell carcinoma of the kidney (40x, H&E). (b) Clear cell carcinoma invading renal vein (10x, H&E).

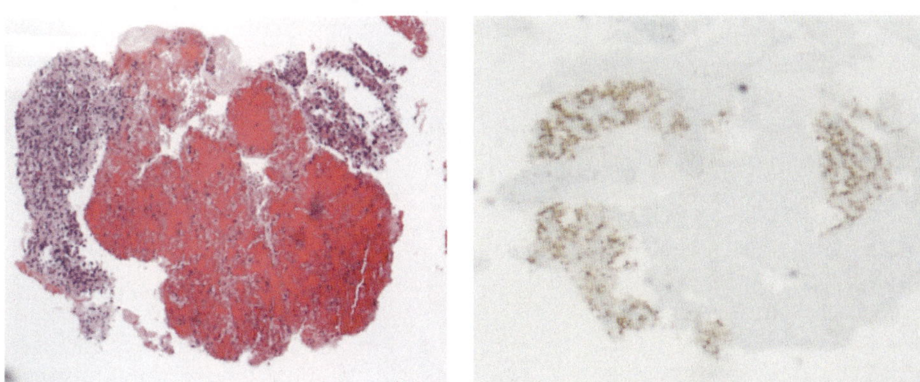

(a) (b)

FIGURE 3: (a) Cell block (4x, H&E) of the thyroid showing atypical cells, which are PAX-8 positive (b) consistent with metastasis of renal origin.

left kidney measuring 3.4 × 2.6 cm in the largest dimension (Figure 1(a)) and a well-defined hypodense nodule in the right lobe of the thyroid gland measuring 2.1 × 2.8 cm in the largest dimension (Figure 1(b)). Biopsy of renal mass was done which showed neoplastic cells with clear cytoplasm arranged in nests and mitotic figures suggesting clear cell carcinoma (Figure 2). Fine-needle aspiration (FNA) from the thyroid nodule also identified neoplastic clear cells on cytology raising possibility of metastasis from RCC (Figure 3(a)). This was confirmed with immunohistochemical stain, which showed atypical cells to be positive for PAX8 (Figure 3(b)) and CAIX while negative for TTF-1. Positron emission tomography (PET) scans showed increased uptake in the distal esophagus, left renal mass, and right thyroid nodule. A diagnosis of concurrent distal esophageal adenocarcinoma along with left renal RCC recurrence and thyroid metastasis was made. The patient was planned for left nephrectomy and thyroidectomy. However, the patient wished to opt out for any surgical intervention or aggressive medical therapy and preferred to be treated with comfort care measures. The patient was treated with palliative intention and died 2 months later.

3. Discussion

RCC accounts for approximately 3-4% of all adult malignancies [6]. It is the most common renal malignancy and the second most common malignancy of urological tract [6, 7]. RCC is more common in males compared to females (ratio of 2 : 1) and occurs predominantly in the 6th to 8th decade of life with a median age of 64 years [6]. Major histopathological subtypes include clear cell carcinoma, papillary carcinoma, chromophobe carcinoma, collecting duct carcinoma, medullary carcinoma, and unclassified categories [8]. Clear cell carcinoma is the most common subtype making up to 75% of cases of RCC [9]. RCC is known to metastasize in unpredictable manner. The metastasis may be detected at the time of diagnosis (synchronous) or may be found years after the diagnosis and treatment (metachronous) [7]. The most common route of metastasis is hematogenous and likely involves lung, liver, bone, lymph nodes, adrenal gland, and brain. Head and neck metastasis are less frequent and of which thyroid is the most commonly involved site. Late recurrences and distant metastasis ranging from few months to several years after initial diagnosis are a notable feature of RCC. It has been estimated that 20–30% of patients including those who have undergone nephrectomy with curative intent will develop recurrence and out of these 50% will relapse distantly [7, 10]. Most of the recurrences are within 3 years of surgery, but delayed recurrences even after decades have been reported [11]. The longer the recurrence-free time from surgery, the more likelihood is of a true cure.

In majority of cases, thyroid metastasis is metachronous with average time of development being 9.4 years following resection of primary RCC [12]. But cases of RCC recurring with thyroid metastasis have been reported as late as 26 years [1]. These metastatic thyroid lesions may pose diagnostic challenge since they often occur years after treatment of primary lesion. RCC metastasis to thyroid can be asymptomatic and may be detected incidentally or may present with symptoms of palpable neck swelling, thyroid enlargement, dysphagia, dysphonia, or dyspnea [3]. Although metastasis to the thyroid gland may be suspected in patients with history of RCC, it is difficult to make a definitive preoperative diagnosis. Metastatic thyroid lesions usually appear as solid, hypoechoic, well-demarcated nodules with irregular border and increased vascularity on ultrasound imaging [13] and cold nodules on radioisotope uptake studies. These radiological features are nonspecific, and it is not possible to distinguish between primary and secondary thyroid neoplasms on imaging. FNA cytology serves as a reliable tool for establishing preoperative diagnosis. However, sometimes it is difficult to distinguish metastasis from tumors of thyroid, which can have clear cell component on FNA cytology alone. In these cases, immunohistochemistry is helpful and aids in differential diagnosis. Some of the traditional immunohistochemical markers for renal cell carcinoma are cytokeratin, vimentin, and CD10 [14]. However, recently novel markers for RCC have been identified which have increased sensitivity and specificity for identifying RCC. These include anti-carbonic anhydrase IX (CAIX), anti-human kidney injury molecule-1 (hKIM-1), and PAX8 [15]. The immunohistochemical markers used for identifying primary thyroid malignancies are thyroglobulin, thyroid transcription factor-1 (TTF-1), and calcitonin. In our case, immunohistochemical stains were positive for CAIX and PAX-8 and negative for TTF-1.

Definitive diagnosis of metastatic RCC is usually made by histopathological examination after thyroidectomy. Surgical resection with either partial or total thyroidectomy should be performed if thyroid gland is the only site for metastasis. Prognosis is good in this group [3, 16]. Patients with disseminated disease have poor prognosis and should undergo thyroidectomy only for palliation for compressive symptoms [16].

4. Conclusion

A thyroid nodule in a patient with a history of renal malignancy should be considered as potentially metastatic. Clinical manifestation and radiographic findings are nonspecific and are unable to distinguish between primary and secondary thyroid neoplasms. FNA cytology and immunohistochemistry are helpful in establishing diagnosis and should be obtained in suspected cases.

References

[1] M. K. Nakhjavani, H. Gharib, J. R. Goellner, and J. A. van Heerden, "Metastasis to the thyroid gland. A report of 43 cases," *Cancer*, vol. 79, no. 3, pp. 574–578, 1997.

[2] H. Chen, T. L. Nicol, and R. Udelsman, "Clinically significant, isolated metastatic disease to the thyroid gland," *World Journal of Surgery*, vol. 23, no. 2, pp. 177–180, 1999.

[3] A. Y. Chung, T. B. Tran, K. T. Brumund, R. A. Weisman, and M. Bouvet, "Metastases to the thyroid: a review of the literature from the last decade," *Thyroid*, vol. 22, no. 3, pp. 258–268, 2012.

[4] L. Hegerova, M. L. Griebeler, J. P. Reynolds, M. R. Henry, and H. Gharib, "Metastasis to the thyroid gland: report of a large series from the Mayo Clinic," *American Journal of Clinical Oncology*, vol. 38, no. 4, pp. 338–342, 2015.

[5] R. A. Willis, "Metastatic tumours in the thyroid gland," *American Journal of Pathology*, vol. 7, no. 3, pp. 187–208, 1931.

[6] R. L. Siegel, K. D. Miller, and A. Jemal, "Cancer statistics, 2016," *CA: A Cancer Journal for Clinicians*, vol. 66, no. 1, pp. 7–30, 2016.

[7] R. J. Motzer, N. H. Bander, and D. M. Nanus, "Renal-cell carcinoma," *New England Journal of Medicine*, vol. 335, no. 12, pp. 865–875, 1996.

[8] G. Kovacs, M. Akhtar, B. J. Beckwith et al., "The Heidelberg classification of renal cell tumours," *Journal of Pathology*, vol. 183, no. 2, pp. 131–133, 1997.

[9] J. J. Hsieh, M. P. Purdue, S. Signoretti et al., "Renal cell carcinoma," *Nature Reviews Disease Primers*, vol. 3, p. 17009, 2017.

[10] R. C. Flanigan, S. C. Campbell, J. I. Clark, and M. M. Picken, "Metastatic renal cell carcinoma," *Current Treatment Options in Oncology*, vol. 4, no. 5, pp. 385–390, 2003.

[11] S. E. Eggener, O. Yossepowitch, J. A. Pettus, M. E. Snyder, R. J. Motzer, and P. Russo, "Renal cell carcinoma recurrence after nephrectomy for localized disease: predicting survival from time of recurrence," *Journal of Clinical Oncology*, vol. 24, no. 19, pp. 3101–3106, 2006.

[12] C. S. Heffess, B. M. Wenig, and L. D. Thompson, "Metastatic renal cell carcinoma to the thyroid gland: a clinicopathologic study of 36 cases," *Cancer*, vol. 95, no. 9, pp. 1869–1878, 2002.

[13] K. Kobayashi, M. Hirokawa, T. Yabuta et al., "Metastatic carcinoma to the thyroid gland from renal cell carcinoma: role of ultrasonography in preoperative diagnosis," *Thyroid Research*, vol. 8, no. 1, p. 4, 2015.

[14] L. D. Truong and S. S. Shen, "Immunohistochemical diagnosis of renal neoplasms," *Archives of Pathology & Laboratory Medicine*, vol. 135, no. 1, pp. 92–109, 2011.

[15] A. R. Sangoi, M. Fujiwara, R. B. West et al., "Immunohistochemical distinction of primary adrenal cortical lesions from metastatic clear cell renal cell carcinoma: a study of 248 cases," *American Journal of Surgical Pathology*, vol. 35, no. 5, pp. 678–686, 2011.

[16] R. De Stefano, R. Carluccio, E. Zanni et al., "Management of thyroid nodules as secondary involvement of renal cell carcinoma: case report and literature review," *Anticancer Research*, vol. 29, no. 2, pp. 473–476, 2009.

27

Primary Diaphragmatic Dedifferentiated Liposarcoma in a Young Female Patient after Delivery

Shinya Sakata, Chieko Yoshida, Sho Saeki, Susumu Hirosako, Hidenori Ichiyasu, and Hirotsugu Kohrogi

Department of Respiratory Medicine, Kumamoto University Hospital, 1-1-1 Honjo, Chuo-ku, Kumamoto 860-8556, Japan

Correspondence should be addressed to Hirotsugu Kohrogi; kohrogi@kumamoto-u.ac.jp

Academic Editor: Jose I. Mayordomo

A 26-year-old woman was admitted with the chief complaint of chest pain. She had delivered her first child 9 months before admission. Computed tomography showed a bulky mass in her left chest, and histopathological analysis revealed it to be dedifferentiated liposarcoma. We initiated doxorubicin chemotherapy, and the tumor mass reduced. After that, we performed vascular embolization along with chemotherapy, but tumor size did not reduce. On the 160th day of illness, the patient died. This is the first report of a primary diaphragmatic dedifferentiated liposarcoma diagnosed after delivery. Establishment of a regimen of chemotherapy for bulky unresectable liposarcoma is necessary.

1. Introduction

Intrathoracic liposarcoma is a very rare tumor. About 90%–95% of liposarcomas occur in the retroperitoneum and femoral regions. Liposarcoma does not show predominance in any one sex and occurs most commonly in individuals in their 40s and 50s. Liposarcoma occurring in young patients is rare, and no cases of primary diaphragmatic dedifferentiated liposarcoma diagnosed after delivery have been reported. Here, we present the case of a young 26-year-old woman with primary diaphragmatic dedifferentiated liposarcoma diagnosed after delivery.

2. Case Report

A 26-year-old woman was admitted to our hospital with left-sided chest pain and a 4-month history of exertional dyspnea. She had delivered her first child 9 months before admission. Physical examination showed decreased breath sounds in the left lung field. Blood tests showed elevated serum lactate dehydrogenase (343 IU/L) and C-reactive protein (4.28 mg/dL). Serum tumor markers carcinoembryonic antigen (0.5 ng/mL), alpha-fetoprotein (1.9 ng/mL), and soluble interleukin-2 receptor (401 U/mL) were all within normal range.

Contrast-enhanced computed tomography (CT) showed a bulky mass with heterogeneous enhancement (Figure 1(a)). We performed CT-guided needle biopsy of the mass, and subsequent histopathology revealed dense growth of atypical cells, differentiated fat cells, and atypical cells with a clear nucleolus and weak acidophilic foamy cytoplasm (Figure 2(a)). Histopathology also revealed differentiated cartilage cells buried among clear cartilage tissues with a dense growth of fusiform immature undifferentiated mesenchymal cells with a high nucleocytoplasmic ratio (Figure 2(b)). Thus, we diagnosed dedifferentiated liposarcoma. Because the inferior phrenic artery was the main nutrient vessel of the tumor, we determined the tumor to be of diaphragmatic origin (Figure 1(b)). Fluorodeoxyglucose positron emission tomography showed no distant metastases (Figure 3), and contrast-enhanced magnetic resonance imaging confirmed the absence of brain metastases. Although left pleural dissemination was found by contrast-enhanced chest CT, surgical resection was planned for the purpose of volume reduction. However, circulation was disturbed due to compression of the heart and mediastinum by the bulky tumor mass, leading to postponement of the planned surgical resection.

Treatment was begun with doxorubicin (25 mg/m^2, days 1, 2, and 3, every 3 weeks) for tumor reduction, which

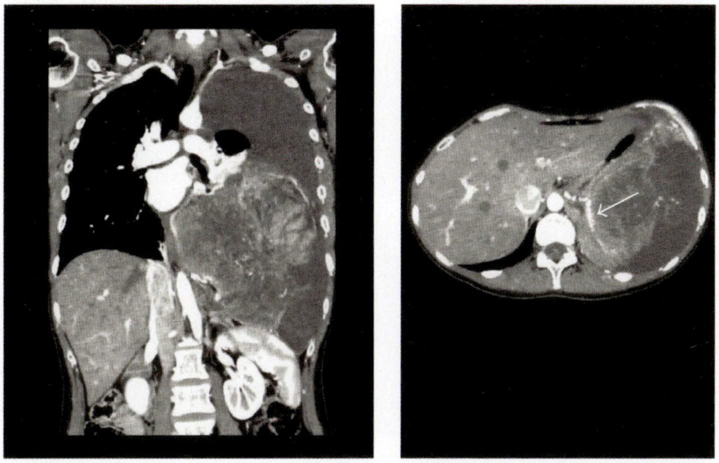

(a) (b)

FIGURE 1: (a) Chest contrast-enhanced computed tomography (CT) showing the bulky intrathoracic mass opacity on the left. (b) The inferior phrenic artery was found to be the main nutrient vessel in the contrast-enhanced CT (arrow).

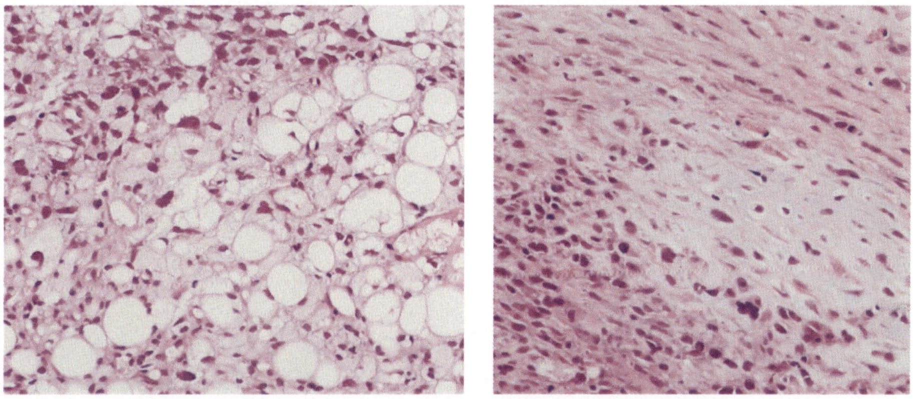

(a) (b)

FIGURE 2: (a) Pathology (hematoxylin and eosin staining, 400x) showing a dense growth of atypical cells indicating differentiation of fat cells; the atypical cells had a clear nucleolus with weakly acidophilic foamy cytoplasm. (b) Pathology (hematoxylin and eosin staining, 400x) showing differentiation of cartilage cells buried among clear cartilage tissues with the dense growth of fusiform immature undifferentiated mesenchymal cells with a high nucleocytoplasmic ratio.

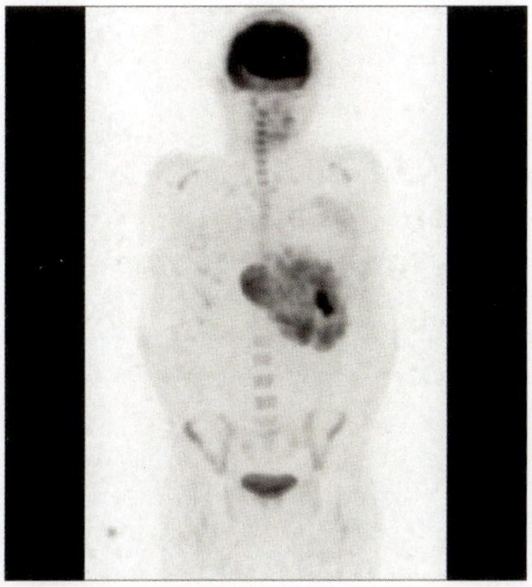

FIGURE 3: Fluorodeoxyglucose positron emission tomography showing no distant metastases.

was obtained after 2 cycles of chemotherapy (Figure 4). Surgical resection was then planned again; however, the tumor showed rapid growth causing congestive heart failure, leading to another postponement of resection. We tried combination chemotherapy with ifosfamide (1200 mg/m^2, days 1, 2, 3, 4, and 5, every 3 weeks) and doxorubicin (25 mg/m^2, days 1, 2, and 3, every 3 weeks), but her pulmonary congestion worsened by excessive fluid transfused to prevent ifosfamide toxicity (3750 mL/day of saline), and the treatment was stopped. We next performed vascular embolization of the main nutrient vessel. Subsequently, we tried chemotherapy with single agent of docetaxel (60 mg/m^2, day 1, every 3 weeks, 1 cycle), doxorubicin (25 mg/m^2, days 1, 2, and 3, every 3 weeks, 1 cycle), and pazopanib (800 mg/day); however, no treatment effects were observed. On the 160th day of illness, the patient died due to progression of her dedifferentiated liposarcoma.

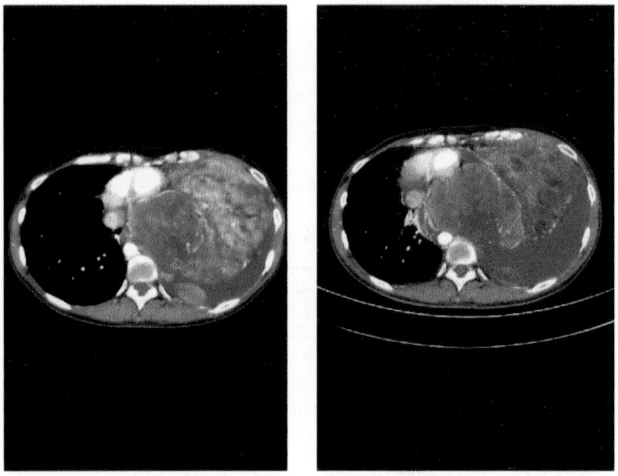

(a) (b)

FIGURE 4: (a) Chest contrast-enhanced computed tomography (CT) before treatment showing a bulky mass in the left chest; pleural dissemination is seen. (b) Chest contrast-enhanced CT after 2 cycles of chemotherapy with doxorubicin showing reduction of the tumor.

3. Discussion

Intrathoracic liposarcoma is a very rare tumor [1], with 90%–95% occurring in the retroperitoneum and femoral regions [2]. Shmookler and Enzinger reported a frequency of intrathoracic liposarcoma of 2.7% at all sites [3]. Recently, Chen et al. reported 23 cases of intrathoracic liposarcoma. This report included 4 cases (17%) of dedifferentiated liposarcoma, with a median overall survival (OS) of 11 months and a median disease-free survival of 6 months. The report showed inferior OS in dedifferentiated, myxoid, and pleomorphic liposarcomas relative to well-differentiated liposarcomas [4]. In the World Health Organization classification of 2013, liposarcoma can be classified as a histologically intermediate malignant well-differentiated liposarcoma, a histologically malignant myxoid liposarcoma, a pleomorphic liposarcoma, a dedifferentiated liposarcoma, or a liposarcoma not otherwise specified. These classifications are associated with their prognosis [5]. In the present case, a dedifferentiated liposarcoma was mixed with a well-differentiated liposarcoma. Thus, the present case is dedifferentiated liposarcoma of *de novo* development.

Myxoid liposarcoma is the most common type (approximately 50% of all liposarcomas), and the next most common type is well-differentiated liposarcoma. Well-differentiated liposarcoma has a good prognosis, with 5-year survival rates of 80%. Meanwhile dedifferentiated liposarcoma has a poor prognosis, with a recurrence rate of 40%–50%, a metastasis rate of 20%, and a 5-year survival rate of 28% [6, 7]. The dedifferentiated liposarcoma is defined as a high-grade sarcoma that does not form fat and developed from a well-differentiated liposarcoma. In the present case, sites indicating adipogenesis and dedifferentiation were observed by biopsy specimens, respectively. Saito et al. have also reported a case of dedifferentiated liposarcoma of *de novo* development [8].

Small specimens such as those obtained by needle biopsy are insufficient to determine the histologic type of liposarcoma, so tissue diagnosis by surgical resection is preferable. However, in cases where surgical resection is difficult, such as the present case, it is important to biopsy from multiple sites of tumor in order to obtain a correct pathological diagnosis. As a result, we are able to predict a prognosis and a therapeutic effect.

The principle treatment for liposarcoma is surgical resection. Klimstra et al. reported that the mean size of liposarcoma at surgery is 157 mm (range 60–0400 mm) and the mean tumor weight is 1500 g [9]. Surgical resection is typically performed with positive results even on bulky tumors. In one case, long-term survival was reported for a patient with liposarcoma who underwent repeated surgical resection for recurrent disease [10]. In another case, a bulky retroperitoneal liposarcoma could be resected surgically after vascular embolization [11]. In our patient, however, we tried chemotherapy, embolization of the feeding artery, and molecularly targeted medicine; but we were unable to resect the tumor.

There is no established standard regimen of chemotherapy for dedifferentiated liposarcoma. In myxoid liposarcoma, it was reported that chemotherapy with doxorubicin plus ifosfamide had a response rate of 43.2% [12]. For our patient, we tried combination chemotherapy with ifosfamide and doxorubicin, but exacerbation of her pulmonary congestion was induced by the transfusion load administration of ifosfamide. Thus, we were unable to use this chemotherapy regimen. We note that intrathoracic liposarcomas may cause compression of the heart and mediastinum by their bulky mass, making an ifosfamide regimen more difficult in this tumor type than in liposarcomas of other sites of origin. Dedifferentiated liposarcoma has high rate of recurrence. Therefore, the combined modality therapy including the postoperative adjuvant chemotherapy is necessary.

Here, we present a case of dedifferentiated liposarcoma in a young female patient after delivery. Recently, overexpression of the estrogen receptor and androgen receptor in well-differentiated and dedifferentiated liposarcoma was reported [13]. In the present case, the immunohistochemical staining showed positive for progesterone receptor and androgen receptor. An association between pregnancy and dedifferentiated liposarcoma has not been reported. However, the present case exhibited dedifferentiated liposarcoma in a young female patient after delivery. We could not deny the association between these hormone receptors and pregnancy. Thus, a further study is necessary in future. During pregnancy, it is common to not conduct examinations using X-rays to avoid the effects of radiation exposure on the fetus. Therefore, delay of the diagnosis of dedifferentiated liposarcoma is possible, as seen in the present case.

4. Conclusion

We present the first report of a primary diaphragmatic dedifferentiated liposarcoma diagnosed after delivery. The current standard of treatment for liposarcoma is surgical resection, which, however, is not always possible in bulky intrathoracic liposarcomas. Therefore, we propose that the establishment of a multidisciplinary regimen for bulky unresectable intrathoracic liposarcomas is necessary.

Acknowledgments

The authors would like to thank the patient and her family for permitting our publication of her disease history.

References

[1] F. Carroll, M. D. Kramer, A. J. Acinapura et al., "Pleural liposarcoma presenting with respiratory distress and suspected diaphragmatic hernia," *The Annals of Thoracic Surgery*, vol. 54, no. 6, pp. 1212–1213, 1992.

[2] J. J. Peterson, M. J. Kransdorf, L. W. Bancroft, and M. I. O'Connor, "Malignant fatty tumors: classification, clinical course, imaging appearance and treatment," *Skeletal Radiology*, vol. 32, no. 9, pp. 493–503, 2003.

[3] B. M. Shmookler and F. M. Enzinger, "Liposarcoma occurring in children. An analysis of 17 cases and review of the literature," *Cancer*, vol. 52, no. 3, pp. 567–574, 1983.

[4] M. Chen, J. Yang, L. Zhu, C. Zhou, and H. Zhao, "Primary intrathoracic liposarcoma: a clinicopathologic study and prognostic analysis of 23 cases," *Journal of Cardiothoracic Surgery*, vol. 9, article 119, 2014.

[5] C. D. Fletcher, J. A. Bridge, P. Hogendoorn, and F. Mertens, *World Health Organization. WHO Classification of Tumours of Soft Tissue and Bone*, IARC Press, Lyon, France, 2013.

[6] A. P. Dei Tos, "Liposarcoma: new entities and evolving concepts," *Annals of Diagnostic Pathology*, vol. 4, no. 4, pp. 252–266, 2000.

[7] D. McCormick, T. Mentzel, A. Beham, and C. D. M. Fletcher, "Dedifferentiated liposarcoma: clinicopathologic analysis of 32 cases suggesting a better prognostic subgroup among pleomorphic sarcomas," *The American Journal of Surgical Pathology*, vol. 18, no. 12, pp. 1213–1223, 1994.

[8] D. Saito, M. Oda, T. Yamato, T. Imai, Y. Tatsuzawa, and K. Sato, "Rapidly growing mediastinal dedifferentiated liposarcoma," *Japanese Journal of Lung Cancer*, vol. 53, no. 6, pp. 767–770, 2013.

[9] D. S. Klimstra, C. A. Moran, G. Perino, M. N. Koss, and J. Rosai, "Liposarcoma of the anterior mediastinum and thymus. A clinicopathologic study of 28 cases," *The American Journal of Surgical Pathology*, vol. 19, pp. 782–791, 1995.

[10] S. W. H. Kendall, E. A. Williams, J. B. Hunt, M. C. Fetch, F. C. Wells, and B. B. Milstein, "Recurrent primary liposarcoma of the pericardium: management by repeated resections," *The Annals of Thoracic Surgery*, vol. 56, no. 3, pp. 560–562, 1993.

[11] K. Makiyama, K. Kobayashi, Y. Senga et al., "Surgical removal of retroperitoneal liposarcoma after transarterial embolization: a case report," *Hinyokika Kiyo*, vol. 45, no. 8, pp. 531–533, 1999.

[12] D. Katz, P. Boonsirikamchai, H. Choi et al., "Efficacy of first-line doxorubicin and ifosfamide in myxoid liposarcoma," *Clinical Sarcoma Research*, vol. 2, article 2, 2012.

[13] D. R. Ingram, L. M. Dillon, D. Lev et al., "Estrogen receptor alpha and androgen receptor are commonly expressed in well-differentiated liposarcoma," *BMC Clinical Pathology*, vol. 14, article 42, 2014.

Skeletal Muscle Lymphoma Presenting with Chronic Compartment Syndrome of Leg after Trauma

Jhong-You Li, Chung-Liang Li, and Chun-Kuan Lu

Kaohsiung Medical University Hospital, No. 100 Tzyou 1st Road, Kaohsiung 807, Taiwan

Correspondence should be addressed to Chun-Kuan Lu; 990295@kmuh.org.tw

Academic Editor: Jose I. Mayordomo

Compartment syndrome may be acute or chronic based on the clinical course and etiology. Here, we report the first known case to be diagnosed with skeletal muscle-derived B-cell lymphoma presenting with chronic compartment syndrome after trauma. A 62-year-old woman sought medical attention due to a one-month history of painful left lower leg swelling and paresthesia of the medial side of the foot after falling over. The patient underwent fasciotomy and debridement under the preoperative diagnosis of fasciitis and myositis with associated compressive neuropathy. Preoperative laboratory tests were within normal limits. Postoperative pathologic examination and bone marrow aspiration revealed B-cell lymphoma with bone marrow involvement postoperatively. Tumor lysis syndrome took place, presenting with drowsiness, poor appetite, and oliguria, after the operation along with multiple organ failure. Awareness of the differential diagnoses of compartment syndrome in such clinical situation is crucial because it may lead to different examination and treatment plan preoperatively.

1. Introduction

Compartment syndrome of the leg is a complication caused by fracture, ischemic reperfusion injury, soft tissue trauma, external compression, burn, or even bleeding disorders [1]. The diagnosis is mainly based on history, clinical examination, and occasionally intracompartment pressure (ICP) measurement. Delay in treatment of compartment syndrome may lead to muscle necrosis, limbs amputation, and even worse, rhabdomyolysis, renal failure, and death [2].

Extranodal non-Hodgkin lymphoma (NHL) is well reported with sites involved including the central nervous system, gastrointestinal tract, lung, skin, or bone [3]. Skeletal muscle-derived extranodal NHL is extremely rare [4], and few of the reported cases in the literature present with compartment syndrome. Correct diagnosis may lead to different evaluation and treatment plans.

2. Case Presentation

A 62-year-old woman with underlying disease of hypertension presented with a one-month history of painful left lower leg swelling and paresthesia of the medial side of the foot after falling over. There were no associated B symptoms noted (known as fever, weight loss, or night sweats). Physical examination disclosed an ill-defined, tense, and tender swelling of left calf with local heat. Dorsalis pedis artery and posterior tibial artery pulsations were intact, but there was numbness over the medial sole and medial 3 toes.

The patient was admitted for diagnostic workup, including laboratory examination and contrast-enhanced computed tomography (CT) of the lower extremities. Preoperative liver, renal function, and white blood cell (WBC) count were within normal limits without evidence of blast or atypical lymphocyte. Contrast-enhanced CT showed hypodense lesions and fluid collection in the medial posterior compartment of the left lower leg (Figure 1). Under the tentative diagnosis of fasciitis and myositis with associated compressive neuropathy, scheduled operation with debridement and fasciotomy were performed.

During operation, subcutaneous fatty necrosis with induration was noted and evacuated. Upon dissection into the deep compartment of posterior leg, myonecrosis of nearly the entire compartment was discovered, and the tibial nerve was surrounded by the necrotic soft tissue (Figure 2).

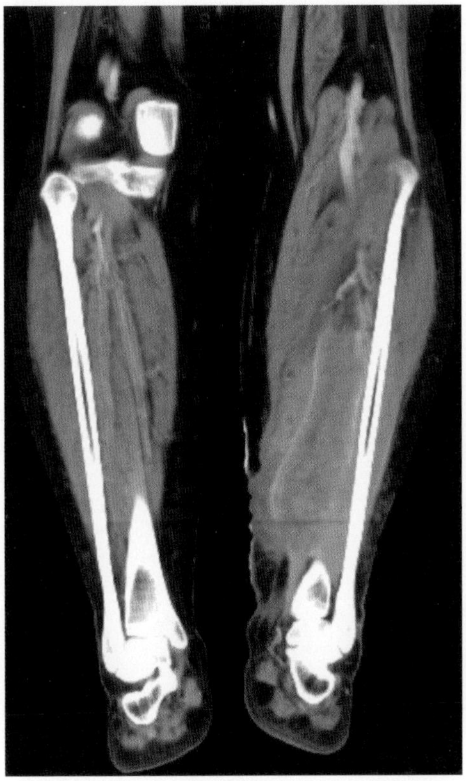

FIGURE 1: Contrast-enhanced CT of lower extremities. CT shows hypodense lesions and fluid collection in the medial aspect of the posterior compartment of the left lower leg.

Fasciotomy and thorough debridement were performed. Microbiology and pathologic studies were done. Skin was approximated, and a Jackson-Pratt drain was inserted into the posterior compartment in order to monitor wound condition and prevent further hematoma formation.

However, drowsiness, poor appetite, and oliguria developed 2 days after the operation while the patient remained afebrile. Repeated laboratory workup revealed leukocytosis with atypical lymphocyte. Abnormal liver function tests and acute renal failure postoperatively suggested the possibility of rhabdomyolysis, severe sepsis, or even tumor lysis syndrome. Additional laboratory studies showed electrolyte imbalance with hypocalcemia, hyperphosphatemia, hyperuricemia, and markedly elevated lactate dehydrogenase (LDH) (19,047 U/L) without significant elevated creatine phosphokinase (CPK) level. Microbiologic examinations were all negative.

Pathologic examination of the deep posterior compartment of the lower leg confirmed the diagnosis of B-cell lymphoma with features intermediate between diffuse large B-cell lymphoma and Burkitt lymphoma (Figure 3). Hematologist and nephrologist were immediately consulted for suspected B-cell lymphoma with tumor lysis syndrome. Bone marrow aspiration on the next day showed abundant blast-like cells (56%) in the smear. Chest CT was arranged for further evaluation, and it revealed probably lymphadenopathy at the right submental area and pretracheal region. Along with the peripheral blood smear and pathologic report, acute lymphoblastic leukemia or lymphoma with

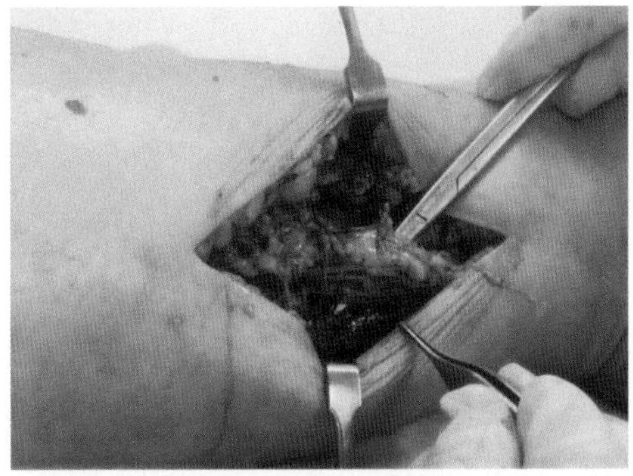

FIGURE 2: Myonecrosis of the left lower leg. Intraoperative finding demonstrated myonecrosis of the deep posterior compartment and the posterior tibial nerve surrounded by necrotizing tissue (status after posterior tibial nerve neurolysis).

secondary muscle involvement was confirmed. Emergent hemodialysis was performed on hospital day 12 due to tumor lysis syndrome with associated electrolyte imbalance. The patient's family members refused chemotherapy. On hospital day 22, the patient died because of intractable gastrointestinal bleeding and multiple organ failure in the intensive care unit (Figure 4).

3. Patient Declaration Statement

The authors certify that they have obtained all appropriate patient consent forms. In the form, the patient has given her consent for her images and other clinical information to be reported in the journal. The patients understand that their names and initials will not be published and due efforts will be made to conceal their identity, but anonymity cannot be guaranteed.

4. Discussion

To date, only few cases of lymphoma originating in the skeletal muscle presenting with compartment syndrome have been reported. During our literature review, 7 cases of compartment syndrome caused by hematologic diseases in the skeletal muscle were found [3–7]. Only two of theses cases had lymphoma and the others had leukemia (Including both acute lymphoblastic leukemia (ALL) and acute myeloid leukemia (AML)). Over half of the patients were either children or teenagers (aged 9, 11, 11, and 20 years). The most commonly involved sites were the forearm (three cases) and legs (two cases). A case with buttock and thigh involvement was also reported [8]. To the best of our knowledge, this is the first case of skeletal muscle-derived B-cell lymphoma that presents with compartment syndrome after trauma.

Compartment syndrome may be acute or chronic based on the clinical course and etiology. Acute compartment syndrome is a limb-threatening and potentially life-threatening condition caused by fracture, ischemic reperfusion injury, soft tissue trauma, external compression, burn, or even bleeding disorders [1, 2]. Chronic compartment syndrome is a relative medical nonemergency and mostly common in athletes with repetitive motions [9]. The characteristics of chronic compartment

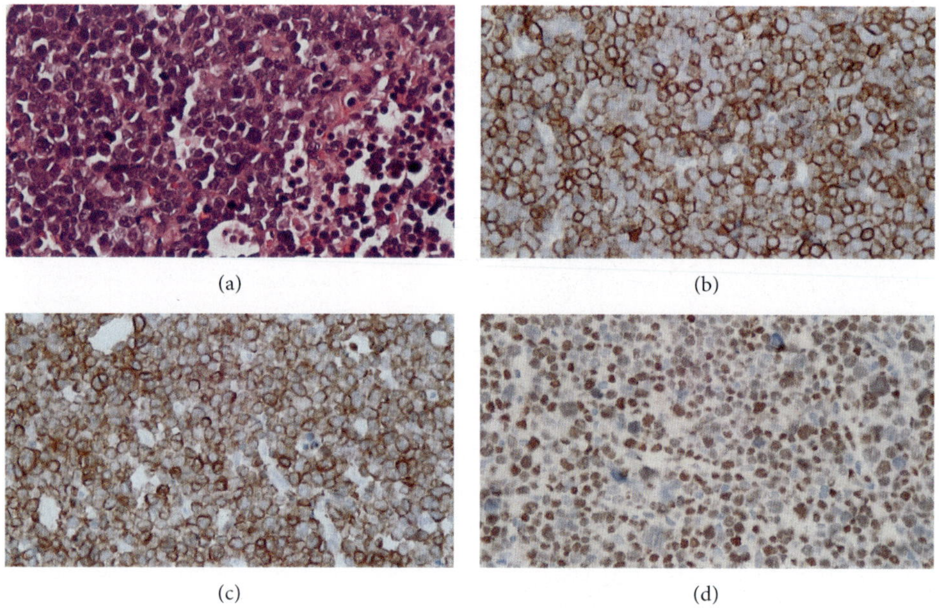

Figure 3: Microscopic view of intraoperative soft tissue specimen. (a) Infiltration of neoplastic cells in the soft tissue, characterized by high nuclear-to-cytoplasmic ratio in hematoxylin and eosin (H&E) stain. Positive in immunochemical stain: CD20 (b), bcl-2 (c), and c-myc (d) in immunochemical stain.

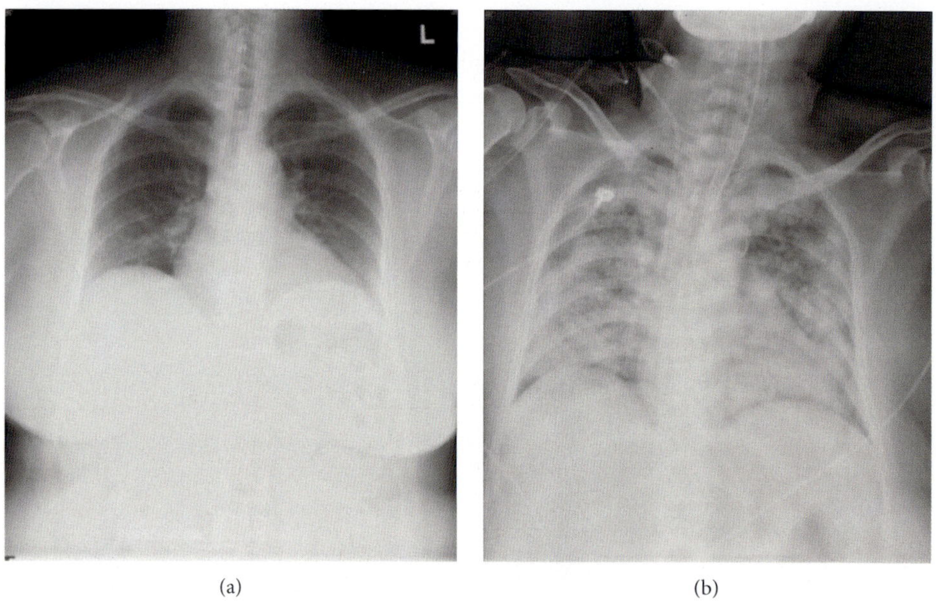

Figure 4: Chest radiograph revealed ARDS lung. (a) preoperative; (b) postoperative.

syndrome are pain, cramping, or even numbness with exercise that are relieved with rest. The anterior and deep posterior compartments of lower extremities are the most frequently affected sites, and fracture or other types of trauma are the precipitating factors [9].

We propose an idea that apart from repetitive exercise, chronically increased intracompartment pressure may also induce symptoms and signs of chronic compartment syndrome in this case. Chronic compartment syndrome gradually developed due to chronic bleeding and poor healing secondary to lymphoma infiltration after the trauma. Additional studies such as muscle biopsy, CT, or magnetic resonance imaging (MRI) should be considered if the disease course is prolonged or disproportionate lesion. Although surgical debridement and fasciotomy is widely recommended in the presence of compartment syndrome [1–3, 5–9], muscle biopsy for pathology proof is crucial before or during the operation. Definite treatment of lymphoma/leukemia usually required systemic chemotherapy that may be contraindicated in the acute setting of compartment syndrome as it might worsen the tissue swelling [6]. Moreover, there is a risk of tumor lysis syndrome whether chemotherapy or surgery is instituted.

Close monitoring of urine output and renal function along the treatment course is needed.

5. Conclusion

Primary skeletal muscle lymphoma is extremely rare, accounting for approximately 1.5% of NHLs. And they usually have large cell histology features and have been associated with a poor prognosis [10]. We have reported a post-traumatic compartment syndrome secondary to primary muscle lymphoma. The case highlights the possibility of malignancy-related compartment syndrome even after a specific trauma history.

References

[1] E. Cohen, J. Truntzer, S. Klinge, K. Schwartz, and J. Schiller, "Acute pediatric leg compartment syndrome in chronic myeloid leukemia," *Orthopedics*, vol. 37, no. 11, pp. e1036–e1039, 2014.

[2] S. Gourgiotis, C. Villias, S. Germanos, A. Foukas, and M. P. Ridolfini, "Acute limb compartment syndrome: a review," *Journal of Surgical Education*, vol. 64, no. 3, pp. 178–186, 2007.

[3] C. S. Chim, C. Choy, and R. Liang, "Primary anaplastic large cell lymphoma of skeletal muscle presenting with compartment syndrome," *Leukemia & Lymphoma*, vol. 33, no. 5-6, pp. 601–605, 1999.

[4] M. Katsura, H. Nishina, Y. Shigemori, and T. Nakanishi, "Extranodal lymphoma originating in the gluteal muscle with adjacent bone involvement and mimicking a soft tissue sarcoma," *International Journal of Surgery Case Reports*, vol. 7, pp. 161–164, 2015.

[5] B. Warme, J. Sullivan, D. Y. Tigrani, and D. M. Fred, "Chloroma of the forearm: a case report of leukemia recurrence presenting with compression neuropathy and tenosynovitis," *Iowa Orthopaedic Journal*, vol. 29, pp. 114–116, 2009.

[6] R. S. Veeragandham, I. B. Paz, and A. Nadeemanee, "Compartment syndrome of the leg secondary to leukemic infiltration: a case report and review of the literature," *Journal of Surgical Oncology*, vol. 55, no. 3, pp. 198–200, 1994.

[7] T. Trumble, "Forearm compartment syndrome secondary to leukemic infiltrates," *Journal of Hand Surgery*, vol. 12, no. 4, pp. 563–565, 1987.

[8] D. K. Lee, W. K. Jeong, D. H. Lee, and S. H. Lee, "Multiple compartment syndrome in a pediatric patient with CML," *Journal of Pediatric Orthopedics*, vol. 31, no. 8, pp. 889–892, 2011.

[9] N. McLaughlin, H. Heard, and S. Kelham, "Acute and chronic compartment syndromes: know when to act fast," *JAAPA*, vol. 27, no. 6, pp. 23–26, 2014.

[10] A. Alamdari, N. Naderi, S. Peiman, and F. Shahi, "Non-Hodgkin lymphoma with primary involvement of skeletal muscle," *International Journal of Hematology-Oncology and Stem Cell Research*, vol. 8, no. 3, pp. 55–57, 2014.

29

Rare Presentation of Primary Extramedullary Plasmacytoma as Lip Lesion

Mali Him,[1] Maggie Meier,[2] and Vikas Mehta[1]

[1] *Mount Sinai Hospital, Chicago, IL, USA*
[2] *St. Luke's Hospital St. Louis, MO, USA*

Correspondence should be addressed to Mali Him; malihim@students.rossu.edu

Academic Editor: Ossama W. Tawfik

Malignant plasma cell proliferation can be presented as part of disseminated disease of multiple myeloma, as solitary plasmacytoma of bone, or in soft tissue as extramedullary plasmacytoma. Extramedullary plasmacytomas represented approximately 3% of all plasma cell proliferation. Approximately 80% of extramedullary plasmacytomas occur in the head and neck region while the other 4% occur in the skin and to a lesser extent in the lip. In this paper, we report a rare case of primary cutaneous plasmacytoma involving the lip in a 65-year-old male. The patient presented with a nonhealing lower lip sore for the past 3 years. Upon further workup, there was no evidence of multiple myeloma or light chain disease. The patient was treated with radiation therapy and his last follow-up revealed no evidence of multiple myeloma or light chain disease.

1. Introduction

A plasmacytoma is a tumor of plasma cells which often develops as a systemic spread of multiple myeloma, in bone as a solitary plasmacytoma of bone, or in soft tissue as extramedullary plasmacytoma (EMP). Extramedullary plasmacytomas are rare, comprising about 3% of all plasma cell neoplasms with bone marrow plasma cell infiltration <5% of nucleated cells and demonstrating no evidence of myeloma [1]. While solitary bone plasmacytomas reveal single tumor inside the bone comprising of abnormal plasma cells. The majority (60%–80%) of extramedullary plasmacytomas are found in the head and neck region, particularly in the upper respiratory tract, and to a lesser extent in gastrointestinal tract. Cases of primary cutaneous plasmacytoma are comprised of 2–4% of extramedullary plasmacytomas. It is unusual to have a primary cutaneous plasmacytoma present as a lip lesion, as only 5 cases have been reported in the literature [2]. The first case reported was by Volk in 1936 [2].

Primary cutaneous plasmacytomas present as relatively slow growing papules or plaques or an erythematous-violaceous nodule either existing in solitary tumor (62%) or possibly involving multiple sites (38%). Patients usually present with a benign past medical history. Symptoms are dependent on location and size of lesion. Rarely, patients present with fever, malaise, night sweats, or weight loss. Other features that may be present are lymphadenopathy and hepatosplenomegaly. The lesion may be ulcerated and necrotic. The skin lesions range in diameter from 1 to 5 cm and the shape may vary. Histologically, it shows a nonepidermotropic dermal infiltrate of plasma cells at different stages of maturation. The plasma cells often show atypical, binucleation, and increased mitotic activity. The epidermis is generally spared. The mean age at diagnosis is 60 years with a male to female predominance of 3 : 1 and it is commonly reported in Asian men. The incidence rate increased with advancing age.

Treatment for solitary or a few lesions can be treated with radiotherapy or surgical excision. Chemotherapy or intralesional corticosteroid therapy may be provided for multiple skin lesions.

Due to this rarity, we feel the need to present this case in order to increase the awareness of the disease to better serve our patients. The clinicopathological features, prognostic factors, and treatment options with its unusual presentation of lip involvement is being discussed in this report.

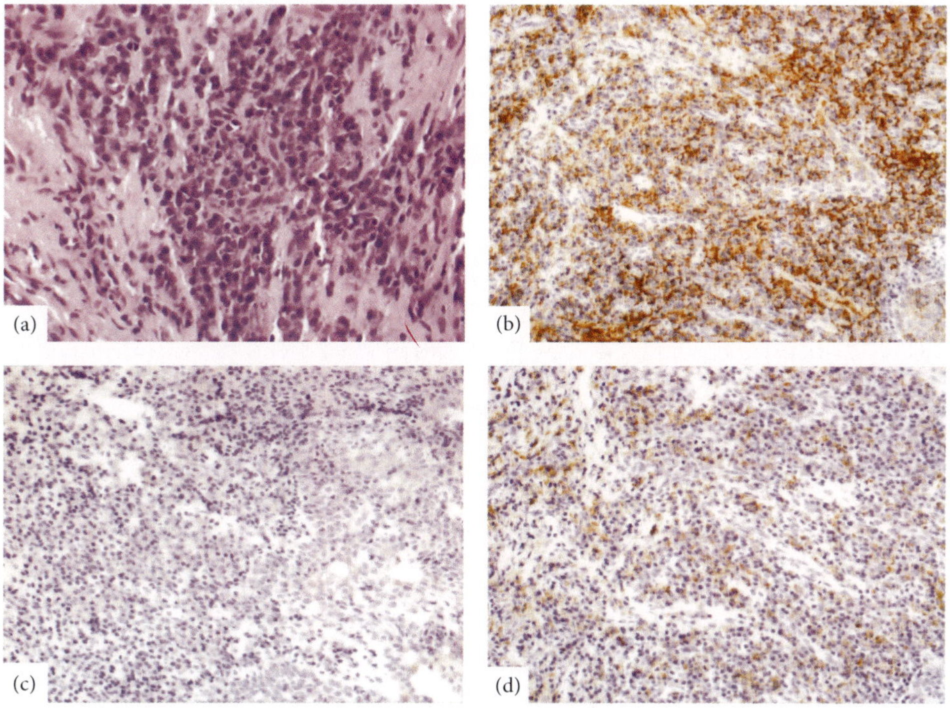

FIGURE 1: (a) Dense plasma cell infiltrate, H&E, 40x; (b) CD138 immunostain labeling plasma cells, IHC 40x; (c) Kappa in situ hybridization with only rare plasma cell labeling, ISH, 40x; (d) Lambda in situ hybridization with most plasma cells labeling, ISH, 40x.

2. Case Description

A 65-year-old male presented to the Ears, Nose, and Throat clinic in September 2015 with complaints of a nonhealing lower lip sore for the past 3 years. The slow growing lesion was described as a burning sensation with scabbing and occasional bleeding. It was slowly increasing in size. The patient had a greater than 50-year history of smoking tobacco (not chewing) which he quit about 7 months prior to his visit. He also complained of unintentionally losing 3 lbs in the last 2 weeks. He denied any fevers or chills. He had no other complaints.

Physical examination was significant for a single lesion on the lower lip 1.5 × 1 cm. A biopsy was performed and sent to pathology. The patient was worked up thoroughly for evidence of multiple myeloma/light chain disease. Laboratory testing was significant for no anemia, normal serum calcium, normal serum albumin, normal total protein, and normal creatinine. There was no Bence Jones protein in urine. Bone survey was done which was negative. Bone marrow biopsy showed <5% plasma cells, ruling out plasmacytoma of the bone. No monoclonal gammopathy was seen, which precluded immunofixation order. Kappa to lambda ratio was normal.

Hematoxylin-eosin staining of the lip biopsy revealed a dense plasmacytic infiltration in the deep dermis (see Figure 1(a)). Immunohistochemical panel included CD3, CD20, and CD138 immunohistochemical stains as well as kappa and lambda light chain in situ hybridization. The superficial dermis and the epidermis were not seen to be involved. Immunohistochemistry was positive for CD138 (see Figure 1(b)) and revealed that most plasma cells were lambda positive and with rare kappa-positive plasma cells (see Figures 1(c) and 1(d)).

Based on the ISCL/EORTC Proposed on TNM Classification of Cutaneous Lymphoma our patient was staged at T1aN0M0. The patient was treated in November 2015 with radiation therapy as follows: 3000 cGy in 15 fractions using 3D conformal technique to his lower lip and level I lymph nodes and he received 2000 cGy boost bringing his total dose to 5000 cGy in 25 fractions. He responded well to treatment. At his last follow-up, there was no evidence of multiple myeloma or light chain disease.

3. Discussion

Primary cutaneous plasmacytoma is a rare diagnosis that represents approximately 4% of extramedullary plasmacytoma cases. Of the 4% cases, only a few cases have been reported to be associated with lip lesions. In the latest comprehensive literature review by Tsang et al. in 2016, there are 5 case reports of primary cutaneous plasmacytomas of the lip [2]. Primary cutaneous plasmacytomas without underlying multiple myeloma is included in the 2005 WHO/EORTC classification among the primary cutaneous marginal zone B-cell lymphoma due to considerable overlapping features [3]. Primary cutaneous marginal zone B-cell lymphoma is considered as part of extranodal marginal zone lymphoma of MALT type [3]. Due to the infrequent and nonspecific presentation of cutaneous plasmacytomas, a clinical diagnosis is not sufficient. Diagnosis is based on clinical, histopathological, and immunohistochemical findings, and multiple myeloma must be ruled out by laboratory, radiologic, and bone marrow studies [4]. After ruling out multiple myeloma, the only findings will be a histopathologic dense monomorphic dermal plasmacytic infiltrate and a monoclonal immunohistochemistry.

Consistent with published literatures, our male patient in this case, at the age of 65, presented with a slow growing lesion and insignificant systemic review. Tissue biopsy immunohistochemically shows cytoplasmic expression of immunoglobulins that are restricted to one immunoglobulin chain. Histopathologic finding of diffuse or nodular dermal and subcuticular infiltrate of plasma cells, displaying varying degrees of maturation and atypia but no epidermotropism, are findings that are consistent with our patient. The immunophenotype demonstrates plasma cells positive for CD138, CD38, and CD79a, but generally not CD20 and leukocyte common antigen, and shows monotypic cytoplasmic immunoglobulin light chain expression on paraffin sections [3]. On the other hand, cutaneous marginal zone B cells express CD 20. Our patient was positive for CD138 and negative for CD20. While 30% of all marrow-based myelomas are lysozyme positive, lysozyme is not expressed by cutaneous plasmacytomas.

Laboratory, radiological, and bone marrow investigations must be done to exclude multiple myeloma. Laboratory studies include but are not limited to complete blood count, blood smear, blood sedimentation rate, renal function, electrolyte (calcium), serum and urine protein electrophoresis, quantitative Ig determination in serum, immunoelectrophoresis in serum and urine, and B-2 microglobulin determination in serum. All laboratory findings will be normal except for quantitative Ig elevation. Radiological studies include a full skeletal X-ray to rule out any osteolytic lesions that are consistent with multiple myeloma. A bone marrow biopsy will demonstrate plasma cell infiltration less than 5% of all nucleated cells. Plasma cells infiltration is common in reactive lesion and must be ruled out with staining for kappa or lambda light chain. In contrast to multiple myeloma, extramedullary plasmacytoma showed absence of cyclin D1 and infrequent expression of CD56.

Other differential diagnoses included secondary cutaneous plasmacytoma in the setting of systemic disease, mucosal extramedullary plasmacytoma with secondary skin involvement, marginal zone B-cell lymphoma, plasma cell granuloma, non-Hodgkin lymphoma, high-grade malignant immunoblastic lymphoma, and poorly differentiated neoplasms, as well as infectious diseases that cause infiltration of plasma cells.

Currently, there are approximately 50 cases of primary cutaneous plasmacytomas that have been reported in the literature [2]. Due to its rarity, little is known about its treatment. Treatment options include surgery, radiation, chemotherapy, and intralesional corticosteroid therapy. Type of treatment depends on the numbers (solitary versus multiple) and location of lesions. Most patients with solitary primary cutaneous plasmacytoma received radiotherapy as a component of treatment. Radiotherapy with curative intent (>4000 cGy) is the standard of care and provides promising result since the tumor is radiosensitive. The optimal dose for local control is 40–50 Gy in 20 fractions delivered over 4–6 weeks. However, caution should be considered when using radiotherapy as local recurrence or lymph node metastases could develop thereafter [2]. In addition to high dose radiotherapy and fractions, adjuvant chemotherapy may also be considered for lesions with high-grade histology or tumors >5 cm or for patients with multiple lesions. Palliative irradiation may also be used for the most symptomatic and large lesions. At the time when this case was written, the patient was in remission with no evidence of multiple myeloma or light chain disease. As reported in previous literatures, patient with solitary lesions received better outcomes than patient with multiple lesions at presentation. They tend to have less local regional or distant dissemination and remained confined to the skin. As a note, large solitary lesions might have a higher risk of progression to metastatic disease, although a size cut-off had not been determined [2].

The main prognostic factor seems to be the clinical presentation with more aggressive cases associated with multiple lesions, larger size, and IgA secretion by neoplastic cells. Multiple myeloma has been estimated to develop in one-third of patients [5]. It is found that progression to multiple myeloma is lower in soft-tissue plasmacytomas compared to osseous plasmacytomas [2]. Patients may also develop local recurrence and distant skin recurrence. Patients with multiple lesions had a higher likelihood of progression to multiple myeloma and subsequent death [2]. From previous case reported, recurrent-free survival increases from 1.4 years to 11 years and overall survival rate increases from 4.3 years to 17 years in patients with solitary primary cutaneous plasmacytomas compared to those with multiple primary cutaneous plasmacytomas lesions [2].

Currently, the pathophysiology is unknown; however there are a few developing hypothesis. Of all up to date cases of primary cutaneous plasmacytoma, five have been described in which local triggering stimulus from trauma may have contributed to the development of plasma cell proliferation. One of these cases reported a primary cutaneous plasmacytoma localized to the lower lip, which had been affected with recurrent herpes simplex virus-1 for 15 years. It was postulated that chronic stimulation of keratinocytes by herpes simplex virus-1, possibly through toll-like receptors, may have favored the release of interleukin-6 able to induce plasma cell proliferation, transformation, and survival [6]. Interleukin-6 may also have some oncogenic effects via enhancement of C-MYC and is antiapoptotic [7]. In the second hypothesis, it is thought that plasma cells expressing CXCR4 cytokine receptor can interact with the inflammatory cascade released due to tissue injury, facilitating the migration of neoplastic plasma cells into the skin [8].

Genetically, extramedullary plasmacytomas share many features of other plasma cell disorders, such as recurrent losses in chromosome 13, chromosome arm 1p, and chromosome arm 14q, as well as gain in chromosome arms 19p, 9q, and 1q [9].

According to the International Society for Cutaneous lymphoma (ISCL) and the cutaneous lymphoma task force of the European Organization of Research and Treatment of Cancer (EORTC), TNM classification system (see the list below) had been proposed to primarily document disease extension and to a lesser extent for prognostic guide [10].

ISCL/EORTC Proposed TNM Classification of Cutaneous Lymphoma Other Than Mycosis Fungoides and Sezary Syndrome

(T)

- (T1) Solitary skin involvement
  - (T1a) A solitary lesion <5 cm diameter
  - (T1b) A solitary >5 cm diameter
- (T2) Regional skin involvement of multiple lesions limited to 1 body region or 2 contiguous body regions
  - (T2a) All-disease encompassing in a <15 cm diameter circular area
  - (T2b) All-disease encompassing in >15 and <30 cm diameter circular area
  - (T2c) All-disease encompassing in a 30 cm diameter circular area
- (T3) Generalized skin involvement
  - (T3a) Multiple lesions involving 2 noncontiguous body regions
  - (T3b) Multiple lesions involving equal to or greater than 3 body regions

(N)

- (N0) No clinical or pathologic lymph node involvement
- (N1) Involvement of 1 peripheral lymph node region that drains an area of current or prior skin involvement
- (N2) Involvement of 2 or more peripheral lymph node regions or involvement of any lymph node region that does not drain an area of current or prior skin involvement
- (N3) Involvement of central lymph nodes

(M)

- (M0) No evidence of extracutaneous non-lymph node disease
- (M1) Extracutaneous non-lymph node disease present

In order to stage the disease, patients should undergo the following testing: a complete history and physical examination, complete blood count with differential count, chemistry panel with LDH, flow cytometry on peripheral blood, and imaging with computed tomography scan of the chest, abdomen, and pelvis with contrast or positron emission-tomography/CT as it can visualize metabolically active disease in relatively small lesions [10].

According to this classification, our patient was stage T1aN0M0 disease. As for treatment management, clinicians are recommended to follow the WHO-EORTC cutaneous lymphoma classification to understand the clinical behavior and prognostic variables in the heterogeneous group of cutaneous lymphomas in order to provide optimal care. Due to its shortcomings, the proposed TNM system will be reexamined as more data are obtained.

4. Conclusion

With few cases in the literature reported, this case is an example of a primary cutaneous lesion in an unusual location with no systemic disease. Follow-up care includes continual monitoring for progression to multiple myeloma. This consists of M-protein measurements and complete blood counts at six-week intervals for the first 6 months. This rarer and nonspecific presentation of a primary extramedullary plasmacytoma is important to keep in mind when evaluating lip lesions.

References

[1] P. Galienia, M. Cavi, S. Pulsoni et al., "Clinical outcome of extramedullary plasmacytoma," *Haemtologica*, vol. 85, no. 1, pp. 47–51, 2000.

[2] D. S. Tsang, L. W. Le, V. Kukreti, and A. Sun, "Treatment and outcomes for primary cutaneous extramedullary plasmacytoma: a case series," *Current Oncology*, vol. 23, no. 6, pp. e630–e646, 2016.

[3] R. Willemze, E. S. Jaffe, G. Burg et al., "WHO-EORTC classification for cutaneous lymphomas," *Blood*, vol. 105, no. 10, pp. 3768–3785, 2005.

[4] C. Prada-García, M. Lamoca-Martín, and M. Rodríguez-Prieto, "Nódulo de crecimiento progresivo localizado en el labio inferior," *Actas Dermo-Sifiliográficas*, vol. 103, no. 4, pp. 325–326, 2012.

[5] A. Wuu, S. D. Bangert, D. M. Weber, and S. R. Hymes, "Primary cutaneous plasmacytoma," *Cutis*, vol. 93, no. 6, pp. E19–E21, 2014.

[6] E. Zendri, C. Venturi, R. Ricci, G. Giordano, and G. De Panfilis, "Primary cutaneous plasmacytoma: a role for a triggering stimulus?" *Clinical and Experimental Dermatology*, vol. 30, no. 3, pp. 229–231, 2005.

[7] M. Magro Cynthia, "Marginal zone lymphoma and other low-grade B cell lymphoproliferative disorders of the skin," in *The Cutaneous Lymphoid Proliferation: A Comprehensive Textbook of Lymphocytic Infiltrates of the Skin*, pp. 149–171, John Wiley & Sons, 2007.

[8] A. Mosea and M. Millwaters, "Cutaneous plasmacytoma adjacent to Bowenoid actinic keratosis on the scalp: is there a link?" *International Journal of Surgery Case Reports*, vol. 21, pp. 52–54, 2016.

[9] V. Aalto, S. Nordling, A. H. Kivioja, E. Karaharju, I. Elomaa, and S. Knuutila, "Among numerous DNA copy number changes, losses of chromosome 13 are highly recurrent in plasmacytoma," *Genes Chromosomes and Cancer*, vol. 25, no. 2, pp. 104–107, 1999.

[10] L. Sokol, M. Naghashpour, and L. Frank Glass, "Primary cutaneous B-cell lymphomas: recent advances in diagnosis and management," *Cancer Control*, vol. 19, no. 3, pp. 236–244, 2012.

30

Alveolar Rhabdomyosarcoma in a 69-Year-Old Woman Receiving Glucagon-Like Peptide-2 Therapy

Laura E. Zyczynski,[1] Jonathan B. McHugh,[2] Thomas E. Gribbin,[3] and Scott M. Schuetze[1]

[1]*Department of Internal Medicine, University of Michigan Health System, 1500 E. Medical Center Drive, Ann Arbor, MI 48109, USA*
[2]*Department of Pathology, University of Michigan Health System, 1500 E. Medical Center Drive, Ann Arbor, MI 48109, USA*
[3]*Mercy Health Lacks Cancer Center, 250 Cherry Street SE, Grand Rapids, MI 489503, USA*

Correspondence should be addressed to Laura E. Zyczynski; lnielsen@med.umich.edu

Academic Editor: Francesco A. Mauri

A 69-year-old woman was diagnosed with alveolar rhabdomyosarcoma (ARMS) of the nasopharynx. She has a history of catastrophic thromboembolic event in the abdomen that caused short-gut syndrome and dependence on total parenteral nutrition (TPN) twelve hours per day. She was treated for short-gut syndrome with teduglutide, a glucagon-like peptide-2 (GLP-2) analog, which led to reduction of TPN requirements. However, a few months later, she developed metastatic alveolar rhabdomyosarcoma. Though a causative relationship is unlikely between the peptide and ARMS due to the brief time course between teduglutide therapy and sarcoma diagnosis, neoplastic growth may have been accelerated by the GLP-2 analog, causing release of IGF-1. The transmembrane receptor for IGF-1 is frequently overexpressed in ARMS and is implicated in cell proliferation and metastatic behavior. This case describes a rare incidence of metastatic alveolar rhabdomyosarcoma in a sexagenarian and possibly the first case reported associated with the use of teduglutide. Teduglutide was discontinued due to a potential theoretical risk of acceleration of sarcoma growth, and the patient's rhabdomyosarcoma is in remission following sarcoma chemotherapy.

1. Introduction

Soft tissue sarcomas are a heterogeneous group of mesenchymal neoplasms that affect patients of all ages. The incidence of soft tissue sarcoma is about 30 per million persons per year; in the United States about 12,000 people are diagnosed with soft tissue sarcoma each year [1]. Rhabdomyosarcoma (RMS) is the most common malignant soft tissue tumor of childhood, comprising approximately 50% of all pediatric soft tissue sarcomas, or about 5% of childhood cancers, but is rare in adults occurring in fewer than 5% of soft tissue sarcoma cases [2, 3]. Males are more likely than females to develop RMS. Rhabdomyosarcoma is most often sporadic, but certain cases are associated with familial syndromes, including Li-Fraumeni syndrome, neurofibromatosis type I, and hereditary retinoblastoma [4]. The two major histologic subtypes of RMS in children are embryonal RMS (ERMS) and alveolar RMS (ARMS). Embryonal RMS has a bimodal age distribution, with more than half of the cases arising before the age of 5 years and a smaller peak in adolescence, whereas ARMS is more likely to occur in adolescence [2].

Treatment of rhabdomyosarcoma is based on risk stratification at the time of diagnosis, which is based on several criteria developed by the Soft Tissue Sarcoma Committee (previously the Intergroup Rhabdomyosarcoma Study Group (IRSG)) of the Children's Oncology Group (COG). Treatment is multidisciplinary in nature, including surgery, radiation therapy, and chemotherapy. Favorable prognostic indicators include gross complete surgical removal of the tumor at the time of diagnosis, tumor size <5 cm, and age older than 1 but less than 10 years at diagnosis. Regional lymph node involvement in patients with alveolar rhabdomyosarcoma and distant metastasis is associated with a less favorable prognosis compared with those patients with localized disease [3].

In adults, soft tissue sarcomas comprise about 1% of solid tumor malignancies, and RMS makes up about only 3% of adult soft tissue sarcomas. If a patient over the age of 18 years is diagnosed with rhabdomyosarcoma, it is much more likely

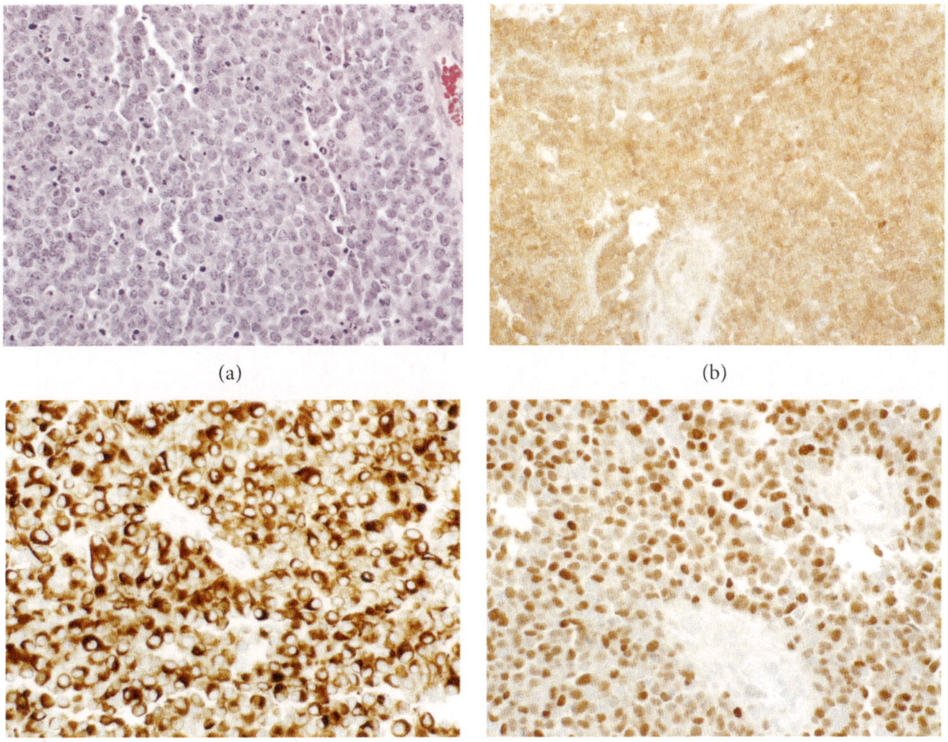

(a) (b) (c) (d)

Figure 1: Photomicrographs of diagnostic biopsy demonstrating rhabdomyosarcoma. (a) 40x magnification of hematoxylin- and eosin-stained section demonstrating diffuse small round cells with a high nuclear to cytoplasmic ratio. (b) 40x magnification of horseradish peroxidase immunohistochemical stain for IGF1-R demonstrating uniform expression. (c) 40x magnification of horseradish peroxidase immunohistochemical stain for desmin demonstrating cytoplasmic expression. (d) 40x magnification of horseradish peroxidase immunohistochemical stain for myogenin demonstrating nuclear localization.

to be pleomorphic (adult-type) RMS than one of the pediatric iterations of the disease. There are case reports in the medical literature about adults with ARMS, but cases are exceedingly rare. Adults with ARMS have a very high risk of developing metastases and usually die from the disease [5]. This report details a case report of an adult woman with alveolar rhabdomyosarcoma of the nasopharynx and discusses the possible role of teduglutide in growth of the sarcoma.

2. Clinical Presentation

The patient is a 69-year-old woman who presented with a chief complaint of unilateral clear rhinorrhea for two weeks. She was treated with steroid nasal spray without benefit. Due to persistent symptoms, she was treated with antibiotics for acute sinusitis, again without improvement. A few weeks later, she noted left-sided nasal occlusion with difficulty breathing through her nose and an enlarging left neck mass. She underwent computed tomography scanning of the neck that showed a left nasopharyngeal mass measuring 3 × 2.4 × 2.6 cm, extending from the skull base along the anterior inferior aspect of the left clivus inferiorly through the level of C1-C2. The mass encased the left upper internal carotid artery. A second mass was in the midline on the posterior choana abutting the nasal septum, measuring 2.2 × 2.2 × 1.8 cm, and a mass-like area between the nasal septum and the left middle turbinate was present, measuring 1.7 × 1.6 × 0.5 cm. Left submandibular and upper deep cervical chain adenopathy and a soft tissue mass in the flank detected on fluorodeoxyglucose-positron-emission tomography (FDG-PET) suggested metastatic cancer.

An excisional biopsy of the nasopharyngeal mass was performed. Pathology was consistent with ARMS. Immunohistochemical staining was notable for diffuse and strong positivity for CD56, vimentin, desmin, and myogenin (see Figure 1). There was patchy positivity for S-100. Tumor was negative for melan-A, HMB45, and cytokeratin cocktail. An antibody to the insulin-like growth factor-1 receptor reacted with tumor cells. The patient had a fine needle aspiration biopsy performed on the left neck and left flank masses, both of which were positive for metastatic ARMS. A portion of the nasopharyngeal mass biopsy was sent for reverse transcriptase-polymerase chain reaction (RT-PCR) for PAX3/FOX01 translocation chimeric transcript, and this was present, confirming the diagnosis.

The patient has a past medical history of a catastrophic thromboembolic event in the abdomen that resulted in necrotic bowel. She had a partial small bowel resection and subtotal colectomy with placement of ileostomy about 15 months prior to presentation to our medical center. This

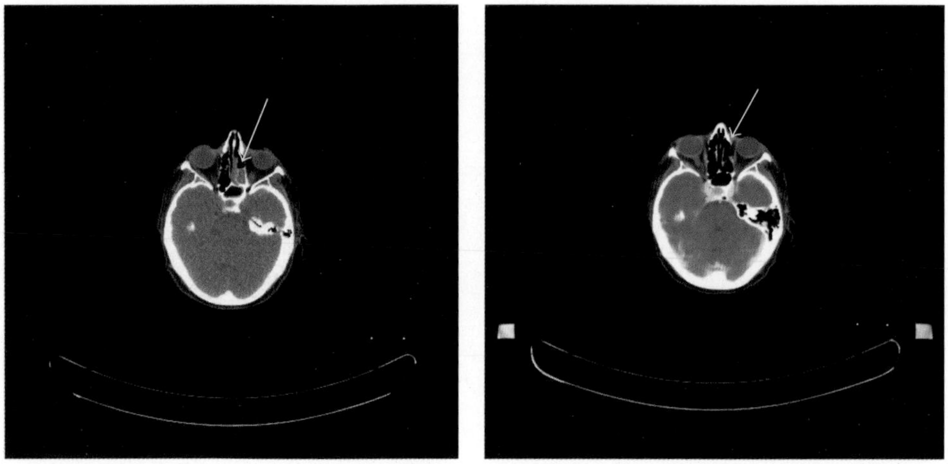

(a) (b)

Figure 2: Images from computed tomography scanning prior to starting chemotherapy and after three cycles, showing resolution of left nasopharyngeal mass.

resulted in short bowel syndrome (SBS) and dependence on total parenteral nutrition (TPN) 12 hours per day. About three months prior to diagnosis of RMS, the patient was started on the recently approved medication, teduglutide (rDNA origin) (Gattex^{R}), which is indicated for the treatment of adult patients with SBS who are dependent on parenteral support [6–8]. Teduglutide is an analog of human glucagon-like peptide-2 (GLP-2) that is resistant to cleavage and inactivation by dipeptidyl peptidase IV, which increases intestinal and portal blood flow and induces intestinal growth. In a randomized, placebo-controlled phase III trial, a significantly greater proportion of patients with SBS receiving teduglutide were able to reduce weekly TPN volume requirements >20% and experienced gain in weight compared to patients treated with placebo; however, none of the patients was able to wean off TPN [7].

3. Treatment

Once the diagnosis was established, teduglutide was discontinued due to the potential risk of acceleration of neoplastic growth. The patient began combination chemotherapy with doxorubicin, vincristine, and cyclophosphamide. Early cycles were complicated by neutropenic fever, oral stomatitis, and pancytopenia; all toxicities were managed with supportive measures and the patient completed a total of 9 months of therapy. Positron-emission tomography-CT scan after 3 cycles of chemotherapy showed dramatic improvement in multiple FDG-avid lesions, consistent with response to therapy. Rhinorrhea and nasal congestion resolved, and multiple masses including the left nasopharyngeal sarcoma regressed (Figure 2). After 9 months of chemotherapy, the patient had a clinical and radiographic complete response.

4. Discussion

The alveolar subtype of rhabdomyosarcoma is uncommon in adults and rarely occurs past the age of 65 years [9]. Chromosomal translocation involving PAX3 and FOXO1 is seen in about 70% of ARMS; a less frequent variant translocation (PAX7/FOX01) is present in 10–15% of ARMS [2, 10]. These reciprocal translocations fuse DNA-binding domains of PAX3 or PAX7 with the transactivation domain of FOX01, and the resultant novel products function as oncogenic proteins by promoting cell transformation and inhibiting apoptosis and myogenic differentiation. The fusion proteins and insulin-like growth factor-2 may cooperate in ARMS to promote a malignant phenotype [11]. The transmembrane receptor for insulin-like growth factor-1 (IGF-1) is frequently overexpressed in ARMS and is implicated in cell proliferation and metastatic behavior [12]. About 80% of ARMS express IGF-1 receptor, and *in vitro* studies suggest IGF-1 induces expression of myogenin, promotes cell proliferation, and prevents terminal muscle differentiation [13]. Inhibition of signaling through the IGF-1 receptor has been associated with significant reduction in ARMS growth *in vitro* [14, 15].

Teduglutide binds to GLP-2 receptors located in intestinal enteroendocrine cells, subepithelioid myofibroblasts, and enteric neurons of the submucosal and myenteric plexus [8]. Activation of these receptors causes local release of insulin-like growth factor- (IGF-) 1, nitric oxide, and keratinocyte growth factor (KGF) which promotes growth of intestinal epithelium [8]. GLP-2 indirectly stimulates intestinal growth through the IGF-1 pathway; both secretion of IGF-1 and expression of the IGF-1 receptor in intestinal epithelium are required for the proliferative effects of teduglutide on intestine [16, 17].

Common side effects of teduglutide occurring in more than 10% of patients include abdominal pain, abdominal distention, nausea, vomiting, change in gastrointestinal stoma, fluid overload, and upper respiratory tract infection [7]. The full prescribing information for teduglutide contains a warning about the potential for acceleration of neoplastic growth. In a 2-year carcinogenicity study in rats at subcutaneous doses of 3, 10, and 35 mg/kg/day (about 60, 200, and 700 times the recommended daily human dose of 0.05 mg/kg, resp.), teduglutide caused statistically significant increases in the incidences of adenomas in the bile duct and jejunum of male rats [8]. However, no dysplastic transformation was seen in intestinal tissue in patients treated in the phase III trial [18]. In a long-term follow-up study of teduglutide, 3 patients were diagnosed with cancer (adenocarcinoma of unknown primary, lung adenocarcinoma, and squamous cell lung cancer), but all three had predisposing risk factors for malignancy [18].

To our knowledge, we describe the first case of ARMS associated with the use of teduglutide. A causative role for the peptide in development of ARMS is unlikely because of the relatively short interval between initiation of teduglutide and diagnosis of sarcoma. Use of teduglutide may have contributed to growth of the malignancy, indirectly, through release of IGF-1, although a causative role for teduglutide in ARMS growth has not, to our knowledge, been established. As more biologic agents and mimetics become available to treat benign disease, physicians need to consider the potential roles of these agents in the pathogenesis of malignancy or acceleration of a previously existing or undiagnosed cancer. For example, a high density of GLP-2 receptors has been detected in the majority of gastrointestinal stromal tumors (GIST) in contrast to a wide range of cancers examined [19]. The biologic and pathologic implications of activation of GLP-2 in GIST need to be established to determine if teduglutide is contraindicated in patients with GIST. In summary, we present a case of metastatic ARMS occurring in a sexagenarian that underwent complete regression following cessation of teduglutide and treatment with sarcoma chemotherapy.

References

[1] R. Siegel, J. Ma, Z. Zou, and A. Jemal, "Cancer statistics, 2014," *CA: Cancer Journal for Clinicians*, vol. 64, no. 1, pp. 9–29, 2014.

[2] D. Egas-Bejar and W. W. Huh, "Rhabdomyosarcoma in adolescent and young adult patients: current perspectives," *Adolescent Health, Medicine and Therapeutics*, vol. 5, pp. 115–125, 2014.

[3] D. A. Rodeberg, N. Garcia-Henriquez, E. R. Lyden et al., "Prognostic significance and tumor biology of regional lymph node disease in patients with rhabdomyosarcoma: a report from the children's oncology group," *Journal of Clinical Oncology*, vol. 29, no. 10, pp. 1304–1311, 2011.

[4] C. M. Coffin, J. L. Davis, and S. C. Borinstein, "Syndrome-associated soft tissue tumours," *Histopathology*, vol. 64, no. 1, pp. 68–87, 2014.

[5] A. Ferrari, P. Dileo, M. Casanova et al., "Rhabdomyosarcoma in adults: a retrospective analysis of 171 patients treated at a single institution," *Cancer*, vol. 98, no. 3, pp. 571–580, 2003.

[6] P. B. Jeppesen, R. Gilroy, M. Pertkiewicz, J. P. Allard, B. Messing, and S. J. O'Keefe, "Randomised placebo-controlled trial of teduglutide in reducing parenteral nutrition and/or intravenous fluid requirements in patients with short bowel syndrome," *Gut*, vol. 60, no. 7, pp. 902–914, 2011.

[7] P. B. Jeppesen, M. Pertkiewicz, B. Messing et al., "Teduglutide reduces need for parenteral support among patients with short bowel syndrome with intestinal failure," *Gastroenterology*, vol. 143, no. 6, pp. 1473.e3–1481.e3, 2012.

[8] GATTEX prescribing information, 2014, https://www.gattex.com/assets/pdf/PIIFU.pdf.

[9] I. Sultan, I. Qaddoumi, S. Yaser, C. Rodriguez-Galindo, and A. Ferrari, "Comparing adult and pediatric rhabdomyosarcoma in the surveillance, epidemiology and end results program, 1973 to 2005: an analysis of 2,600 patients," *Journal of Clinical Oncology*, vol. 27, no. 20, pp. 3391–3397, 2009.

[10] S. Gallego Melcón and J. Sánchez de Toledo Codina, "Molecular biology of rhabdomyosarcoma," *Clinical and Translational Oncology*, vol. 9, no. 7, pp. 415–419, 2007.

[11] W. Wang, M. Slevin, S. Kumar, and P. Kumar, "The cooperative transforming effects of PAX3-FKHR and IGF-II on mouse myoblasts," *International Journal of Oncology*, vol. 27, no. 4, pp. 1087–1096, 2005.

[12] A. S. Martins, D. Olmos, E. Missiaglia, and J. Shipley, "Targeting the insulin-like growth factor pathway in rhabdomyosarcomas: rationale and future perspectives," *Sarcoma*, vol. 2011, Article ID 209736, 11 pages, 2011.

[13] K. Tsuchiya, H. Hosoi, A. Misawa-Furihata, P. J. Houghton, and T. Sugimoto, "Insulin-like growth factor-I has different effects on myogenin induction and cell cycle progression in human alveolar and embryonal rhabdomyosarcoma cells," *International Journal of Oncology*, vol. 31, no. 1, pp. 41–47, 2007.

[14] T. Kalebic, M. Tsokos, and L. J. Helman, "In vivo treatment with antibody against IGF-1 receptor suppresses growth of human rhabdomyosarcoma and down-regulates p34cdc2," *Cancer Research*, vol. 54, no. 21, pp. 5531–5534, 1994.

[15] D. N. Shapiro, B. G. Jones, L. H. Shapiro, P. Dias, and P. J. Houghton, "Antisense-mediated reduction in insulin-like growth factor-I receptor expression suppresses the malignant phenotype of a human alveolar rhabdomyosarcoma," *The Journal of Clinical Investigation*, vol. 94, no. 3, pp. 1235–1242, 1994.

[16] P. E. Dubé, C. L. Forse, J. Bahrami, and P. L. Brubaker, "The essential role of insulin-like growth factor-1 in the intestinal tropic effects of glucagon-like peptide-2 in mice," *Gastroenterology*, vol. 131, no. 2, pp. 589–605, 2006.

[17] K. J. Rowland, S. Trivedi, D. Lee et al., "Loss of glucagon-like peptide-2-induced proliferation following intestinal epithelial insulin-like growth factor-1-receptor deletion," *Gastroenterology*, vol. 141, no. 6, pp. 2166.e7–2175.e7, 2011.

[18] C. B. Burness and P. L. McCormack, "Teduglutide: a review of its use in the treatment of patients with short bowel syndrome," *Drugs*, vol. 73, no. 9, pp. 935–947, 2013.

[19] M. Körner, R. Rehmann, and J. C. Reubi, "GLP-2 receptors in human disease: high expression in gastrointestinal stromal tumors and Crohn's disease," *Molecular and Cellular Endocrinology*, vol. 364, no. 1-2, pp. 46–53, 2012.

Durable Clinical Benefit of Pertuzumab in a Young Patient with BRCA2 Mutation and HER2-Overexpressing Breast Cancer Involving the Brain

Anna Koumarianou,[1] Christina Kontopoulou,[2] Vassilis Kouloulias,[3] and Christina Tsionou[4]

[1]*Hematology-Oncology Unit, Fourth Department of Internal Medicine, National and Kapodistrian University of Athens, Attikon University Hospital, Rimini 1, Haidari, 12462 Athens, Greece*
[2]*Second Radiology Department, Attikon University Hospital, National and Kapodistrian University of Athens, Rimini 1, Haidari, 12462 Athens, Greece*
[3]*Radiotherapy Unit, Second Radiology Department, Attikon University Hospital, National and Kapodistrian University of Athens, Rimini 1, Haidari, 12462 Athens, Greece*
[4]*Maternity-Health, 30 Papanikoli Street, Halandri, 15232 Athens, Greece*

Correspondence should be addressed to Anna Koumarianou; akoumari@yahoo.com

Academic Editor: Guido Fadda

Patients with HER2-positive breast cancer and brain metastases have limited treatment options, and, as a result of their poor performance status and worse prognosis, they are underrepresented in clinical trials. Not surprisingly, these patients may not be fit enough to receive any active treatment and are offered supportive therapy. BRCA2 mutations are reported to be rarely associated with HER2-overexpressing advanced breast cancer and even more rarely with brain metastases at diagnosis. We report on a BRCA2-positive breast cancer patient with metastatic disease in multiple sites, including the brain, and poor performance status who exhibited an extraordinary clinical and imaging response to the novel anti-HER2 therapy pertuzumab after multiple lines of therapy including anti-HER2 targeting. To our knowledge, the clinicopathologic and therapeutic characteristics of this patient point to a unique case and an urgent need for further investigation of pertuzumab in patients with brain metastases.

1. Introduction

Brain involvement of metastatic breast cancer is largely dependent on the molecular subtype of the disease, and in the case of HER2-overexpressing tumors, it affects 30% of patients and is associated with devastating symptoms and quality of life [1, 2].

Several studies confirm that the median survival from diagnosis of brain metastases is from 6 months for patients who do not receive trastuzumab to 13 months for those who receive trastuzumab [1, 3, 4]. With few exceptions, there are hardly any prospective phases II-III clinical studies interrogating the role of anti-HER2 drugs in brain involvement [5, 6]. A plausible explanation for such a serious underrepresentation of patients in clinical trials is the poor performance status of this patient subgroup due to the tumoral involvement of the central nervous system. A recent study combining trastuzumab and pertuzumab for patients with metastatic disease resulted in survival improvement of 15.7 months [7]. Because this study did not include patients with brain metastases, there is no established experience about such anti-HER2 therapy's potential administration and benefit in patients relapsing after trastuzumab and lapatinib. With regard to patients with HER2-overexpressing metastatic breast cancer who are BRCA2 carriers, there is a scarcity of information in the published literature [8], so there is not much data on their survival and responses to the available treatments. However, a recent meta-analysis including breast

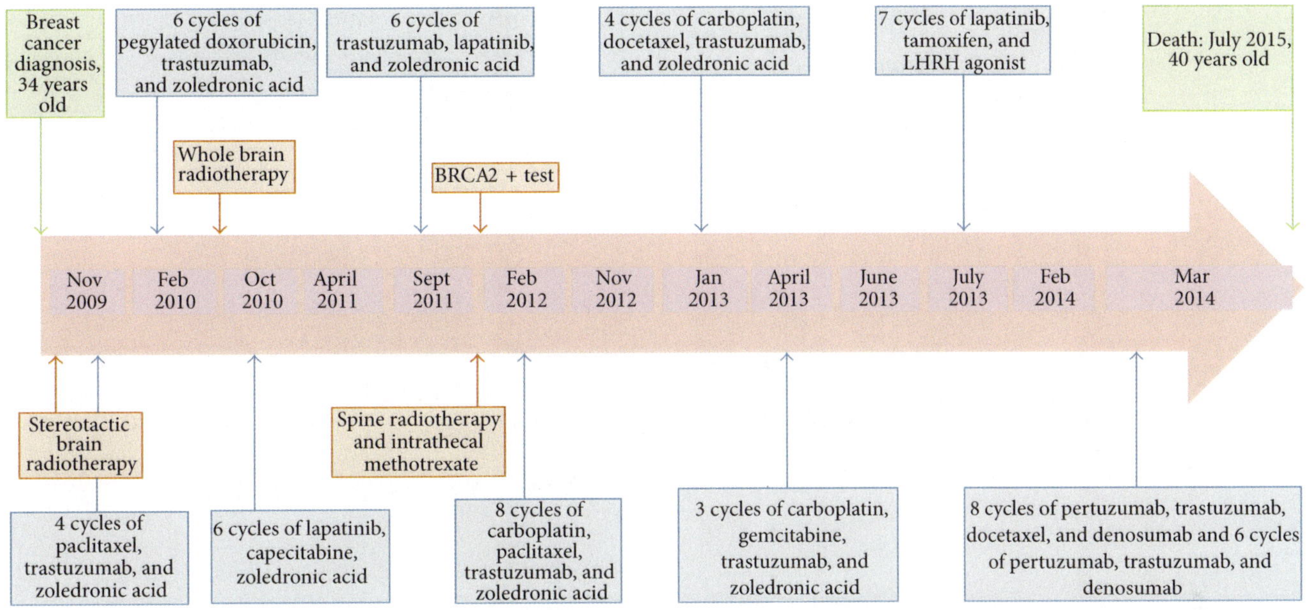

FIGURE 1: Timeline of patient's diagnosis and treatments.

cancer patients who are BRCA2 mutation carriers indicated no survival differences compared to patients without BRCA2 mutations [9].

2. Case Presentation

A 34-year-old female with abdominal pain and headache presented at the emergency department in November 2009. Upon clinical examination, she had a red, hard, fixed right breast with a fixed lymph nodal mass in the right axilla. She was living in the outskirts of Sparta with her husband and two children. She was never a smoker or an alcohol drinker.

Her past medical history included a pituitary adenoma; she had no brothers or sisters, but she had a remarkable family history, as her father and uncle died of metastatic breast cancer.

Her imaging with computed tomography (CT) and laboratory investigations revealed a single brain and multiple lung, liver, and bone metastases. A full blood count and biochemistry were normal except for the following: hemoglobin: 9.8 g/dL (normal value; nv 12–16); aspartate aminotransferase: 78 U/L (nv 5–40); alanine aminotransferase: 96 U/L (nv 5–35); gamma-glutamyl transferase: 216 U/L (nv 7–49); alkaline phosphatase: 261 U/L (nv 25–125); lactic acid dehydrogenase: 778 U/L (<250); and tumor markers: Ca 15-3 >1000 U/mL (nv < 31) and CEA > 50 ng/mL (nv < 5).

Histologic and immunohistochemical examination of a true-cut biopsy revealed an invasive ductal adenocarcinoma, grade III differentiation, estrogen receptor (ER) strong nuclear positivity in 70% of cells, progesterone receptor (PR) nuclear positivity in less than 3%, HER2 strongly positive (+3), Ki-67 nuclear positivity in 40% of cells, and p53 nuclear positivity in 60% of cells according to the histopathology.

Following stereotactic brain radiotherapy to the single lesion, the patient was treated according to the 2009 NCCN first-line strategy recommendations, which included paclitaxel, trastuzumab, and zoledronic acid [10]. Reevaluation after four cycles revealed disease progression (PD) in the lung and liver according to the RECIST criteria of response. A second line of therapy was initiated and included pegylated doxorubicin, trastuzumab, and zoledronic acid [11]. The choice of this combination was primarily based on patient's desire to avoid further alopecia. The first reevaluation at 3 months indicated partial response (PR) at all sites, including the breast, but a second assessment at 6 months revealed a relapse in the brain and lung. Following whole brain radiation, the patient was treated with a third-line therapy consisting of combination therapy with lapatinib, capecitabine, and zoledronic acid [12]. At CT reevaluation at 6 months, there was leptomeningeal dissemination and a vertebral thoracic mass (T12). After cytologic confirmation of leptomeningeal disease by lumbar puncture, the patient was treated with three courses of intrathecal methotrexate and radiotherapy to the spine (T12 level). The reevaluation showed a negative cerebrospinal fluid cytology but PD at all other sites: brain, lung, and liver. The patient received three further lines of combination chemotherapy including carboplatin, following a positive BRCA2 test [13–16], experiencing brief responses as described in Figure 1.

Following PD after the seventh line of therapy based on the combination of carboplatin, gemcitabine, and trastuzumab [16], the patient was physically and psychologically exhausted and willing to proceed with some form of active treatment. Thus, an eighth line of orally administered therapy at home was initiated and included lapatinib and hormonal therapy. Seven months later, the patient deteriorated clinically (PS ECOG/WHO: 3-4) and arrived at the outpatient department in a wheelchair. Total body CT scans revealed PD in all sites, including the brain. Based on new NCCN guidelines and following discussion with the patient and her family, a ninth

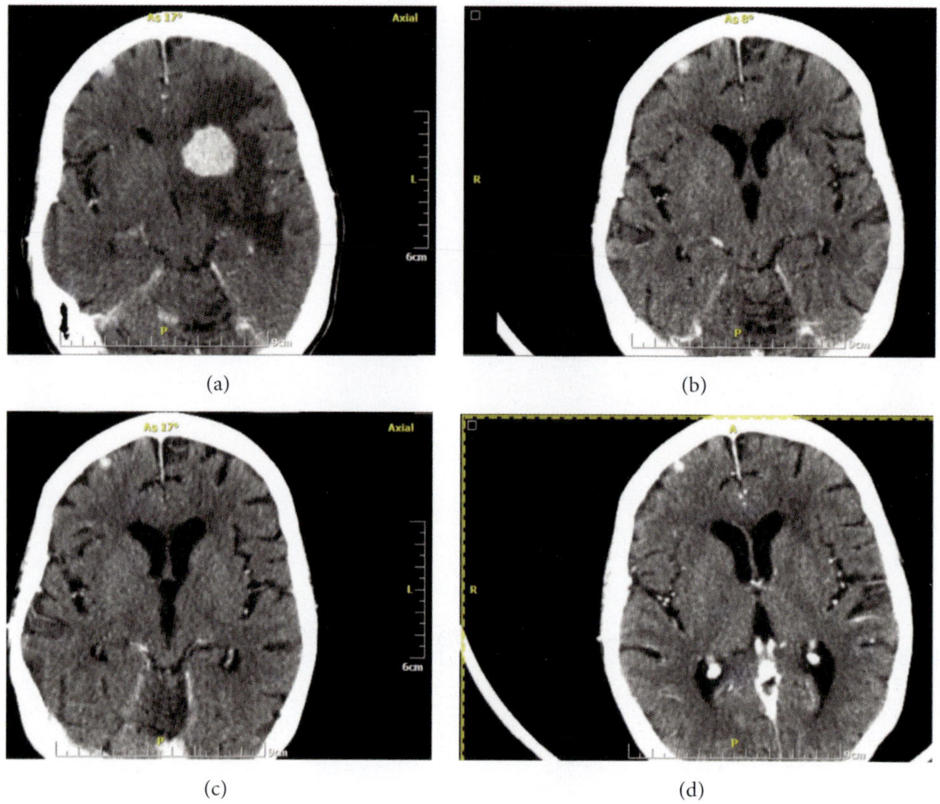

FIGURE 2: Brain computed tomography at baseline (a) and after 3 (b), 9 (c), and 12 (d) months of treatment with pertuzumab, trastuzumab, and taxane-based chemotherapy.

line of therapy was initiated, including the novel combination of pertuzumab/trastuzumab, docetaxel, and denosumab [17]. The patient's performance status gradually improved with CT reevaluation at 4 months, revealing a PR at all sites, including the brain (Figure 2). The clinical and imaging response continued to improve until 12 months later when a "plateau" was achieved. The patient continued on maintenance therapy with pertuzumab/trastuzumab/denosumab without chemotherapy for further six months. During all this time, she was walking and active at home taking care of her children, but when this time elapsed the patient rapidly deteriorated and succumbed to her disease.

3. Discussion

We report on a young patient who is a BRCA2 mutation carrier diagnosed with HER2-positive breast cancer with visceral and brain metastases. Having received nine lines of anti-HER2 treatment, including a platinum agent, and radiotherapy to the brain, there were only two available options: referral to the supportive care team or a tenth line of treatment with the recently approved pertuzumab. The CLEOPATRA trial had indicated an excellent survival benefit for patients with HER2-positive metastatic disease treated with pertuzumab but provided no data on patients with brain metastases, as these were excluded [7]. At that time, the EMILIA trial on TMD-1 had just been completed, and the treatment was shown to result in very good response rates [18], but it was not yet locally approved or readily available for the patient. A recently reported phase II trial on pertuzumab/trastuzumab combination without chemotherapy in patients who had progressed under trastuzumab based regimen indicated a 50% clinical benefit rate and a 5.5-month median progression-free survival [19]. Our patient received one cycle of pertuzumab, trastuzumab, and docetaxel and experienced rapid symptomatic relief, indicating the need for continuation.

Patients with HER2-positive breast cancer are living longer due to effective treatment, and as a result, brain metastases are now most common [3]. Patients like ours are usually not involved in clinical trials due to their poor performance status that is allegedly related to bad prognosis, and the optimal therapy remains an open question. Until today, only one case with brain metastases has been reported to experience complete response under second-line combination of pertuzumab-trastuzumab and docetaxel [20]. A retrospective study including patients rechallenged with trastuzumab after second-line lapatinib therapy for CNS involvement indicated a rather poor median OS of 17.3 (3.4–32.2) months [21]. Although monoclonal antibody penetration in the CNS has been questioned [22, 23], recently, a TDM-1 study [24] and a PET imaging analysis employing a radiolabeled trastuzumab-DOTA conjugate [25] have indicated indirectly and directly that monoclonal antibody targeting of brain metastases occurs effectively.

There are only a few studies available evaluating the role of anti-HER2 treatments in patients with disease metastasized to the brain, and these include small numbers of patients. Among these is one retrospective exploratory analysis of the phase III EMILIA study including 92 patients, of whom 43 were treated with T-DM1 and had an overall survival time of 26.8 months, compared to 12.9 months in the lapatinib/capecitabine group (49 patients) [24]. Additional studies include a multicenter phase II study including 242 patients treated with lapatinib [6], one phase III study of 36 patients with brain metastases treated with trastuzumab and lapatinib [5], one retrospective analysis of 432 patients, indicating that patients treated with both trastuzumab and lapatinib after developing metastases had significantly longer survival than patients treated with either agent alone [26], and one retrospective study including 79 patients treated with trastuzumab [27]. Based on the clinical activity observed in the EGF104900, LANDSCAPE, and EMILIA studies, the most active treatment options for HER2-positive breast cancer patients with brain metastases include trastuzumab/lapatinib [28], capecitabine/lapatinib [29], and TDM-1 [24].

A major challenge faced in patients with metastatic disease, including those with breast cancer, is whether metastases develop according to a linear or a metastatic cascade model, which could lead to a separate molecular profile with important therapeutic implications [30].

4. Conclusions

Brain metastases are increasingly being acknowledged as the next major step to prolong survival in HER2-positive breast cancer. Our patient, combining systemic and local therapies, lived 67 months from the diagnosis of brain disease. The effectiveness observed in our patient indicated that the combination of pertuzumab/trastuzumab deserves further investigation in the context of larger studies. Nevertheless, it is necessary to assess the optimal anti-HER2 drug sequence in conjunction with efforts to redefine the role of radiotherapy and surgery in breast cancer patients with metastatic disease in the brain.

Authors' Contributions

All the authors have contributed to the paper preparation.

Acknowledgments

The costs of this paper were deducted from a donation of the Hellenic Study Group of Psychoneuroimmunology in Cancer.

References

[1] J. C. Bendell, S. M. Domchek, H. J. Burstein et al., "Central nervous system metastases in women who receive trastuzumab-based therapy for metastatic breast carcinoma," *Cancer*, vol. 97, no. 12, pp. 2972–2977, 2003.

[2] N. U. Lin, L. Amiri-Kordestani, D. Palmieri, D. J. Liewehr, and P. S. Steeg, "CNS metastases in breast cancer: old challenge, new frontiers," *Clinical Cancer Research*, vol. 19, no. 23, pp. 6404–6418, 2013.

[3] A. M. Brufsky, M. Mayer, H. S. Rugo et al., "Central nervous system metastases in patients with HER2-positive metastatic breast cancer: incidence, treatment, and survival in patients from registHER," *Clinical Cancer Research*, vol. 17, no. 14, pp. 4834–4843, 2011.

[4] S. Dawood, K. Broglio, F. J. Esteva et al., "Defining prognosis for women with breast cancer and CNS metastases by HER2 status," *Annals of Oncology*, vol. 19, no. 7, pp. 1242–1248, 2008.

[5] K. L. Blackwell, H. J. Burstein, A. M. Storniolo et al., "Randomized study of lapatinib alone or in combination with trastuzumab in women with ErbB2-positive, trastuzumab-refractory metastatic breast cancer," *Journal of Clinical Oncology*, vol. 28, no. 7, pp. 1124–1130, 2010.

[6] N. U. Lin, V. Diéras, D. Paul et al., "Multicenter phase II study of lapatinib in patients with brain metastases from HER2-positive breast cancer," *Clinical Cancer Research*, vol. 15, no. 4, pp. 1452–1459, 2009.

[7] S. M. Swain, J. Baselga, S.-B. Kim et al., "Pertuzumab, trastuzumab, and docetaxel in HER2-positive metastatic breast cancer," *The New England Journal of Medicine*, vol. 372, no. 8, pp. 724–734, 2015.

[8] B. Arun, S. Bayraktar, D. D. Liu et al., "Response to neoadjuvant systemic therapy for breast cancer in BRCA mutation carriers and noncarriers: a single-institution experience," *Journal of Clinical Oncology*, vol. 29, no. 28, pp. 3739–3746, 2011.

[9] E.-H. Lee, S. K. Park, B. Park et al., "Effect of BRCA1/2 mutation on short-term and long-term breast cancer survival: a systematic review and meta-analysis," *Breast Cancer Research and Treatment*, vol. 122, no. 1, pp. 11–25, 2010.

[10] D. J. Slamon, B. Leyland-Jones, S. Shak et al., "Use of chemotherapy plus a monoclonal antibody against HER2 for metastatic breast cancer that overexpresses HER2," *The New England Journal of Medicine*, vol. 344, no. 11, pp. 783–792, 2001.

[11] E. Stickeler, M. Klar, D. Watermann et al., "Pegylated liposomal doxorubicin and trastuzumab as 1st and 2nd line therapy in her2/neu positive metastatic breast cancer: a multicenter phase II trial," *Breast Cancer Research and Treatment*, vol. 117, no. 3, pp. 591–598, 2009.

[12] C. E. Geyer, J. Forster, D. Lindquist et al., "Lapatinib plus capecitabine for HER2-positive advanced breast cancer," *The New England Journal of Medicine*, vol. 355, no. 26, pp. 2733–2743, 2006.

[13] M. Kriege, C. Seynaeve, H. Meijers-Heijboer et al., "Sensitivity to first-line chemotherapy for metastatic breast cancer in BRCA1 and BRCA2 mutation carriers," *Journal of Clinical Oncology*, vol. 27, no. 23, pp. 3764–3771, 2009.

[14] N. Robert, B. Leyland-Jones, L. Asmar et al., "Randomized phase III study of trastuzumab, paclitaxel, and carboplatin compared with trastuzumab and paclitaxel in women with HER-2-overexpressing metastatic breast cancer," *Journal of Clinical Oncology*, vol. 24, no. 18, pp. 2786–2792, 2006.

[15] V. Valero, J. Forbes, M. D. Pegram et al., "Multicenter phase III randomized trial comparing docetaxel and trastuzumab with docetaxel, carboplatin, and trastuzumab as first-line chemotherapy for patients with HER2-gene-amplified metastatic breast cancer (BCIRG 007 study): two highly active therapeutic regimens," *Journal of Clinical Oncology*, vol. 29, no. 2, pp. 149–156, 2011.

[16] F. Nelli, L. Moscetti, G. Natoli et al., "Gemcitabine and carboplatin for pretreated metastatic breast cancer: the predictive value of immunohistochemically defined subtypes," *International Journal of Clinical Oncology*, vol. 18, no. 2, pp. 343–349, 2013.

[17] J. Baselga, J. Cortés, S.-B. Kim et al., "Pertuzumab plus trastuzumab plus docetaxel for metastatic breast cancer," *The New England Journal of Medicine*, vol. 366, no. 2, pp. 109–119, 2012.

[18] S. Verma, D. Miles, L. Gianni et al., "Trastuzumab emtansine for HER2-positive advanced breast cancer," *New England Journal of Medicine*, vol. 367, no. 19, pp. 1783–1791, 2012.

[19] J. Baselga, K. A. Gelmon, S. Verma et al., "Phase II trial of pertuzumab and trastuzumab in patients with human epidermal growth factor receptor 2-positive metastatic breast cancer that progressed during prior trastuzumab therapy," *Journal of Clinical Oncology*, vol. 28, no. 7, pp. 1138–1144, 2010.

[20] N. Senda, A. Yamaguchi, H. Nishimura, T. Shiozaki, and S. Tsuyuki, "Pertuzumab, trastuzumab and docetaxel reduced the recurrence of brain metastasis from breast cancer: a case report," *Breast Cancer*, vol. 23, no. 2, pp. 323–328, 2016.

[21] S. Gori, F. Montemurro, S. Spazzapan et al., "Retreatment with trastuzumab-based therapy after disease progression following lapatinib in HER2-positive metastatic breast cancer," *Annals of Oncology*, vol. 23, no. 6, pp. 1436–1441, 2012.

[22] P. S. Steeg, K. A. Camphausen, and Q. R. Smith, "Brain metastases as preventive and therapeutic targets," *Nature Reviews Cancer*, vol. 11, no. 5, pp. 352–363, 2011.

[23] H.-J. Stemmler, M. Schmitt, A. Willems, H. Bernhard, N. Harbeck, and V. Heinemann, "Ratio of trastuzumab levels in serum and cerebrospinal fluid is altered in HER2-positive breast cancer patients with brain metastases and impairment of blood-brain barrier," *Anti-Cancer Drugs*, vol. 18, no. 1, pp. 23–28, 2007.

[24] I. E. Krop, N. U. Lin, K. Blackwell et al., "Trastuzumab emtansine (T-DM1) versus lapatinib plus capecitabine in patients with HER2-positive metastatic breast cancer and central nervous system metastases: a retrospective, exploratory analysis in EMILIA," *Annals of Oncology*, vol. 26, no. 1, pp. 113–119, 2015.

[25] H. Kurihara, A. Hamada, M. Yoshida et al., " ^{64}Cu-DOTA-trastuzumab PET imaging and HER2 specificity of brain metastases in HER2-positive breast cancer patients," *EJNMMI Research*, vol. 5, article 8, 2015.

[26] N. Hayashi, N. Niikura, N. Masuda et al., "Prognostic factors of HER2-positive breast cancer patients who develop brain metastasis: a multicenter retrospective analysis," *Breast Cancer Research and Treatment*, vol. 149, no. 1, pp. 277–284, 2015.

[27] S. Dawood, A. M. Gonzalez-Angulo, C. Albarracin et al., "Prognostic factors of survival in the trastuzumab era among women with breast cancer and brain metastases who receive whole brain radiotherapy: a single-institution review," *Cancer*, vol. 116, no. 13, pp. 3084–3092, 2010.

[28] K. L. Blackwell, H. J. Burstein, A. M. Storniolo et al., "Overall survival benefit with lapatinib in combination with trastuzumab for patients with human epidermal growth factor receptor 2-positive metastatic breast cancer: final results from the EGF104900 study," *Journal of Clinical Oncology*, vol. 30, no. 21, pp. 2585–2592, 2012.

[29] T. Bachelot, G. Romieu, M. Campone et al., "Lapatinib plus capecitabine in patients with previously untreated brain metastases from HER2-positive metastatic breast cancer (LANDSCAPE): a single-group phase 2 study," *The Lancet Oncology*, vol. 14, no. 1, pp. 64–71, 2013.

[30] K. Naxerova and R. K. Jain, "Using tumour phylogenetics to identify the roots of metastasis in humans," *Nature Reviews Clinical Oncology*, vol. 12, no. 5, pp. 258–272, 2015.

32

Successful Outcome of Low-Dose S-1 Used to Treat Buccal Squamous Cell Carcinoma

Kazuyuki Yusa,[1] Hideyuki Yamanouchi,[2] Ayako Sugano,[2] and Mitsuyoshi Iino[1]

[1] *Department of Dentistry, Oral and Maxillofacial, Plastic and Reconstructive Surgery, Yamagata University Faculty of Medicine, Yamagata, Japan*
[2] *Department of Dentistry and Oral Surgery, Shinjo Tokushukai Hospital, Yamagata, Japan*

Correspondence should be addressed to Kazuyuki Yusa; k-yusa@med.id.yamagata-u.ac.jp

Academic Editor: Constantine Gennatas

This case report describes an 86-year-old woman with dormant right buccal squamous cell carcinoma who was able to maintain a reasonable quality of life after being treated with oral low-dose S-1 (80 mg/day). The treatment regimen started in April 2014 and consisted of two weeks of S-1 followed by a one-week interval. The patient remains on this regimen while maintaining her quality of life and she has been under follow-up as an outpatient for 36 months. The outcomes for this patient indicated that low-dose S-1 is a valid anticancer therapy that may help maintain quality of life for some patients with incurable or dormant cancers.

1. Introduction

The destruction of normal tissues by head and neck cancers often results in dysfunction, and postoperative sequelae such as speech disorders, pain, depression, dysphagia, and xerostomia are common and often significant [1, 2]. Hence, the approach to treating cancers of the head and neck should be selected depending on the age, general health status, and prognosis of patients, as well as their comprehension. Fundamental treatment strategies such as tumor resection or chemoradiotherapy are not usually the first choice for treating elderly patients with head and neck carcinoma. Also, whether intensive chemotherapy using platinum drugs, taxanes, methotrexate, or bleomycin can improve the quality of life of such patients is doubtful [3, 4].

Although its effectiveness as chemotherapy for head and neck carcinoma has not been fully demonstrated, S-1 might be safe and effective for treating elderly patients with head and neck carcinoma. This case report describes an elderly patient with dormant buccal squamous cell carcinoma who could maintain a reasonable quality of life with long-term low-dose S-1.

2. Case Presentation

A family dentist referred an 86-year-old woman to us in March 2014 with a complaint of contact pain in the right buccal mucosa. Her medical history revealed hyperlipidemia and diabetes mellitus, which were controlled with medication. She had a gastric carcinoma that was resected in 2011, and she has remained free of postoperative recurrence and lymph node metastasis. She denied difficulty with swallowing, chewing, speech, and breathing. The findings of a general physical examination were unremarkable. An intraoral examination showed an ulcerated mass around the right buccal mucosa at a right angle to the mouth (Figure 1(a)), and CT imaging revealed a 31×18 mm enhanced lesion around the right buccal region (Figure 1(b)) and an enlarged submandibular lymph node (Figure 1(c)). A biopsy confirmed the lesion as well-differentiated squamous cell carcinoma classified as T2N1M0, stage III.

Neither the patient nor her family wished to consider radical therapy such as tumor resection, considering her advanced age. Therefore, we obtained written, informed consent from the patient and her family for oral administration of low-dose S-1 (80 mg/day) starting in April 2014. The regimen

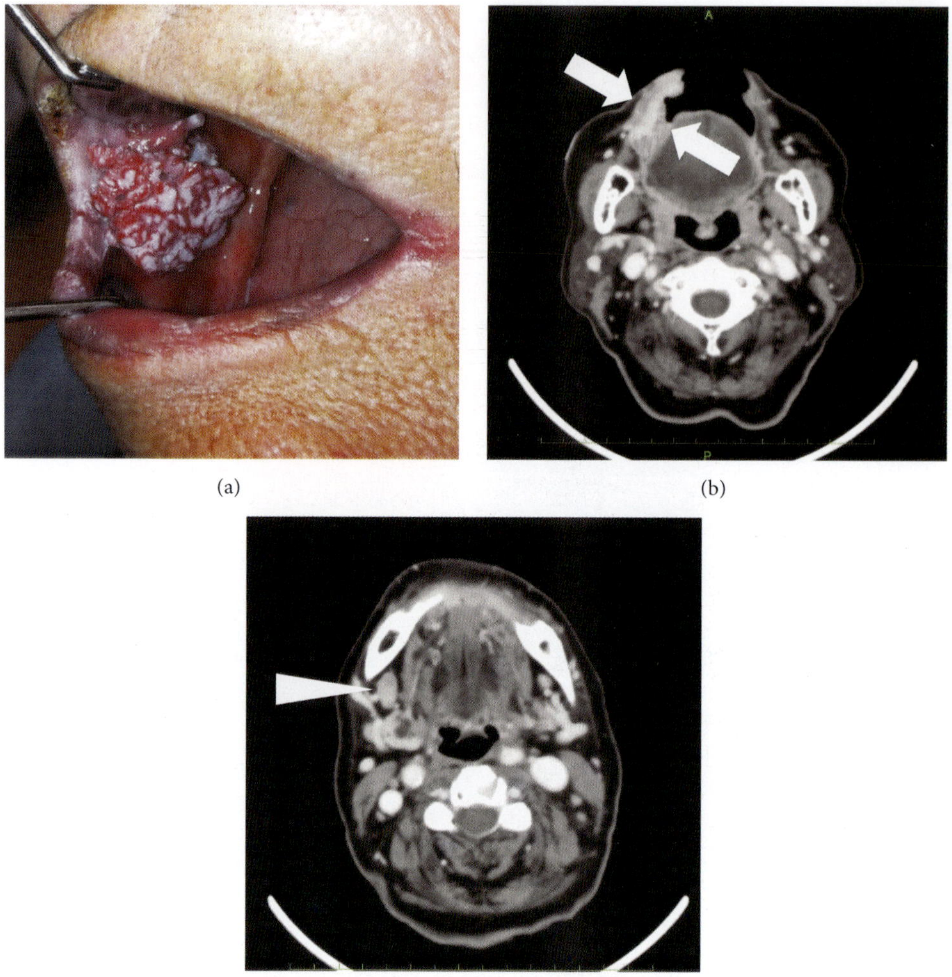

(a) (b) (c)

FIGURE 1: *Intraoral findings at initial presentation.* Ulcerated lesion in the right buccal area (a). CT images in the right buccal area show an enhanced lesion ((b), arrow) and enlarged submandibular lymph node ((c), arrow head).

consisted of two weeks of S-1 therapy followed by a one-week interval. This regimen is ongoing and she has remained free of adverse reactions defined in the National Cancer Institute Common Toxicity Criteria version 4.0 toxicity scale.

Figure 2 shows that the size of the tumor had decreased to 12 × 6 mm, both clinically (Figure 2(a)) and radiographically (Figure 2(b)) and that the size of the metastatic submandibular lymph node had also decreased (Figure 2(c)) at the time of the last follow-up. The patient has survived for 36 months since she was initially referred to us, and her quality of life has not decreased.

3. Discussion

S-1 is an oral anticancer agent containing tegafur, a prodrug of 5-fluorouracil (5-FU), and two modulators. One is 5-chloro-2,4-dihydroxypyridine, which causes prolonged retention of 5-FU in the bloodstream and enhances the pharmacological actions of 5-FU by competitively inhibiting its degradation. The other is potassium oxonate, which localizes in the mucosa of the gastrointestinal tract after oral administration and alleviates gastrointestinal toxicities induced by 5-FU [5, 6]. S-1 monotherapy is considered a second- or third-line chemotherapy for unresectable cancer [7]. Although response rates are modest, S-1 monotherapy is safe and well tolerated by elderly patients [8], and it can be administered over the long term in the outpatient setting. Thus, patients can undergo S-1 chemotherapy while maintaining a reasonable quality of life. The original S-1 regimen comprised four weeks of chemotherapy followed by two weeks of rest. However, Itoi et al. [9] reported that a regimen comprising two weeks of S-1 followed by one week of rest is less likely to be interrupted by side effects and is safer for outpatients.

Some studies of models have found that continuous low-dose chemotherapy can cause the long-term suppression of tumor proliferation in vitro and in vivo and that one of the action mechanisms involves antiangiogenic effects [10, 11]. Recently, much attention has been focused on metronomic chemotherapy; some successful drug combinations for several cancers have been reported [12]. Allegrini et al. [13] reported metronomic chemotherapy regimen including

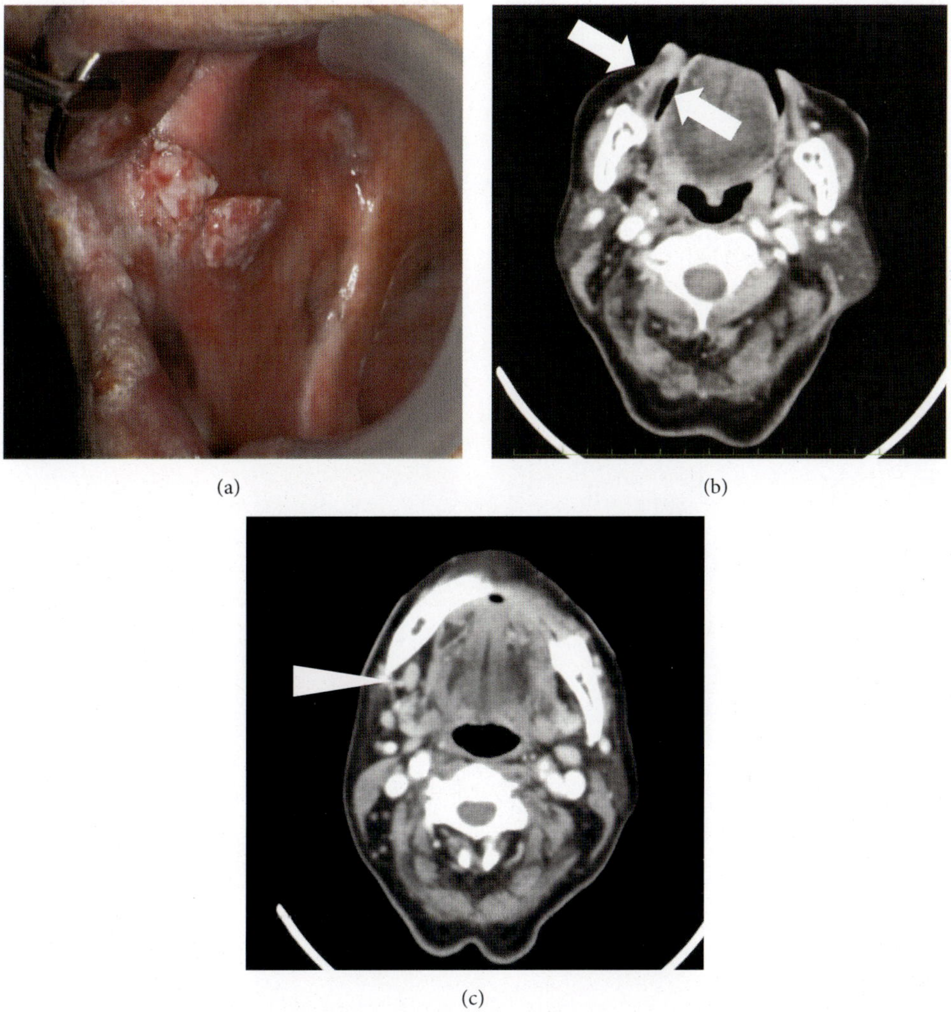

FIGURE 2: *Intraoral findings at most recent follow-up*. Intraoral findings (a) and CT images of the right buccal region (b, arrow) and submandibular lymph node (c, arrow head).

UFT plus cyclophosphamide (CTX) and celecoxib (CXB) in patients with advanced refractory gastrointestinal cancers. The results of this study suggested a possible antitumor activity of this metronomic regimen, comparable with those observed in the same setting patients treated with other chemotherapy. Tumor vasculatures instead of tumor cells were main target of these chemotherapy regimens, and the same mechanisms might have been involved in the outcome for our patient.

Low-dose S-1 chemotherapy for elderly patients with head and neck carcinoma appears to be safe in the outpatient setting and might be an effective strategy with which to maintain the quality of life of patients who have incurable and dormant tumors.

References

[1] B. R. Pauloski, J. A. Logemann, A. W. Rademaker et al., "Speech and swallowing function after oral and oropharyngeal resections: One-year follow-up," *Head & Neck*, vol. 16, no. 4, pp. 313–322, 1994.

[2] N. P. Nguyen, S. Sallah, U. Karlsson, and J. E. Antoine, "Combined chemotherapy and radiation therapy for head and neck malignancies: Quality of life issues," *Cancer*, vol. 94, no. 4, pp. 1131–1141, 2002.

[3] M. Clavel, J. B. Vermorken, F. Cognetti et al., "Randomized comparison of cisplatin, methotrexate, bleomycin and vincristine (CABO) versus cisplatin and 5-fluorouracil (CF) versus cisplatin (C) in recurrent or metastatic squamous cell carcinoma of the head and neck: A phase III study of the EORTC head and neck cancer cooperative group," *Annals of Oncology*, vol. 5, no. 6, pp. 521–526, 1994.

[4] E. Guardiola, F. Peyrade, L. Chaigneau et al., "Results of a randomised phase II study comparing docetaxel with methotrexate in patients with recurrent head and neck cancer," *European Journal of Cancer*, vol. 40, no. 14, pp. 2071–2076, 2004.

[5] T. Shirasaka, Y. Shimamato, H. Ohshimo et al., "Development of a novel form of an oral 5-fluorouracil derivative (S-1) directed to the potentiation of the tumor selective cytotoxicity of 5-fluorouracil by two biochemical modulators," *Anti-Cancer Drugs*, vol. 7, no. 5, pp. 548–557, 1996.

[6] T. Shirasaka, K. Nakano, T. Takechi et al., "Antitumor activity of 1 M tegafur-0.4 M 5-chloro-2,4-dihydroxypyridine-1 M potassium oxonate (S-1) against human colon carcinoma orthotopically implanted into nude rats," *Cancer Research*, vol. 56, no. 11, pp. 2602–2606, 1996.

[7] Y. Akutsu, T. Kono, M. Uesato et al., "S-1 monotherapy as second- or third-line chemotherapy for unresectable and recurrent esophageal squamous cell carcinoma," *Oncology (Switzerland)*, vol. 84, no. 5, pp. 305–310, 2013.

[8] W. Koizumi, H. Narahara, T. Hara et al., "S-1 plus cisplatin versus S-1 alone for first-line treatment of advanced gastric cancer (SPIRITS trial): a phase III trial," *The Lancet Oncology*, vol. 9, no. 3, pp. 215–221, 2008.

[9] A. Itoi, M. Takashima, H. Ishimasa, H. Murata, and K. Tomoda, "Adjuvant chemotherapy with TS-1 for head and neck cancer—side effect of two-week application followed by one-week rest regimen," *Gan to Kagaku Ryoho. Cancer & Chemotherapy*, vol. 33, no. 5, pp. 617–620, 2006.

[10] T. Browder, C. E. Butterfield, B. M. Kräling et al., "Antiangiogenic scheduling of chemotherapy improves efficacy against experimental drug-resistant cancer," *Cancer Research*, vol. 60, no. 7, pp. 1878–1886, 2000.

[11] G. Klement, S. Baruchel, J. Rak et al., "Continuous low-dose therapy with vinblastine and VEGF receptor-2 antibody induces sustained tumor regression without overt toxicity," *Journal of Clinical Investigation*, vol. 105, no. 8, pp. R15–R24, 2000.

[12] G. Bocci and R. S. Kerbel, "Pharmacokinetics of metronomic chemotherapy: a neglected but crucial aspect," *Nature Reviews Clinical Oncology*, vol. 13, no. 11, pp. 659–673, 2016.

[13] G. Allegrini, T. Di Desidero, M. T. Barletta et al., "Clinical, pharmacokinetic and pharmacodynamic evaluations of metronomic UFT and cyclophosphamide plus celecoxib in patients with advanced refractory gastrointestinal cancers," *Angiogenesis*, vol. 15, no. 2, pp. 275–286, 2012.

33

Rituximab Monotherapy in the Management of a Rare Case of an HIV Associated Lymphoproliferative Disorder

Jason Hew, Fauzia Rana, and Louise Zhou

Department of Internal Medicine, Division of Medical Oncology, University of Florida COM, Jacksonville, FL, USA

Correspondence should be addressed to Jason Hew; tharkur@yahoo.com

Academic Editor: Jose I. Mayordomo

Background. Castleman's disease (CD), also known as angiofollicular node hyperplasia, is a rare heterogenous lymphoproliferative disorder. This disease exists as two distinct entities: a localized or unicentric CD (UCD) which has a more benign clinical course and multicentric CD (MCD) which is a systemic disease and carries a worse prognosis. MCD is often associated with human immunodeficiency virus (HIV) infection and these patients are usually coinfected with human herpes virus-8 (HHV-8). Rituximab is an anti-CD20 monoclonal antibody that has become integral to the management of this disease. It is used alone or in combination with chemotherapy to treat MCD. *Case Report.* We describe a case of a 58-year-old man with HIV and HHV-8 MCD and evidence of organ failure with a poor performance status that went into complete remission after four cycles of therapy with weekly rituximab. *Conclusion.* HIV-MCD can be challenging to diagnose and to manage. Early recognition can reduce morbidity and mortality associated with the disease. Rituximab monotherapy can be used as a safe and effective treatment option in patients with a poor performance status.

1. Background

CD was first described in 1956 at the Massachusetts General Hospital by the pathologist Benjamin Castleman [1, 2]. The initial cases described were localized or UCD, and it was thought to be a nonneoplastic disorder which presented as a mediastinal mass in young adults [1]. MCD is an aggressive disease which usually presents in the sixth decade of life and if left untreated is associated with a high risk of mortality [3]. Clinically, patients can present with generalized lymphadenopathy, hepatosplenomegaly, fevers, and night sweats. The diagnosis of MCD requires pathological confirmation typically through an excisional lymph node biopsy [1, 4]. In addition, patients should have fever, elevated C-reactive protein, and other signs of active disease. MCD has three major histological subtypes; these are hyaline vascular, plasma cell, and mixed variants. The plasma cell variant is the most common subtype of MCD seen in up to 80–90% of cases while the hyaline vascular subtype occurs more frequently in UCD [1].

Most of the cases of MCD are associated with HIV infection and these patients are universally coinfected with HHV-8 [1]. Although the pathogenesis of MCD is not well understood, it appears that HHV-8 has a key role in the development of this disease. HHV-8 is a gamma herpes virus which has been linked to acquired immunodeficiency syndrome (AIDS) defining illnesses such as Kaposi sarcoma (KS) as well as primary effusion lymphoma (PEL) [4]. The presence of HHV-8 is known to cause cytokine dysregulation leading to excessive release of interleukin-6 (IL-6). This occurs particularly during viral replication where the HHV-8 infected B-cells release the virally encoded form of IL-6 (vIL-6) that subsequently activates the human IL-6 receptor which causes the systemic inflammatory response seen in MCD. Although both MCD and KS are associated with the presence of HHV-8, elevations of vIL-6 are rarely seen in KS [1, 4, 5]. Since the advent of highly active retroviral therapy (HAART), the incidence of KS has declined while the MCD incidence has risen from 2.3 per 10,000 patient-years in the pre-HAART era prior to 1996 to 8.3 per 10,000 patient-years since the year 2000. There also seems to be no direct correlation between the degree of immunodeficiency or Cluster of Differentiation 4 (CD4) count and the incidence of MCD [6, 7].

Optimal management strategies for MCD are not well defined and clinical practice varies. To date, there has only been one randomized clinical controlled trial evaluating treatment in MCD. Due to the rarity of this disease, the majority of the data comes from systematic literature reviews, case series, and case reports. Based on several published reports, high rates of response are seen with the use of rituximab by itself or in combination with chemotherapy in HIV-MCD. This case highlights and confirms the efficacy of this drug [7, 8].

2. Case

A 58-year-old Caucasian man presented with a one-month history of fever, night sweats, progressive fatigue, dyspnea, abdominal pain, and swelling. He had a past medical history of chronic hepatitis C and HIV disease/AIDS which was found 8 months prior to his presentation. He was started on HAART prior to this hospital visit and had a CD4 count of 83 cells/μL and a viral load of 214 copies/mL at the time of his presentation. His initial examination findings were significant for a middle-aged Caucasian male in moderate distress that was tachycardic at rest with a heart rate of 110 beats/min and febrile with a temperature of 101.6°F with generalized peripheral adenopathy, anasarca, and splenomegaly and decreased breath sounds in bilateral lung bases. Initial laboratory investigations revealed that he was pancytopenic with hemoglobin of 6.7 g/dL, white blood cell (WBC) count of 2700/μL, and a platelet count of 64000/μL. His complete metabolic panel showed that he was hypoalbuminemic with albumin of 2.3 g/dL; the remainder of his panel was within normal limits. Computerized Tomography (CT) imaging was performed on his chest, abdomen, and pelvis with contrast which showed diffuse bulky adenopathy, marked splenomegaly with evidence of portal hypertension, moderate ascites, and bilateral pleural effusions (Figure 1). The initial management was directed at treating him for possible sepsis and he was placed on broad-spectrum empiric antibiotics which did not improve his symptoms and blood and urine cultures returned negative.

A core needle biopsy was performed on an enlarged left axillary lymph node on the third day of hospitalization which demonstrated features consistent with MCD with focal features of early development of a plasmablastic microlymphoma. The pathology report highlighted the presence of numerous plasma cells seen mainly in the mantle zone and interfollicular area showing nuclear HHV-8 positivity. The plasma cells were evaluated using mRNA in situ hybridization (ISH) studies which were polyclonal for kappa/lambda. CD staining was performed which demonstrated a background of T-cells with occasional microscopic foci of lambda restricted plasmablast (HHV-8+), variably expressing CD20 seen invading follicles. A unilateral bone marrow aspirate and biopsy was subsequently done which showed a hypercellular marrow with evidence of hemophagocytosis in a background of plasma cell infiltration consistent with involvement by MCD. Additional laboratory studies revealed markedly elevated C-reactive protein (CRP) of 229 mg/L (reference range: <5 mg/L) and an elevated lactate dehydrogenase (LDH) and β2 microglobulin which were 282 U/L (reference range: 126–266 U/L) and 9.7 mg/L (reference range:

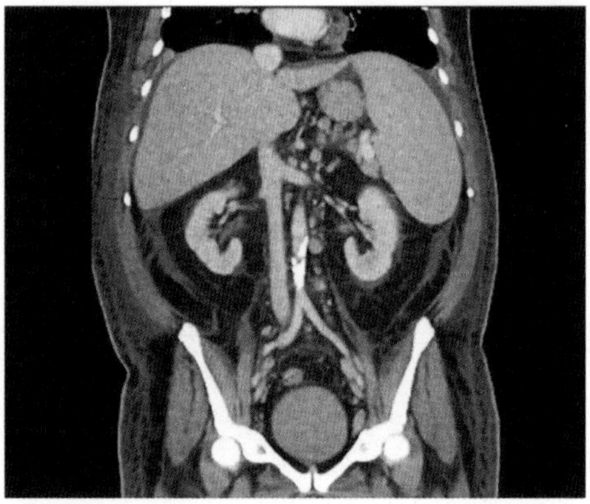

Figure 1: Pretreatment CT with contrast showing enlarged intra-abdominal nodes and splenomegaly.

0.6–2.4 mg/L), respectively. His serum protein electrophoresis showed hypergammaglobulinemia and hepatitis B was found to be negative.

Prior to starting treatment, this patient was evaluated for skin lesions suggestive of Kaposi's sarcoma and no lesions were identified. He was also started on treatment with ganciclovir for HHV-8 but this was subsequently discontinued due to worsening cytopenias. His laboratory studies suggested worsening of his organ function since his admission with a decrease in his platelet count to 10000/μL; his albumin was further decreased to 1.7 g/dL; both his creatinine and his bilirubin had risen from previous normal values to 1.39 mg/dL and 1.5 mg/dL, respectively. He required multiple transfusions while in hospital and had a total of 9 units of packed red blood cells and 4 units of platelets. Given his declining performance status (PS) which was considered to be Eastern cooperative oncology group PS grade 3 (ECOG PS grade 3), he was not considered to be a candidate for chemotherapy and was offered treatment with rituximab only.

On day 10 of his hospitalization, treatment with rituximab was initiated at 375 mg/m^2 with plans for weekly administration for a total of 4 cycles. This patient tolerated treatment with rituximab without any adverse effects. Within days of completing therapy, there was an observed clinical response with the resolution of his fever, night sweats, and anorexia as well as rapid improvement of his cytopenias. He completed all 4 cycles of rituximab in hospital. His posttreatment CT with contrast of the abdomen showed a marked reduction in the size of his enlarged intra-abdominal lymph nodes and splenic size (Figure 2). A follow-up PET (positron emission tomography)/CT study was done 2 months after completing therapy with rituximab which showed complete resolution of his previously seen bulky adenopathy and pleural effusions. Clinically, his performance status improved to ECOG PS grade 0 with no limitations in his activity level. Laboratory studies demonstrated resolution of his pancytopenia and hypoalbuminemia. Approximately 8 months after completing his treatment with rituximab, he remains in clinical remission.

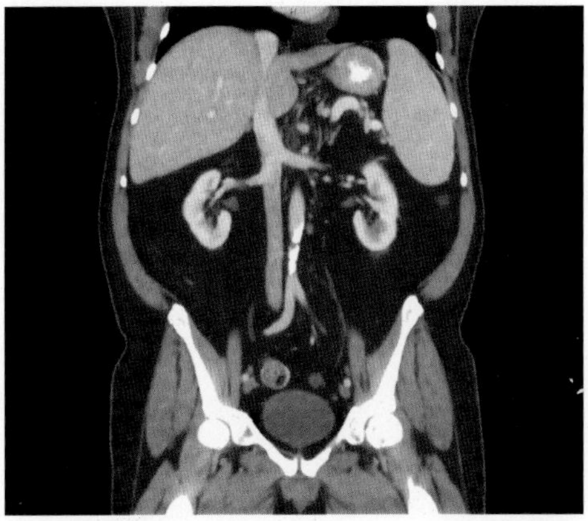

FIGURE 2: Posttreatment CT with contrast of the abdomen showing resolution of the enlarged intra-abdominal lymph nodes and reduction in splenic size.

3. Discussion

MCD continues to present a challenge for clinicians despite being discovered over fifty years ago. Ideal management strategies are not known and there is still a limited understanding of its pathogenesis [3, 7]. In the era of HAART, the incidence of HIV associated MCD continues to rise while other HHV-8 associated diseases are now seen less frequently. Patients with HIV-MCD tend to present more often with fulminant disease as compared to their idiopathic counterparts and can be a diagnostic dilemma at the time of presentation. As seen in this case, delays in making the diagnosis and initiating management may prove to be costly to patients as this disease can be rapidly progressive and even fatal. Clinicians should still evaluate these patients for opportunistic infections and lymphomas which may present similarly and can coexist with MCD [1, 3, 7].

Clinical practice in the management of HIV-MCD varies, but there appears to be a growing body of evidence supporting the use of rituximab by itself or in combination with chemotherapy. Rituximab is a monoclonal antibody directed against CD20 positive cells. Although the HHV-8 infected plasmablasts do not highly express CD20, it has been suggested that this drug is effective in eliminating the affected B-cells in the mantle zone of the lymph node and this decreases the inflammatory response and reduces the HHV-8 viremia. Two pilot trials have been completed which show the benefit of rituximab in HIV-MCD. Gerard et al. conducted a phase II open label study evaluating the effect of rituximab given at 375 mg/m^2 weekly for 4 weeks on 24 stable patients with HIV-MCD previously maintained on single agent chemotherapy. 17 of 24 patients (71%) were alive in sustained remission at day 365 without specific treatment, and the overall survival rate was 92% (95% CI: 71% to 98%). There were no severe adverse effects reported [7]. Three of five patients however had flares of their Kaposi's sarcoma but did not require additional treatment. Similarly, in another open label phase II study by Bower et al., rituximab was shown to be efficacious. This study enrolled 21 treatment naive patients with HIV-MCD to receive 4 weeks of weekly rituximab, The results showed overall and disease-free survival rates at 2 years of 95% (95% CI: 86% to 100%) and 79% (CI: 49% to 100%), respectively. The main adverse effect reported was reactivation of Kaposi's sarcoma [4, 7, 9]. Other reports of prolonged remission have been seen when rituximab has been combined with chemotherapy [7, 9, 10]. In a retrospective multicenter analysis evaluating therapy in HIV-MCD conducted by Hoffman et al., there was a statistically significant survival benefit observed with using rituximab based therapy versus chemotherapy and antiviral therapy only [10].

Alternative treatment options have been used in the management of HIV-MCD often with temporary and partial results. Glucocorticoids have been reported to be effective in providing symptom control and short-term responses [1, 7]. Historically, prior to the introduction of rituximab, single agent chemotherapy and combination chemotherapy regimens were used such as cyclophosphamide/vincristine/doxorubicin and prednisone (CHOP) and other lymphoma regimens with more durable responses being reported with the use of combined agents [1–3]. Antiherpes virus agents have been explored as a treatment option that would target HHV-8, the implicated pathogen in this disease during its lytic replication. Uldrick and colleagues conducted a pilot study on 14 patients with HIV-MCD who were treated with a combination of zidovudine and valganciclovir. The results were that 86% of these patients attained a clinical response and the median progression-free survival was 6 months. Another observation noted in the study was that reductions in the HHV-8 viral load, IL-6, and CRP levels correlated with an improved clinical response. Bortezomib, a drug frequently employed in the management of multiple myeloma, has also been reported anecdotally to be efficacious in the management of MCD and in some instances provided a durable response. Bortezomib is a proteasome inhibitor which acts on plasma cells and is believed to decrease the production of IL-6 through the nuclear factor kappa blockade [1, 7].

At present, there has only been one randomized double blinded placebo control trial evaluating drug therapy in MCD. Siltuximab which is a monoclonal antibody to the IL-6 receptor was tested in 79 patients with HIV negative, HHV-8 negative MCD compared to placebo. The primary endpoint of the study was a durable radiological and clinical response lasting at least 18 weeks. Treatment with siltuximab was associated with a higher rate of achieving the primary endpoint (34% versus 0%). Radiographic tumor response rates were seen in 38% and 4% of patients, favoring the siltuximab arm, and symptomatic response rates were 57% and 19% [11]. Siltuximab has been US Food and Drug Administration (FDA) approved for the treatment of HIV and HHV-8 negative MCD based on the results of this study. Tocilizumab which is a humanized antibody to the IL-6 receptor has also been shown to be active in the management of HIV negative MCD in a phase 2 trial; however, it has not been approved for use in the treatment of MCD. It is uncertain whether IL-6 receptor antibodies will provide similar results in patients with HIV-MCD [1, 7, 12].

Nagao et al. reported on 2 patients with HIV-MCD who were treated with tocilizumab and received rapid but short-term benefit from this treatment with relapses occurring at 15 and 22 weeks. These patients were subsequently treated with rituximab and achieved durable and complete remission [12].

4. Conclusion

MCD continues to be a rare lymphoproliferative disorder despite a rising incidence in HIV patients. There is no well-defined treatment strategy and clinical practice varies. The HIV-MCD patient is clinically challenging as these patients can present with fulminant disease. The management of immunodeficiency as well as concomitant opportunistic infections and other lymphomas needs to be incorporated in the treatment plan. Rituximab appears to be safe, effective, and less toxic than traditional cytotoxic chemotherapy and can result in durable remission. It is not known whether rituximab as a single agent is as effective as when it is combined with chemotherapy. There remain several unanswered questions with regard to the treatment of MCD and further studies are warranted.

Acknowledgments

The authors of this manuscript would like to acknowledge the Southern Medical Association 2016 scientific assembly where the abstract of this case was presented.

References

[1] J. D. Soumerai, A. R. Sohani, and J. S. Abrahamson, "Diagnosis and management of Castleman disease," *Cancer Control*, vol. 21, no. 4, pp. 266–278, Oct 2014.

[2] M. Flejsierowicz, M. Ahmed, P. Kotov, and C. Cheng, "Successful treatment of aggressive HIV associated multicentric Castlemans Disease: a case report," *Wis Med J.*, vol. 107, no. 4, pp. 191–194, 2008.

[3] E. E. Mylona, I. G. Baraboutis, L. J. Lekakis, O. Georgiou, V. Papastamopoulos, and A. Skoutelis, "Multicentric castlemans disease in HIV infection a systematic review of the literature," *AIDS Reviews*, vol. 10, no. 1, pp. 25–35, 2008.

[4] A. Waterston and M. Bower, "Fifty years of multicentric Castleman disease," *Acta Oncol*, vol. 43, no. 8, pp. 698–704, 2004.

[5] D. C. Fajgenbaum, F. Rhee, and C. S. Nabel, "Idiopathic multicentric Castleman disease: novel insights into biology, pathogenesis and therapy," *Blood*, vol. 123, no. 19, pp. 2924–2933, Mar 2014.

[6] T. S. Uldrick, M. N. Polizzotto, K. Aleman et al., "High-dose zidovudine plus valganciclovir for Kaposi sarcoma herpesvirus-associated multicentric Castleman disease: a pilot study of virus-activated cytotoxic therapy," *Blood*, vol. 117, no. 26, pp. 6977–6986, 2011.

[7] C. Rokx, B. J. Rijnders, and J. A. van Laar, "Treatment of multicentric Castlemans disease in HIV-1 infected and uninfected patients: a systematic review," *Neth J Med*, vol. 73, no. 5, pp. 202–210, Jun 2015.

[8] P. Nicoli, U. Familiari, M. Bosa, T. Allice, F. Mete, A. Morotti et al., "HHV8-positive, HIV-negative multicentric Castlemans disease: early and sustained complete remission with rituximab therapy without reactivation of Kaposi sarcoma," *Int J Hematol.*, vol. 90, pp. 392–396, 2009.

[9] M. Bower, T. Powles, S. Williams, T. N. Davis, M. Atkins, S. Montoto et al., "Rituximab in HIV associated multicentric Castleman disease," *Ann Intern Med.*, vol. 147, no. 12, pp. 836–839, 2007.

[10] C. Hoffman, H. Schmid, M. Moller, C. Chris Teutsch, J. Lunzen, and S. Esser, "Improved outcome with Rituximab in patients with HIV – associated multicentric Castleman disease," *Blood*, vol. 118, no. 13, pp. 3499–3503, Sep 2011.

[11] F. Van Rhee, R. S. Wong, M. Munshi, J. F. Rossi, K. e. XY, A. Fossa et al., "Siltuximab for multicentric Castleman's disease: a randomised, double-blind, placebo-controlled trial," *Lancet Oncol*, vol. 15, no. 9, pp. 966–974, Aug 2014.

[12] A. Nagao, S. Nakazawa, and H. Hanabusa, "Short term efficacy of the IL6 receptor antibody Tocilizumab in patients with HIV – associated multicentric Castleman disease: report of two cases," *Journal of Hematology and Oncology*, vol. 7, p. 10, 2014.

34

Primary Malignant Neuroendocrine Tumour of Pleura: First Case Report

Anirban Das[1] and Abhishek Pratap[2]

[1]*Department of Pulmonary Medicine, Murshidabad Medical College, Berhampore, West Bengal 742101, India*
[2]*Department of Pulmonary Medicine, Medical College, Kolkata, West Bengal 700 073, India*

Correspondence should be addressed to Anirban Das; dranirbandas¯chest@rediffmail.com

Academic Editor: Jose I. Mayordomo

Metastatic tumours of pleura are the most common malignant tumours causing malignant pleural effusion. Lungs are the most common primary sites. Primary pleural tumours are rarely seen and diffuse malignant mesothelioma is the most common malignant tumour of pleura. Primary malignant neuroendocrine tumour of pleura is not reported in the literature. Here, we report a rare case of primary malignant neuroendocrine tumour of pleura in a fifty-two-year-old, nonsmoker female who presented with right-sided pleural effusion and ipsilateral, dull aching chest pain. Clinical presentations of inflammatory lesions like tuberculous pleuritis and benign and malignant neoplasms of pleura are indistinguishable; hence, fluid cytology, pleural biopsy, and immunohistochemistry are necessary for exact tissue diagnosis of the tumours, which is mandatory for correct treatment and prognostic assessment.

1. Introduction

Metastatic pleural tumours are by far the most common malignant neoplasms of the pleura and greatly outnumbering the primary pleural tumours. Lungs, breasts, and hematological malignancies are the most common primary sites for pleural metastasis. Among the primary pleural malignancies, diffuse malignant mesothelioma is the most common primary malignant tumour of the pleura. Primary pleural tumours other than mesothelioma account for less than 1% of all pleural tumours and are rarely reported in the literature, hence causing diagnostic and management dilemma [1]. In most cases, they are diagnosed as incidental during histopathological examination of pleural tissue, obtained by closed pleural biopsy or obtained under thoracoscopic visualization. Immunohistochemistry (IHC) further helps to establish the diagnosis of exact tissue type of pleural neoplasms. Besides malignant pleural mesothelioma, other primary malignancies of pleura are malignant solitary fibrous tumour, fibrosarcoma, liposarcoma, primary pleural lymphoma, synovial sarcoma, desmoplastic round cell tumours, primitive neuroectodermal tumours, blastoma, and so forth [2]. But after extensive search of literature in English, we do not find any report of primary malignant neuroendocrine tumour of pleura. Here, we report the first case of primary malignant neuroendocrine tumour of pleura in a fifty-two-year-old female, presenting with isolated right-sided pleural effusion.

2. Case Report

A fifty-two-year-old, nonsmoker female presented with right-sided severe dull aching chest pain, dry cough, and exertional dyspnoea for four months. Severity of chest pain was gradually increasing and disturbs her sleep at night. Shortness of breath was initially of mMRC grading 2; later it was increased to grade 3. There was no history of hemoptysis, fever, weight loss, and loss of appetite. There was no past history of pulmonary tuberculosis.

On examination, general survey revealed no abnormality. Her temperature was 97.2°F, pulse rate, 84 beats/minute, respiratory rate, 24 beats/minute, and blood pressure, 124/80 mmHg. Examination of respiratory system revealed diminished movement of chest wall on right side, tracheal shifting to left, apical impulse in left fifth intercostal space, 1.5 cm lateral to the left midclavicular line, stony

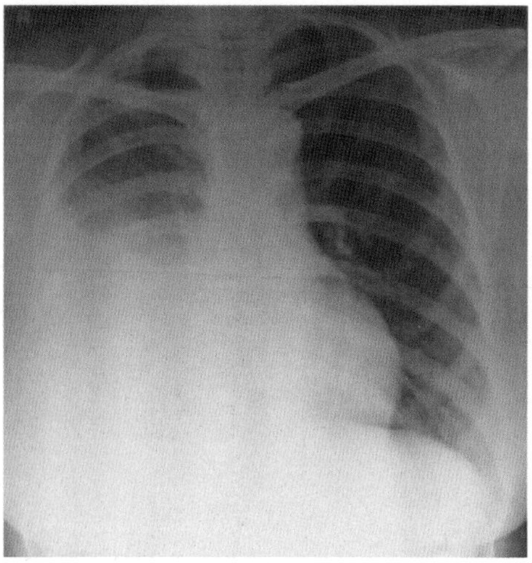

Figure 1: CXR, PA view showing right-sided pleural effusion.

dull percussion note over right chest wall, absent vesicular breath sound, and diminished vocal resonance on right side, suggestive of right-sided pleural effusion. Examination of other systems revealed no abnormality.

Complete hemogram and blood biochemistry (including serotonin, gastrin, somatostatin, and glucagon) were within normal limit. Chest X-ray posteroanterior view (CXR, PA view) revealed right-sided pleural effusion (Figure 1). Ultrasound of abdomen revealed no abnormality. Pleural fluid was aspirated from right hemithorax and its analysis showed haemorrhagic, exudative, and lymphocyte predominant pleural effusion with adenosine deaminase level 16 U/L. No malignant cell or acid fast bacilli were seen in pleural fluid. Contrast enhanced computed tomography (CECT) of thorax showed only right-sided pleural effusion (Figure 2). No mass lesion or mediastinal lymphadenopathy was detected on CECT thorax. Closed pleural biopsy was done with Abram's needle and histopathological examination of biopsy tissue taken from right parietal pleura showed diffuse sheets of round to oval cells with hyperchromatic nuclei and scant to moderate amount of cytoplasm. Few scattered large cells with abundant eosinophilic cytoplasm were present. Focally spindle cells with hyperchromatic nuclei were seen. Focal micropapillae formation was also noted; features were suggestive of a poorly differentiated malignant tumour (Figure 3). Immunohistochemistry of pleural tissue showed that majority of tumour cells were positive for synaptophysin and a few cells were positive for Ki-67 (2%) and negative for pan-cytokeratin, calretinin, Wilm's tumour protein 1 (WT1), desmin, vimentin, carcinoembryonic antigen (CEA), thyroid transcription factor 1 (TTF1), and CD 56 (Figure 4). Hence, tissue diagnosis was well-differentiated malignant neuroendocrine tumour of pleura. Histopathology and IHC findings were reviewed by another pathologist of different centre, and the diagnosis was confirmed. Fibreoptic bronchoscopy (FOB) was normal. CECT of abdomen and brain revealed no abnormality. No abnormality was detected on endoscopic examination of upper gastrointestinal tract and on colonoscopy. Radionuclide bone scan did not show any metastatic deposit in bones. So, final diagnosis was primary, well-differentiated, malignant neuroendocrine tumour of pleura, presenting as isolated right-sided pleural effusion.

Six cycles of cytotoxic chemotherapy comprising of intravenous infusion of carboplatin (at an area under the concentration-time curve 6.0 on day 1, 450 mg in this case) and etoposide (100 mg/m^2/day, 130 mg in this case on days 1, 2, and 3) were given. Along with chemotherapy, intercostal tube drainage under water seal was given in right hemithorax through fifth intercostal space at right midaxillary line, as recurrent and rapid collection of massive amount of pleural fluid occurred and repeated aspiration of pleural fluid failed to reduce the volume of pleural fluid. When there was clinicoradiological evidence of complete expansion of right lung parenchyma, chemical pleurodesis with 20 mL of 10% povidone-iodine was done. On one-year follow-up, progressive regression of pleural effusion with alleviation of chest pain was documented.

3. Discussion

Diffuse malignant mesothelioma is the most common primary malignant tumour of pleural tissue [3]. Metastatic carcinoma of pleura is the most common neoplastic lesions of pleura [4]. Malignant pleural tumours mainly present with pleural effusion or pleural nodules. But, it is needless to say that clinical manifestations of inflammatory lesions of pleura, benign tumours, metastases, and primary malignant tumours of pleura are indistinguishable. Hence, cytological and biochemical analysis of pleural fluid, histopathology of pleural biopsy tissue, and immunohistochemistry are essential to establish the exact etiology of pleural pathology. Presence of primary tumour in other body sites definitely indicates the metastatic pleural lesion, but primary tumours cannot always be detected.

In India, which is tuberculosis endemic zone, the most common cause of pleural effusion is tuberculosis and TB is one of the important causes of exudative, lymphocyte predominant pleural effusion. If there is evidence of rapid and recurrent collection of haemorrhagic pleural effusion, malignancy should be ruled out especially in elderly individuals, and when adenosine deaminase value is extremely low, as in our case. In these cases, CECT thorax, FOB, pleural fluid cytology, closed pleural biopsy or thoracoscopic biopsy, and immunohistochemistry are a must to confirm the diagnosis.

Lungs are the most common primary sites for metastatic pleural effusion [5]. In our case, there was no evidence of primary tumour in other body sites which were confirmed by different investigations, available in our institution. Although F-18 fluorodeoxyglucose labeled positron emission tomography (FDG-PET)-CT scan with Ga68-SSA or octreoscan is the best investigation to detect any occult primary tumour, it cannot be done in our case due to financial constraint and unavailability of the facility in our institution [6]. As lung malignancy was almost ruled out in CECT thorax and FOB, closed pleural biopsy by Abram's needle was done in our case. Closed pleural biopsy or thoracoscopic biopsy should be done in cytology negative pleural effusion, when malignancy is strongly suspected. But it is well known that

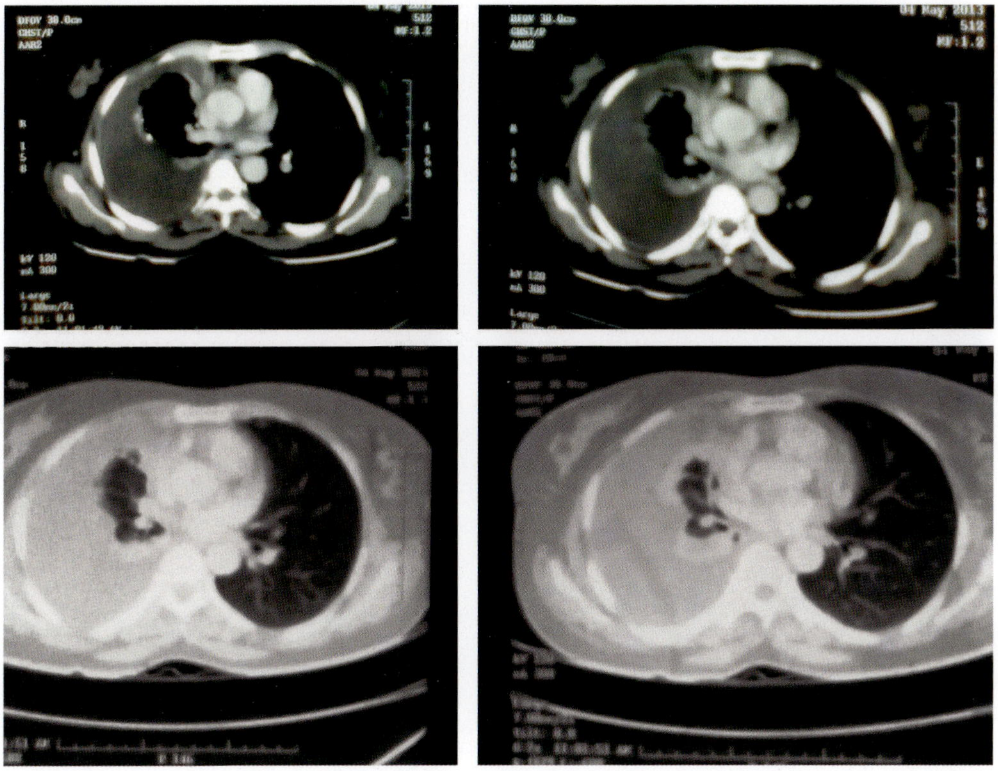

FIGURE 2: CECT of thorax showing right-sided pleural effusion.

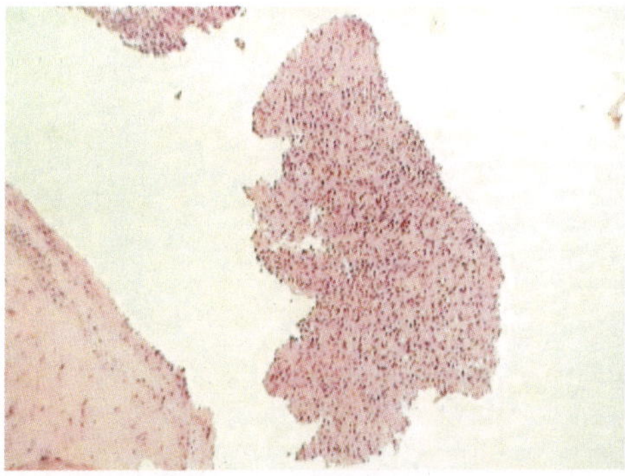

FIGURE 3: Microphotograph of histopathology of pleural biopsy tissue showing diffuse sheets of round to oval cells with hyperchromatic nuclei and scant to moderate amount of cytoplasm, focal spindle cells with hyperchromatic nuclei, and focal micropapillae formation, suggestive of a poorly differentiated malignant tumour (H&E stain, 40x).

diagnostic yield of closed pleural biopsy is poor in malignant pleural effusion due to predominance of malignant deposits in mediastinal and diaphragmatic surfaces of pleura which are unapproachable by Abram's needle and also due to skip lesions, characteristic of malignant effusion [7]. Hence, thoracoscopic biopsy is better as biopsy tissue is taken under direct visualization, but again it could not be done in our case due to financial constraint and unavailability of the facility in our institution.

Among the primary malignancies of the pleura, malignant solitary fibrous tumour, synovial sarcoma, fibrosarcoma, and liposarcoma are reported in the literature, beside the diffuse malignant mesothelioma. But, primary neuroendocrine tumour of the pleura is not reported till date, although there are a few reports of metastatic neuroendocrine tumours (like carcinoids) of pleura. Neuroendocrine tumours originate from hormone producing cells of neuroendocrine system and are most commonly seen in gastrointestinal tract, brain, and lungs [8, 9]. Neuroendocrine tumors of the lungs arise from Kulchitzky cells of the bronchopulmonary mucosa [10]. They comprise typical carcinoid, atypical carcinoid, large cell neuroendocrine carcinoma (LCNEC), and small cell lung cancer (SCLC) [11]. Neuroendocrine differentiation is considered if at least one of the following features is present: argyrophilia the demonstration of neuron-specific enolase or other neuropeptides like synaptophysin or chromogranin A by immunohistochemistry or the demonstration of numerous dense-core membrane-bound granules by electron microscopy [12]. The atypical carcinoids are distinguished by the presence of tumor necrosis, anaplastic large cell nuclei with numerous mitotic figures, and have a worse prognosis. Small cell carcinoma is characterized by finely granular chromatin pattern and is associated with extremely poor prognosis. Most of the small cell carcinomas share the neuroendocrine differentiation which produces different ectopic neuropeptides. In our case, histopathology of pleural biopsy tissue showed round to oval cells with hyperchromatic nuclei majority which were positive for synaptophysin and occasionally for Ki-67 but negative for pan-cytokeratin, CD56, TTF-1, desmin, vimentin, and calretinin on immunohistochemistry. Desmin, vimentin, and

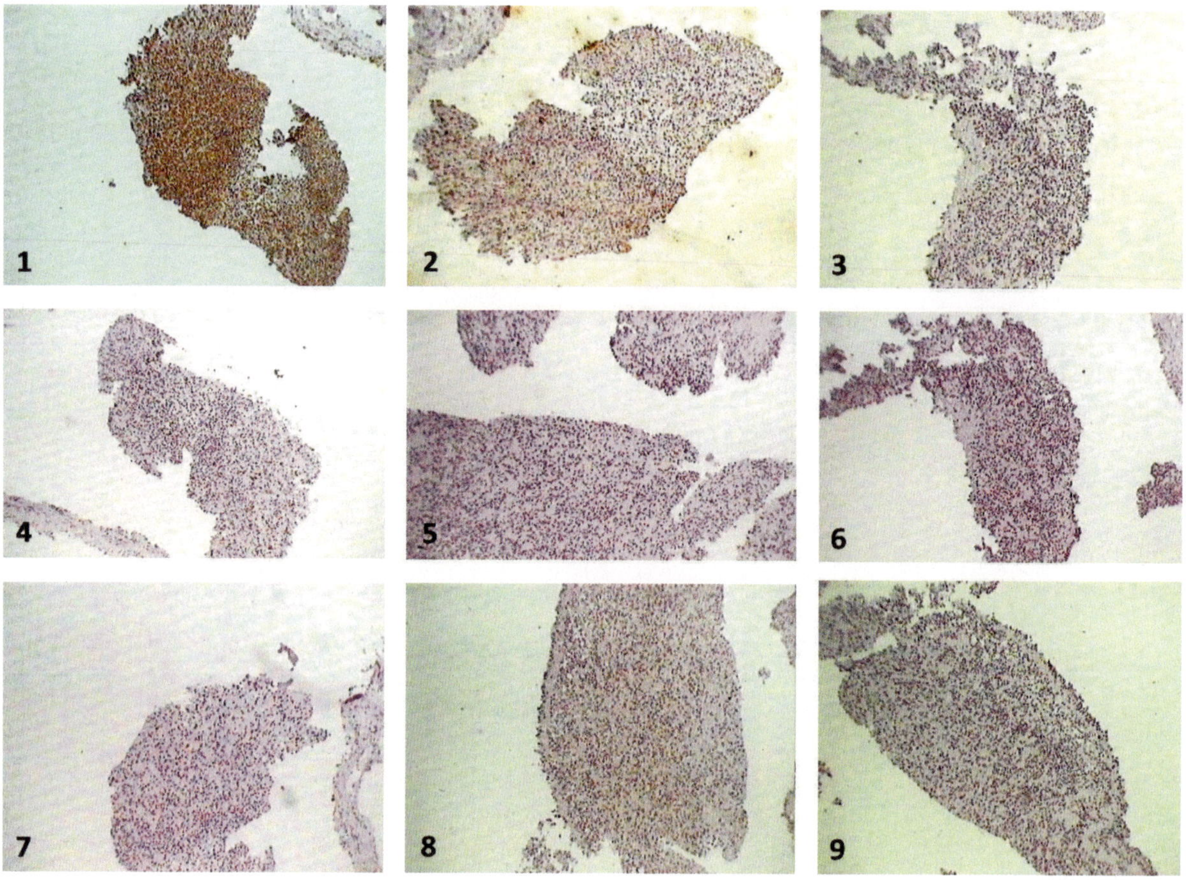

FIGURE 4: Microphotograph of immunohistochemistry showing tumour cells positive for synaptophysin (1) and occasionally for Ki-67 (2) and negative for CEA (3), CD 56 (4), calretinin (5), desmin (6), pan-cytokeratin (7), TTF1 (8), and WT1 (9) (40x).

calretinin are characteristic immunohistochemical markers of mesenchymal tumours which were negative in our case on IHC [13]. CD56 and TTF-1 positivity are seen in small cell carcinoma and carcinoids [14, 15]. Hence, the tumour was malignant and of neuroendocrine origin (as synaptophysin positive round to oval cells) without any evidence of primary tumour in other body sites, so the diagnosis was primary malignant neuroendocrine tumour of pleura. Platinum-based cytotoxic chemotherapy comprises carboplatin or cisplatin and etoposide is useful in the treatment of neuroendocrine tumour of pleura [16]. Intercostal tube drainage and chemical pleurodesis were successful in our case and on two-year follow-up the patient was asymptomatic and pleural fibrosis was developed on affected side.

Disclosure

The current address of Abhishek Pratap is Murshidabad Medical College, Berhampore, West Bengal, India.

References

[1] C. T. Erb, K. M. Johnson, and A. W. Kim, "Rare Pleural Tumors," *Clinics in Chest Medicine*, vol. 34, no. 1, pp. 113–136, 2013.

[2] L. Granville, A. C. Laga, T. C. Allen et al., "Review and update of uncommon primary pleural tumors: a practical approach to diagnosis," *Archives of Pathology and Laboratory Medicine*, vol. 129, no. 11, pp. 1428–1443, 2005.

[3] T. J. Barreiro and P. J. Katzman, "Malignant mesothelioma: a case presentation and review," *The Journal of the American Osteopathic Association*, vol. 106, no. 12, pp. 699–704, 2006.

[4] H.-S. Nam, "Malignant pleural effusion: medical approaches for diagnosis and management," *Tuberculosis and Respiratory Diseases*, vol. 76, no. 5, pp. 211–217, 2014.

[5] D. K. Muduly, S. V. S. Deo, T. S. Subi, A. A. Kallianpur, and N. K. Shukla, "An update in the management of malignant pleural effusion," *Indian Journal of Palliative Care*, vol. 17, no. 2, pp. 98–103, 2011.

[6] G. Pereira, G. C. Silva, and E. Monteiro, "Positron emission tomography in the detection of occult primary head and neck carcinoma: a retrospective study," *Head & Neck Oncology*, vol. 4, article 34, 2012.

[7] N. van Zandwijk, C. Clarke, D. Henderson et al., "Guidelines for the diagnosis and treatment of malignant pleural mesothelioma," *Journal of Thoracic Disease*, vol. 5, no. 6, pp. E254–E307, 2013.

[8] B. I. Gustafsson, M. Kidd, A. Chan, M. V. Malfertheiner, and I. M. Modlin, "Bronchopulmonary neuroendocrine tumors," *Cancer*, vol. 113, no. 1, pp. 5–21, 2008.

[9] S. Massironi, V. Sciola, M. Peracchi, C. Ciafardini, M. P. Spampatti, and D. Conte, "Neuroendocrine tumors of the gastro-entero-pancreatic system," *World Journal of Gastroenterology*, vol. 14, no. 35, pp. 5377–5384, 2008.

[10] A. Fisseler-Eckhoff and M. Demes, "Neuroendocrine tumors of the lung," *Cancers*, vol. 4, no. 3, pp. 777–798, 2012.

[11] W. D. Travis, "Advances in neuroendocrine lung tumors," *Annals of Oncology*, vol. 21, supplement 7, pp. vii65–vii71, 2010.

[12] A. Kasprzak, M. Zabel, and W. Biczysko, "Selected markers (chromogranin A, neuron-specific enolase, synaptophysin, protein gene product 9.5) in diagnosis and prognosis of neuroendocrine pulmonary tumours," *Polish Journal of Pathology*, vol. 58, no. 1, pp. 23–33, 2007.

[13] A. Bahrami, L. D. Truong, and J. Y. Ro, "Undifferentiated tumor: true identity by immunohistochemistry," *Archives of Pathology and Laboratory Medicine*, vol. 132, no. 3, pp. 326–348, 2008.

[14] L. Verset, M. Arvanitakis, P. Loi et al., "TTF-1 positive small cell cancers: don't think they're always primary pulmonary!," *World Journal of Gastrointestinal Oncology*, vol. 3, no. 10, pp. 144–147, 2011.

[15] E. Z. Du, P. Goldstraw, J. Zacharias et al., "TTF-1 expression is specific for lung primary in typical and atypical carcinoids: TTF-1-positive carcinoids are predominantly in peripheral location," *Human Pathology*, vol. 35, no. 7, pp. 825–831, 2004.

[16] J. S. de Cos Escuín, "Diagnosis and treatment of neuroendocrine lung tumors," *Archivos de Bronconeumología*, vol. 50, no. 9, pp. 392–396, 2014.

35

Solitary Skull Metastasis as the First Presentation of a Metachronous Primary Lung Cancer in a Survivor from Pancreatic Cancer

Ali Altalhy,[1] Yazid Maghrabi,[1] Zuhoor Almansouri,[2] and Saleh S. Baeesa[1]

[1] *Division of Neurosurgery, Department of Surgery, Faculty of Medicine, King Abdulaziz University, Jeddah, Saudi Arabia*
[2] *Department of Pathology and Laboratory Medicine, King Faisal Specialist Hospital and Research Center, Jeddah, Saudi Arabia*

Correspondence should be addressed to Saleh S. Baeesa; sbaeesa@kau.edu.sa

Academic Editor: Jose I. Mayordomo

Skull metastasis from lung cancer is relatively common, yet the first presentation for this malignant disease is a rare occurrence. We herein report a case of a 54-year-old female, who had a good outcome following Whipple procedure for periampullary adenocarcinoma five years before her current presentation. During a routine follow-up, she was found to have a slowly progressive painless right parietal swelling. The systemic screening workup revealed no abdominal disease, but a solitary pulmonary nodule was identified. The presence of these two lesions raised the diagnosis of metastases from a previously treated pancreatic adenocarcinoma. The patient underwent complete excision of the skull lesion and subsequent lung biopsy, both of which proved on histopathological examination to be consistent with a primary lung cancer. This case emphasizes the importance of imaging and histopathological correlation in the diagnosis of solitary skull metastases and their effect on the subsequent management.

1. Introduction

Certain types of cancers such as carcinoma of the breast, lung, and kidney are associated with the highest rate of metastatic bone lesions, which approximately account for more than 75% of all patients affected by these types of cancers [1, 2]. It is known that many patients diagnosed with lung carcinoma are in an advanced stage of their disease at the time of diagnosis, and the presence of metastatic lesions is sign of poor prognosis of such cancer [1].

Bony metastases in lung carcinoma are the most common type of metastases associated with such malignant disease, accounting for 36% of affected patients [2]. Moreover, bone metastatic lesions are by far the most common reason for patients to seek medical advice since they result in severe pain [2]. Pain usually results from pathological fractures, which subsequently result from metastatic bony deposits [2].

A metachronous tumor is defined as the development of two primary malignant lesions usually with lag time, often years, between the first and second lesion [3]. Although rare, there have been many reports of metachronous pancreatic and lung adenocarcinoma [4–6]. Metachronous malignant lesions pose diagnostic dilemma since they are hard to differentiate from other metastatic lesions [4–6].

Skull metastases from breast, lung, and prostate carcinoma are relatively common accounting for 15–25% of all cancer patients [7, 8]. Primary malignancy in other sites such as renal, uterine, or hepatocellular sites has rarely been reported in the literature [9–12]. Skull metastasis is usually discovered as an incidental finding since it is asymptomatic in most cases [13]. Sometimes, metastatic lesions can produce mild pain or, with dural sinuses involvement, an increase in intracranial pressure (ICP), leading patients to seek medical advice [13].

Nevertheless, only one reported case in literature has presented a case of solitary skull mass as the first presentation of lung adenocarcinoma, in which a patient, with no history of a previous malignant disease, presented with a skull swelling that proved later to be the first presentation of lung malignancy [2]. Moreover, it differs from our current case, since the same presentation happened in our patient, who survived previously treated malignancy. Herein, we present a case of single skull metastasis as the first presentation of metachronous lung adenocarcinoma, in a 54-year-old carcinoma of the head of the pancreas survivor following Whipple procedure performed five years before this presentation. Therefore, we aim in this report to describe this unusual case and raise the awareness of the development of metachronous primary lung cancer.

2. Case Report

The patient, a 54-year-old female, is a known case of carcinoma of the head of the pancreas, which revealed being a periampullary pancreatic adenocarcinoma after histopathological examination. She underwent uneventful Whipple's procedure in September 2010 followed by adjuvant chemotherapy (carboplatin and methotrexate), with the last cycle being five years before her presentation. She has been on regular follow-up with oncology department without local or systemic recurrence.

In November 2015, she presented with a progressive painless swelling in the right parietal region of six-month duration. There was no history of trauma or previous head radiation. Before the presentation, patient overall health condition was stable with unremarkable history. Her social history was unremarkable and specifically negative for smoking.

Her physical exam and vital signs were within normal. Local examination revealed a hard mass of 5 × 6 cm in diameter with distinct edges, fixed to the skull.

The scalp over it was mobile and with no discoloration or discharges and no regional cervical lymphadenopathy. Neurological examination revealed a conscious, alert, and oriented patient without a focal neurological deficit.

Laboratory workup including CBC, renal, hematology, and hepatic profiles was within normal. Chest X-ray identified a small nodule in the left upper lobe.

Investigations also included CT brain, which demonstrated a lytic bony lesion with classic sunburst periosteal reaction measuring 4.3 × 3.1 × 5.4 cm (Figure 1(a)). The lesion was causing mild displacement of the adjunct cortex with no detected calcifications. There was no underlying vasogenic edema, and no other osseous skull lesions were detected. The cerebral and cerebellar parenchyma showed preserved gray-white matter differentiation, with no evidence of acute territorial infarction and no evidence of abnormally enhancing cerebral parenchyma or meninges. There was no midline shift, and ventricular system, basal cistern, and cortical sulci are within normal limits.

Magnetic resonance imaging (MRI) demonstrated a right parietal hyperintense lesion in nonenhanced T1- and T2-weighted image sequences which involved full skull thickness and has an epidural extension. The lesion demonstrates significant heterogenous enhancement after gadolinium administration, with adjunct focal dural enhancement. The gradient echo sequences demonstrate some areas of susceptibility artifacts within the lesion representing calcification (Figures 1(b), 1(c), and 1(d)). Further screening with CT scan of the chest and abdomen did not reveal any lesions aside from the lung nodule, which was malignant, looking like pleural-based lobulated left upper lobe soft tissue mass, with central necrosis measuring 4.1 × 5.3 cm (Figures 2(a) and 2(b)). Moreover, there were no additional lung lesions and no pleural effusion. Bone scan showed no evidence of other osseous metastases.

The provisional diagnosis was that the skull lesion was probably a metastatic deposit of the previously resected pancreatic cancer. Thus, surgery was planned to excise the skull lesion and send for histopathology, followed by CT guided biopsy of the lung nodule in a later date.

Under general anesthesia, the patient was placed in a supine position, with the head fixed using three-pin Mayfield clamp. The patient was registered using neuronavigation, and anatomical marking of the tumor was achieved. After usual draping under aseptic condition, an incision was made in a straight fashion. The skull flap was reflected, and the lesion was identified without scalp involvement (Figure 3(a)). Two burr holes were created, and free craniotomy flap was raised with the precise demarcation of 2 cm from the tumor edges using the navigation. The entire lesion was excised; it was brown in color, slippery, and with high viscosity (Figures 3(b), 3(c), and 3(d)). The dura was excised up to the healthy looking edges of the craniotomy; after that, a dural graft measuring 4 × 4 cm was used to fill the dural defect created. The underlying brain tissue was normal without infiltration from the lesion. Titanium mesh was fixed, and cement was applied to fill the bony defect resulting from the craniotomy (Figures 3(e) and 3(f)). The excised lesion was sent for histopathology. The patient tolerated the procedures and the postoperative period was unremarkable.

Histopathological examination of the lesion revealed a piece of bone (5.5 cm × 5 cm × 1 cm) almost entirely replaced by a bulging mass that measures 1.5 cm in thickness. The cut surface is bone with cystic contents filled with mucinous material. Sections from bone revealed that a neoplastic growth was destructing and infiltrating in between bone trabeculae. The tumor infiltrated in form of glands lined by columnar epithelial cells with intracytoplasmic mucin. The nuclei are hyperchromatic and mildly pleomorphic with some showing prominent nucleoli (Figure 4). Immunohistochemistry is positive for Napsin A with basal cytoplasmic granular positivity pattern. It is also positive for cytokeratins CK7 and CK19 but negative for CK20, caudal type homeobox 2 (CDX2), and thyroid transcription factor-1 (TTF1) (Figure 5).

An issue was raised after histopathological examination that the skull lesion is mucinous in type, unlike the resected pancreatic adenocarcinoma, which was nonmucinous, raising the possibility that the solitary lung nodule is the source of this lesion as a second primary cancer.

The patient has been admitted again for CT guided biopsy of the lung nodule. Surprisingly, the obtained biopsy, after histopathological examination, showed infiltrative glandular epithelium with intracytoplasmic mucin, hyperchromatic nuclei, and prominent nucleoli, which is identical to the histopathological morphology of skull lesion, thus proving lung nodule to be a metachronous adenocarcinoma presenting initially with a skull metastasis. The sample of lung biopsy

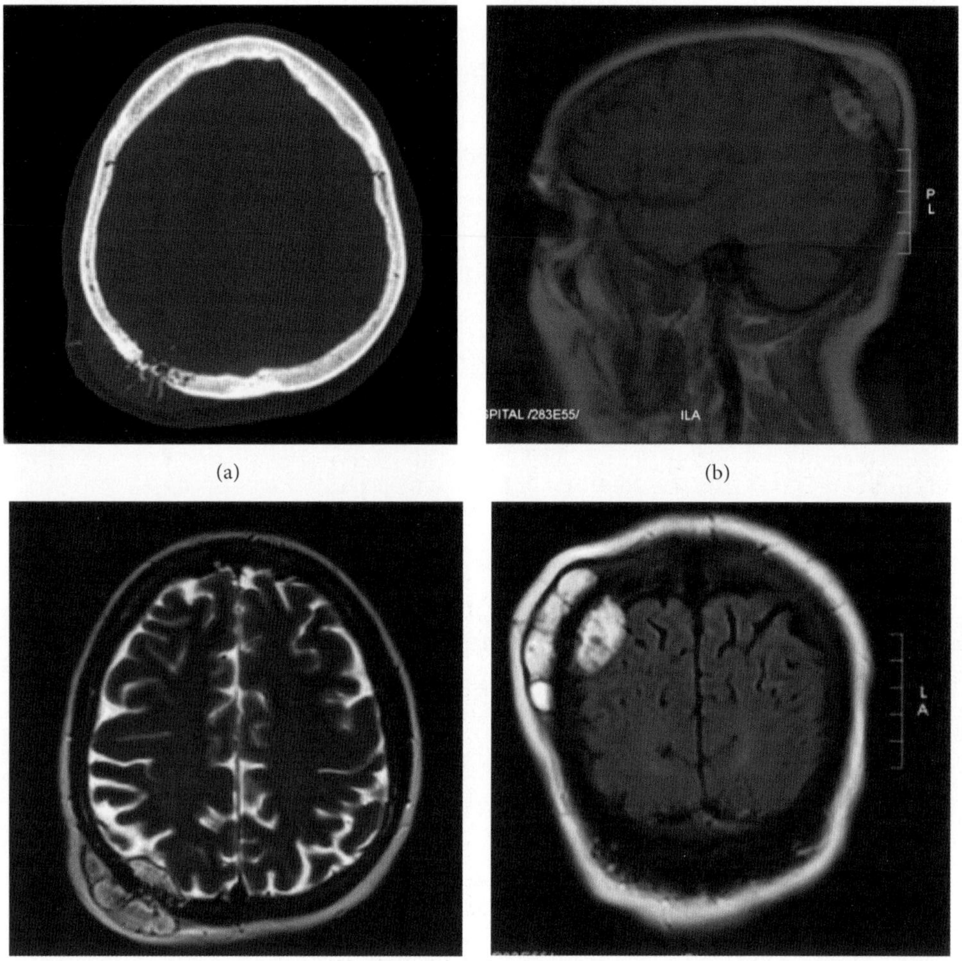

(a) (b) (c) (d)

Figure 1: (a) Preoperative axial CT scan of the brain (bone window) showing osteolytic changes with associated soft tissue swelling. (b) Preoperative unenhanced parasagittal T1-weighted MRI image showing hyperintense epidural cystic mass compressing the cortex underlying. (c) Preoperative axial T2-weighted MRI image showing mildly hyperintense mass on the right parietal region. (d) Preoperative FLAIR coronal MRI showing hyperintense mass that traverses the skull.

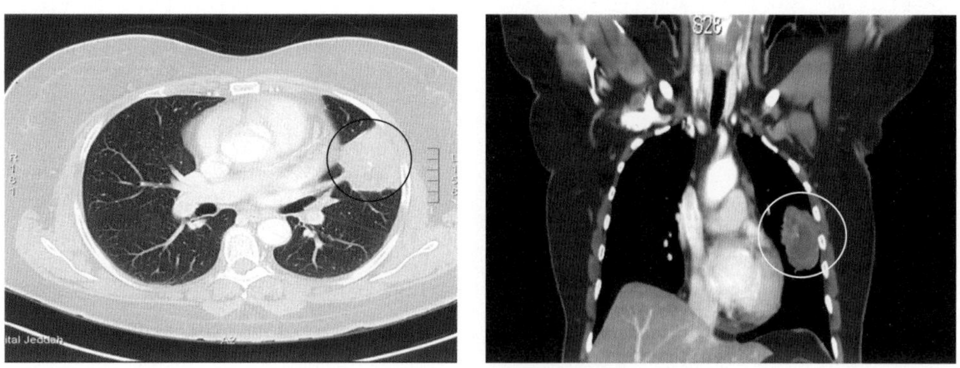

(a) (b)

Figure 2: (a) Axial and (b) coronal contrast-enhanced chest CT scan showing malignant looking pleural-based lobulated left upper lobe soft tissue.

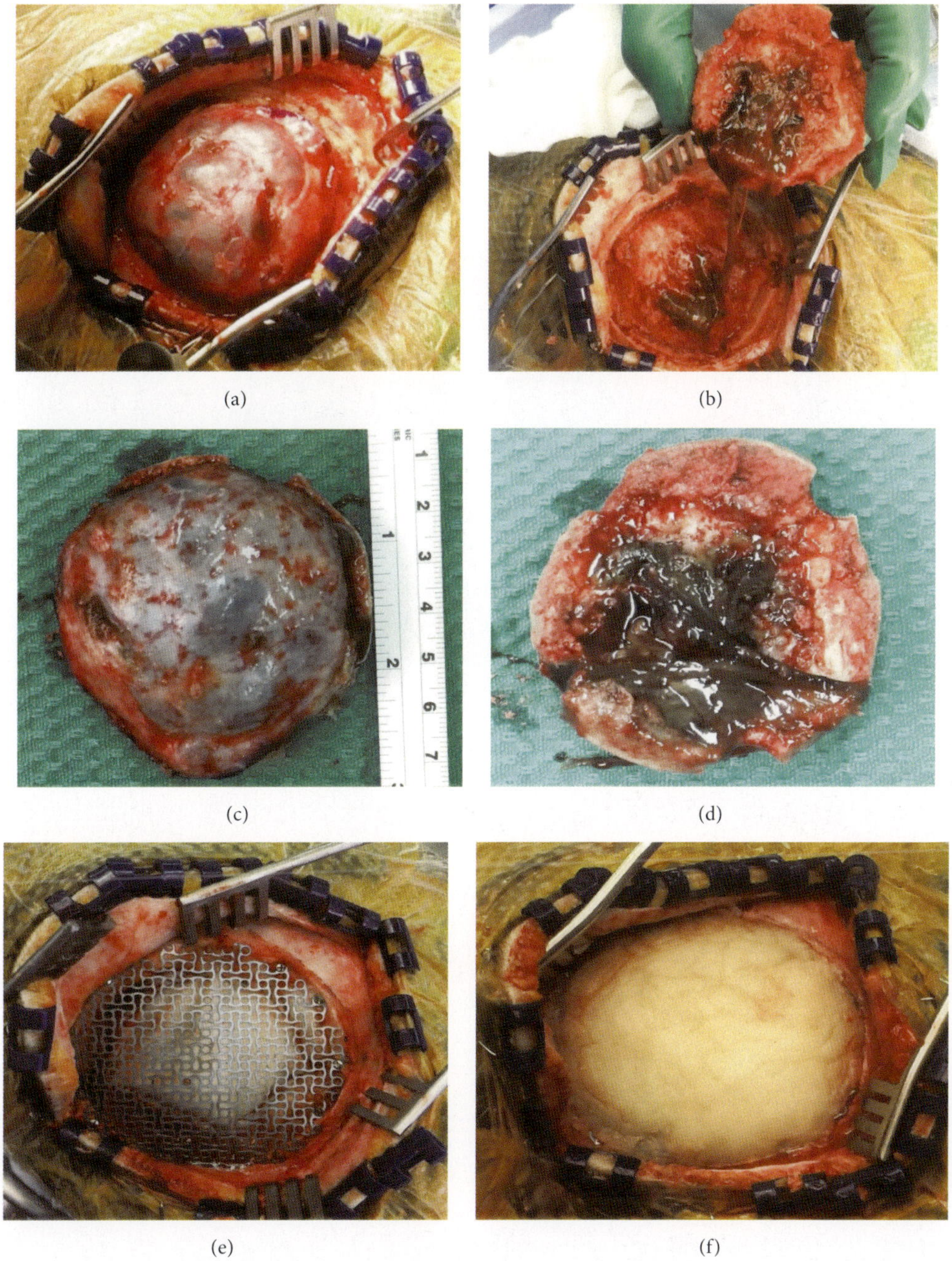

Figure 3: Intraoperative photographs showing (a) the cystic destructive skull lesion, (b) inner side of the lesion after reflection of bone flap, (c) outer side of lesion after excision, and (d) inner side of the lesion after excision. Duraplasty and the application of titanium mesh (e) followed by the application of cement (f).

was tested for Epidermal Growth Factor Receptor (EGFR) status, and it was found to be of the wild type.

The patient had unremarkable recovery and received whole brain radiation 2 weeks later. The follow-up CT scan (Figure 6) revealed good reconstruction, and MRI scan revealed no recurrence at one-year follow-up. In regard to the treatment of the lung lesion, the patient received six cycles of chemotherapy (carboplatin and pemetrexed) for the primary lung adenocarcinoma, which failed to provide a tumor response. Then, she received three cycles of Docetaxel, which also failed too. Due to the poor response to chemotherapy, she underwent palliative radiotherapy for the lung mass, and she survives as of her last follow-up in June 2017 with stable lung disease.

3. Discussion

Certain types of cancers such as breast, prostate, and lung cancers are associated with high rate of metastatic deposits to other sites in the body [1]. A retrospective cohort study of

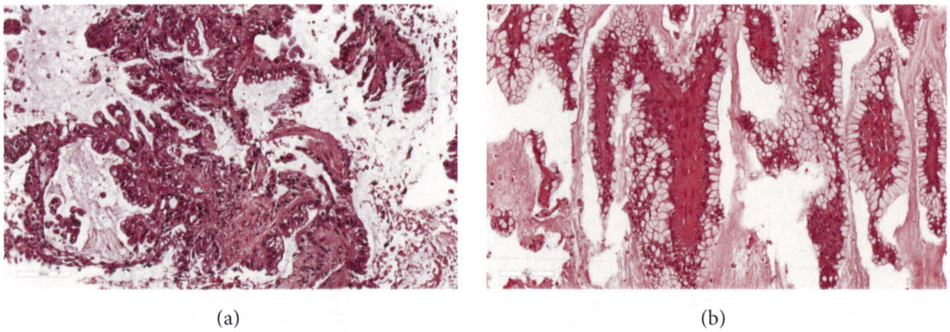

FIGURE 4: Both lung (a) and (b) skull bone and dura specimens demonstrating infiltrative glandular epithelium with intracytoplasmic mucin and hyperchromatic nuclei, some showing prominent nucleoli (hematoxylin & eosin, magnification ×200).

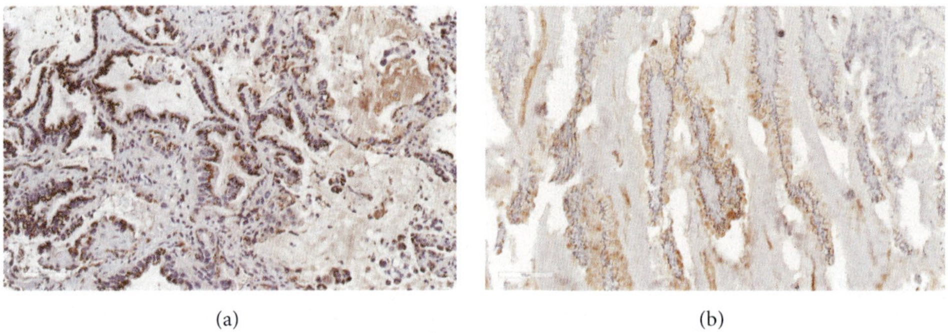

FIGURE 5: Tumor cells are positive for Napsin A staining in (a) lung and (b) skull bone and dura specimens (immunohistochemistry, magnification ×200).

175 patients has found that 55% of skull metastases originated from breast origin, 14% from lung carcinoma, 6% from prostate cancer, and 25% from other origins [14].

Patients presenting with lung carcinoma are usually in an advanced primary disease stage, and survival of such population is poor and can be as low as 10–20% as reported by Stanley and his colleagues [1, 15]. Moreover, lung carcinoma usually metastasizes to bone rather than other sites, and rate of bone metastases can reach up to 36% comparing to metastases in other locations [2]. However, a small number of lung carcinomas metastasize to the skull, and they constitute, according to Turner et al., around 3% of total lung carcinoma bone metastases [2]. There is only one case reporting skull mass as the first presentation of lung adenocarcinoma in the literature [2], and, to our best knowledge, our reported case is considered the second. The uniqueness of our case from the previously mentioned similar reported case arises in that the skull swelling gave a hint about the development of rare entity such metachronous lung adenocarcinoma in a pancreatic cancer survivor, which had not been reported in the literature before.

Another unique feature found in the currently reported case is that the skull metastasis was originated from a metachronous lung adenocarcinoma that appeared after five years of carcinoma of the head of the pancreas resection. Such entity is rare in literature, and Schwarz et al. have reported three cases of secondary metachronous lung adenocarcinoma; in those cases, the time interval between the primary pancreatic carcinoma and secondary metachronous lung adenocarcinoma ranged from 16 to 66 months [16]. In our case, the patient developed secondary metachronous lung adenocarcinoma after 61 months of carcinoma of the head of the pancreas resection, which is considered a late metachronous adenocarcinoma, which falls into the time frame proposed by Schwarz et al.

Studies concerning genetic mutations that occur in such cases are lacking in the literature. However, there have been extensive reports discussing metachronous multiple primary tumors in the lung [17, 18]. Isaka et al. have demonstrated in their case report that epidermal growth factor receptor (EGFR) mutation status is an important indicator of determining the metachronous lung carcinoma, assisting in differentiating primary disease versus metastasis [17]. In a study including 59 sections of metachronous and synchronous lung carcinoma, it was found that 66% of the sections demonstrated mutations in *p53* gene, raising the possibility of an association between such mutations and the development of metachronous carcinoma [18]. Talbott and his colleagues, in their case series studying synchronous and metachronous cancer of the pancreas, have argued that K-ras mutations can play a role in the development of such circumstances [19]. Evidence in literature is still inconsistent, and other factors should be taken into account in determining genetic mutation abnormalities such types of cancers, although, with the limited occurrence of metachronous cancerous lesions,

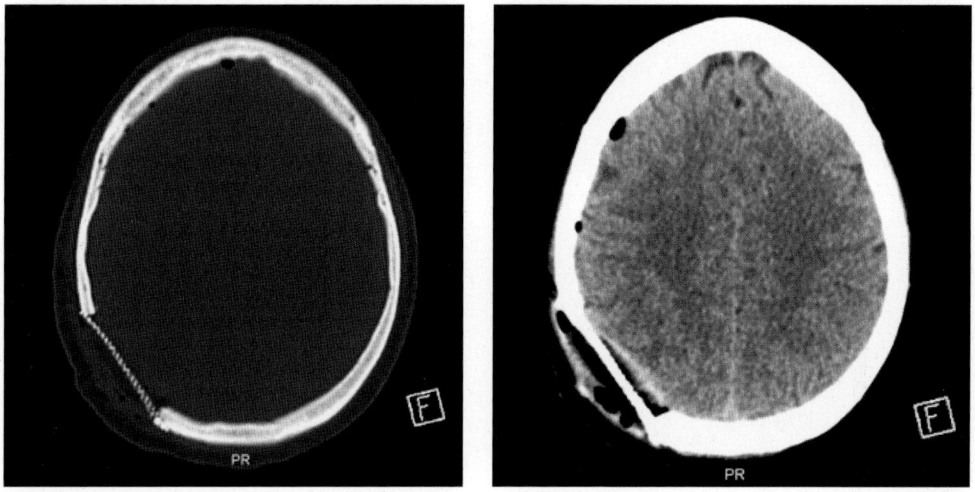

(a) (b)

FIGURE 6: Postoperative nonenhanced (a) bone window and (b) brain window axial CT showing a metallic mesh over the site of bony resection, with no associated intracranial hemorrhage or residual bony lesion.

larger studies are required to provide a firm basis for profiling the genetic abnormalities of such cases.

Our case did not demonstrate the mode of spread of the skull metastasis from the lung adenocarcinoma. Even though metastases of lung carcinoma are widespreadly known to occur through the hematogenous spread, sometimes they appear in locations that are not predictable as a direct spread from the primary focus. Batson has proposed that vertebral veins could explain the appearance of cranial metastases from a lung origin, according to animal and cadaveric experimentation [20].

Skull metastases are usually small and asymptomatic and are discovered incidentally, thus posing a diagnostic difficulty. However, sometimes they are associated with pain, hemorrhage, or intracranial extension leading to focal neurological deficits [13, 21]. In some instances, dural sinuses become involved leading to rising in the ICP [13, 21].

Metastatic deposits to the skull are initially diagnosed by imaging such as CT and MRI [13, 22]. Usually, metastases from the lungs to the skull are lytic in nature causing bone destruction, same as lesions from breast, kidneys, and thyroid gland [13, 22]. In MRI, these lesions appear to be hypointense on T1-weighted images and with variable signal intensities in T2 images and variable enhancement by contrast injection [13, 22]. A study by Nemeth et al. has demonstrated that diffusion-weighted magnetic resonance imaging (DWI-MRI) is superior to routine MRI in detecting skull metastases from lung or breast origin [23]. Yohena and his colleagues argue that brain MRI is not to be done routinely in all lung carcinoma patients [24].

The definitive diagnosis is only available via histopathological examination coupled with immunohistochemistry (tissue diagnosis), as illustrated in our case since it can reveal an underlying, undiagnosed malignant disease [13]. The pathological specimen is usually taken after surgical excision, and sometimes due to the small size of the lesion or the presence of multiple lesions, fine-needle aspiration (FNA) is carried out [13, 25].

A significant number of patients with skull metastasis are not suitable for surgical intervention, owing in large part to the behavior of the primary malignancy and number of lesions [13, 26]. The difficulty of surgery depends on the involvement of vital structures such as the dural sinuses [13, 21]. Nevertheless, the surgical technique is straightforward involving the complete removal of the lesion and cranioplasty [13, 21]. In some instances, total excision of the lesion is not possible. Thus, radiotherapy is the another option for treatment [13, 26].

In a case of lung carcinoma, it has been suggested that lung carcinoma with distant metastasis is identified as a poor predictor of survival [1]. However, there have been many reports in which patients with solitary metastasis had an excellent increased rate of survival, with excision of the metastatic lesion and aggressive chemotherapy and radiotherapy [27, 28].

4. Conclusion

Skull metastasis from lung cancer is not uncommon, yet the first presentation for this malignant disease is a rare instant. The definitive diagnosis of the origin of metastasis is through tissue diagnosis. However, imaging has to be carried out to detect the primary malignancy and other metastases to guide surgical resection and subsequent treatment.

Ethical Approval

All procedures were in accordance with the ethical standards at the authors' institution and with the 1964 Helsinki declaration and its later amendments or comparable ethical standards.

Consent

A written consent was obtained from the patient for reproduction of the information appearing in this report.

Authors' Contributions

Saleh S. Baeesa and Ali Altalhy participated in the whole diagnostic and treatment process of the described patients. Saleh S. Baeesa, Ali Altalhy, and Yazid Maghrabi conceived the concept of the study. Ali Altalhy and Yazid Maghrabi collected the data. Yazid Maghrabi wrote the article. Saleh S. Baeesa, Ali Altalhy, Zuhoor Almansouri, and Yazid Maghrabi participated in the sequence alignment and helped to draft the manuscript. Zuhoor Almansouri dealt with pathological aspects of the lesion. All authors read and approved the final manuscript.

References

[1] H. Sugiura, K. Yamada, T. Sugiura, T. Hida, and T. Mitsudomi, "Predictors of survival in patients with bone metastasis of lung cancer," *Clinical Orthopaedics and Related Research*, vol. 466, no. 3, pp. 729–736, 2008.

[2] R. C. Turner, B. P. Lucke-Wold, R. Hwang, and B. D. Underwood, "Lung cancer metastasis presenting as a solitary skull mass," *Journal of Surgical Case Reports*, vol. 2016, no. 6, 2016.

[3] N. Tziris, J. Dokmetzioglou, K. Giannoulis et al., "Synchronous and metachronous adenocarcinomas of the large intestine," *Hippokratia*, vol. 12, no. 3, pp. 150–152, 2008.

[4] Y. Kitasato, M. Nakayama, G. Akasu et al., "Metastatic pulmonary adenocarcinoma 13 years after curative resection for pancreatic cancer: Report of a case and review of Japanese literature," *Journal of the Pancreas*, vol. 13, no. 3, pp. 296–300, 2012.

[5] S. Pericleous, S. Mukherjee, and R. R. Hutchkins, "Lung adenocarcinoma presenting as obstructive jaundice: a case report and review of literature," *World Journal of Surgical Oncology*, vol. 6, article no. 120, 2008.

[6] R. F. Falkenstern-Ge, M. Wohlleber, M. Kimmich et al., "Pulmonary adenocarcinoma occurring 5 years after resection of a primary pancreatic adenocarcinoma: a relevant differential diagnosis," *Case Reports in Oncological Medicine*, vol. 2014, Article ID 841907, 4 pages, 2014.

[7] C.-T. Hsieh, J.-M. Sun, W.-C. Tsai, T.-H. Tsai, Y.-H. Chiang, and M.-Y. Liu, "Skull metastasis from hepatocellular carcinoma," *Acta Neurochirurgica*, vol. 149, no. 2, pp. 185–190, 2007.

[8] J. Shen, S. Wang, X. Zhao, X. Shao, X. Jiang, and Y. Dai, "Skull metastasis from follicular thyroid carcinoma: report of three cases and review of literature," *International Journal of Clinical and Experimental Pathology*, vol. 8, no. 11, pp. 15285–15293, 2015.

[9] N. Barbetakis, D. Paliouras, C. Asteriou et al., "Cutaneous skull metastasis from uterine leiomyosarcoma: a case report," *World Journal of Surgical Oncology*, vol. 7, article 45, 2009.

[10] H. Yeh, S. Yang, H. Ke, K. Lee, C. Huang, and W. Wu, "Renal cell carcinoma presenting with skull metastasis: a case report and literature review," *The Kaohsiung Journal of Medical Sciences*, vol. 23, no. 9, pp. 475–479, 2007.

[11] KW. Lee, DS. Chung, PW. Huh, YK. Hong, HK. Rha, and JK. Kang, "Intracranial metastasis of hepatocellular carcinoma associated with epidural hematoma: a case report," *Journal of Korean Neurosurgical Society*, vol. 25, pp. 1738–1742, 1996.

[12] M. V. Aydin, M. Cekinmez, O. Kizilkilic, F. Kayaselcuk, O. Sen, and N. Altinors, "Unusual case of skull metastasis secondary to pancreatic adenocarcinoma," *Pathology and Oncology Research*, vol. 11, no. 3, pp. 182-183, 2005.

[13] E. G. Clair and I. E. McCutcheon, "Skull tumors," in *Youmans Neurological Surgery*, H. R. Winn and R. Julian, Eds., Saunders, Philadelphia, Pa, USA, 2011.

[14] K. Mitsuya, Y. Nakasu, S. Horiguchi et al., "Metastatic skull tumors: MRI features and a new conventional classification," *Journal of Neuro-Oncology*, vol. 104, no. 1, pp. 239–245, 2011.

[15] K. E. Stanley, "Prognostic factors for survival in patients with inoperable lung cancer," *Journal of the National Cancer Institute*, vol. 65, no. 1, pp. 25–32, 1980.

[16] R. E. Schwarz, P. G. Chu, and F. W. Grannis Jr., "Pancreatic tumors in patients with lung malignancies: a spectrum of clinicopathologic considerations," *Southern Medical Journal*, vol. 97, no. 9, pp. 811–815, 2004.

[17] T. Isaka, T. Yokose, H. Ito et al., "Diagnosis of metachronous multiple lung adenocarcinoma at the cut-end by epidermal growth factor receptor mutation status discordance 4 years after sublobar resection for adenocarcinoma in situ: report of a case," *Surgery Today*, vol. 45, no. 10, pp. 1330–1334, 2015.

[18] M. T. M. Van Rens, E. J. E. Eijken, J. R. J. Elbers, J.-W. J. Lammers, M. G. J. Tilanus, and P. J. Slootweg, "p53 mutation analysis for definite diagnosis of multiple primary lung carcinoma," *Cancer*, vol. 94, no. 1, pp. 188–196, 2002.

[19] V. A. Talbott, C. J. Yeo, J. R. Brody, and A. K. Witkiewicz, "Molecular profiling of synchronous and metachronous cancers of the pancreas reveal molecular mimicry between samples from the same patient," *Journal of Surgical Research*, vol. 176, no. 1, pp. 154–158, 2012.

[20] O. V. Batson, "The function of the vertebral veins and their role in the spread of metastases," *Annals of Surgery*, vol. 112, no. 1, pp. 138–149, 1940.

[21] C. B. Michael, Z. L. Gokaslan, F. DeMonte, I. E. McCutcheon, R. Sawaya, and F. F. Lang, "Surgical resection of calvarial metastases overlying dural sinuses," *Neurosurgery*, vol. 48, no. 4, pp. 745–755, 2001.

[22] F. Laigle-Donadey, S. Taillibert, N. Martin-Duverneuil, J. Hildebrand, and J.-Y. Delattre, "Skull-base metastases," *Journal of Neuro-Oncology*, vol. 75, no. 1, pp. 63–69, 2005.

[23] A. J. Nemeth, J. W. Henson, M. E. Mullins, R. G. Gonzalez, and P. W. Schaefer, "Improved detection of skull metastasis with diffusion-weighted MR imaging," *American Journal of Neuroradiology*, vol. 28, no. 6, pp. 1088–1092, 2007.

[24] T. Yohena, I. Yoshino, M. Kitajima et al., "Necessity of preoperative screening for brain metastasis in non-small cell lung cancer patients without lymph node metastasis," *Annals of Thoracic and Cardiovascular Surgery*, vol. 10, no. 6, pp. 347–349, 2004.

[25] D. A. Wecht and R. Sawaya, "Lesions of the calvaria: surgical experience with 42 patients," *Annals of Surgical Oncology*, vol. 4, no. 1, pp. 28–36, 1997.

[26] F. DeMonte, F. Hanbali, and M. T. Ballo, "Skull base metastasis," in *Textbook of Neuro-Oncology*, Berger M. S. and Prados M. D., Eds., Saunders, Philadelphia, Pa, USA, 2005.

[27] A. K. Agarwala and N. H. Hanna, "Long-term survival in a patient with stage IV non-small-cell lung carcinoma after bone metastasectomy," *Clinical Lung Cancer*, vol. 6, no. 6, pp. 367-368, 2005.

[28] Y. Hirano, M. Oda, Y. Tsunezuka, N. Ishikawa, and G. Watanabe, "Long-term survival cases of lung cancer presented as solitary bone metastasis," *Annals of Thoracic and Cardiovascular Surgery*, vol. 11, pp. 401–404, 2005.

36

Cytomegalovirus Colitis Masquerading as Apple-Core Lesion after Systemic Chemotherapy in a Patient with Relapsed Acute Myeloid Leukemia

Jong An,[1] Jason Brownell,[2] Darrell Barker,[3] Theresa Stockinger,[4] Robert Brady,[4] Katherine Cebe,[4] and Russell Baur[1]

[1]*Department of Hematology and Oncology Service, San Antonio Military Medical Center, Fort Sam Houston, San Antonio, TX 78234, USA*
[2]*Department of Internal Medicine, San Antonio Military Medical Center, Fort Sam Houston, San Antonio, TX 78234, USA*
[3]*Department of Gastroenterology, San Antonio Military Medical Center, Fort Sam Houston, San Antonio, TX 78234, USA*
[4]*Department of Pathology, San Antonio Military Medical Center, Fort Sam Houston, San Antonio, TX 78234, USA*

Correspondence should be addressed to Jong An; jong.w.an.mil@mail.mil

Academic Editor: Jeanine M. Buchanich

We report the case of a 71-year-old male with relapsed acute myeloid leukemia who developed cytomegalovirus (CMV) colitis presenting as an apple-core lesion during induction chemotherapy. CMV infection occurs rarely during induction chemotherapy for acute myeloid leukemia. CMV infection is usually observed in patients with acquired immune deficiency syndrome (AIDS) and in those on immunosuppressive agents following bone marrow transplant. Although rare, CMV colitis should be considered in patients who are critically ill after systemic chemotherapy as it can cause significant morbidity and mortality.

1. Introduction

CMV colitis typically occurs in severely immunocompromised patients with AIDS and in those on immunosuppressive agents after allogenic stem cell transplant or solid organ transplant. Infection in immunocompetent patients is generally asymptomatic or may present as transient symptoms consisting of fever, myalgias, and cervical lymphadenopathy. In recent years, however, there have been a rising number of cases of severe CMV infections in immunocompromised elderly patients with malignancies [1]. Given that CMV seroprevalence rates rise with age, there is a higher risk of reactivation in the setting of chemotherapy among elderly patients leading to significant morbidity and mortality.

This report documents an incidental finding of CMV colitis presenting as an apple-core lesion after chemotherapy in a patient with acute myeloid leukemia.

2. Case Presentation

A 71-year-old man, with a past medical history significant for acute myeloid leukemia, underwent induction with cytarabine and idarubicin followed by consolidation with three cycles of high-dose cytarabine. After one year of achieving remission, he was found to have relapsed leukemia during workup for anemia. He was admitted to the hospital for salvage chemotherapy with cytarabine and mitoxantrone. Ten days after salvage chemotherapy, he developed a neutropenic fever, diarrhea, abdominal pain, and elevated total bilirubin. Abdominal ultrasound showed no signs of biliary obstruction. CT scan of the abdomen and pelvis showed pericecal inflammatory stranding without pneumatosis concerning cecal typhlitis as well as an "apple-core mass" of the ascending colon near the hepatic flexure concerning colon cancer (Figure 1).

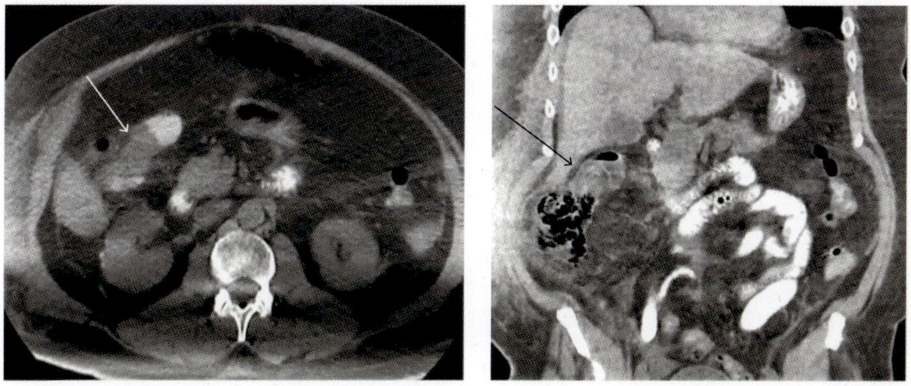

(a) (b)

FIGURE 1: Abdominal computed tomography (CT) demonstrating apple-core mass of the ascending colon.

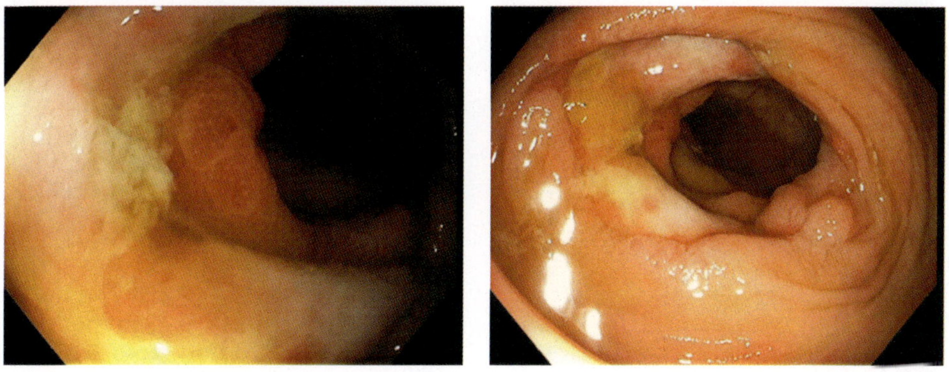

(a) (b)

FIGURE 2: Colonoscopy showing a mass in the proximal transverse colon. Mucosa presents with nodularity, loss of vascular pattern, and diffuse exudates.

Colonoscopy was deferred because he was critically ill with neutropenic enterocolitis. Despite initiation of broad-spectrum antibiotics consisting of vancomycin and piperacillin-tazobactam, his clinical condition deteriorated. He was transferred to the medical intensive care unit with acute respiratory failure requiring assisted ventilation for several days. Blood cultures revealed *Granulicatella adjacens* and transthoracic echocardiogram revealed an aortic valve vegetation consistent with endocarditis requiring 6 weeks treatment with intravenous vancomycin. Additionally, he was noted to have hyperbilirubinemia secondary to hepatic veno-occlusive disease for which he completed a course of defibrotide with eventual normalization of liver enzymes. The patient improved clinically, and subsequent bone marrow biopsy obtained 7 weeks after induction chemotherapy showed no evidence of leukemia. After six weeks of inpatient treatment and subsequent clinical improvement, a colonoscopy was performed to rule out colon cancer given the suspicious apple-core lesion noted on the CT at the hepatic flexure. It revealed diffuse friable changes of the colonic wall extending from the cecum to the hepatic flexure and the transverse colon (Figure 2). Biopsies of the ascending colon, cecum, hepatic flexure, and transverse colon were taken. He was discharged to acute rehabilitation due to deconditioning and a 55 pound weight loss after 7 weeks of inpatient hospitalization.

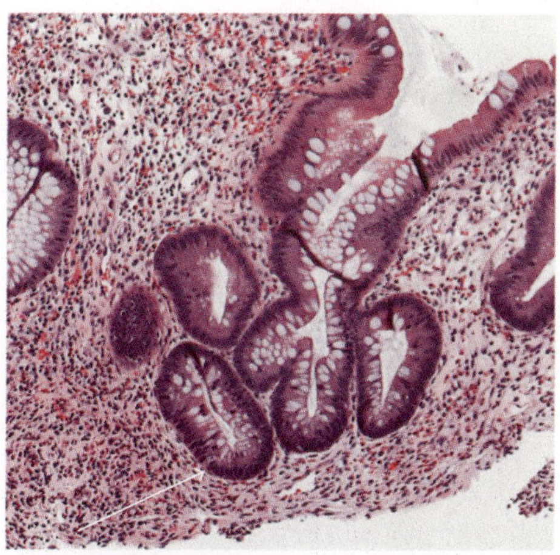

FIGURE 3: H&E, 126x magnification, showing changes of chronic, active colitis including crypt architectural distortion (branching) and focal active cryptitis (white arrow).

Final pathology from the cecal biopsy specimens showed chronic active colitis with cryptitis, ulceration, and architectural

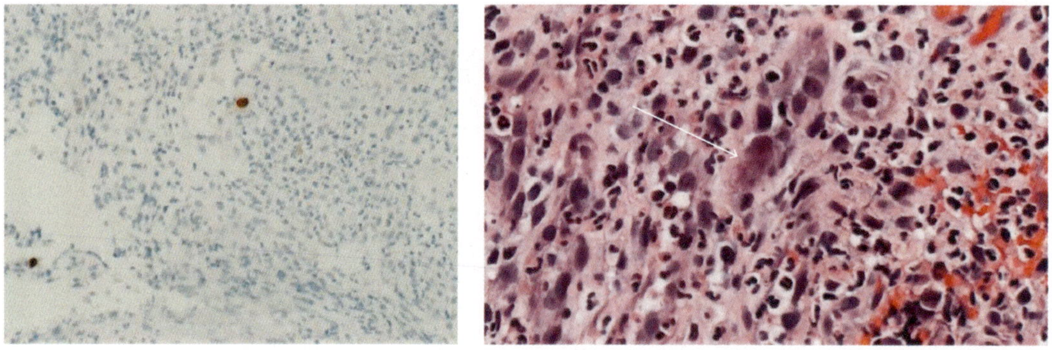

(a) (b)

Figure 4: (a) CMV immunohistochemical stain, 200x magnification, highlighting both nuclear and cytoplasmic staining (brown chromogen) within the ulcerated granulation tissue. (b) H&E stain, 400x magnification, showing a CMV-infected endothelial cell with dot-like cytoplasmic inclusions (white arrow).

distortion (Figure 3). CMV immunohistochemical staining was positive for CMV type inclusions compatible with CMV colitis (Figure 4). The biopsies were negative for dysplasia and malignancy. The ascending colon, hepatic flexure mass, and transverse colon mass were negative for CMV inclusions on immunohistochemical stains but showed features consistent with chronic active colitis with cryptitis and architectural distortion.

Our patient remained asymptomatic, without recurrence of diarrhea, fever, or abdominal pain.

3. Discussion

We describe a rare case of CMV colitis in a 71-year-old male treated with salvage chemotherapy consisting of cytarabine and mitoxantrone for relapsed acute myeloid leukemia.

CMV remains latent within the host after initial infection and can reactivate later in life. Clinically significant CMV disease is typically seen in profound immunocompromised state such as in AIDS and bone marrow transplant patients. Although CMV status among AIDS and transplant patients is closely monitored with the subsequent initiation of preemptive treatment using antiviral therapy if needed, similar monitoring and treatment plans are not routinely implemented for cancer patients receiving standard chemotherapy. Generally, conventional chemotherapy does not lead to significant alterations in lymphocyte function which is thought to be considered a high risk for the development of CMV disease. However, this paradigm may be changing.

There is increasing incidence of CMV reactivation in patients undergoing conventional chemotherapy. In our literature review, the earliest reported case of CMV colitis after standard chemotherapy was in a patient receiving azacitidine, published in 2011 [2]. A recent study involving 15 cancer patients with 11 head and neck cancers, two lung cancers, one lymphoma, and one rectal cancer showed that all but one patient experienced CMV reactivation during the course of chemotherapy [3]. Ten of the 15 participants had no detectable viral DNA before starting chemotherapy, but the viral load increased in 14 of 15 patients after chemotherapy. The highest CMV viral loads were >100,000 copies/mL in two patients who died. As viral loads increased, patients experienced an increase in symptoms as well as abnormal liver function tests. Another study showed that CMV viremia predicts high mortality rate in cancer patients. The retrospective analysis of cancer patients with CMV viremia showed overall mortality rate of 56% (60/107). This study recommended preemptive antiviral therapy for cancer patients with positive serum CMV PCR results, especially those requiring mechanical ventilation [4]. It is not known in our case whether infection with CMV was present prior to or after the initiation of chemotherapy, as we did not obtain CMV serology.

Because CMV infections commonly occur after allogenic stem cell transplant, these serologic tests are used pretransplant to establish the serostatus which predicts the risk of developing disease, and guides the use of preemptive antiviral therapy. The exact mechanism of the reactivation of CMV is not well established. However, disturbance of the host's immune defenses are thought to play an important role. Male sex, lower body mass index, lymphopenia, hematological malignancy, steroid use, and red blood cell transfusion within one month prior to CMV disease were risk factors for the development of CMV gastrointestinal infection in adult patients with cancer [5]. Our patient possessed several risk factors to include male sex, lymphopenia, and hematological malignancy.

An apple-core lesion of the colon is most frequently associated with obstruction of the colon lumen by colorectal carcinoma but can also be seen in setting of lymphomas, Crohn's disease, ulcerative colitis, ischemic colitis, chlamydia infection, colonic tuberculosis, helminthoma, colonic amoebiasis, villous adenoma, and colonic cytomegalovirus [6]. Thus, tissue biopsy remains the keystone in obtaining the definitive diagnosis.

The gold standard for diagnosing CMV tissue invasive disease is the identification of CMV inclusion or positive CMV immunohistochemistry staining on histopathology [7]. CMV gastrointestinal disease cannot be excluded based on negative blood tests. In a retrospective study of 81 solid organ transplant recipients, 20 cases of biopsy-proven gastrointestinal disease were identified. The sensitivity of

PCR for diagnosing CMV gastrointestinal disease was only 85 percent [8]. Plasma CMV DNA was undetectable in three patients with biopsy-proven CMV gastrointestinal disease. Also, gastrointestinal disease may be focal, as seen in this patient. Therefore, multiple biopsies may be needed to confirm the diagnosis of CMV colitis.

Individuals suspected to have CMV colitis should have plasma or whole blood PCR testing since PCR results are often available prior to biopsy results and may influence the decision to initiate antiviral therapy. Furthermore, the early PCR detection can prompt earlier treatment when "gold standard" testing is not available as colonoscopy is relatively contraindicated in the presence of neutropenia. Our patient's CMV infection resolved without the use of antivirals, which we attribute to recovery of the immune system. However, it is possible that the use of early antiviral treatment could have led to shorter hospitalization and reduced complications.

Given the high morbidity and mortality associated with reactivated CMV disease, physicians may consider CMV testing, monitoring, and preemptive treatment in leukemic patients with high risk features who are undergoing chemotherapy. A high index of suspicion for CMV disease may be beneficial in those cancer patients who clinically deteriorate and may benefit from early antiviral therapy to improve prognosis.

References

[1] S. Jacob and N. Zayyani, "Cytomegalovirus colitis masquerading as rectal malignancy in an immunocompetent patient," *Indian Journal of Pathology and Microbiology*, vol. 58, no. 1, pp. 80–82, 2015.

[2] R. Khan, P. Rudkin, K. Grewal et al., "Cytomegalovirus colitis following azacitidine therapy," *Canadian Journal of Infectious Diseases and Medical Microbiology*, vol. 22, no. 3, pp. e21–e23, 2011.

[3] C. P. Kuo, C. L. Wu, H. T. Ho, C. G. Chen, S. I. Liu, and Y. T. Lu, "Detection of cytomegalovirus reactivation in cancer patients receiving chemotherapy," *Clinical Microbiology and Infection*, vol. 14, no. 3, pp. 221–227, 2008.

[4] Y. Wang, N. Wang, J. Lin et al., "Risk factors and outcomes of cytomegalovirus viremia in cancer patients: a study from a medical center in northern Taiwan," *Journal of Microbiology, Immunology and Infection*, vol. 44, no. 6, pp. 442–448, 2011.

[5] J. H. Ko, K. R. Peck, W. J. Lee et al., "Risk factors for cytomegalovirus gastrointestinal disease in adult patients with cancer," *European Journal of Clinical Microbiology & Infectious Diseases*, vol. 33, no. 10, pp. 1847–1853, 2014.

[6] P. Paolantonio and C. Dromain, *Imaging of Small Bowel Colon and Rectum*, Vol. 1, p. 15, Springer, Berlin, Germany, 2014.

[7] P. Ljungman, M. Boeckh, H. H. Hirsche et al., "Definitions of cytomegalovirus infection and disease in transplant patients for use in clinical trials," *Clinical Infectious Diseases*, vol. 64, no. 1, pp. 87–91, 2017.

[8] C. M. Durand, K. A. Marr, C. A. Arnold et al., "Detection of cytomegalovirus DNA in plasma as an adjunct diagnostic for gastrointestinal tract disease in kidney and liver transplant recipients," *Clinical Infectious Diseases*, vol. 57, no. 11, pp. 1550–1559, 2013.

Solitary Plasmacytoma of the Mesentery: A Systematic Clinician's Diagnosis

Georgia Mitropoulou,[1] Adamantia Zizi-Sermpetzoglou,[2] Hippokrates Moschouris,[3] Athanasios Kountourogiannis,[2] Despoina Myoteri,[2] and Dionysios Dellaportas[4]

[1] *Pathology Department, "Agia Sofia" Children's Hospital, Athens, Greece*
[2] *Pathology Department, "Tzaneion" General Hospital, Piraeus, Greece*
[3] *Radiology Department, "Tzaneion" General Hospital, Piraeus, Greece*
[4] *2nd Department of Surgery, University Hospital "Aretaieion", Athens, Greece*

Correspondence should be addressed to Despoina Myoteri; dmyoteri@gmail.com

Academic Editor: Ossama W. Tawfik

Introduction. Plasmacytoma is an uncommon plasma cell neoplasm and its localized form is solitary plasmacytoma of the bone and solitary extramedullary plasmacytoma. Solitary plasmacytoma of the mesentery is extremely rare, reported only in a handful of cases. *Case Presentation*. A 47-year-old man with nonspecific abdominal complains was found to have an ill-defined mass on his mesenteric root. Laparoscopic biopsy and stepwise histopathological examination revealed a mesenteric plasmacytoma, and extensive imaging and laboratory investigations led to the diagnosis of the solitary mesenteric plasmacytoma. The patient underwent definitive radiotherapy and remains under remission one year later. *Discussion*. Plasma cell dyscrasias include a variant of proliferative disease, characterized by clonal expansion of bone marrow plasma cells, producing a massive quantity of monoclonal immunoglobulin called paraprotein or M-protein. Solitary extramedullary plasmacytoma accounts for only 3–5% of all plasma cell neoplasms. Meticulous adherence to the established diagnostic criteria helps the clinician to set the correct, yet very unusual and unexpected diagnosis.

1. Introduction

Plasma cell neoplasms result from clonal expansion of plasma cells which produce large amount of M-protein, with plasma cell myeloma being the most common disorder of plasma cell dyscrasias [1]. Plasmacytoma is an uncommon plasma cell neoplasm and its localized form is solitary plasmacytoma of the bone and solitary extramedullary plasmacytoma (SEP). The latter is extremely rare with a reported incidence less than 5% of plasma cell dyscrasias, affecting mostly the upper aerodigestive tract [2].

SEP of the mesentery has only been reported in a handful of cases, to the best of our knowledge [3]. A case of mesenteric plasmacytoma in a 47-year-old man is presented herein, initially managed as a pancreatic tumor, and the clinical and histopathological stepwise diagnosis is highlighted.

2. Case Presentation

A 47-year-old Caucasian male was admitted with nonspecific abdominal pain, vomiting, weight loss, and early satiety. The patient had no significant past medical history, and physical examination was inconclusive, apart from noting slight abdominal distension, with routine observations within normal limits. Laboratory investigations including complete blood count, biochemical and coagulation tests, and urinalysis examinations were unremarkable as well. Subsequently, a computed tomography (CT) of his abdomen was performed, revealing a multilobulated and ill-defined, soft tissue mass, arising from the root of the mesentery, compressing the posterior wall of the stomach (Figure 1(a)). To characterize the mass further an abdominal MRI was performed, showing peripheral enhancement and a likely necrotic center, with

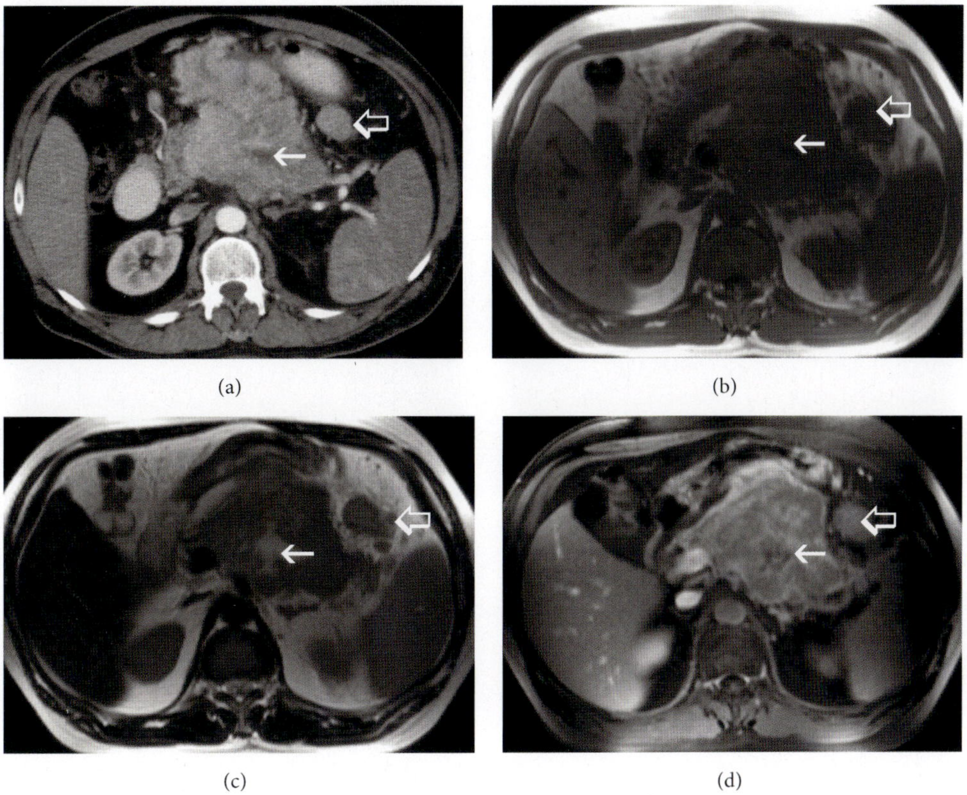

FIGURE 1: (a) Contrast-enhanced CT, (b) T1 weighted MR (c) T2 weighted MR, and (d) T1 weighted, contrast-enhanced MR. Arrows: the central part of the lesion lacks enhancement- necrotic part. Open arrows: satellite lesions are evident at the periphery of the mass.

satellite lesions evident at the periphery of the mass (Figures 1(b), 1(c), and 1(d)). Radiological evaluation opted towards a lymph nodal mass of unknown origin. After multidisciplinary meeting team discussion (MDT) a laparoscopic biopsy was decided and performed, deemed to be the safest approach. Histopathological examination revealed a $3 \times 1 \times 0{,}4$ cm solid, soft, and tan mass. On microscopic examination, the neoplasm was composed of neoplastic plasma cells showing variable degree of maturation. Some of the cells were oval with round eccentric nucleus, "spoke wheel" chromatin, and no nucleoli. Other cells appeared with prominent nucleoli and occasional multinucleated. Mitotic figures were also apparent (Figure 2). Immunohistochemically these cells were positive for CD138 (Figure 3(a)) and CD38 (Figure 3(b)) while CD56 was expressed in a small percentage of neoplastic cells. Other markers such CD20, CD79a, CD3, CK20, CK7, chromogranin, synaptophysin, and HHV8 were negative, whereas proliferative index MIB-1 was high. The neoplastic cells also showed cytoplasmic monotypic IgA and κ-light chain restriction (Figure 4).

All the above set the diagnosis of mesentery plasmacytoma, which was finally classified as SEP of the mesentery, since bone marrow examination was normal with less than 5% of plasma cells and concentrated urine was negative of Bence-Jones protein, while no other site of disease was revealed on additional imaging investigations, and renal parameters and calcium levels were normal. Moreover, serum protein electrophoresis did not show any monoclonal protein spike. The final diagnosis was IgA- κ type solitary extramedullary plasmacytoma of mesentery. The patient was treated with 50 Gy of radiotherapy, delivered over six weeks, and developed mild radiation related diarrhea. The tumor responded very well, with complete radiological response, and the patient remains disease free one year later, on follow-up visits.

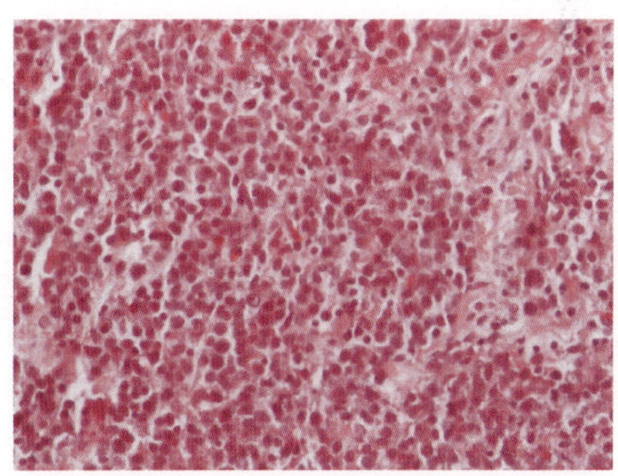

FIGURE 2: The neoplastic plasma cells showed variable degree of maturation with some of them being oval with round eccentric nucleus, "spoke wheel" chromatin, and no nucleoli, while others have prominent nucleoli or are occasional multinucleated (H-E ×200).

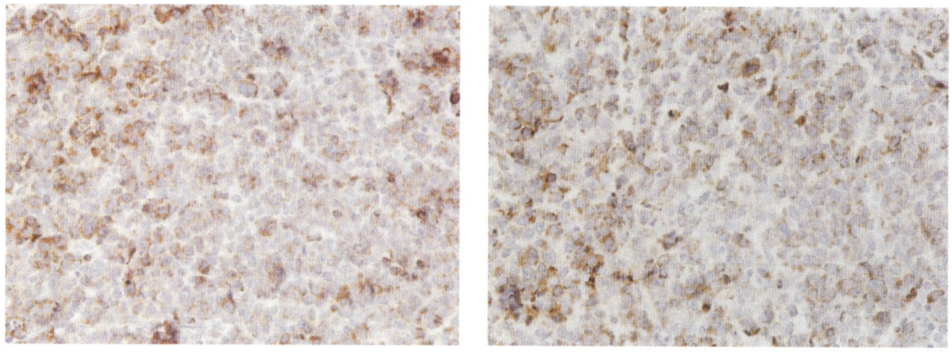

(a) (b)

Figure 3: (a) The neoplastic cells were positive for CD138 (CD138 ×200). (b) The neoplastic cells were positive for CD38 (CD38 ×400).

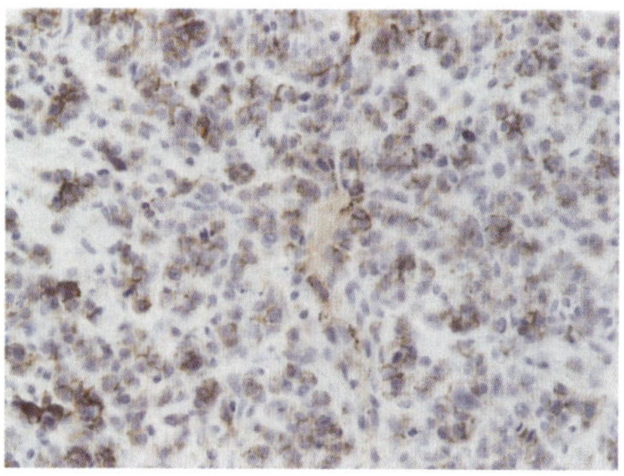

Figure 4: The neoplastic cells showed cytoplasmic monotypic IgA and κ-light chain restriction (κ ×400).

3. Discussion

Plasma cell dyscrasias include a variant of proliferative disease, characterized by clonal expansion of plasma cells in the bone marrow or other tissues, producing a massive quantity of monoclonal immunoglobulin called paraprotein or M-protein [4]. The main disorders of this group are plasma cell myeloma, plasmacytoma, and conditions which result from immunoglobulin deposits in tissues. Plasma cell myeloma, characterized by disseminated proliferation of plasma cells, is a bone marrow origin neoplasm. In contrast plasmacytoma, which is quite rare, appears as a unique focus of neoplastic plasma cells, occurring either in bone (solitary plasmacytoma of bone) or in soft tissue (solitary extramedullary plasmacytoma). Immunoglobulin deposition diseases include primary amyloidosis and light and heavy chain deposition diseases [5].

Solitary extramedullary plasmacytoma (SEP) is a rare tumor accounting for only 3–5% of all plasma cell neoplasms [6]. It is defined as either primary, when it occurs as isolated mass, or secondary, when it is associated with generalized multiple myeloma. Although SEP can occur in almost any tissue, it mostly involves the upper aerodigestive tract [7]. Other sites of involvement include the gastrointestinal tract, breast, thyroid, skin, urinary bladder, lymph nodes, testis, and CNS [8]. It affects more frequently males than females in the sixth decade of life [1].

The clinical features are related to the anatomic site that is involved. The diagnosis of SEP is based upon the following recommended diagnostic criteria compiled by Soutar et al. [9]: (1) histopathological tissue evidence of single area of extramedullary involvement of monoclonal plasma cells; (2) normal marrow without clonal involvement; (3) normal results on skeletal imaging survey; (4) no anemia, hypercalcemia, or renal impairment, attributable to plasma cell dyscrasias; and (5) no or low serum or urinary levels of monoclonal immunoglobulins.

In the case reported above these criteria were fulfilled.

Serum protein electrophoresis should be performed whenever multiple myeloma or related disorders are suspected, and this can be used as a prognostic marker if positive at presentation [10].

On histopathological examination SEP is straightforward to diagnose, except for cases where the tumor cells are poorly differentiated. Microscopically, the neoplasm consists of plasma cells of variable degree of plasmacytic maturation. Mature cells usually have clumped nuclear chromatin, abundant cytoplasm, and no nucleoli. Immature cells often have large nuclei with prominent nucleoli. In some cases, multinucleated and pleomorphic plasma cells may be present. Amyloid may also be present in 10% of the cases. Immunohistochemical examination with antibodies to kappa and lambda light chains is essential to confirm the diagnosis. The immunophenotypic features are similar to those of plasma cell myeloma. The cells usually express CD138 and are strongly positive for CD38. The differential diagnosis of plasmacytoma includes plasma cell granuloma, plasmacytoid lymphoma, large cell lymphoma, and marginal zone lymphoma of MALT type [11]. Supplementary laboratory and radiologic examinations are useful in order to exclude remote disease sites [12].

SEP is considered radiosensitive and therefore the treatment of choice is radiation therapy [13]. Despite surgical resection is thought to be equally effective to radiotherapy, their combination is preferred for large masses that can be surgically resected safely [14].

The radiotherapy field in the case presented above was indeed large, and it was very challenging to manage the patient's postradiation enteritis. Radiotherapy delivered in fields involving the small bowel can cause significant short- and long-term side-effects, which can be equally troublesome to manage [15]. The optimal radiotherapy dose is not accurately defined, due to the rarity of the disease. Doses below 20 Gy were used as palliative and between 25 and 50 Gy were used for cutaneous lesions in a recent case series, with mixed results [13].

The effectiveness of adjuvant chemotherapy is not thoroughly investigated and is used for refractory or relapsed disease. However, chemotherapy is considered in the adjuvant setting for tumors larger than 5 cm and high-grade histology [16]. Regional recurrence and distant metastasis may develop in 22% of patients and 15% will develop generalized myeloma [8]. SEP prognosis is considered good with a median survival of approximately 10 years [6].

The follow-up has no established protocols or guidelines and it has to be mentioned that our patient's follow-up is short, compared to reported survival from SEP [13].

In conclusion, osseous and extraosseous plasmacytomas are localized tumors of monoclonal plasma cell origin. Although extramedullary plasmacytomas occur mainly in the upper aerodigestive tract, mesentery may also be involved with very few case reports in current literature. The sound combination of radiological, laboratory, and histopathological work-up leads to the correct diagnosis, and subsequent treatment is highly effective, for a disease with impressive and diverse initial presenting features.

References

[1] V. D. Dayton, S. J. Williams, R. W. McKenna, and M. A. Linden, "Unusual extramedullary hematopoietic neoplasms in lymph nodes," *Human Pathology*, vol. 62, pp. 13–22, 2017.

[2] E. G. de Waal, M. Leene, N. Veeger et al., "Progression of a solitary plasmacytoma to multiple myeloma. A population-based registry of the northern Netherlands," *British Journal of Haematology*, vol. 175, no. 4, pp. 661–667, 2016.

[3] R. Galhotra, K. Saggar, K. Gupta, and P. Singh, "Primary isolated extramedullary plasmacytoma of mesentry: a rare case report," *The Gulf journal of oncology*, no. 12, pp. 81–84, 2012.

[4] M. Boccadoro and A. Pileri, "1Plasma cell dyscrasias: classification, clinical and laboratory characteristics, and differential diagnosis," *Bailliere's Clinical Haematology*, vol. 8, no. 4, pp. 705–719, 1995.

[5] J. Weisberger, C. D. Wu, Z. Liu et al., "Differential diagnosis of malignant lymphomas and related disorders by specific pattern of expression of immunophenotypic markers revealed by multiparameter flow cytometry (Review)," *International Journal of Oncology*, vol. 17, pp. 1165–1177, 2000.

[6] P. Finsinger, S. Grammatico, M. Chisini, A. Piciocchi, R. Foà, and M. T. Petrucci, "Clinical features and prognostic factors in solitary plasmacytoma," *British Journal of Haematology*, vol. 172, no. 4, pp. 554–560, 2016.

[7] P. Galieni, M. Cavo, A. Pulsoni et al., "Clinical outcome of extramedullary plasmacytoma," *Haematologica*, vol. 85, no. 1, pp. 47–51, 2000.

[8] C. Alexiou, R. J. Kau, H. Dietzfelbinger et al., "Extramedullary plasmacytoma: tumor occurrence and therapeutic concepts," *Cancer*, vol. 85, no. 11, pp. 2305–2314, 1999.

[9] R. Soutar, H. Lucraft, G. Jackson et al., "Guidelines on the diagnosis and management of solitary plasmacytoma of bone and solitary extramedullary plasmacytoma," *British Journal of Haematology*, vol. 124, no. 6, pp. 717–726, 2004.

[10] R. A. Kyle, J. A. Child, K. Anderson et al., "Criteria for the classification of monoclonal gammopathies, multiple myeloma and related disorders: a report of the International Myeloma Working Group," *British Journal of Haematology*, vol. 121, no. 5, pp. 749–757, 2003.

[11] E. Katodritou, E. Terpos, A. S. Symeonidis et al., "Clinical features, outcome, and prognostic factors for survival and evolution to multiple myeloma of solitary plasmacytomas: a report of the Greek myeloma study group in 97 patients," *American Journal of Hematology*, vol. 89, no. 8, pp. 803–808, 2014.

[12] B. Amini, S. Yellapragada, S. Shah, E. Rohren, and R. Vikram, "State-of-the-art imaging and staging of plasma cell dyscrasias," *Radiologic Clinics of North America*, vol. 54, no. 3, pp. 581–596, 2016.

[13] D. S. Tsang, L. W. Le, V. Kukreti, and A. Sun, "Treatment and outcomes for primary cutaneous extramedullary plasmacytoma: a case series," *Current Oncology*, vol. 23, no. 6, pp. e630–e646, 2016.

[14] T. Skóra, K. Pudełek, J. Nowak-Sadzikowska, M. Pietrasz, B. Szyszka-Charewicz, and J. Jakubowicz, "Effect of definitive radiotherapy on the long-term outcome in patients with solitary extramedullary plasmacytoma," *Hematological Oncology*, 2015.

[15] T. Zimmerer, U. Böcker, F. Wenz, and M. V. Singer, "Medical prevention and treatment of acute and chronic radiation induced enteritis—is there any proven therapy? a short review," *Zeitschrift fur Gastroenterologie*, vol. 46, no. 5, pp. 441–448, 2008.

[16] R. Soutar, H. Lucraft, G. Jackson et al., "Guidelines on the diagnosis and management of solitary plasmacytoma of bone and solitary extramedullary plasmacytoma," *Clinical Oncology*, vol. 16, no. 6, pp. 405–413, 2004.

Malignant Pleural Mesothelioma with Marked Lymphatic Involvement: A Report of Two Autopsy Cases

Reiko Ideguchi,[1] Kazuto Ashizawa,[2] Saori Akashi,[1] Michiko Shindo,[1] Kazunori Minami,[1] Toshio Fukuda,[1] Junji Irie,[3] Minoru Fukuda,[4] and Masataka Uetani[5]

[1] *Department of Radiology, Nagasaki Harbor Medical Center City Hospital, Nagasaki, Japan*
[2] *Department of Clinical Oncology, Nagasaki University Graduate School of Biomedical Sciences, Nagasaki, Japan*
[3] *Department of Pathology, Nagasaki Harbor Medical Center City Hospital, Nagasaki, Japan*
[4] *Department of Internal Medicine, Nagasaki Harbor Medical Center City Hospital, Nagasaki, Japan*
[5] *Department of Radiological Sciences, Nagasaki University Graduate School of Biomedical Sciences, Nagasaki, Japan*

Correspondence should be addressed to Kazuto Ashizawa; ashi@nagasaki-u.ac.jp

Academic Editor: Jeanine M. Buchanich

We herein report two cases of malignant pleural mesothelioma with marked lymphangiosis. The patients included a 68-year-old man and a 67-year-old man who both had a history of exposure to asbestos. Computed tomography (CT) on admission showed pleural effusion with pleural thickening. In both cases, a histopathological examination of the pleura confirmed the diagnosis of epithelioid malignant mesothelioma. They received chemotherapy, but the treatment was only palliative. The chest CT assessments during admission revealed marked pleural effusion and mediastinal lymphadenopathy. CT also showed a consolidative mass with bronchovascular bundle and septal thickening in the lungs suggesting pulmonary parenchymal involvement and the lymphangitic spread of the tumor. These CT findings mimicked lung cancer with pleuritis and lymphangitic carcinomatosis. Autopsy was performed in both cases. Macroscopically, the tumor cells infiltrated the lung with the marked lymphatic spread of the tumor. Microscopy also revealed that the tumor had invaded the pulmonary parenchyma with the marked lymphatic spread of the tumor. Although this growth pattern is unusual, malignant pleural mesothelioma should be considered as the differential diagnosis, especially in patients with pleural lesions.

1. Introduction

Malignant mesothelioma is a rare neoplasm that arises from the pleura or, rarely, the pericardium or peritoneum [1]. The prognosis is poor due to the diffuse nature of the tumor, with the involvement of the surrounding structures and local progression of the disease generally leading to death within 9–17 months after diagnosis [2]. Extrapleural metastases are present at autopsy in 87.7% of cases [3]. Major sites for metastases are regional lymph nodes, lung, adrenal glands, liver, and kidneys.

Lymphatic spread is known to occur as a microscopic phenomenon. Nind et al. reported that lymphatic spread was seen in 27 cases (13.5%) among a series of 200 patients with malignant pleural mesothelioma pathologically [4], while lymphatic spread is rare even in advanced cases clinically. To the best of our knowledge, the bilaterally diffuse lymphatic spread of malignant pleural mesothelioma has been reported as the predominant radiographic finding in at least one case in the last 20 years [5]. We herein report two autopsy cases of treated pleural mesothelioma in which marked lymphatic involvement was identified based on the radiologic-pathologic correlation.

2. Case Presentation

2.1. Clinical Summary

2.1.1. Case 1. A 67-year-old male patient presented to us with a history of pleural effusion. He had a medical history of hypertension, cardiac arrhythmia, and acute hepatitis.

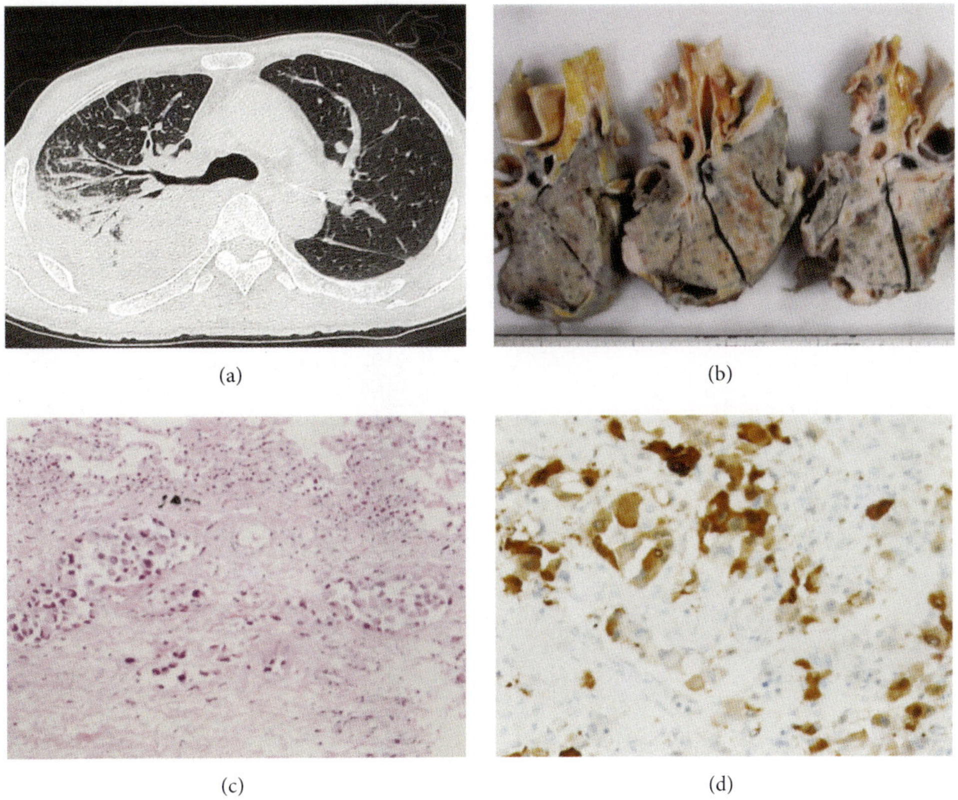

FIGURE 1: (a) An axial high-resolution chest CT scan showed extensive bronchovascular bundle and septal thickening and a consolidative mass in the upper lobe of the right lung; these findings are consistent with the lymphangitic spread of the tumor. (b) The gross pathological findings of the lung and pleura at autopsy showing multiple pleural nodules and masses on the pleural surface. The lung parenchyma is encased by tumor growth and the lymphatic spread of the tumor is observed. (c) Light microscopy of the resected pleural tumor. The lesion was histologically diagnosed as epithelioid-type malignant pleural mesothelioma. The marked invasion of the lymphatic vessel by tumor cells was observed (hematoxylin and eosin staining, ×100). (d) On immunohistochemical staining, the tumor cells were positive for calretinin, a mesothelial cell marker.

Prior to being referred to our institution for further treatment, he had been evaluated at another institute. A presumptive diagnosis of lung adenocarcinoma was made and he was treated with chemotherapy. A computed tomography (CT) scan showed right-sided pleural effusion with pleural thickening. Biopsies of the pericardium and pleura were performed, and the patient was diagnosed with epithelioid malignant mesothelioma. The patient had been regularly exposed to asbestos during 10 years of employment as a seaman. Because the patient did not wish to undergo surgery, he subsequently received three cycles of chemotherapy including cisplatinum and pemetrexed. Two cycles of chemotherapy with pemetrexed and carboplatin were administered; however, his condition did not improve.

A CT scan showed marked right pleural effusion and mediastinal lymphadenopathy in addition to a consolidative mass of the upper lobe with bronchovascular bundle and septal thickening, suggesting lung parenchymal involvement and the lymphangitic spread of the tumor (Figure 1(a)). The bilateral pleural effusion increased in volume, and the patient ultimately died of respiratory failure at 16 months after the diagnosis.

2.1.2. Case 2. A 68-year-old male presented with a cough and dyspnea approximately 4 months prior to his admission. She had no significant past medical history. A cytological examination performed in another institute suggested malignant pleural mesothelioma or adenocarcinoma. He was referred to our institution for further treatment. A CT scan showed left-sided pleural effusion and pleural thickening, some of which contained calcification. A histopathological examination of the pleura confirmed the diagnosis of epithelioid malignant mesothelioma. The patient had been regularly exposed to asbestos during 25 years of employment as a seaman.

A CT scan performed after four cycles of chemotherapy with the combination of cisplatinum and pemetrexed revealed left-sided pleural effusion, a consolidative mass with bronchovascular bundle, and septal thickening, suggesting lung parenchymal involvement and the lymphatic spread of the tumor (Figures 2(a) and 2(b)). Metastasis to the mediastinal lymph nodes with peritoneal metastasis and ascites were also present (Figure 2(b)). The patient ultimately died of respiratory failure at 18 months after the diagnosis.

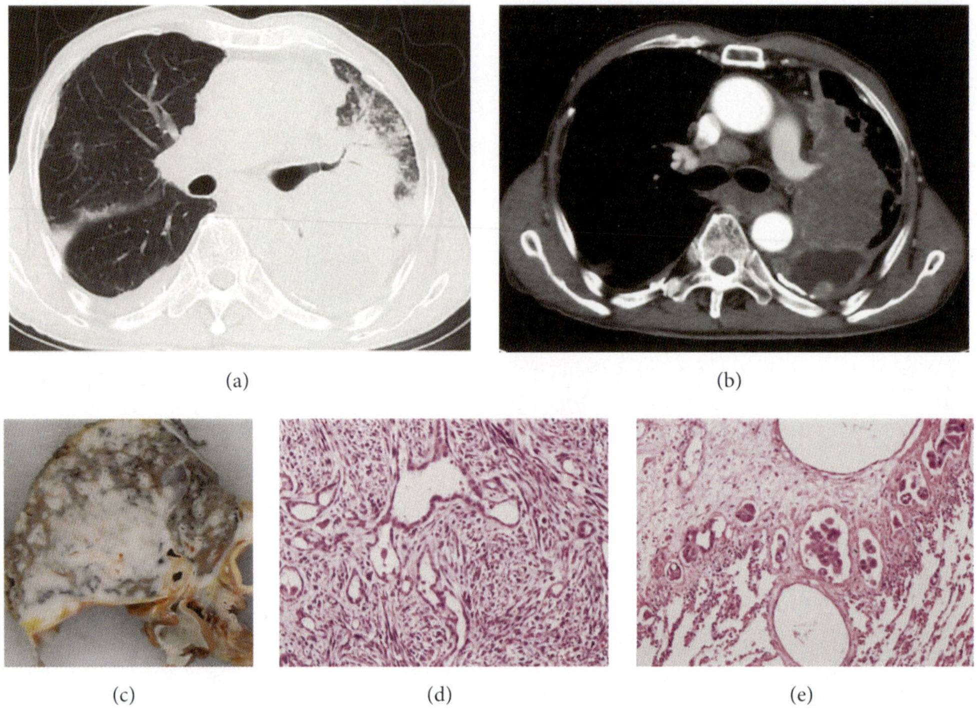

FIGURE 2: (a) An axial chest CT scan showed extensive bronchovascular bundle and septal thickening, an upper lobe consolidative mass, and perilymphatic nodules in the left lung; these findings are consistent with the lymphangitic spread of the tumor. (b) A contrast-enhanced chest CT scan showing a left upper lobe consolidative mass, left-sided pleural effusion, and pleural thickening with mediastinal lymph node swelling. (c) The gross pathological findings of the lung and pleura at autopsy. The lung parenchyma is encased by tumor growth and the lymphatic spread of the tumor is observed. (d) A low-power magnification view of the pleural tumor. The tumor is composed of epithelioid and spindle cells (hematoxylin and eosin staining, ×100). (e) Low-power magnification of the pleural tumor. The lesion was histologically diagnosed as biphasic-type malignant pleural mesothelioma. The photomicrograph shows invasion of the lymphatic channels by the tumor (hematoxylin and eosin staining, ×100).

2.2. Pathological Findings

2.2.1. Case 1. At autopsy, the right whole lung showed severe adhesion to the right pleural cavity. The right parietal and visceral pleura had thickened and surrounded the right lung. The tumor was found to be primarily located in the right pleura invading the pulmonary parenchyma (Figure 1(b)). On the cut surface, the tumor was white in color and solid and firm in consistency. The tumor also invaded the peritoneal cavity, diaphragm, and trachea. Microscopically, the tumor cells showed a glandular pattern and were suggestive of malignant epithelioid mesothelioma. The tumor cells were epithelioid cells with eosinophilic cytoplasm infiltrating the pulmonary parenchyma with the lymphatic spread of the tumor (Figure 1(c)). An immunohistochemical examination was positive for calretinin and D2-40 and negative for TTF-1, SP-A, Ber-EP4, and carcinoembryonic antigen (CEA) (Figure 1(d)). Immunohistochemical markers are used to differentiate malignant mesothelioma from adenocarcinoma. Epithelioid-type malignant mesothelioma is positive for calretinin and D2-40 and negative for the TTF-1, SP-A, Ber-EP4, and CEA. Thus, the definite diagnosis was epithelioid-type malignant pleural mesothelioma.

2.2.2. Case 2. At autopsy, the whole left lung showed severe adhesion to the left pleural cavity. The left parietal and visceral pleura had thickened and surrounded the left lung. The properties of the cut surface were similar to case 1. The tumor was found to be primarily located in the left pleura invading the lung parenchyma (Figure 2(c)). The tumor spread across the mediastinum and involved the opposite pleural cavity. The penetration of the diaphragm was also observed. Microscopically, the tumor cells were a biphasic lesion of malignant pleural mesothelioma (Figure 2(d)) and invaded the pulmonary parenchyma with the marked lymphatic spread of the tumor (Figure 2(e)). Immunohistochemically, the epithelioid tumor cells were positive for calretinin and D2-40 and AE1/AE3 and negative for TTF-1, Napsin A, Ber-EP4, and CEA. The spindle-shaped cells were also similar. Thus, the definite diagnosis was biphasic-type malignant pleural mesothelioma.

3. Discussion

Malignant mesothelioma is a rare neoplasm that arises from the pleura or, rarely, the pericardium or peritoneum. Microscopically, malignant mesothelioma is classified into

3 histologic subtypes that determine prognosis and therapy. These subtypes are epithelial, sarcomatoid, and mixed or biphasic. Malignant pleural mesothelioma, unlike lung cancer, progresses in a locally aggressive manner via invasion into the chest wall, mediastinum, and diaphragm. In the largest postmortem case series of patients with malignant plural mesothelioma, extrapleural dissemination was seen in 87.7% and extrathoracic metastasis in 55.4% [3]. Major sites for metastases are regional lymph nodes, lung, adrenal glands, liver, and kidneys.

Previous studies have reported that lymph node metastasis was significantly more common in epithelial and biphasic containing tumors than in sarcomatoid mesotheliomas. The rate of any extrapleural spread was high across all tumor types, with no statistically significant differences [3]. Lymphatic spread may occur in advanced cases of malignant pleural mesothelioma, such as the present cases, and has been well documented in histopathological studies. Nind et al. showed that the patterns of pulmonary parenchymal growth of malignant pleural mesothelioma were directly subpleural, lymphangitic, and other [4]. They described the histological patterns of lung parenchymal involvement with diffuse pleural mesothelioma. The lymphangitic involvement of the lung parenchyma was seen in 27 cases among a series of 200 cases of malignant pleural mesothelioma, including 16 epithelioid lesions, 3 biphasic lesions, and 8 sarcomatoid lesions. Our cases included 1 epithelioid type and 1 biphasic type.

Kadota et al. [6] correlated the histologic subtypes of epithelioid diffuse malignant pleural mesothelioma with the clinicopathological features. Five histological subtypes (tubulopapillary, trabecular, solid, micropapillary, and pleomorphic) were evaluated, and lymphatic invasion, which was detected in 44% of cases, was associated with the micropapillary (95%) and pleomorphic (68%) subtypes.

Although malignant lymphangiosis is known to occur as a microscopic phenomenon, as mentioned above, mesothelioma presenting as malignant lymphangiosis with a clear clinical and radiological picture is rare. To the best of our knowledge, the diffuse lymphatic spread of malignant pleural mesothelioma has been previously reported as the predominant radiographic finding in at least one case in the last 20 years [5]. Edde et al. [5] demonstrated a case of right pleural mesothelioma in which neoadjuvant chemotherapy was administered prior to right extrapleural pneumonectomy followed by adjuvant chemotherapy. After 21 months, CT showed diffuse parenchymal infiltration and lymphangitic spread over the contralateral lung. Similarly to our cases, this case resulted in a quick progression to respiratory failure and death.

Kim et al. analyzed multidetector CT images of 103 patients with malignant pleural mesothelioma and 24 patients with metastatic pleural disease from extrathoracic malignancy. They reported lymphangitic metastases were observed in 6 patients (5.8%) of the malignant pleural mesothelioma and 2 patients (8.3%) of the metastatic pleural disease [7]. In this way, the frequency of lymphatic involvement in malignant pleural mesothelioma differs between the histopathology and radiology.

In the present cases, CT showed a consolidative mass with bronchovascular bundle and septal thickening, mimicking lung cancer with lymphangitic carcinomatosis. The features of lymphangitic carcinomatosis are infiltration of cancer cells and interstitial edema in and around lymphatic vessels caused by lymph node metastasis in the lung. The metastatic cancer in the mediastinal and hilar lymph nodes may obstruct lymphatic drainage, resulting in retrograde spread of tumor into terminal lung tissues via lymphatic vessels. In addition, tumor microemboli may form in the terminal vessels of the lung due to hematogenous metastasis, which can invade the interstitium surrounding lymphatic vessels [8].

According to the TNM classification, ipsilateral parietal pleura is involved in early stage and later visceral pleura is involved [9]. The lymphatic drainage system of the pleura is complex and is important in the assessment of the spread of malignant mesothelioma. The visceral pleura drains to the same nodal groups as the lung parenchyma: bronchopulmonary, hilar, mediastinal, supraclavicular, and scalene. However, the parietal pleura has a different drainage into internal mammary, cardiophrenic, extrapleural, and intercostal nodes [10, 11].

Kadota et al. showed that lymphatic invasion showed a strong association with lymph node metastasis and an increased risk of death [6]. In the present cases, metastasis to the mediastinal lymph nodes was also present. The two cases were similar in that both patients had advanced-stage disease. In both cases, the pathological findings also showed the involvement of the lung parenchyma with the marked lymphatic spread of the tumor. We should keep this growth pattern in mind when treating patients with advanced-stage malignant pleural mesothelioma.

In conclusion, we reported two cases of malignant pleural mesothelioma with marked lung parenchymal and lymphatic involvement of the tumor. Although this growth pattern is unusual, malignant pleural mesothelioma should be considered as the differential diagnosis, especially in patients with pleural lesions.

Disclosure

Reiko Ideguchi present address is Department of Radioisotope Medicine, Atomic Bomb Disease and Hibakusha Medicine Unit, Atomic Bomb Disease Institute, Nagasaki University Graduate School of Biomedical Sciences. Saori Akashi present address is Department of Radiology, Sasebo City General Hospital, Sasebo, Nagasaki, Japan. Michiko Shindo present address is Department of Radiology, Omura City Municipal Hospital, Omura, Nagasaki, Japan. Minoru Fukuda present address is Clinical Oncology Center, Nagasaki University Hospital, Nagasaki, Japan.

References

[1] Z. J. Wang, G. P. Reddy, M. B. Gotway et al., "Malignant pleural mesothelioma: evaluation with CT, MR imaging, and PET," *Radiographics*, vol. 24, no. 1, pp. 105–119, 2004.

[2] A. S. Tsao, I. Wistuba, J. A. Roth, and H. L. Kindler, "Malignant pleural mesothelioma," *Journal of Clinical Oncology*, vol. 27, no. 12, pp. 2081–2090, 2009.

[3] R. S. Finn, F. J. H. Brims, A. Gandhi et al., "Postmortem findings of malignant pleural mesothelioma: A two-center study of 318 patients," *Chest*, vol. 142, no. 5, pp. 1267–1273, 2012.

[4] N. R. Nind, R. L. Attanoos, and A. R. Gibbs, "Unusual intraparenchymal growth patterns of malignant pleural mesothelioma," *Histopathology*, vol. 42, no. 2, pp. 150–155, 2003.

[5] P. Edde, N. Romy, and C. Mirna, "Pulmonary lymphangitic mesotheliomatosis," *Journal of Pulmonary & Respiratory Medicine*, vol. 3, article 136, 2013.

[6] K. Kadota, K. Suzuki, C. S. Sima, V. W. Rusch, P. S. Adusumilli, and W. D. Travis, "Pleomorphic epithelioid diffuse malignant pleural mesothelioma: a clinicopathological review and conceptual proposal to reclassify as biphasic or sarcomatoid mesothelioma," *Journal of Thoracic Oncology*, vol. 6, no. 5, pp. 896–904, 2011.

[7] Y. K. Kim, J. S. Kim, K. W. Lee, C. A. Yi, J. M. Koo, and S.-H. Jung, "Multidetector CT findings and differential diagnoses of malignant pleural mesothelioma and metastatic pleural diseases in Korea," *Korean Journal of Radiology*, vol. 17, no. 4, pp. 545–553, 2016.

[8] A. Nair, M. J. Klusmann, K. H. Jogeesvaran, S. Grubnic, S. J. Green, and I. Vlahos, "Revisions to the TNM staging of non-small cell Lung Cancer: Rationale, clinicoradiologic implications, and persistent limitations," *Radiographics*, vol. 31, no. 1, 2011.

[9] International Mesothelioma Interest Group, "A proposed new international TNM staging system for malignant pleural mesothelioma," *Chest*, vol. 108, no. 4, pp. 1122–1128, 1995.

[10] E. J. Helm, T. N. Matin, and F. V. Gleeson, "Imaging of the pleura," *Journal of Magnetic Resonance Imaging*, vol. 32, no. 6, pp. 1275–1286, 2010.

[11] M. T. Truong, C. Viswanathan, M. B. C. Godoy, B. W. Carter, and E. M. Marom, "Malignant pleural mesothelioma: Role of CT, MRI, and PET/CT in staging evaluation and treatment considerations," *Seminars in Roentgenology*, vol. 48, no. 4, pp. 323–334, 2013.

Fatal Outcome of Imatinib in a Patient with Idiopathic Hypereosinophilic Syndrome

Ashraf Abugroun, Ahmed Chaudhary, and Gabriel Rodriguez

Advocate Illinois Masonic Medical Center, Chicago, IL, USA

Correspondence should be addressed to Ashraf Abugroun; ashraf.abugroun@advocatehealth.com

Academic Editor: Peter F. Lenehan

Cytokine storm is a poorly explained clinical entity caused by an undesired and aggrandized immune system response leading to unregulated activation of the proinflammatory cascade, often contributing to multisystem organ failure and even death. Its potentially diverse etiologies and sepsis-like presentation have made it even more challenging to diagnose, and so far, no well-established treatment protocol has been proposed. Its association with certain medications, especially with monoclonal antibodies, has well been reported in literature. To the best of our knowledge, so far, no previous case of cytokine storm associated with imatinib has been reported. We herein present a case report of a 77-year-old male with a past medical history of hypereosinophilic syndrome who developed acute fatal cytokine storm following treatment with imatinib. This study highlights a life-threatening complication of the medication that may be underrecognized.

1. Introduction

Imatinib is a tyrosine kinase inhibitor that is used in various hematologic malignancies, including idiopathic hypereosinophilic syndrome (IHES) which is a myeloproliferative disorder characterized by sustained, nonreactive, unexplained persistent hypereosinophilia that commonly results in multiorgan dysfunction. This case highlights the development of a cytokine storm with severe uncontrolled systemic inflammatory response with a fatal outcome following the initiation of imatinib in a patient with IHES.

2. Case Presentation

A 77-year-old male with a history of IHES, COPD, CKD stage III, and active *Mycobacterium avium* complex (MAC) infection on treatment with rifampin, azithromycin, and levofloxacin was sent to the ER from oncology clinic for evaluation of progressive weakness, lethargy, and hyperkalemia.

The patient had outpatient workup for unexplained hypereosinophilia. He underwent lymph node biopsy which showed no evidence of lymphoma (Figure 1). Peripheral blood flow cytometry showed myeloid and lymphoid cells with unremarkable immunophenotypic expression. Bone marrow biopsy showed eosinophilia that varied from approximately 25% in the aspirate smears to 60% in the core biopsy (Figure 2). The infiltrate of eosinophils consisted of eosinophilic myelocytes and mature eosinophils. There were no increase in blasts and no morphologic evidence of lymphoma. The patient had negative fluorescence in situ hybridization (FISH) results using a panel for hypereosinophilia containing probes for 4q12 (SCFD2, LNX, and PDGFRA) rearrangement, 5q32 (PDGFRB) rearrangement, 8p11.2 (FGFR1) rearrangement, and 9q34 and 22q11.2 (BCR/ABL1) rearrangement on a bone marrow specimen. He had normal cytogenetic studies and male-type karyotype. A final diagnosis of idiopathic hypereosinophilic syndrome was made. His disease was resistant to steroids and brief course of chemotherapy with methotrexate.

On his current admission, he was lethargic and cachectic. Vital signs were normal. Skin examination showed widespread erythroderma, scaling, and excoriations. Initial laboratory workup revealed potassium 6.9 mmol/L, creatinine

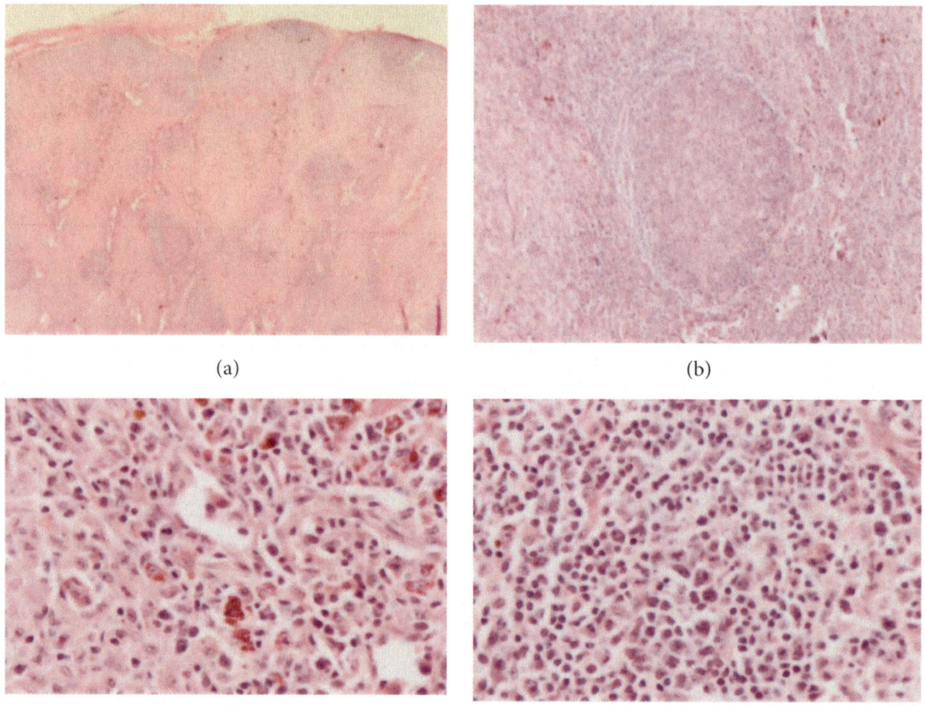

FIGURE 1: Lymph node biopsy. H&E stain. Low-power view (a). Paracortical (T-zone) hyperplasia (b). At higher magnification (c, d), this zone contains interdigitating dendritic cells, Langerhans cells, and melanin-containing histiocytes. There are also scattered immunoblasts in the paracortex of unknown significance.

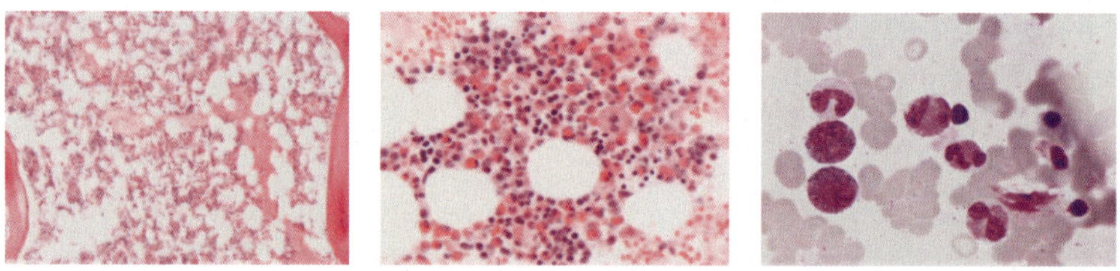

FIGURE 2: The bone marrow shows eosinophilia. Low-power H&E of the core (a), a high-power H&E from the clot section (b), and an oil immersion image from the aspirate (Giemsa stain) (c).

1.3 mg/dL, alkaline phosphatase 671 unit/L, and WBC 18,000 cells/mcL with 58% eosinophils. Hyperkalemia resolved on the third day of admission. Subsequently, a decision was made to start imatinib at a lower than recommended dose due to the high risk of developing tumor lysis syndrome. Shortly after initiation of imatinib, the patient developed acute restlessness, agitation, shortness of breath, and acute urinary retention. His condition rapidly deteriorated and progressed to acute respiratory failure requiring intubation and mechanical ventilation. He also developed distributive shock with hypothermia and non-anion gap metabolic acidosis. Absolute eosinophil count dropped dramatically from 9,500 cells/mcL to 0 cells/mcL within less than 24 hours following administration of imatinib (Figure 3). Given the dramatic decline in clinical condition, imatinib was immediately discontinued, and the patient was treated empirically with methylprednisolone and broad-spectrum antibiotics. The patient had normal echocardiogram and brain CT scan. On the next day, chest X-ray showed patchy airspace infiltrates in the left lower lobe suggestive of pneumonia (Figure 4). Blood cultures showed no microbial growth, and respiratory culture eventually grew multidrug-resistant organisms (MDROs) *Klebsiella pneumoniae* and moderate *Pseudomonas aeruginosa*. A CT abdomen and pelvis showed prominent bowel loops with wall thickening, suggestive of bowel ischemia (Figure 5). The patient condition dramatically declined and died following acute cardiac arrest on the sixth day of admission.

3. Discussion

According to the World Health Organization (WHO) classification, hypereosinophilic syndrome (HES) is classified into three distinct subsets caused by different

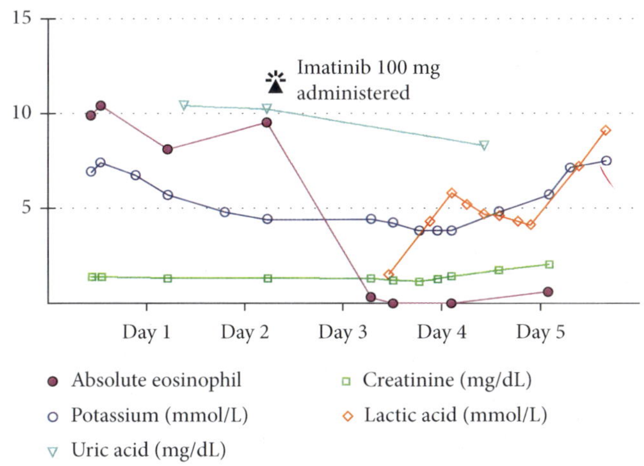

FIGURE 3: Timeline summarizes the laboratory changes on daily follow-up throughout admission. Rapid decline of eosinophil count from 9,500/mcl to zero levels within less than 24 hours from administration of imatinib is noted. Uric acid level slightly declined and potassium level remained stable except for the last day during which it raised progressively to the level of 7.5 mmol/L.

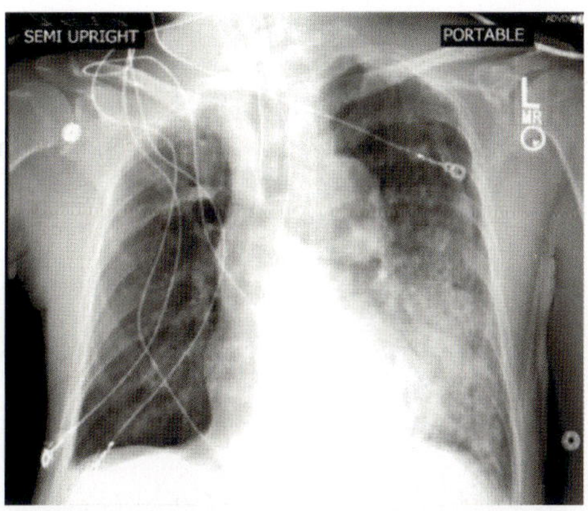

FIGURE 4: Chest X-ray showed patchy airspace infiltrates in the left lower lobe suggestive of pneumonia.

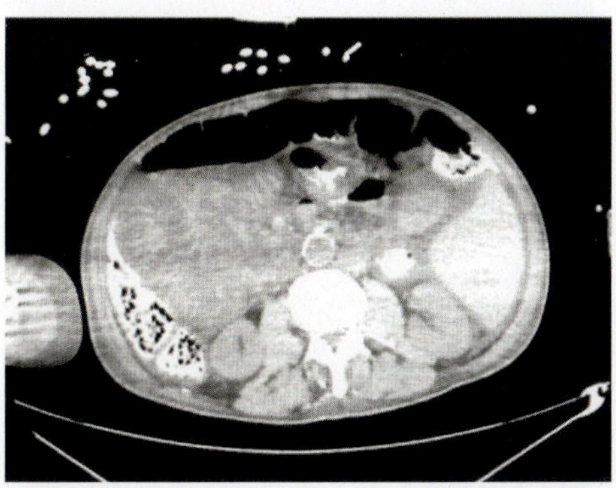

FIGURE 5: CT abdomen and pelvis showed prominent bowel loops with wall thickening, suggestive of bowel ischemia.

pathogenic mechanisms including chronic eosinophilic leukemia caused by fusion protein (FIP1L1-PDGFRA) with tyrosine kinase activities, lymphoproliferative HES caused by clonal IL-5/Th2 lymphocyte-mediated hypereosinophilia, and idiopathic or myeloproliferative HES where no evidence of clonal hypereosinophilia is identified [1]. Patients with HES present with variable clinical manifestations related to the target organ involved by eosinophils. Although all body parts can be involved, the disease commonly involves the skin, heart, digestive tract, and nervous system [1]. The pathogenesis of HES is related to various molecular and cytogenetic abnormalities that ultimately result in overactivity of tyrosine kinase causing dysregulated clonal overproduction of eosinophils [2].

The goal of therapy in HES is to prevent eosinophil-induced progressive end-organ damage and irreversible complications of sustained hypereosinophilia. Available therapeutic options include corticosteroids, hydroxyurea, interferon-alpha, bone marrow transplant, and other cytotoxic and immunomodulatory agents [1, 3]. Due to low incidence of HES and increased heterogeneity of presenting symptoms, there are paucity of available data and limited numbers of studies on treatment options. Most studies on treatment are restricted to case reports and case series. The tyrosine kinase inhibitor imatinib was recently proposed as a rescue medication with high response rate among patients with HES refractory to medical therapy [4]. Imatinib was found to be particularly useful among patients with positive (FIP1L1-PDGFRA) phenotypes. In few cases, some reported therapeutic effect with the use of imatinib in idiopathic HES with negative (FIP1L1-PDGFRA) phenotypes [5–9]. The mechanism of action through which imatinib achieved success in these patients remains unknown [9].

Cytokine storm syndrome refers to massive release of cytokines from an undesired activation of the immune system by various factors that lead to uncontrolled systemic inflammatory response causing multiple organ dysfunction and often death. Cytokines are glycoproteins that are produced by leukocytes. They may have autocrine, paracrine, and endocrine actions, which explains both local and systemic response seen in cytokine storm. Under normal circumstances, cytokine causes monitored release of proinflammatory mediators, which not only helps the body mount response to any threat but also prevents any further injury to local tissue and helps in the process of healing. Contrarily, in cytokine storm, unregulated and robust activation of proinflammatory mediators aggrandized immune cellular lineages with enhanced activity, resulting in the unregulated cascade of acute inflammatory response. This all contributes to endothelial cell dysfunction that leads to increased capillary permeability/leak, which has been postulated as a mechanism for parenchymal injury and end-organ damage. As expected, organs susceptible to the worst injuries are the ones with stronger immune defense mechanisms, notably the lungs and gut [10].

Cytokine storm has been attributed to certain medications and treatments. Of note, monoclonal antibodies have long been associated with cytokine storm. In 2006, the first human clinical trial of TGN1412 monoclonal antibody to treat rheumatologic disease was conducted, and it was proposed that all 6 volunteers participated had fatal outcome from TGN1412-induced cytokine storm [11]. Alemtuzumab, another monoclonal antibody used in treatment of chronic lymphocytic leukemia, has been well known to be associated with cytokine release [12]. Unfortunately, no clear guidelines are available on how to approach cytokine storm. The primary goal of suggested treatments is to prevent end-organ damage and multiorgan failure through adequate resuscitative measure, use of broad-spectrum antibiotics, fluid resuscitation, and vasopressors if indicated. Anti-inflammatory medications including steroids and nonsteroidal medications have also been proposed but have been shown to have limited benefit/efficacy.

Imatinib, a monoclonal antibody, which acts as a tyrosine kinase inhibitor is FDA approved for treatment of hematological malignancies. It is considered to be a safe and effective drug and is on the WHO's list of essential medicines. Imatinib has well tolerability with a low incidence of toxicities [13]. Common side effects reported include nausea, diarrhea, visual disturbance, itchy rash, fluid retention, weight gain, and pancytopenia. On rare instances, some of the adverse effects reported with the use of imatinib include tumor lysis syndrome, hepatotoxicity, dermatological manifestations, left ventricular dysfunction, and cardiogenic shock [14–16]. Unexpectedly, our patient developed acute distributive shock and multiorgan failure immediately following the first dose of imatinib. The pathogenesis of such acute clinical decline is explained by the massive histamine release and cytokine storm, and this hypothesis is evident by the temporal relation between the initiation of imatinib therapy and the dramatic decline of eosinophilic count to zero within hours of therapy. The clinical presentation and laboratory data did not support a diagnosis of tumor lysis syndrome. His uric acid level dropped from the initial level of 10.4 gm/dl to 8.3 gm/dl following imatinib administration. Unfortunately, further laboratory tests including the level of plasma interleukins which could have further supported the diagnosis of cytokine storm were not performed.

Given the nonspecific presentation of cytokine storm, possibility of coexisting septicemia cannot be ruled; although the patient had left lower lobe infiltrates and positive respiratory cultures, it is worth mentioning that prior to imatinib administration, there was no clinical or radiological suspicion of the acute infectious process. Moreover, the patient had two blood cultures taken following the onset of distributive shock, and both did not show any bacterial growth. Though negative blood cultures cannot rule out septicemia as a cause of death, the timeline of events and the clinical, laboratory, and radiological findings that developed as a consequence of initiation of imatinib therapy pointed towards a massive cytokine storm (Figure 3).

4. Conclusion

In this case, imatinib caused severe acute distributive shock and multiorgan failure secondary to massive histamine release and cytokine storm evident by the temporal relation with initiation of therapy and dramatic decline of eosinophilic count to zero. Such an observation has not been documented in the past. This study highlights a life-threatening complication of the medication that may be underrecognized. HES remains a therapeutic challenge. The choice of therapy for HES should be carefully guided based on the balance between therapeutic benefit and potential for side effects. More research on safety of use of imatinib on a wide scale of patients with HES is needed.

References

[1] E. Cogan and F. Roufosse, "Clinical management of the hypereosinophilic syndromes," *Expert Review of Hematology*, vol. 5, no. 3, pp. 275–289, 2012.

[2] A. M. S. Müller, U. M. Martens, S. C. Hofmann, L. Bruckner-Tuderman, R. Mertelsmann, and M. Lübbert, "Imatinib mesylate as a novel treatment option for hypereosinophilic syndrome: two case reports and a comprehensive review of the literature," *Annals of Hematology*, vol. 85, no. 1, pp. 1–16, 2006.

[3] S. A. Antoniu, "Novel therapies for hypereosinophilic syndromes," *Netherlands Journal of Medicine*, vol. 68, no. 1, pp. 304–310, 2010.

[4] J. L. Schaller and G. A. Burkland, "Case report: rapid and complete control of idiopathic hypereosinophilia with imatinib mesylate," *Medscape General Medicine*, vol. 3, no. 5, p. 9, 2001.

[5] P. Ault, J. Cortes, C. Koller, E. S. Kaled, and H. Kantarjian, "Response of idiopathic hypereosinophilic syndrome to treatment with imatinib mesylate," *Leukemia Research*, vol. 26, no. 9, pp. 881–884, 2002.

[6] D. Wolf, G. Gastl, and H. Rumpold, "Complete remission of an idiopathic hypereosinophilic syndrome while using imatinib," *Deutsche Medizinische Wochenschrift*, vol. 129, no. 40, pp. 2104–2106, 2004.

[7] Z. Salem, P. A. Zalloua, A. Chehal et al., "Effective treatment of hypereosinophilic syndrome with imatinib mesylate," *Hematology Journal*, vol. 4, no. 6, pp. 410–412, 2003.

[8] G. Anghel, L. De Rosa, C. Ruscio et al., "Efficacy of imatinib mesylate in a patient with idiopathic hypereosinophilic syndrome and severe heart involvement," *Tumori*, vol. 91, no. 1, pp. 67–70, 2005.

[9] J. Cortes, P. Ault, C. Koller et al., "Efficacy of imatinib mesylate in the treatment of idiopathic hypereosinophilic syndrome," *Blood*, vol. 101, no. 12, pp. 4714–4716, 2003.

[10] S. W. Canna and E. M. Behrens, "Making sense of the cytokine storm: a conceptual framework for understanding, diagnosing and treating hemophagocytic syndromes," *Pediatric Clinics of North America*, vol. 59, no. 2, pp. 329–344, 2012.

[11] G. Suntharalingam, M. R. Perry, S. Ward et al., "Cytokine storm in a phase 1 trial of the anti-CD28 monoclonal antibody TGN1412," *New England Journal of Medicine*, vol. 355, no. 10, pp. 1018–1028, 2006.

[12] T. T. Hansel, H. Kropshofer, T. Singer, J. A. Mitchell, and A. J. T. George, "The safety and side effects of monoclonal antibodies," *Nature Reviews Drug Discovery*, vol. 9, no. 4, pp. 325–338, 2010.

[13] G. Metzgeroth, C. Walz, P. Erben et al., "Safety and efficacy of imatinib in chronic eosinophilic leukaemia and hypereosinophilic syndrome–a phase-II study," *British Journal of Haematology*, vol. 143, no. 5, pp. 707–715, 2008.

[14] A. Garcia-Alvarez, M. Sitges, X. Garcia-Albeniz, A. Sionis, P. Loma-Osorio, and X. Bosch, "Atypical cardiac manifestation

of hypereosinophilic syndrome and reversible cardiotoxicity to imatinib," *International Journal of Cardiology*, vol. 139, no. 2, pp. e29–e31, 2010.

[15] E. Ridruejo, R. Cacchione, A. G. Villamil, S. Marciano, A. C. Gadano, and O. G. Mandó, "Imatinib-induced fatal acute liver failure," *World Journal of Gastroenterology*, vol. 13, no. 48, pp. 6608–6111, 2007.

[16] E. Bois, L. M. Holle, and U. Farooq, "Late onset imatinib-induced Stevens-Johnson syndrome," *Journal of Oncology Pharmacy Practice*, vol. 20, no. 6, pp. 476–478, 2014.

An Extremely Rapid Case of Pneumonitis with the Use of Nivolumab for Pancreatic Adenocarcinoma

Rubens Barros Costa,[1,2] Al Benson,[2] Vahid Yaghmai,[3] Ricardo L. B. Costa,[4] Haijun Zhou,[5] Amir Behdad,[5] Jason B. Kaplan,[1,2] Maureen Sadim,[1,2] Sarah Talamantes,[6] and Aparna Kalyan[1,2]

[1]*Developmental Therapeutics Program, Feinberg School of Medicine and Robert H. Lurie Comprehensive Cancer Center of Northwestern University, 233 East Superior Street, Chicago, IL 60611, USA*
[2]*Division of Hematology and Oncology, Robert H. Lurie Comprehensive Cancer Center, Northwestern University, 676 North Clair Street, Chicago, IL 60611, USA*
[3]*Department of Radiology, Northwestern University Feinberg School of Medicine, 676 North Saint Clair Street, Chicago, IL 60611, USA*
[4]*Department of Breast Oncology, Lee Moffitt Cancer Center, Moffitt McKinley Outpatient Center, 10920 North McKinley Drive, BR-Program, Tampa, FL 33612, USA*
[5]*Department of Pathology, Northwestern University Feinberg School of Medicine, 251 East Huron Street, Chicago, IL 60611, USA*
[6]*Northwestern University Feinberg School of Medicine, 420 East Superior Street, Chicago, IL 60611, USA*

Correspondence should be addressed to Rubens Barros Costa; barros4@yahoo.com

Academic Editor: Katsuhiro Tanaka

Pancreatic cancer is the fourth most common cancer death in the United States despite comprising a small percentage of the total number of cancer cases. The estimated 5-year overall survival (OS) for patients with distant metastatic disease is approximately 3%. New treatment options are an unmet need and remain an area of active investigation. A 53-year-old male with metastatic pancreatic cancer presented to the hospital with acute-on-chronic respiratory failure approximately 24 hours after receiving a novel therapeutic combination. Chest imaging showed marked changes as concerning for pneumonitis. Infectious workup was negative. The patient had initial clinical improvement after receiving initial intravenous steroids and oxygen support but eventually deteriorated later opting for supportive measures only. With infection ruled out, drug-induced pneumonitis was felt to be the likely cause of the radiologic and clinical changes. The rapidity of onset of symptoms is the aspect being highlighted in this case.

1. Introduction

Pancreatic cancer is the fourth leading cause of cancer death in the United States and is expected to become the second leading cause of cancer death by 2020. It is estimated that approximately 53,670 patients will be diagnosed and 43,090 will die of pancreatic cancer in 2017. The estimated 5-year overall survival (OS) for patients with distant metastatic disease is approximately 3% [1].

Gemcitabine has historically been the backbone in the treatment of metastatic pancreatic cancer. In a randomized phase 3 clinical trial, gemcitabine was compared to 5-fluorouracil (5-FU) for the treatment of previously untreated metastatic pancreatic adenocarcinoma. The median OS and 12-month survival rate were 5.6 months and 18% for patients who received gemcitabine. These results led to FDA approval of gemcitabine for the treatment of metastatic pancreatic cancer in 1996 [2].

In a more recent phase II/III randomized trial, gemcitabine was compared to the combination regimen FOLFIRINOX (fluorouracil, irinotecan, and oxaliplatin). The median OS was 11.1 months for the combination compared

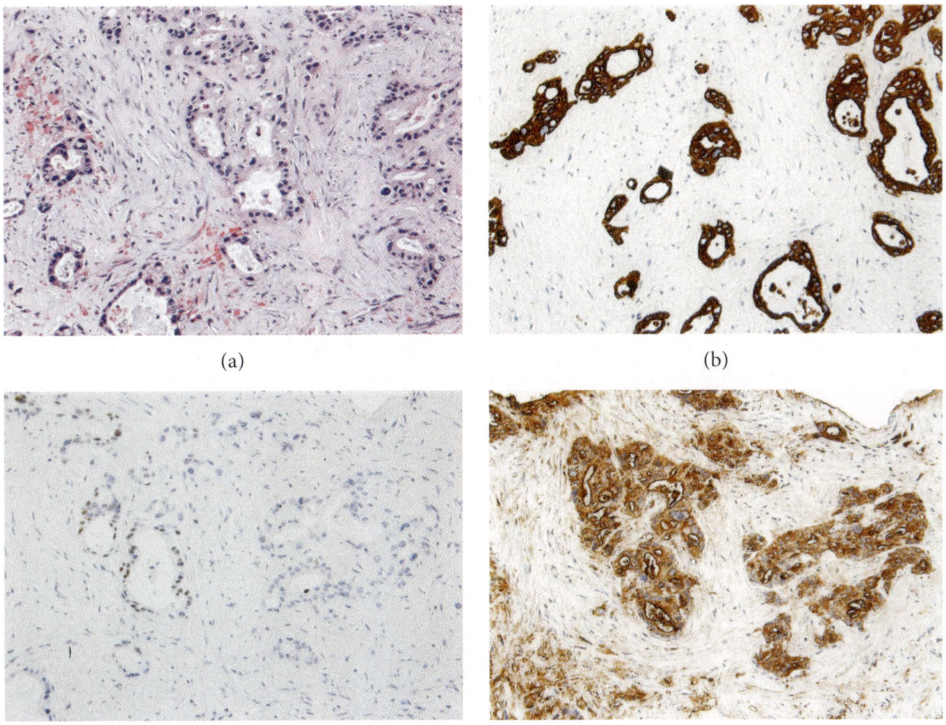

Figure 1: (a) Lung lesion histology (H&E, 200x); (b) cytokeratin-7 immunohistochemical stain; (c) immunohistochemical stain; (d) CA19-9 immunohistochemical stain (200x for all IHC stains).

with 6.8 months with gemcitabine monotherapy. Median progression-free survival (PFS) and objective response rate (RR) favored FOLFIRINOX compared with gemcitabine alone: 6.4 months and 31.6% versus 3.3 months and 9.4%, respectively ($p < 0.001$) [3].

The MPACT gemcitabine was also compared to the combination of gemcitabine and nab-paclitaxel in a large randomized phase III trial. The combination regimen improved RR (23 versus 7%), median PFS (5.5 versus 3.7 months), and OS (8.5 versus 6.7 months) but at the expense of increased toxicity [4].

These two combinations are widely used across the US for the treatment of metastatic/advanced pancreatic adenocarcinoma [5]. Despite representing incremental progress in this field, prognosis remains poor. Therefore, new therapeutic agents and combinations are urgently needed.

Herein, we present a case of fulminant and fatal pneumonitis in a patient who received a novel combination of nivolumab, gemcitabine, and nab-paclitaxel for the treatment of metastatic pancreatic carcinoma.

2. Case Report

The patient was a 53-year-old male with no past medical history who presented to the Emergency Department for evaluation of abdominal pain of one-month duration. His physical examination and vital signs were unremarkable. All his laboratory data were within normal limits.

A contrast-enhanced computed tomography (CT) of the abdomen and pelvis showed multiple pulmonary nodules, a small left pleural effusion, a cystic lesion in tail of the pancreas measuring $4.2 \times 2.7 \times 3.2$ cm, and cystic hepatic lesions. Nonenhanced CT of the chest demonstrated a 4 cm pleural-based lung mass along the anterior medial aspect of the left upper lobe and innumerable indistinct nodular densities in both lungs and hepatic metastases.

A left upper lobe lung fine-needle aspirate and core biopsy revealed a malignant infiltrative proliferation of epithelial cells forming glands, indicating adenocarcinoma. The cells displayed nuclear enlargement, hyperchromasia, marked anisonucleosis, scant eosinophilic cytoplasm, and mitotic activity. The background stroma was fibrotic displaying desmoplasia and areas of necrosis. Immunohistochemical stains were as follows: CK7 positive, CA19-9 positive, CDX2 weakly focal positive, CK20 negative, and TTF1 negative. The cytomorphologic results were consistent with a metastatic process of pancreatic origin (Figure 1). The serum CA19-9 was elevated at 737 U/mL.

He was evaluated by the medical oncology service who recommended treatment with the FOLFIRINOX regimen. Three weeks later, he was seen at our institution for a second opinion and consideration of a clinical trial. After further discussion, he opted to participate in a clinical trial utilizing gemcitabine, nab-paclitaxel, and the antiprogrammed cell death 1 (PD1) inhibitor nivolumab. A repeat CT of the chest, abdomen, and pelvis prior to starting therapy showed worsening bilateral pleural effusions and peritoneal carcinomatosis compared to previous study.

While waiting for treatment initiation, he developed severe and rapid onset dyspnea which brought him in to the

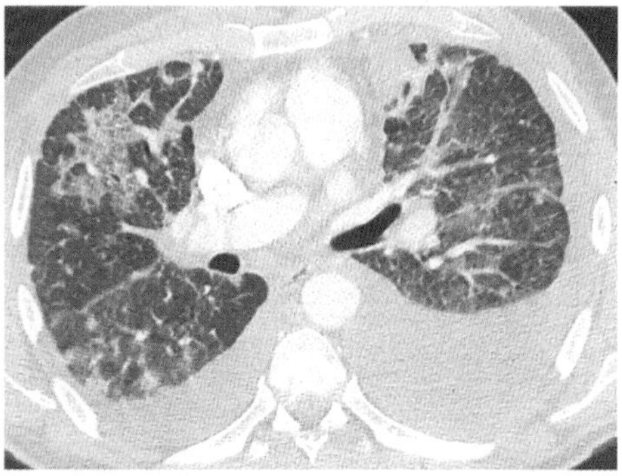

Figure 2: Chest CT showing scattered ground glass opacities and bilateral pleural effusions.

Emergency Department. An enhanced CT of the chest showed no evidence of acute pulmonary embolism, but innumerable soft tissue masses throughout both lungs with accompanying interlobular septal thickening were noted suggesting the possibility of lymphangitic spread. Bilateral pleural effusions with overlying atelectasis compared to the previous study. Axillary and mediastinal lymphadenopathy and hepatic metastases were unchanged from 10 days priorly (Figure 2). He was admitted to our hospital for further management and evaluation. He was empirically treated with antimicrobials to cover for a possible pneumonia. All infectious workup including blood cultures, *Streptococcus* antigen, and legionella testing were negative. Due to the size of the effusion, a left-sided thoracentesis was performed. The pleural fluid showed vacuolated tumor cells with hyperchromatic irregular nuclei with anisonucleosis and prominent nucleoli consistent with adenocarcinoma (Figure 3). On cell count, numerous lymphocytes were noted. An infectious workup of the pleural fluid, including gram stain and cultures, was negative. While hospitalized, it was decided that he should start on treatment promptly, as his clinical deterioration was likely due to disease progression.

He was discharged from the hospital to receive his first treatment with gemcitabine, nab-paclitaxel, and nivolumab as an outpatient. On that day, his transaminase and bilirubin levels were within normal range. Alkaline phosphatase was slightly elevated, and the serum albumin was slightly decreased. The white blood cell count was 20.1K/μL (upper limit of normal 10.5K/μL). CA19-9 was 4537 U/mL. Treatment was started as planned.

Approximately eighteen hours after receiving his therapy, he woke up from sleep with increased dyspnea which prompted a visit to the ED. He was found to be hypoxemic with oxygen saturation around 80%. He was placed on BIPAP and transferred to the intensive care unit for further management. A CT angiogram of the chest revealed no pulmonary embolism at the lobar pulmonary artery branch level. There were progressive extensive ground glass opacities and interlobular septal thickening throughout the lungs compared to the previous study performed just four days priorly. There was a focal new airspace opacity in the posterior right upper lobe. The size of the pleural effusion was decreased on the left and stable on the right. There was no change in the extensive thoracic and abdominal metastatic lymphadenopathy (Figure 4). He was empirically treated with methylprednisolone and piperacillin/tazobactam for possible pneumonitis and infection. The steroids were continued throughout his hospital stay. On admission to the ICU, his labs were as follows: sodium 130 mEq/L (upper limit of normal (ULN) 135 mEq/L), potassium 5.6 mEq/L (ULN 5 mEq/L), creatinine 1.5 mg/dl (ULN 1.3 mg/dl), AST 3534 U/L (ULN 39 U/L), ALT 3206 U/L (ULN 52 U/L), total bilirubin within normal limits, INR 1.7, and WBC 21.9 (ULN 3.5K/μL). A panel for respiratory viruses including influenza types A and B, RSV types A and B, parainfluenza types 1, 2, and 3, rhinovirus, metapneumovirus, and adenovirus types B, C, and E was negative. Blood cultures showed no growth. A viral hepatitis panel was negative. Four days later, his lab work was as follows: ALT 990 U/L, AST 173 U/L, albumin 2.5 g/dl, alkaline phosphatase 171, and total bilirubin 1.9 mg/dl. Six days from admission, his labs ALT 605 U/L, AST 83 U/L, albumin 2.4 g/dl, alkaline phosphatase 164 U/L, total bilirubin 2.5 mg/dl, INR 1.2, and creatinine 0.54 mg/dl.

After initial improvement, he had acute respiratory decompensation and opted for supportive care only. The family declined to have an autopsy performed.

3. Discussion

Pancreatic cancer is an aggressive neoplasm with a dismal prognosis as most patients present with metastatic disease. Despite recent therapeutic advances, one of its main characteristics is resistance to current therapies. The majority build upon chemotherapy backbones with other novel therapeutic strategies including immune and targeted therapies [6, 7].

Immunotherapy has shown promising activity for other neoplasms including lung, melanoma, bladder, and kidney [8–11]. Additionally, the toxicity profile of this class of drugs has consistently been shown to be acceptable. Grade 3-4 adverse events (AEs) occur in 7% to 12% with single-agent antiprogrammed cell (PD-1) monoclonal antibodies such as nivolumab. The most common AE is fatigue with an estimated rate of 16%–24% and grade 3-4 severity of 1-2%. Dermatological toxicity including rash, pruritus, and vitiligo has been reported in 34% of patients with a very low rate of grade 3-4 events with patients receiving nivolumab. Grade 3-4 colitis and hepatitis occur in approximately 1–3% of the cases. The incidence of grade 3-4 thyroid disorder is approximately 0.1%. Neurologic symptoms, ocular, pancreatic, and renal toxicity are rare events. Thus, toxicity rates have not been a major barrier for further development of this drug class [12–14].

Preliminary data with the use of the immune checkpoint inhibitor ipilimumab suggested that this approach could be further explored for the treatment of pancreatic adenocarcinoma [15]. Tumor shrinkage was documented in at least one patient with pancreatic cancer treated with the anti PDL1 antibody MEDI4376 after 6 weeks of treatment [16]. Clinical trials testing the combination of checkpoint inhibitors and chemotherapy are underway [7].

This patient was in excellent health and performance prior to his diagnosis of pancreatic cancer. Given previous

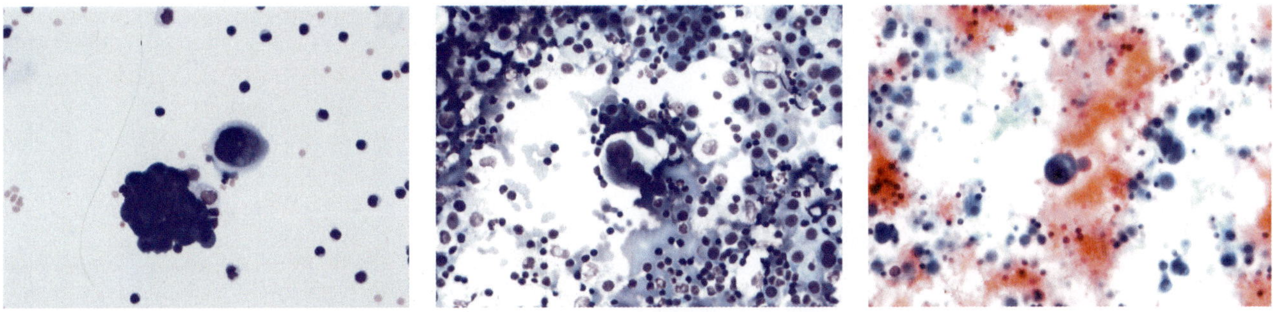

(a) (b) (c)

FIGURE 3: Pleural fluid involved by pleomorphic tumor cells. (a) Wright–Giemsa stain; (b) Romanowsky stain; (c) Papanicolaou stain, 400x.

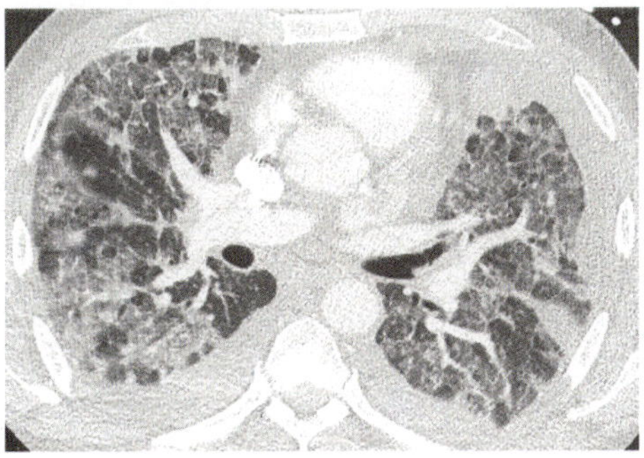

FIGURE 4: Chest CT showing diffuse ground glass opacities and new interlobular interstitial thickening.

results with standard therapy, enrollment in a clinical trial using a combination strategy was considered a reasonable option. Unfortunately, he developed acute severe respiratory failure after one single treatment despite meeting strict criteria for protocol initiation.

While an autopsy was not performed in this case, treatment-related lung injury was likely the cause of his hypoxemic respiratory failure. Viral or bacterial infection seems unlikely given results of cultures and previous evaluation. Decompensated heart failure was not diagnosed. The numerous lymphocytes in his pleural fluid after treatment with nivolumab may indicate an inflammatory response accounting for the acute presentation. Furthermore, his transaminases elevation is another substrate to support this diagnostic possibility.

One of the confounding factors here is that drug-induced lung injury has been well described with the use gemcitabine alone or in combination with taxanes. In a large database, the median time of diagnosis of severe lung toxicity was 48 days. However, symptoms were also seen within 1 day of administration of the drug [17]. Albeit uncommon, drug-related pneumonitis has also been reported with the use of single-agent nab-paclitaxel [18].

Pneumonitis has also been described with the use of checkpoint inhibitors including nivolumab with an estimated rate of approximately 2.5% for all grade toxicity and 0.8% for grade 3-4 toxicity. Its incidence appears to be higher with the use of combination treatment. The median time of onset is 2.5 months. It may present with different radiologic patterns. Initial treatment with methylprednisolone is usually successful [12, 19, 20]. Unfortunately, this patient received a combination of three drugs concurrently making it impossible to determine if a single, a doublet, or triplet combination were the culprit. The radiologic findings are nondiagnostic in this setting. Furthermore, the treatment of severe drug-induced pneumonitis usually consists of steroids with improvement. The lack of a specific radiologic pattern is also a characteristic of either immune- or chemotherapy-related pneumonitis. However, the fact that the transaminases promptly improved after institution of steroids also favors toxicity related to the immune checkpoint inhibitors. Severe transaminase elevations are scarce with the use of gemcitabine [21]. It is also possible that bronchoalveolar lavage and or transbronchial biopsy could have had elucidated the cause of respiratory failure. The fact that the previous cultures and infectious workup were previously negative made a weaker case for further interventions/procedures making the diagnosis elusive.

In summary, this case illustrates that pneumonitis with an immune checkpoint inhibitor-based combination may happen very rapidly despite careful selection of patients. Clinicians and patients should have a low threshold in considering pneumonitis with new respiratory symptoms.

References

[1] R. L. Siegel, K. D. Miller, and A. Jemal, "Cancer statistics, 2017," *CA: A Cancer Journal for Clinicians*, vol. 67, no. 1, pp. 7–30, 2017.

[2] H. A. Burris III, M. J. Moore, J. Andersen et al., "Improvements in survival and clinical benefit with gemcitabine as first-line therapy for patients with advanced pancreas cancer: a randomized trial," *Journal of Clinical Oncology*, vol. 15, no. 6, pp. 2403–2413, 1997.

[3] T. Conroy, F. Desseigne, M. Ychou et al., "FOLFIRINOX versus gemcitabine for metastatic pancreatic cancer," *New England Journal of Medicine*, vol. 364, no. 19, pp. 1817–1825, 2011.

[4] D. D. Von Hoff, T. Ervin, F. P. Arena et al., "Increased survival in pancreatic cancer with nab-paclitaxel plus gemcitabine,"

New England Journal of Medicine, vol. 369, no. 18, pp. 1691–1703, 2013.
[5] NCC Network, *Pancreatic Adenocarcinoma Version 3.2017*, October 2017, https://www.nccn.org/professionals/physician_gls/f_guidelines.asp.pancreatic.
[6] G. A. Manji, K. P. Olive, Y. M. Saenger, and P. Oberstein, "Current and emerging therapies in metastatic pancreatic cancer," *Clinical Cancer Research*, vol. 23, no. 7, pp. 1670–1678, 2017.
[7] F. Aroldi and A. Zaniboni, "Immunotherapy for pancreatic cancer: present and future," *Immunotherapy*, vol. 9, no. 7, pp. 607–616, 2017.
[8] A. Krishnamurthy and A. Jimeno, "Atezolizumab: a novel PD-L1 inhibitor in cancer therapy with a focus in bladder and non-small cell lung cancers," *Drugs of Today*, vol. 53, no. 4, pp. 217–237, 2017.
[9] R. J. Motzer, B. I. Rini, D. F. McDermott et al., "Nivolumab for metastatic renal cell carcinoma: results of a randomized phase II trial," *Journal of Clinical Oncology*, vol. 33, no. 13, pp. 1430–1437, 2015.
[10] J. Brahmer, K. L. Reckamp, P. Baas et al., "Nivolumab versus docetaxel in advanced squamous-cell non-small-cell lung cancer," *New England Journal of Medicine*, vol. 373, no. 2, pp. 123–135, 2015.
[11] C. Robert, G. V. Long, B. Brady et al., "Nivolumab in previously untreated melanoma without BRAF mutation," *New England Journal of Medicine*, vol. 372, no. 4, pp. 320–330, 2015.
[12] R. Costa, B. A. Carneiro, M. Agulnik et al., "Toxicity profile of approved anti-PD-1 monoclonal antibodies in solid tumors: a systematic review and meta-analysis of randomized clinical trials," *Oncotarget*, vol. 8, no. 5, pp. 8910–8920, 2017.
[13] J. Naidoo, D. B. Page, B. T. Li et al., "Toxicities of the anti-PD-1 and anti-PD-L1 immune checkpoint antibodies," *Annals of Oncology*, vol. 26, no. 12, pp. 2375–2391, 2015.
[14] R. Barroso-Sousa, W. T. Barry, A. C. Garrido-Castro et al., "Incidence of endocrine dysfunction following the use of different immune checkpoint inhibitor regimens: a systematic review and meta-analysis," *JAMA Oncology*, vol. 4, no. 2, pp. 173–182, 2018.
[15] R. E. Royal, C. Levy, K. Turner et al., "Phase 2 trial of single agent Ipilimumab (anti-CTLA-4) for locally advanced or metastatic pancreatic adenocarcinoma," *Journal of Immunotherapy*, vol. 33, no. 8, pp. 828–833, 2010.
[16] N. H. Segal, S. J. Antonia, J. R. Brahmer et al., "Preliminary data from a multi-arm expansion study of MEDI4736, an anti-PD-L1 antibody," *Journal of Clinical Oncology*, vol. 32, no. 15, p. 3002, 2014.
[17] S. M. Belknap, T. M. Kuzel, P. R. Yarnold et al., "Clinical features and correlates of gemcitabine-associated lung injury: findings from the RADAR project," *Cancer*, vol. 106, no. 9, pp. 2051–2057, 2006.
[18] P. F. Peddi, M. Cho, J. Wang, F. Gao, and A. Wang-Gillam, "Nab-paclitaxel monotherapy in refractory pancreatic adenocarcinoma," *Journal of Gastrointestinal Oncology*, vol. 4, no. 4, pp. 370–373, 2013.
[19] M. Nishino, A. Giobbie-Hurder, H. Hatabu, N. H. Ramaiya, and F. Stephen Hodi, "Incidence of programmed cell death 1 inhibitor-related pneumonitis in patients with advanced cancer: a systematic review and meta-analysis," *JAMA Oncology*, vol. 2, no. 12, pp. 1607–1616, 2016.
[20] S. Chuzi, F. Tavora, M. Cruz et al., "Clinical features, diagnostic challenges, and management strategies in checkpoint inhibitor-related pneumonitis," *Cancer Management and Research*, vol. 9, pp. 207–213, 2017.
[21] H. Saadati, J. Peccerillo, K. Kaley, M. L. Schilsky, and M. W. Saif, "Gemcitabine-induced hepatitis in a pancreatic cancer patient receiving adjuvant therapy following metastasectomy," *Journal of Periodontology*, vol. 10, no. 5, pp. 573–575, 2009.

41

A Rare Thyroid Metastasis from Uveal Melanoma and Response to Immunotherapy Agents

Dearbhaile Catherine Collins,[1] Ruben Yela,[2] Noel Horgan,[3] and Derek Gerard Power[1]

[1] *Department of Medical Oncology, Cork University Hospital, Wilton, Co. Cork, Ireland*
[2] *Department of Histopathology, Cork University Hospital, Wilton, Co. Cork, Ireland*
[3] *Department of Ophthalmology, Royal Victoria Eye and Ear Hospital, Dublin 2, Ireland*

Correspondence should be addressed to Dearbhaile Catherine Collins; collinsdearbhaile1@gmail.com

Academic Editor: Raffaele Palmirotta

Thyroid metastasis is a rare occurrence with cutaneous melanoma and even more uncommon with uveal melanoma. The management of such metastasis is uncertain due to its infrequency and, in the era of immunotherapy, the effect of these novel drugs on uncommon metastasis, such as to the thyroid, is unknown. We report the rare case of a thyroid metastasis in a patient diagnosed with ocular melanoma initially managed with enucleation. Metastatic disease developed in the lung and thyroid gland. The case patient received the immunotherapy ipilimumab with stable disease in the thyroid and progressive disease elsewhere. The patient was then further treated with a second immunotherapy agent, pembrolizumab, and remains with stable disease one year later. We discuss the current literature on thyroid metastases from all causes and the optimal known management strategies. Furthermore, we provide an original report on the response of this disease to the novel immunomodulators, ipilimumab, and pembrolizumab with stable disease four years after initial diagnosis of ocular melanoma.

1. Introduction

Thyroid metastases are an uncommon occurrence. Reported incidence ranges from 0.5% to 24.2% in autopsy studies [1–5]. They most often arise from renal, breast, and lung primaries; however cutaneous melanoma is also a common site [1, 2, 6]. Diagnosis is most commonly made with ultrasonography and fine needle aspiration cytology (FNAC). Systemic management of the primary disease is the optimal treatment strategy, although thyroidectomy may be necessary for palliative symptom control and, in some malignancies, resection may improve survival [7]. Ocular melanoma comprises 3 to 4% of all malignant melanoma and most commonly metastasizes to the liver [8, 9]. It has only been reported once before in the literature as giving rise to thyroid metastases in 1986 [10]. To add to this scant literature, we report a rare case of thyroid metastasis from uveal melanoma and furthermore report a disease response to the systemic immunotherapies in the form of ipilimumab and pembrolizumab.

2. Case Presentation

We present the case of a 63-year-old French national who was residing in Ireland. He was diagnosed with right ocular melanoma and underwent enucleation in a specialist institution in February 2011. Histopathology at this time revealed a superonasal posterior pole uveal melanoma measuring 17 × 12 × 10 millimeters. There was histopathological evidence of extrascleral extension, spindle B cell morphology, and considered stage pT4e. There were no mitoses in 40 high power fields. Tumour involved the overlying retina and 17% of cell revealed monosomy of chromosome 3 using fluorescence in situ hybridisation (FISH) analysis. FISH also indicated normal results for chromosome 8 and MYC abnormalities. At time of initial staging and workup our patient was found to have subcentimetre lung nodules on computed tomography (CT) scanning. These were biopsied and on histopathological assessment were identified as benign on both FNAC and core biopsy. Follow-up scanning with annual CT and positron

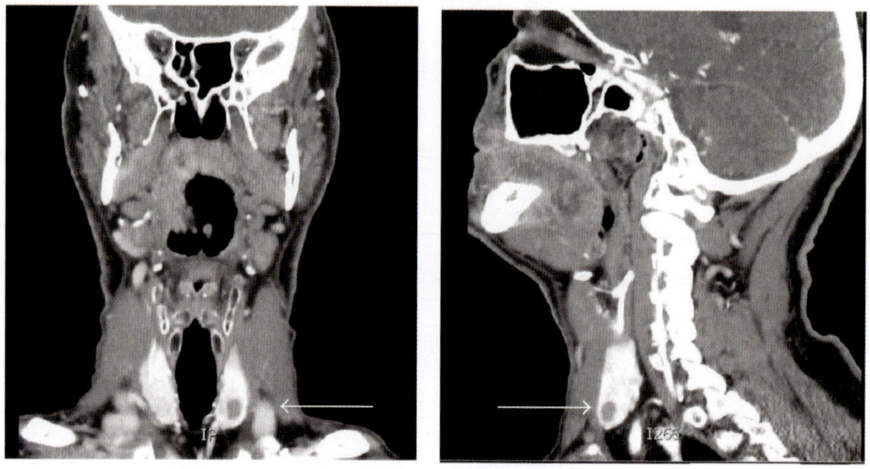

Figure 1: CT neck image of thyroid nodules (identified by white arrows).

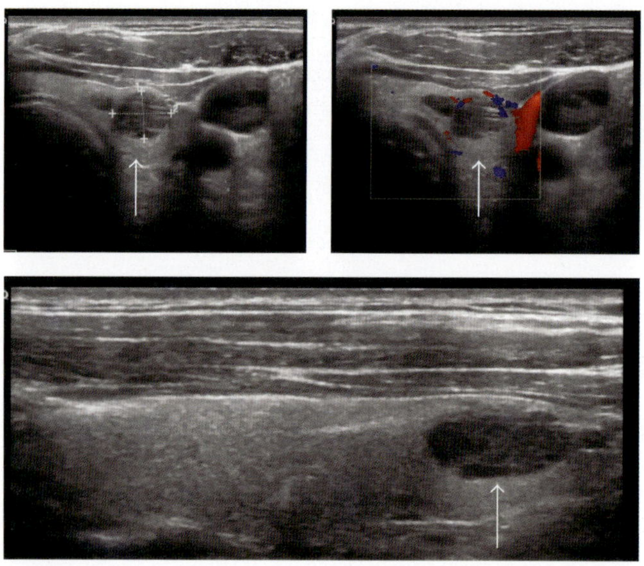

Figure 2: Ultrasound images of thyroid metastasis (identified by white arrows).

emission tomography- (PET-) CT revealed stable cold lung nodules and no evidence of metastatic melanoma over a thirty-two-month period.

In October 2013, he underwent a routine surveillance CT neck, thorax, abdomen, and pelvis, which noted increased size of all lung nodules. For instance, a nodule in the right middle pulmonary lobe measured 8 mm from previous 3 mm. It also identified two new solid lesions in the thyroid, the largest of which was 8 mm in diameter (Figure 1).

Ultrasound guided biopsy of the largest lesion revealed metastatic melanoma (Figure 2).

Pathological examination showed the presence of metastatic spindle and epithelioid malignant melanoma cells (positive staining for HMB45, MelanA, and S100 immunocytochemistry (ICC)) amongst residual thyroid follicles (positive staining for TTF-1 ICC). Some of the metastatic melanoma cells showed fine intracytoplasmic pigment and prominent nucleoli (Figure 3).

The case patient was of protooncogene *braf* mutation wild type and went on to receive four cycles of the immunotherapy, ipilimumab in early 2014, which were tolerated well. Restaging CT one month after the final cycle revealed progressive disease in the lungs, with new disease in the adrenal gland. The thyroid metastases were considered unchanged from prior imaging. The patient was managed with surveillance and further CT scanning three months and six months later revealed stable disease in the thyroid (Figure 4) with new disease infradiaphragmatically. In January 2015, the novel immunomodulator, pembrolizumab, was prescribed at two milligrams per kilogram every three weeks. The patient continues on regular pembrolizumab with all thyroid, pulmonary, and adrenal metastatic disease stable by immune response criteria (iRECIST) at each three-month CT assessment since commencing this therapy.

3. Discussion

Thyroid metastases are an uncommon occurrence in clinical practice. Autopsy reports vary considerably between 0.5% and 24% in incidence [1–5]. Primary sources most commonly include carcinomas of the breast, lung, kidney, gastrointestinal tract, head and neck, and malignant melanoma [1, 4, 11]. Renal cell carcinoma [12–14] and breast [15] are the most frequent in the literature. Thyroid metastases usually occur in the presence of metastatic disease elsewhere [7, 12, 14] and, if isolated, are often quickly followed by the development of disseminated disease. Their development can be distant from the primary diagnosis. This is particularly in the case of renal cell carcinoma, where there have been multiple cases of metastasis developing over twenty years after diagnosis of the primary malignancy [11, 16]. The published literature on cutaneous melanoma metastatic to the thyroid gland is limited to case reports or small case series [13, 17–19]. Bozbora et al. reported a case of cutaneous malignant melanoma to

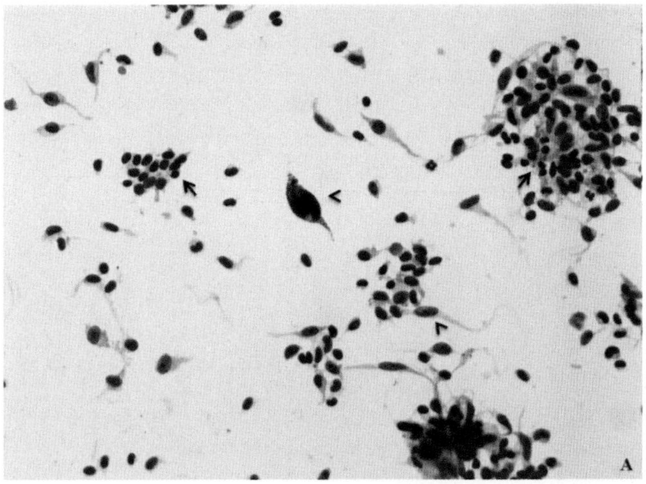

(a)

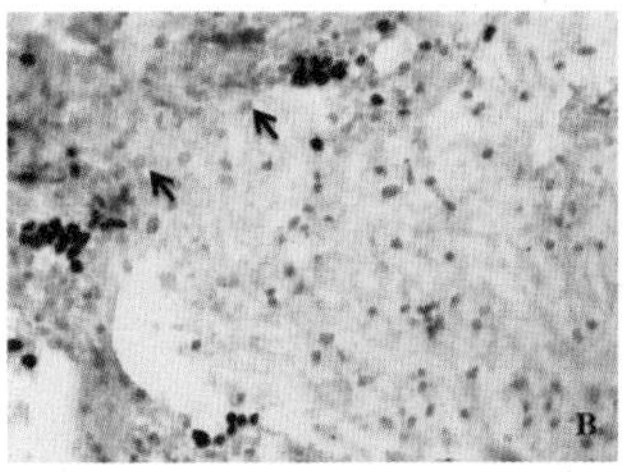

(b)

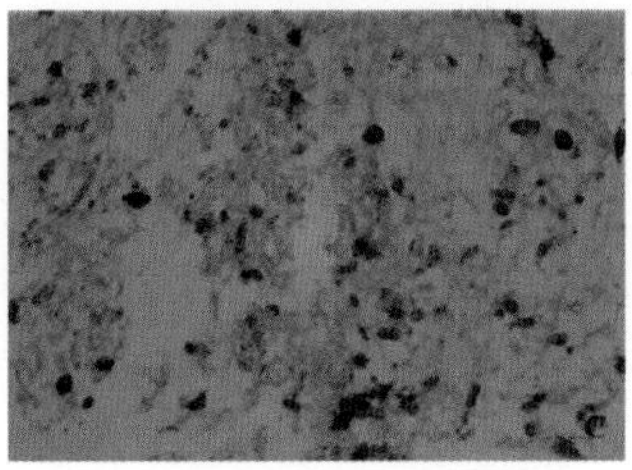

(c)

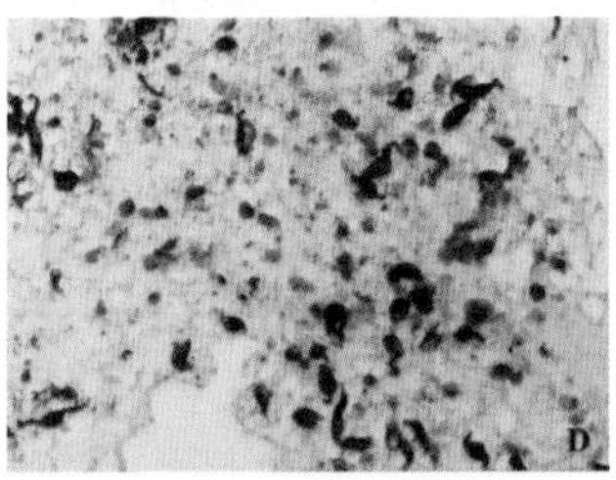

(d)

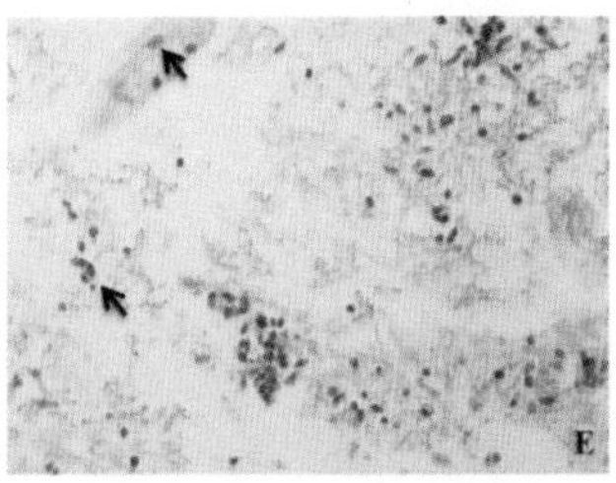

(e)

Figure 3: (a) Spindle and epithelioid malignant melanoma cells (arrowheads) admixed with background residual thyroid follicular cells (arrows). Papanicolaou stain, original magnification ×400. (b) TTF-1 highlights residual thyroid follicular cells and is negative in the lesional cells (arrows). TTF-1 ICC, original magnification ×200. (c) HMB45 and (d) MelanA ICC show strong positivity in the lesional cells. Original magnifications ×200. (e) S100 ICC weakly highlights the fine intracytoplasmic pigment present in the lesional cells (arrows). Original magnification ×100.

thyroid after excision of a two-millimeter melanoma five years before [17]. There is only one cited case report of ocular melanoma metastasising to the thyroid gland [10].

Uveal melanomas differ from cutaneous melanomas in a number of areas. Firstly, ocular melanomas have a predilection to metastasise to the liver along haematogenous drainage pathways although spread can occur to lung, bone, brain, skin, and potentially any site within the body [20]. Factors predictive of metastasis from uveal melanoma include tumour thickness and genetic aberrations. Shields et al. found for each millimeter increase in tumour thickness that there

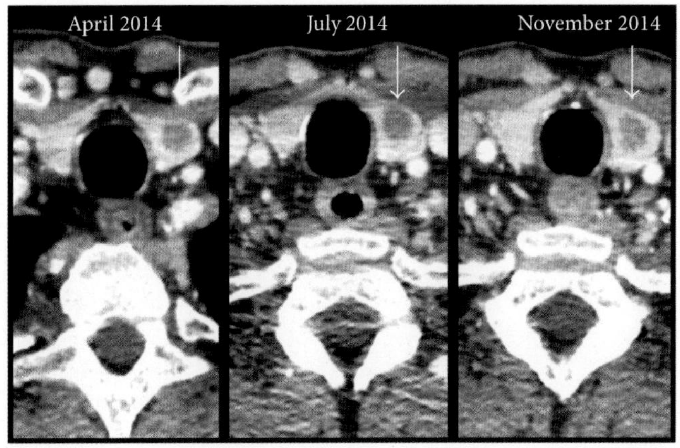

Figure 4: CT neck image of thyroid nodule (identified by white arrows) over time.

was a resultant increased risk of metastasis of 1.06 [21]. The risk of spread is approximately 6% with uveal melanomas less than or equal to one millimeter in thickness and up to 51% for those greater than ten millimeters. Uveal melanomas also differ from cutaneous lesions in their expression of genetic abnormalities, in particular, anomalies of chromosomes 1, 3, 6, and 8. These abnormalities are prognostic as well as predictive for metastasis [22–24]. As, in our case, monosomy of chromosome 3 is the most frequent chromosomal aberration, reported in about half of patients [25, 26]. Its loss is detected in more than 70% of metastasising and only 20% nonmetastasising uveal melanomas and correlated with reduced patient survival [22–24, 27]. A further difference between uveal melanoma and cutaneous melanoma is that the latter frequently carries oncogenic driver mutations in the proteins Raf and Ras, which results in constitutively activated mitogen associated protein kinase (MAPK) pathway signalling and leads to tumorigenesis, cellular proliferation, and dissemination [28–30]. Although MAPK activation also exists in uveal melanoma it is rarely due to mutations in Raf and Ras [31–34]. Other genetic oncogenic drivers include GNAQ [35–37], GNA11 [38], BAP1 mutations [39], and PTEN (phosphatase and tensin homolog) loss [40]. Whether these mutations actually correlate with overall patient outcome is unconfirmed [36, 41].

Management of thyroid metastasis is varied and depends upon symptoms at presentation. Treatment strategies can include surgical resection or debulking by complete or partial thyroidectomy, radiotherapy, and/or systemic therapy. The aim of surgical intervention should be primarily for compressive symptom control such as dysphagia, dyspnea, and stridor [42]. Thyroid metastasis from other malignancies such as renal cell carcinoma, if resected, may have a cytoreductive role and impact positively upon patient outcome [7]. Metastasectomy in melanoma patients has been shown to confer a significant increase in survival for patients in particular with pulmonary and hepatic metastasis [43–45]. This is irrespective of whether the primary melanoma is cutaneous or uveal [46]. It is unknown whether thyroid metastasectomy, specifically, confers any survival benefit on account of the rarity of this occurrence [7, 12].

In this case report, we describe a rare case of uveal melanoma with metastasis to the thyroid gland. To date, the literature only records one such case previously published in 1986 [10]. We also give an account of the response of this metastatic thyroidal disease to immunotherapy. The malignancy, following four cycles of ipilimumab, remained stable within the thyroid gland although new metastatic deposits developed elsewhere. Ipilimumab is an inhibitor of cytotoxic-T-lymphocyte-associated-antigen 4 (CTLA-4) that results in upregulation of the immune system. It is well established as a treatment for metastatic malignant cutaneous melanoma [47]. One year later, he received pembrolizumab, a novel immunomodulator that targets programmed-death-1 (PD-1) receptor and activates T-cell mediated immune responses against tumour cells. Again pembrolizumab is a proven efficacious treatment in metastatic cutaneous melanoma [48]. He remains well with stable metastatic disease almost one year after commencing this second immunotherapy and four years after his initial diagnosis.

In conclusion, unusual metastasis, for instance, to the thyroid should always be considered in the setting of carcinoma, including uveal melanoma. The disease should be managed according to the primary malignancy with appropriate chemotherapy, biological therapy and radiotherapy, and multidisciplinary discussion. Surgical resection of thyroid metastasis can be considered on a case-by-case basis, keeping in mind the natural biology of the primary malignancy as well as available systemic treatment strategies. Although immunotherapies such as ipilimumab and pembrolizumab are frequently used in cutaneous melanoma, they can be efficacious on metastatic uveal melanoma also.

Acknowledgments

The authors would like to acknowledge the patient and his family in permitting our publication of his disease history. They would also like to acknowledge Dr. Emily Harrold for her help in obtaining images.

References

[1] M. K. Nakhjavani, H. Gharib, J. R. Goellner, and J. A. van Heerden, "Metastasis to the thyroid gland. A report of 43 cases," *Cancer*, vol. 79, no. 3, pp. 574–578, 1997.

[2] K. Shimaoka, J. E. Sokal, and J. W. Pickren, "Metastatic neoplasms in the thyroid gland: pathological and clinical findings," *Cancer*, vol. 15, pp. 557–565, 1962.

[3] S. G. Silverberg and R. A. Vidone, "Carcinoma of the thyroid in surgical and postmortem material. Analysis of 300 cases at autopsy and literature review," *Annals of Surgery*, vol. 164, no. 2, pp. 291–299, 1966.

[4] G. Papi, G. Fadda, S. M. Corsello et al., "Metastases to the thyroid gland: prevalence, clinicopathological aspects and prognosis: a 10-year experience," *Clinical Endocrinology*, vol. 66, no. 4, pp. 565–571, 2007.

[5] K. Y. Lam and C. Y. Lo, "Metastatic tumors of the thyroid gland: a study of 79 cases in Chinese patients," *Archives of Pathology and Laboratory Medicine*, vol. 122, no. 1, pp. 37–41, 1998.

[6] B. R. Haugen, S. Nawaz, A. Cohn et al., "Secondary malignancy of the thyroid gland. A case report and review of the literature," *Thyroid*, vol. 4, no. 3, pp. 297–300, 1994.

[7] M. A. Romero Arenas, H. Ryu, S. Lee et al., "The role of thyroidectomy in metastatic disease to the thyroid gland," *Annals of Surgical Oncology*, vol. 21, no. 2, pp. 434–439, 2014.

[8] C. C. McLaughlin, X.-C. Wu, A. Jemal, H. J. Martin, L. M. Roche, and V. W. Chen, "Incidence of noncutaneous melanomas in the U.S.," *Cancer*, vol. 103, no. 5, pp. 1000–1007, 2005.

[9] A. E. Chang, L. H. Karnell, and H. R. Menck, "The national cancer data base report on cutaneous and noncutaneous melanoma. A summary of 84,836 cases from the past decade," *Cancer*, vol. 83, no. 8, pp. 1664–1678, 1998.

[10] G. Gherardi, P. Scherini, and S. Ambrosi, "Occult thyroid metastasis from untreated uveal melanoma," *Archives of Ophthalmology*, vol. 103, no. 5, pp. 689–691, 1985.

[11] A. Y. Chung, T. B. Tran, K. T. Brumund, R. A. Weisman, and M. Bouvet, "Metastases to the thyroid: a review of the literature from the last decade," *Thyroid*, vol. 22, no. 3, pp. 258–268, 2012.

[12] K. Wood, L. Vini, and C. Harmer, "Metastases to the thyroid gland: the Royal Marsden experience," *European Journal of Surgical Oncology*, vol. 30, no. 6, pp. 583–588, 2004.

[13] E. Mirallié, J. Rigaud, M. Mathonnet et al., "Management and prognosis of metastases to the thyroid gland," *Journal of the American College of Surgeons*, vol. 200, no. 2, pp. 203–207, 2005.

[14] H. Chen, T. L. Nicol, and R. Udelsman, "Clinically significant, isolated metastatic disease to the thyroid gland," *World Journal of Surgery*, vol. 23, no. 2, pp. 177–180, 1999.

[15] T. Y. Kim, W. B. Kim, G. Gong, S. J. Hong, and Y. K. Shong, "Metastasis to the thyroid diagnosed by fine-needle aspiration biopsy," *Clinical Endocrinology*, vol. 62, no. 2, pp. 236–241, 2005.

[16] M. Kihara, H. Yokomise, and A. Yamauchi, "Metastasis of renal cell carcinoma to the thyroid gland 19 years after nephrectomy: a case report," *Auris Nasus Larynx*, vol. 31, no. 1, pp. 95–100, 2004.

[17] A. Bozbora, U. Barbaros, H. Kaya et al., "Thyroid metastasis of malignant melanoma," *American Journal of Clinical Oncology*, vol. 28, no. 6, pp. 642–643, 2005.

[18] S. Basu and A. Alavi, "Metastatic malignant melanoma to the thyroid gland detected by FDG-PET imaging," *Clinical Nuclear Medicine*, vol. 32, no. 5, pp. 388–389, 2007.

[19] B. Kung, S. Aftab, M. Wood, and D. Rosen, "Malignant melanoma metastatic to the thyroid gland: a case report and review of the literature," *Ear, Nose & Throat Journal*, vol. 88, no. 1, article E7, 2009.

[20] Collaborative Ocular Melanoma Study Group, "Assessment of metastatic disease status at death in 435 patients with large choroidal melanoma in the Collaborative Ocular Melanoma Study (COMS): COMS report no. 15," *Archives of Ophthalmology*, vol. 119, no. 5, pp. 670–676, 2001.

[21] C. L. Shields, M. Furuta, A. Thangappan et al., "Metastasis of uveal melanoma millimeter-by-millimeter in 8033 consecutive eyes," *Archives of Ophthalmology*, vol. 127, no. 8, pp. 989–998, 2009.

[22] G. Prescher, N. Bornfeld, and R. Becher, "Nonrandom chromosomal abnormalities in primary uveal melanoma," *Journal of the National Cancer Institute*, vol. 82, no. 22, pp. 1765–1769, 1990.

[23] K. Sisley, I. G. Rennie, M. Andrew Parsons et al., "Abnormalities of chromosomes 3 and 8 in posterior uveal melanoma correlate

with prognosis," *Genes, Chromosomes and Cancer*, vol. 19, no. 1, pp. 22–28, 1997.

[24] Y. Aalto, L. Eriksson, S. Seregard, O. Larsson, and S. Knuutila, "Concomitant loss of chromosome 3 and whole arm losses and gains of chromosome 1, 6, or 8 in metastasizing primary uveal melanoma," *Investigative Ophthalmology and Visual Science*, vol. 42, no. 2, pp. 313–317, 2001.

[25] G. Prescher, N. Bornfeld, H. Hirche, B. Horsthemke, K.-H. Jöckel, and R. Becher, "Prognostic implications of monosomy 3 in uveal melanoma," *The Lancet*, vol. 347, no. 9010, pp. 1222–1225, 1996.

[26] A. G. M. Scholes, B. E. Damato, J. Nunn, P. Hiscott, I. Grierson, and J. K. Field, "Monosomy 3 in uveal melanoma: correlation with clinical and histologic predictors of survival," *Investigative Ophthalmology and Visual Science*, vol. 44, no. 3, pp. 1008–1011, 2003.

[27] V. A. White, J. D. Chambers, P. D. Courtright, W. Y. Chang, and D. E. Horsman, "Correlation of cytogenetic abnormalities with the outcome of patients with uveal melanoma," *Cancer*, vol. 83, no. 2, pp. 354–359, 1998.

[28] H. Davies, G. R. Bignell, C. Cox et al., "Mutations of the BRAF gene in human cancer," *Nature*, vol. 417, no. 6892, pp. 949–954, 2002.

[29] J. N. Poynter, J. T. Elder, D. R. Fullen et al., "BRAF and NRAS mutations in melanoma and melanocytic nevi," *Melanoma Research*, vol. 16, no. 4, pp. 267–273, 2006.

[30] L. A. Fecher, R. K. Amaravadi, and K. T. Flaherty, "The MAPK pathway in melanoma," *Current Opinion in Oncology*, vol. 20, no. 2, pp. 183–189, 2008.

[31] W. Zuidervaart, F. van Nieuwpoort, M. Stark et al., "Activation of the MAPK pathway is a common event in uveal melanomas although it rarely occurs through mutation of BRAF or RAS," *British Journal of Cancer*, vol. 92, no. 11, pp. 2032–2038, 2005.

[32] A. Weber, U. R. Hengge, D. Urbanik et al., "Absence of mutations of the *BRAF* gene and constitutive activation of extracellular-regulated kinase in malignant melanomas of the uvea," *Laboratory Investigation*, vol. 83, no. 12, pp. 1771–1776, 2003.

[33] Y. Cohen, N. Goldenberg-Cohen, P. Parrella et al., "Lack of BRAF mutation in primary uveal melanoma," *Investigative Ophthalmology and Visual Science*, vol. 44, no. 7, pp. 2876–2878, 2003.

[34] F. Cruz III, B. P. Rubin, D. Wilson et al., "Absence of BRAF and NRAS mutations in uveal melanoma," *Cancer Research*, vol. 63, no. 18, pp. 5761–5766, 2003.

[35] M. D. Onken, L. A. Worley, M. D. Long et al., "Oncogenic mutations in GNAQ occur early in uveal melanoma," *Investigative Ophthalmology and Visual Science*, vol. 49, no. 12, pp. 5230–5234, 2008.

[36] J. Bauer, E. Kilic, J. Vaarwater, B. C. Bastian, C. Garbe, and A. de Klein, "Oncogenic GNAQ mutations are not correlated with disease-free survival in uveal melanoma," *British Journal of Cancer*, vol. 101, no. 5, pp. 813–815, 2009.

[37] C. D. Van Raamsdonk, V. Bezrookove, G. Green et al., "Frequent somatic mutations of GNAQ in uveal melanoma and blue naevi," *Nature*, vol. 457, no. 7229, pp. 599–602, 2009.

[38] C. D. Van Raamsdonk, K. G. Griewank, M. B. Crosby et al., "Mutations in GNA11 in uveal melanoma," *The New England Journal of Medicine*, vol. 363, no. 23, pp. 2191–2199, 2010.

[39] J. W. Harbour, M. D. Onken, E. D. O. Roberson et al., "Frequent mutation of BAP1 in metastasizing uveal melanomas," *Science*, vol. 330, no. 6009, pp. 1410–1413, 2010.

[40] M. H. Abdel-Rahman, Y. Yang, X.-P. Zhou, E. L. Craig, F. H. Davidorf, and C. Eng, "High frequency of submicroscopic hemizygous deletion is a major mechanism of loss of expression of PTEN in uveal melanoma," *Journal of Clinical Oncology*, vol. 24, no. 2, pp. 288–295, 2006.

[41] A. E. Koopmans, J. Vaarwater, D. Paridaens, N. C. Naus, E. Kilic, and A. de Klein, "Patient survival in uveal melanoma is not affected by oncogenic mutations in GNAQ and GNA11," *British Journal of Cancer*, vol. 109, no. 2, pp. 493–496, 2013.

[42] P. H. Montero, T. Ibrahimpasic, I. J. Nixon, and A. R. Shaha, "Thyroid metastasectomy," *Journal of Surgical Oncology*, vol. 109, no. 1, pp. 36–41, 2014.

[43] U. Pastorino, M. Buyse, G. Friedel et al., "Long-term results of lung metastasectomy: prognostic analyses based on 5206 cases," *Journal of Thoracic and Cardiovascular Surgery*, vol. 113, no. 1, pp. 37–49, 1997.

[44] A. Oliaro, P. L. Filosso, M. C. Bruna, C. Mossetti, and E. Ruffini, "Pulmonary metastasectomy for melanoma," *Journal of Thoracic Oncology*, vol. 5, no. 6, supplement 2, pp. S187–S191, 2010.

[45] D. Van Raemdonck and G. Friedel, "The European society of thoracic surgeons lung metastasectomy project," *Journal of Thoracic Oncology*, vol. 5, no. 6, pp. S127–S129, 2010.

[46] S. W. Ryu, R. Saw, R. A. Scolyer, M. Crawford, J. F. Thompson, and C. Sandroussi, "Liver resection for metastatic melanoma: equivalent survival for cutaneous and ocular primaries," *Journal of Surgical Oncology*, vol. 108, no. 2, pp. 129–135, 2013.

[47] F. S. Hodi, S. J. O'Day, D. F. McDermott et al., "Improved survival with ipilimumab in patients with metastatic melanoma," *The New England Journal of Medicine*, vol. 363, no. 8, pp. 711–723, 2010.

[48] C. Robert, J. Schachter, G. V. Long et al., "Pembrolizumab versus ipilimumab in advanced melanoma," *The New England Journal of Medicine*, vol. 372, no. 26, pp. 2521–2532, 2015.

42

Oral Capecitabine Achieves Response in Metastatic Eccrine Carcinoma

Kristian Larson,[1] **Hani M. Babiker**,[1,2,3] **Andrew Kovoor**,[3] **Joy Liau**,[4] **Jordan Eldersveld**,[5] **and Emad Elquza**[1,3]

[1]*Early Phase Clinical Trial Program, The University of Arizona Cancer Center, 1515 N. Campbell Ave., Tucson, AZ 85724, USA*
[2]*Translational Genomics Research Institute (TGen), 445 N. 5th Street, Phoenix, AZ 85004, USA*
[3]*Division of Hematology and Oncology, University of Arizona College of Medicine, 1515 N. Campbell Ave., Tucson, AZ 85724, USA*
[4]*Department of Medical Imaging, University of Arizona, 1501 N. Campbell Ave., Tucson, AZ 85712, USA*
[5]*Department of Pathology, University of Arizona, 1501 N. Campbell Ave., Tucson, AZ 85712, USA*

Correspondence should be addressed to Kristian Larson; kris7c@email.arizona.edu

Academic Editor: Jose I. Mayordomo

The low prevalence rate and limited literature on eccrine carcinoma (EC) pose a challenge to properly diagnosing and treating this rare malignancy. EC lesions tend to present similarly to other cutaneous neoplasms and dermatitis-like conditions. Efficacious treatment guidelines have not been established for patients diagnosed with EC, and few treatment regimens have demonstrated clinical benefit. Due to the high metastatic potential of EC, recognizing the clinical presentation, properly diagnosing, and utilizing beneficial treatment options are important for managing this disease. We report a case of a 66-year-old female who presented with lesions that her primary care provider misdiagnosed as basal cell carcinoma. The disease responded poorly to taxane- and platinum-based chemotherapies as well as an isolated limb perfusion of an alkylating agent. However, continuous dosing of oral capecitabine achieved an 18-month period of progression free survival (PFS) and ameliorated quality of life. We wish to highlight this rare disease and discuss presentation, diagnosis, and management as it is most often misdiagnosed leading to advanced metastatic disease when patients present to the oncologist. In addition, it is crucial to study and report potentially efficacious regimens considering the lack of clinical trials in this disease.

1. Introduction

Eccrine carcinoma (EC) is an appendageal cancer that originates from the eccrine sweat gland and accounts for an estimated 0.005–0.01% of diagnosed cutaneous malignancies [1]. Histopathologies closely associated with EC include hidroadenocarcinoma, spiradenocarcinoma, and porocarcinoma [1–3]. A consistent clinical presentation of these lesions has not been identified; other authors have reported brown, bluish, and erythematous lesions which may appear papular or ulcerative [1, 4, 5]. Proper recognition and diagnosis of EC prove to be difficult due to its infrequency and similar presentation to basal and squamous cell carcinoma, amelanotic melanoma, seborrheic keratosis, cutaneous lymphoma, and verruca vulgaris [1]. EC lesions are commonly reported in the lower extremities (35%), head and neck (24%), and upper extremities (14%) [1]. Immunohistochemical (IHC) stains and serum cancer markers have also been inconsistently reported, which include but are not limited to carcinoembryonic antigen, epithelial membrane antigen, estrogen receptors, progesterone receptors, cytokeratin 7, and pancytokeratins [2, 6]. Thus, recognizing the pleomorphic features of basaloid cells within the epidermis that infiltrate into the ductal papillary structures of the dermis help diagnose EC [2].

A limited understanding of EC in addition to unestablished treatment guidelines contributes to a relative mortality rate of 80% and a 10-year disease survival rate of 9% when metastatic in stage [1, 7]. Based on the current literature, there seems to be

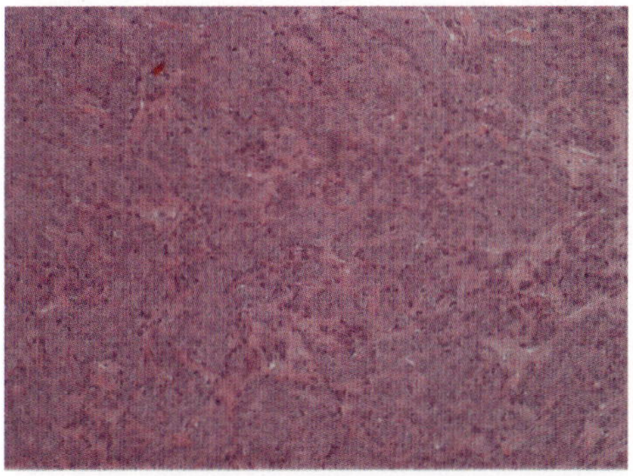

Figure 1: Eccrine carcinoma. Infiltrative, poorly differentiated neoplasm in a nested to trabecular pattern. Nuclei are relatively uniform with notably prominent nucleoli (hematoxylin-eosin, original magnification ×200).

a clinical consensus that wide surgical excision with the goal of clear margins is the most effective treatment for locoregional EC [8]. However, this option is not optimal for metastatic cases [9]. Other cases of metastatic EC have illustrated resistance to radiotherapy as well as a variety of chemotherapies [9]. We describe a case of a patient who continued to progress during treatments with carboplatin, paclitaxel, melphalan, actinomycin D, and radiotherapy but achieved 18 months of progression free survival (PFS) and an improved quality of life with oral capecitabine despite her diffusely metastatic disease.

2. Case Description

A 66-year-old female with a history of ongoing thrombocytosis (platelets at 724×10^3/uL, range: 150–450 $\times 10^3$/uL), emphysema and coronary artery disease visited her primary care physician (PCP) with complaints about pruritic "bumps" on her left calf in 2007. Her PCP noted that the lesions presented as erythematous, 2-3 mm in diameter, and papular. The PCP diagnosed these neoplasms as basal cell carcinoma without further diagnostic testing or intervention. The patient returned in early 2009 with enlarged lesions, increased pruritus, and ulceration. The patient was referred to dermatology and oncology.

She underwent wide surgical excision with clear margins attained, and three lymph nodes from the left inguinal zone were excised in April 2009. One lymph node was positive for disease involvement. A skin graft was placed thereafter. Histopathological analysis of the skin resection (Figure 1) supported the initial diagnosis of EC. Immunohistochemistry (IHC) resulted negative for the expression of estrogen and progesterone receptors and positive for HER-2/neu and EGF-R (2+ on 0–3+ scale). Albeit the aforementioned IHC data have been reported in EC, there are inconsistent and inadequate data in literature confirming it as a diagnostic tool. Unremarkable CT studies warranted no remaining disease.

The patient returned in July 2009 with recurrent erythematous papular lesions throughout the skin graft of the left calf and new multifocal lesions in transit with the left medial thigh. A punch biopsy of the left thigh demonstrated recurrent metastatic EC. The metastatic lesion resulted negative for the aforementioned positive IHC stains on the primary tumor. CT studies indicated no internal organ metastasis. Surgical oncology performed a hypoxic-hyperthermic isolated limb perfusion on the left leg with melphalan and actinomycin D that resulted in a partial response. However, the patient returned in December 2009 with recurrent lesions along her left thigh and calf measuring 1-2 centimeters in diameter and appearing ulcerated. In March 2010, a regimen

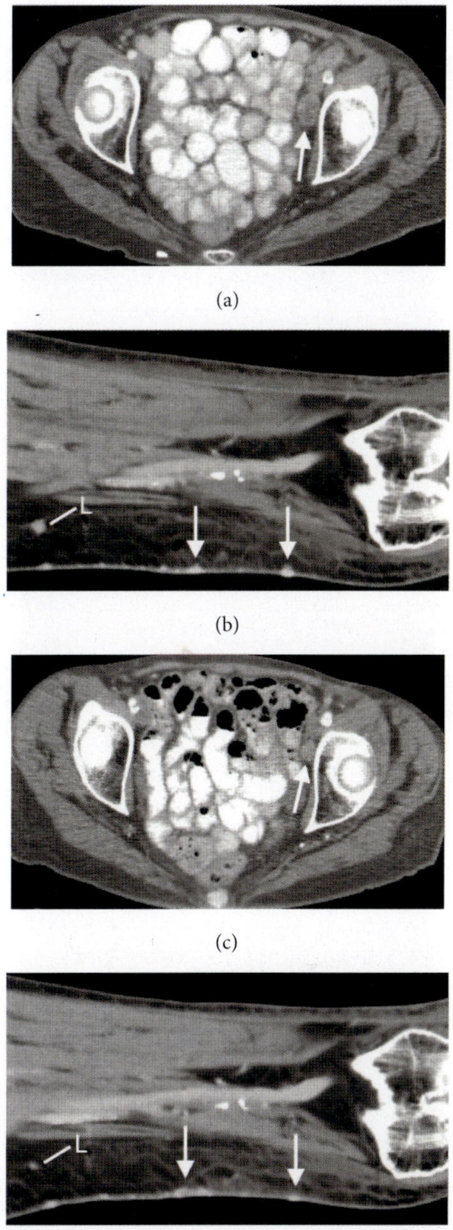

(a) (b) (c) (d)

Figure 2: Progression of the disease despite treatment with carboplatin, paclitaxel, and radiotherapy (a, b), with subsequent partial treatment response two months after starting capecitabine (c, d). Axial postcontrast CTs of the pelvis show metastatic left pelvic lymph nodes, with decrease in size of a metastatic left external iliac chain lymph node from 2.2 × 1.1 cm (white arrow, a) to 1.5 × 0.9 cm (white arrow (c)) with capecitabine treatment. Coronal postcontrast CTs of the left leg (b) before and (d) after capecitabine treatment show similar cutaneous metastases (white arrows) with decreased size of a metastatic lymph node (L).

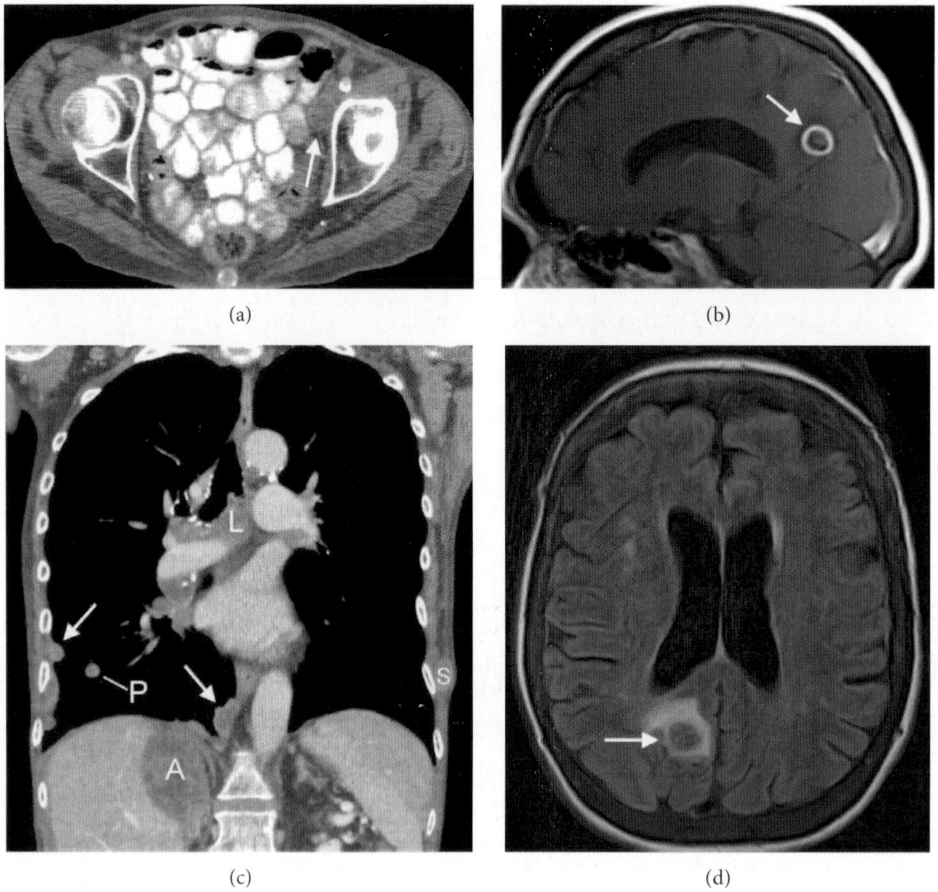

Figure 3: Progression of disease 18 months after starting capecitabine treatment. Axial postcontrast CT of the pelvis (a) shows increased size of a centrally necrotic left external chain lymph node, measuring 2.2 × 1.7 cm (white arrow). Postcontrast sagittal T1 MRI (b) and noncontrast coronal FLAIR MRI (d) of the brain show a new rim enhancing 1.2 cm metastasis in the right posterior parietal lobe with surrounding edema (white arrows). Coronal postcontrast CT of the chest and abdomen (c) shows new right pleural metastasis (arrows), mediastinal and hilar lymph node (L), and left lateral chest wall soft tissue (S) metastases, as well as an enlarging right lower lobe pulmonary metastasis (P) and right adrenal metastasis superimposed on an existing adrenal adenoma (A).

of intravenous carboplatin (AUC of 2) and paclitaxel (45 mg/m^2) given on days 1, 8, and 15 (28-day cycle) concurrent to sensitizing 6 MV external beam radiation (4500 cGy over 25 fractions applied to the left extremity lesions) was performed, and she completed two cycles of therapy by May 2010. CT scans in October 2011 revealed left pelvic lymph node metastases (Figure 2(a)) as well as recurrence in the left leg (Figure 2(b)).

In February 2012, the patient started a capecitabine regimen (1500 mg PO q12h) that followed a 2-week on/1-week off dosing schedule. Due to grade 3 palmar-plantar erythrodysesthesia syndrome occurring 12 months after dosing, the dose was reduced to 1000 mg. The absence of cutaneous lesion recurrence was noted. CT studies (Figure 2) revealed an overall partial response with a decrease in size of the left pelvic lymph node metastases (Figure 2(c)) and cutaneous lesions in the left leg (Figure 2(d)). Capecitabine was continued until August 2013 when new cutaneous metastases appeared in the left gluteus (1.3 cm) and right anterior breast (1.7 cm). CT studies showed interval enlargement of left pelvic lymph node, right adrenal, and pulmonary metastases (Figures 3(a) and 3(c)). New metastatic disease was identified in the thoracic and abdominal lymph nodes, the right pleura, and cutaneous tissue (Figure 3(c)). An MRI of the brain revealed multiple metastases with index lesions in the right posterior parietal lobe (Figures 3(b) and 3(d)). The patient was referred to palliative care and hospice; she expired shortly after.

3. Discussion

Treatment strategies have been reported (Table 1) and illustrate the resistant nature of EC to numerous chemotherapies with only a few options increasing patient survival. Patients treated with platinum-based, taxane-based, and tyrosine kinase inhibitors seem not to derive a substantial therapeutic benefit. The tyrosine kinase inhibitor, sunitinib, achieved 8 months of PFS after a patient progressed through prior platinum-based therapy [10]. Poor outcomes are also noted with the anthracycline antibiotic, doxorubicin, and monotherapy with cyclophosphamide; EC rapidly progressed with metastases into multiple organs and the patients expired soon after [4, 11].

Distinct tumor markers have not been characterized for EC, and other authors have reported a variety of positive IHC stains [2, 6, 13]. Thus, correlative studies of biomarkers can help develop targeted therapies aimed at specific pathways and

Table 1: Demographics, presentations, treatments, and outcomes of reported cases of metastatic EC.

Serial number	Age/sex [reference]	Presentation of primary cutaneous lesion	Metastatic sites	Treatment	Outcome
1	60/F [5]	Ulcerative, nodular, scaly, erythematous	Axillary and subclavicular LNs	Capecitabine	PFS (18 months)
2	73/M [12]	Ulcerative, nodular, erythematous	Parotid gland, cervical LNs, lung	Capecitabine	CR
3	64/F [13]	ND	Intraparotid LN	Tamoxifen	PFS (3 years)
4	43/F [10]	ND	Occipital LNs, cervical nerve root, vertebrae	Sunitinib	PFS (8 months)
5	45/F [11]	ND	Cervical LNs, bone, choroid	Doxorubicin	POD (deceased after 2 months)
6	59/F [4]	Bluish nodule, 2 cm diameter	Mediastinal LNs, lung	Cyclophosphamide	POD (deceased after 1 month)

CR: complete response; F: female; LN: lymph node; M: male; ND: not described; PFS: progression free survival; POD: progression of disease.

genetic mutations [2, 13]. For example, a case was reported of a patient with metastatic EC whose tumor biopsy revealed 100% reactivity for estrogen and progesterone receptors; the patient was started on empirical tamoxifen citrate therapy and achieved 3 years of complete remission [13]. On the other hand, our patient had negative reactivity for both of these receptors, so molecular profiles need to be identified and the prevalence assessed. A study that evaluated the molecular profiles of apocrine-eccrine carcinoma cases found that 6 of the 7 EC cases tested positive for the epidermal growth factor receptor (EGFR) mutant [14]. This highlights a potential role for clinical trials to determine the outcomes of targeted therapies that correspond to pertinent oncogene mutations [14].

To the best of our knowledge, we report the third case of metastatic EC treated with capecitabine [5, 12]. Our patient continued on capecitabine dosing from February 2012 to August 2013 without disease progression. Per RECIST version 1.1 criteria, our patient's follow-up CT study (Figures 2(c) and 2(d)) showed a partial response two months after starting capecitabine treatment. This regimen of oral capecitabine afforded efficacy and improved the patient's quality of life compared to the doublet therapy of carboplatin and paclitaxel which had more toxicities. The high mortality and morbidity rates associated with metastatic EC indicate the necessity for clinical trials to fully delineate safety and efficacy of potential future therapies [1–3, 9].

4. Conclusion

Eccrine carcinoma is an uncommon skin cancer that accompanies a poor prognosis. The clinical presentation of EC can be equivocal and result in misdiagnosis, which adversely affects patient outcomes. Standard of care treatment options for metastatic EC have not yet been developed. Further investigation into the efficacy of capecitabine treatment as monotherapy or in combination with other regimens for metastatic EC is worthwhile to improve the poor outcomes of diagnosed patients. Moreover, correlation of molecular profiles to tumor responses would provide helpful data to identify efficacious treatment regimens in the future.

Acknowledgments

The authors thank oncologic pharmacist, Ali McBride, PharmD, for providing data on drug dosing.

References

[1] A. M. Salih, F. H. Kakamad, R. A. Essa et al., "Porocarcinoma: a systematic review of literature with a single case report," *International Journal of Surgery Case Reports*, vol. 30, pp. 13–16, 2017.

[2] A. Gómez-Zubiaur, S. Medina-Montalvo, M. D. Vélez-Velázquez, and I. Polo-Rodríguez, "Eccrine porocarcinoma: patient characteristics, clinical and histopathologic features, and treatment in 7 cases," *Actas Dermo-Sifiliográficas*, vol. 108, no. 4, pp. e27–e32, 2017.

[3] S. N. Tolkachjov, A. R. Schmitt, J. G. Muzic, A. L. Weaver, and C. L. Baum, "Incidence and clinical features of rare cutaneous malignancies in Olmsted County, Minnesota, 2000 to 2010," *Dermatologic Surgery*, vol. 43, no. 1, pp. 116–124, 2017.

[4] V. K. Dave, "Eccrine sweat gland carcinoma with metastases," *British Journal of Dermatology*, vol. 86, no. 1, pp. 95–97, 1972.

[5] T. Jouary, A. Kaiafa, P. Lipinski et al., "Metastatic hidradenocarcinoma: efficacy of capecitabine," *Archives of Dermatology*, vol. 142, no. 10, pp. 1366-1367, 2006.

[6] G. Sanchez Petitto, N. M. Sarwari, P. Jain, M. Swaby, and M. Bhattacharjee, "FDG PET/CT in malignant eccrine spiradenoma," *Clinical Nuclear Medicine*, vol. 42, no. 2, pp. 125-126, 2017.

[7] Chintamani, R. D. Sharma, R. Badran, V. Singhal, S. Saxena, and A. Bansal, "Metastatic sweat gland adenocarcinoma: a clinicopathological dilemma," *World Journal of Surgical Oncology*, vol. 1, p. 13, 2003.

[8] M. Shaw, P. H. McKee, D. Lowe, and M. M. Black, "Malignant eccrine poroma: a study of twenty-seven cases," *British Journal of Dermatology*, vol. 107, no. 6, pp. 675–680, 1982.

[9] C. J. Coonley, D. P. Kelsen, A. G. Huvos, P. Schauer, and P. Sordillo, "Chemotherapy of metastatic sweat gland carcinoma. A retrospective review," *American Journal of Clinical Oncology*, vol. 8, no. 4, pp. 307–311, 1985.

[10] M. Battistella, C. Mateus, N. Lassau et al., "Sunitinib efficacy in the treatment of metastatic skin adnexal carcinomas: report of two patients with hidradenocarcinoma and trichoblastic carcinoma," *Journal of the European Academy of Dermatology and Venereology*, vol. 24, no. 2, pp. 199–203, 2010.

[11] L. R. Moura, B. Ayres, L. Feijóo, S. Romano, A. N. Odashiro, and M. N. Burnier Jr., "Presumed eccrine carcinoma

metastatic to the choroid," *Clinical and Experimental Ophthalmology*, vol. 34, no. 7, pp. 699-700, 2006.

[12] A. Lerner, A. Beckford, S. Ugent, L. Goldberg, S. Jalisi, and M. F. Demierre, "Complete response of metastatic malignant hidradenocarcinoma to capecitabine treatment," *Archives of Dermatology*, vol. 147, no. 8, pp. 998-999, 2011.

[13] U. Schröder, V. Dries, J. P. Klussmann, C. Wittekindt, and H. E. Eckel, "Successful adjuvant tamoxifen therapy for estrogen receptor-positive metastasizing sweat gland adenocarcinoma: need for a clinical trial?," *Annals of Otology, Rhinology & Laryngology*, vol. 113, no. 3, pp. 242–244, 2004.

[14] L. P. Le, D. Dias-Santagata, A. C. Pawlak et al., "Apocrine-eccrine carcinomas: molecular and immunohistochemical analyses," *PLoS One*, vol. 7, no. 10, article e47290, 2012.

43

Neuroendocrine Cancer of Rectum Metastasizing to Ovary

Sapna Vinit Amin,[1] Aswathy Kumaran,[2] Sunanda Bharatnur,[1] Akhila Vasudeva,[1] Kartik Udupa,[3] Dinesh Bangalore Venkateshiah,[4] and Shaila T. Bhat[5]

[1]*Department of OBG, Kasturba Medical College, Manipal University, Manipal 576104, India*
[2]*IVF and Reproductive Biology Centre, Maulana Azad Medical College, New Delhi 110002, India*
[3]*Department of Medical Oncology, Kasturba Medical College, Manipal University, Manipal 576104, India*
[4]*Department of Surgery, Kasturba Medical College, Manipal University, Manipal 576104, India*
[5]*Department of Pathology, Melaka Manipal Medical College, Manipal University, Manipal 576104, India*

Correspondence should be addressed to Aswathy Kumaran; astra117us@gmail.com

Academic Editor: Jorg Kleeff

Neuroendocrine carcinomas (NECs) are rare malignancies that originate from the hormone-producing cells of the body's neuroendocrine system. Rectal high grade NEC (HG-NEC) constituting less than 1% of colorectal cancers can cause large ovarian metastasis that may be the initial presenting complaint. Ovarian Krukenberg tumor from a primary rectal HG-NEC is a very unusual and exceedingly uncommon differential diagnosis for secondary ovarian malignancy. This case report describes one such extremely rare case of a woman who had presented to the gynecology department with features suggestive of ovarian malignancy and was ultimately diagnosed to have Krukenberg tumor originating from neuroendocrine cancer of rectum. We felt this is a good opportunity to spread more light on neuroendocrine neoplasms that are very rare in gynecological practice.

1. Introduction

Neuroendocrine neoplasms (NENs) are rare and fascinating neoplasms that begin in the hormone-producing cells of the body's neuroendocrine system, which is made up of cells that share the features of traditional endocrine cells (or hormone-producing cells) and nerve cells. They are multifaceted diseases that can primarily localize in many organs like the gastrointestinal tract, lungs, or brain and have various presentations. The most common neuroendocrine neoplasms are gastroenteropancreatic NENs (GEP-NENs). Based on the cell differentiation and immunohistochemistry, the GEP-NENs are differentiated into the slow growing well-differentiated neuroendocrine tumors, or WD-NETs, and the aggressive high grade/poorly differentiated neuroendocrine carcinomas, HG-NECs, that easily metastasize. The HG-NECs comprise less than one percent of the elusive neuroendocrine neoplasms (NENs).

This case report describes a woman with secondary ovarian malignancy that was neuroendocrine in origin, the primary being rectal HG-NEC. The GEP-neuroendocrine cancers metastasizing to ovaries make it extremely uncommon differential diagnosis for secondary ovarian neoplasms and hence the novelty of this case report.

Unfortunately, they have a very poor prognosis. Often only palliative chemotherapy is the therapeutic option, with 5-year survival being 12%.

2. Case Report

A 42-year-old parous woman presented with chief complaints of abdominal distension and abdominal pain over a period of the last six months to the gynecology department of our tertiary level teaching hospital in 2013. General examination yielded nothing significant. On abdominal examination, there was a solid firm mass corresponding to 24 weeks' uterine size with ill-defined borders. Bimanual pelvic examination divulged bilateral forniceal fullness and rectal examination revealed a growth on the left lateral rectal wall. Abdominopelvic ultrasound showed bilateral complex

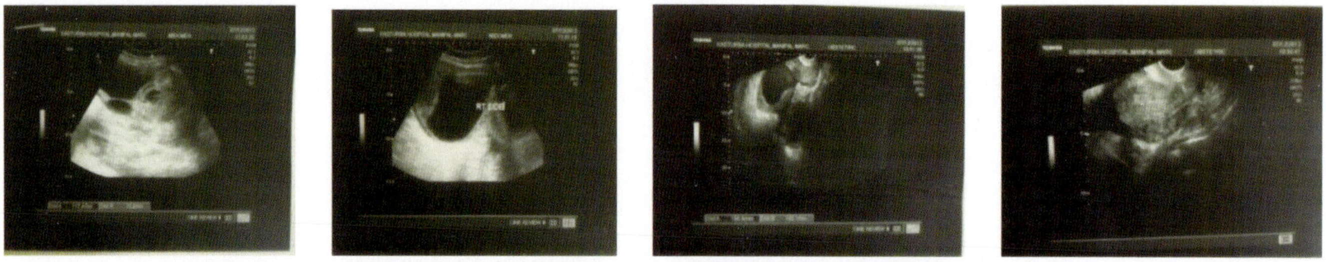

Figure 1: Ultrasonography.

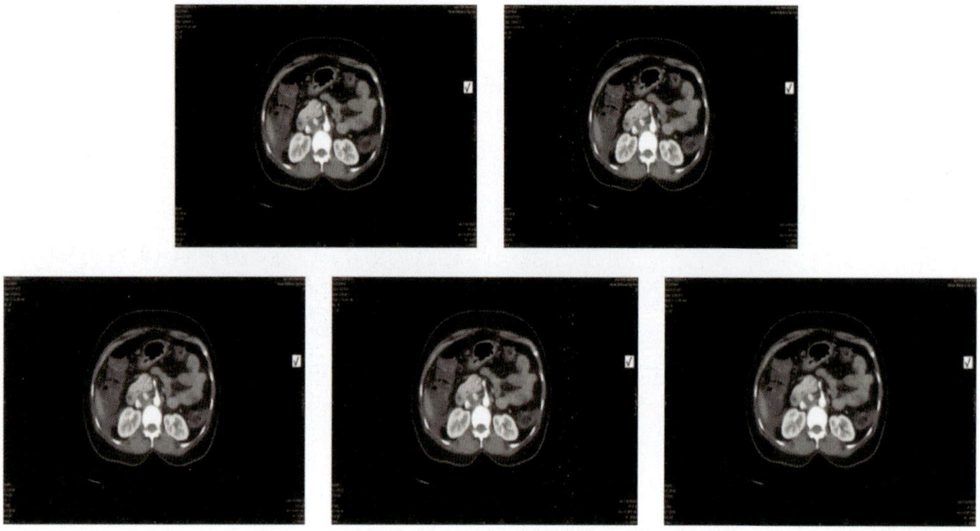

Figure 2: CT scan (abdomen and pelvis).

adnexal masses (Figure 1) as well as moderate ascites. Tumor markers showed an elevated CA 125 of 195.3 U/mL. Liver and renal function tests were normal. Thus, we made a provisional diagnosis of ovarian malignancy.

CT scan done showed two heterogeneously enhancing solid cystic lesions arising from the adnexae on either side measuring 12 × 9 cm on left and 9.7 × 8.5 cm on right, eccentric asymmetric wall thickening along the right posterolateral wall in the anal canal and rectum for a length of approximately 3-4 cm of maximal thickness 1.3 cm, and multiple hepatic metastatic lesions noted (Figure 2). This raised suspicion of primary rectal malignancy with bilateral metastatic ovarian tumor (Krukenberg) and liver metastasis.

The ascitic fluid was positive for malignant cytology. Sigmoidoscopy (Figure 3) showed ulceroproliferative growth 1 cm from anal verge from which multiple biopsies were taken. The endocrine profile was normal and not suggestive of abnormal hormone production.

Rectal and ovarian biopsies were consistent with neuroendocrine carcinoma (Figures 4 and 5). The histopathology showed poorly differentiated cells with mitotic index of 42 per 10 high power fields (HPF). Immunocytochemistry for synaptophysin and chromogranin was positive (Figures 6 and 7) and also immunolabelled as Ki67 antigen positive. The Ki67 index was 76%. Hence, we reached a diagnosis of primary neuroendocrine carcinoma (NEC) of rectum or nonfunctional high grade NEC (NF HG-NEC) of rectum with distant metastasis to ovaries. As there was ovarian and liver metastasis, she had stage IV disease as per the American Joint Committee on Cancer (AJCC) staging for colorectal cancer.

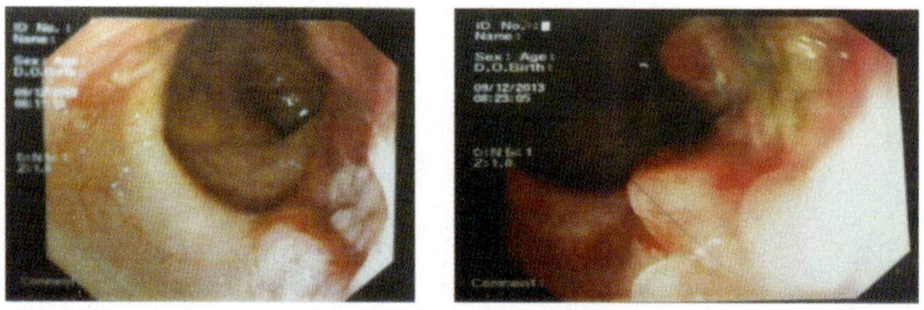

Figure 3: Sigmoidoscopy.

The nature and stage of the disease as well as poor prognosis were explained to the patient and her relatives. She received 3 courses of palliative chemotherapy (etoposide and cisplatin) and pegfilgrastim and underwent paracentesis twice in view of abdominal distension. She subsequently developed pain in right lower limb. Doppler of right lower limb was suggestive of subacute thrombosis of bifurcation of common femoral and entire superficial and popliteal veins. Patient received enoxaparin and warfarin and she recovered. After adjusting the INR, she continued warfarin. She had

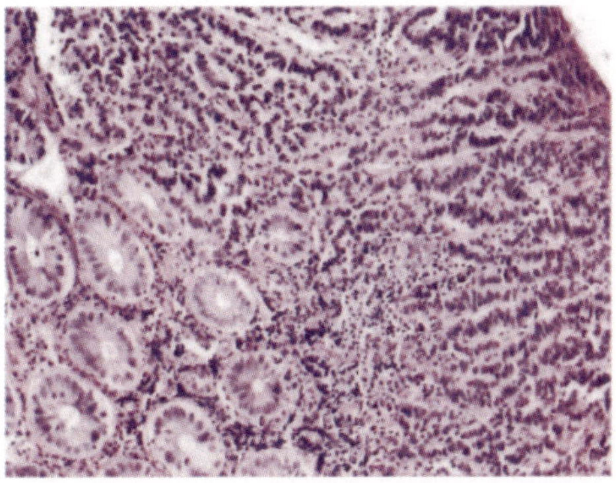

FIGURE 4: Photomicrograph showing neuroendocrine carcinoma involving the rectum.

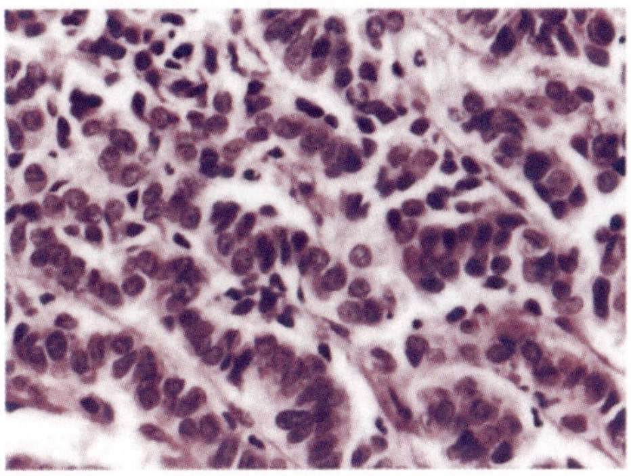

FIGURE 5: Photomicrograph showing tumor composed of cells with round to oval nuclei and stippled chromatin.

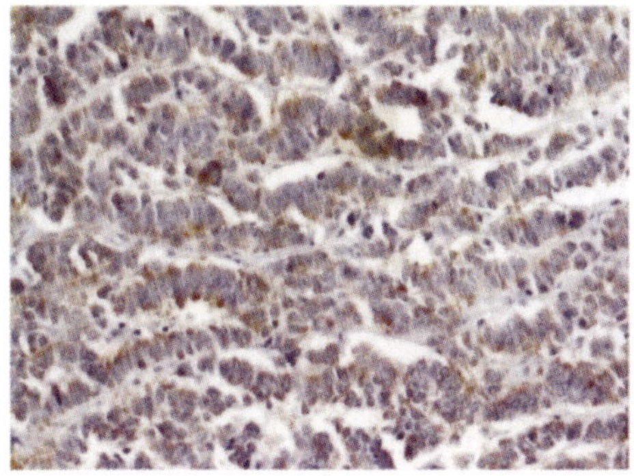

FIGURE 6: Tumor cells showing positivity for synaptophysin (immunohistochemistry for synaptophysin, ×200).

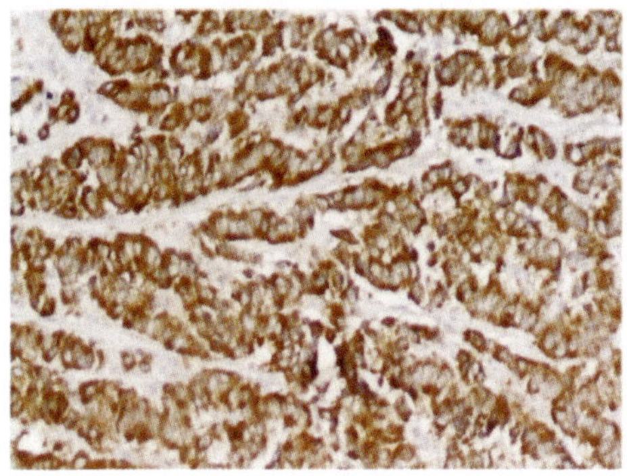

FIGURE 7: Tumor cells showing positivity for chromogranin (immunohistochemistry for chromogranin, ×200).

regular follow-ups with medical oncologists and us, the gynecologists, for one year and has had no evidence of new growths 6 months following treatment.

3. Discussion

First described by Otto Lurbarsch in 1867, the neuroendocrine neoplasms are very rare with incidence around 2.5–5 per 100,000 and prevalence of 35 per 100,000. The diagnosis and monitoring of neuroendocrine neoplasms (NENs) can be challenging [1]. The NENs may form in multiple locations throughout the body, and although they share a number of common features, the clinical presentation may vary according to site of origin, secretory potential, and histological subtype. They are usually named based on their site of origin, the usual sites being intestine, pancreas, or the lung. Neuroendocrine neoplasms may be slow growing neuroendocrine tumors (NETs) or aggressive neuroendocrine cancers (NECs) that often arise in lungs and gastrointestinal tract [1–3].

Patients may be asymptomatic or present episodically with nonspecific symptoms that can be mistaken for other more common conditions, including irritable bowel syndrome (IBS), diabetes, and asthma. Many patients may have NENs for years before they are diagnosed. In fact, the estimated time to diagnosis of certain NENs can reach 5 to 7 years.

3.1. Classification and Staging. Traditionally, the NENs were named after the site of origin, the most common being the gastrointestinal tract (GIT) and the pancreas—the gastroenteropancreatic NENs (GEP-NENs). These are again divided into the foregut, midgut, and hindgut NENs based on the embryological development of the GIT and the arterial supply [2]. Our case study pertains to hindgut NEN, specifically rectal high grade neuroendocrine carcinoma (HG-NEC).

Several organizations like the World Health Organization (WHO), the European Neuroendocrine Tumor Society (ENETS), the American Joint Committee on Cancer (AJCC), and the North American Neuroendocrine Tumor Society (NANETS) have proposed guidelines to arrive at a more specific classification system to accurately assess prognosis of these tumors [2–8].

The World Health Organization (WHO) and the European Neuroendocrine Tumor Society (ENETS) both incorporate mitotic count and Ki-67 proliferation for the classification of gastroenteropancreatic NENs (GEP-NETs). For NENs of the lungs and thymus, the WHO includes mitotic count and assessment of necrosis [2–4].

As shown in Table 1, NENs may be classified based on their histopathology, cell differentiation, mitotic index, and immunohistochemistry into mainly two groups [2–8]:

Table 1: Compiled classification and nomenclatures of NENs.

Traditional nomenclature based on grades of differentiation and histopathology		WHO; ENETs classification of NENs: Types	Mitotic index per 10 high power fields (HPF)	Immunohistochemistry Ki 67 index	Accepted nomenclature
Low	Carcinoid tumor	Neuroendocrine tumor (NET), grade 1	<2	<3%	Well-differentiated neuroendocrine tumor (WD-NET) May be functional (F) or nonfunctional (NF)
Intermediate	Atypical carcinoid tumor	Neuroendocrine tumor (NET), grade 2	2–20	3–20%	
High	Small-cell carcinoma Large-cell neuroendocrine carcinoma (NEC)	NEC grade 3, small-cell carcinoma NEC grade 3, large cell neuroendocrine carcinoma	>20	>20%	High grade neuroendocrine carcinoma (HG-NEC) (F or NF)

(i) Well-differentiated neuroendocrine tumor (WD-NET): slow growing, mostly benign—staged by AJCC/ENETS systems.

(ii) High grade neuroendocrine carcinoma (HG-NEC): poorly differentiated, invasive and highly metastatic—usually staged by AJCC.

Neuroendocrine neoplasms may also be functional (F) or nonfunctional (NF). Functional tumors produce hormones, which exert various clinical manifestations and include insulinomas, gastrinomas, and glucagonomas. Nonfunctional NENs cause symptoms like pain abdomen or bloating related to tumor or due to the presence of metastases [1]. These tumors are aggressive, and even when the primary tumor is small, there can be extensive locoregional spread and bulky metastases [1, 8].

3.2. Neuroendocrine Cancers (NECs). Poorly differentiated (PD) or high grade (HG) neuroendocrine carcinomas (NECs) encompass many NENs including small-cell carcinoma of the lung, large-cell high grade NEC of the lung, extra pulmonary small-cell/large-cell NEC, and high grade NEC with mixed features [9, 10].

Extra pulmonary HG-NECs are very rare and elusive. They may originate anywhere in the GI tract, bladder cervix, or prostate. The prognosis is poor, with median survival periods in patients with localized and distant disease of 34 and 5 months, respectively [11, 12]. The tumor cell type (i.e., small-cell versus large-cell versus mixed) does not predict survival or prognosis.

Hindgut NECs are aggressive tumors with more than 60% having metastatic disease at the time of diagnosis. The median survival interval in affected patients ranges between 5 and 14 months [12]. Rectal HG-NECs comprise less than 1% of colorectal cancers [3].

3.3. Diagnosis. Radio imaging by CT/MRI scan and directed biopsy followed by histopathologic examination and immunohistochemistry help in diagnosing the disease. Endoscopy and directed biopsy play an important role in identifying smaller lesions that are sometimes asymptomatic. Unlike WD-NETs, the HG-NECs have poor somatostatin receptor expression rendering somatostatin receptor scintigraphy useless in assessing NEC. 18F-fluorodeoxyglucose positron emission tomography appears to be the best method of evaluating disease spread and guiding further treatment [13].

NEN can be an incidental finding on routine endoscopy. NENs secrete several biomarkers like chromogranin A, 5-hydroxyindoleacetic acid, neuron specific enolase, and synaptophysin. Chromogranin A is a marker that is elevated in up to 90% of patients with NENs. They have prognostic significance and can be used to help monitor disease progression and to correlate with disease burden and survival. Another marker, synaptophysin, is a membrane component of presynaptic vesicles, found in neurons and neuroendocrine cells. It also acts as a reliable marker for NENs when combined with chromogranin A [14, 15].

The high grade NECs are characterized by a high mitotic rate (more than 20 mitoses per 10 high power fields) and extensive necrosis. In fact, most of the cancers in this family have more mitoses than these values often ranging as high as 40 to 70 mitoses per 10 high power fields. The Ki-67 proliferation index is high in gastrointestinal HG-NEC (more than 20% by definition and usually 50–90%). Sometimes HG-NECs may contain elements of adenocarcinomas or squamous cells. When these components constitute more than 30% of the tumor, we refer to these as combined NECs [8–11].

The biopsies from our patient revealed poorly differentiated cells with mitotic index of 42/10HPF and Ki67 index of 76%, as well as chromogranin and synaptophysin positivity. This led to the diagnosis of high grade neuroendocrine carcinoma, HG-NEC, of rectum, an aggressive NEN that had metastasized to ovaries and liver. The primary site was determined to be the rectum as primary ovarian NEC is usually unilateral. Thus, our patient had stage IV GEP-HG-NEC (gastroenteropancreatic high grade neuroendocrine carcinoma) of rectum. Her disease staging was as per the AJCC staging of colorectal cancer.

3.4. Treatment Modalities for Hindgut NEC. National Comprehensive Cancer Network (NCCN), North American Neuroendocrine Tumor Society (NANETS), and European Neuroendocrine Tumor Society (ENETS) have all proposed management guidelines, whose principles are similar.

3.5. Locoregional Disease Management: Multimodality Approach. The HG-NECs have high proclivity to metastasize even when they are localized, and published research evidence shows that surgery alone is rarely curative [16, 17].

(i) Definitive Chemoradiation Treatment [9]. 4–6 cycles of cisplatin/carboplatin and etoposide chemotherapy and radiation is effective in locoregional disease.

(ii) Surgery with Adjuvant Chemotherapy/Radiation [9]. The recommended regimen is optimal resection of locoregional disease followed by 4–6 cycles of cisplatin/carboplatin and etoposide chemotherapy.

Where the risk of local disease recurrence is higher, the recommended treatment is sequential radiation.

3.6. Metastatic Disease (Stage IV)/Inoperable Cases. More than half of the patients with HG-NEC have advanced metastatic disease at the time of diagnosis. The standard first-line salvage treatment for widespread poorly differentiated neuroendocrine tumors is the combination of cisplatin and etoposide [9, 18]. Palliative chemotherapy with cisplatin and etoposide for metastatic neuroendocrine carcinoma improves the survival duration [18, 19]. The general recommendation is to give 3-4 cycles of salvage chemotherapy [9]. Carboplatin based chemotherapeutic regimens have been proven successful in lung NECS, so it is assumed that they may be useful in advanced hindgut GEP HG-NECs also. Topotecan, paclitaxel, docetaxel, vinorelbine, and gemcitabine are some options for second-line management in relapsed HG-NEC [9].

Our patient had stage IV metastatic extra pulmonary HG-NEC and received 3 cycles of palliative chemotherapy with cisplatin and etoposide. The subsequent evaluation revealed complete regression of lesions and she was doing well 6 months after treatment.

4. Conclusion

High grade neuroendocrine carcinomas (HG-NECs) of rectum are very rare cancers that comprise less than 1% of colorectal cancers. More than half of these patients have metastatic disease at the time of diagnosis and may present with large ovarian Krukenberg tumor. Thus, they form a very rare differential diagnosis for secondary ovarian malignancy. Histopathology (high mitotic rate, presence of necrosis) and immunohistochemical markers like chromogranin, synaptophysin, and high Ki67 index help clinch the diagnosis. Palliative cisplatin-etoposide chemotherapy is the treatment advised in such advanced cases while surgical resection and chemoradiation is the current recommendation in locoregional disease.

Acknowledgments

The authors would like to acknowledge the faculty especially Dr. S. Archana, of the Department of Pathology, Melaka Manipal Medical College, for providing generous academic insight and contributions to this case study. In addition, They would like to acknowledge the faculty from the Surgery Department, Kasturba Medical College, Manipal University, Manipal, for their support and involvement in case management.

References

[1] K. Oberg and D. Castellano, "Current knowledge on diagnosis and staging of neuroendocrine tumors," *Cancer and Metastasis Reviews*, vol. 30, supplement 1, pp. 3–7, 2011.

[2] J. D. Smith and G. Nandakumar, "Hindgut neuroendocrine neoplasia," *Indian Journal of Surgical Oncology*, vol. 7, no. 1, pp. 73–78, 2016.

[3] J. D. Smith, D. L. Reidy, K. A. Goodman, J. Shia, and G. M. Nash, "A retrospective review of 126 high-grade neuroendocrine carcinomas of the colon and rectum," *Annals of Surgical Oncology*, vol. 21, no. 9, pp. 2956–2962, 2014.

[4] F. T. Bosman, F. Carneiro, R. H. Hruban, and N. D. Theise, *World Health Organization Classification of Tumours of the Digestive System*, IARC, Lyon, France, 2010.

[5] G. Rindi, G. Klöppel, H. Alhman et al., "TNM staging of foregut (neuro)endocrine tumors: a consensus proposal including a grading system," *Virchows Archiv*, vol. 449, no. 4, pp. 395–401, 2006.

[6] W. D. Travis, E. Brambilla, H. K. Muller-Hermelink, and C. C. Harris, *World Health Organization Classification of Tumours of the Lung, Pleura, Thymus and Heart*, IARC, Lyon, France, 2004.

[7] M. H. Kulke, L. B. Anthony, D. L. Bushnell et al., "NANETS treatment guidelines: Well-differentiated neuroendocrine tumors of the stomach and pancreas," *Pancreas*, vol. 39, no. 6, pp. 735–752, 2010.

[8] V. T. DeVita, T. S. Lawrence, and S. A. Rosenberg, *Cancer—Principles and Practice of Oncology*, Lippincott Williams and Wilkins, 8th edition, 2008.

[9] J. R. Strosberg, D. Coppola, D. S. Klimstra et al., "The NANETS consensus guidelines for the diagnosis and management of poorly differentiated (high-grade) extrapulmonary neuroendocrine carcinomas," *Pancreas*, vol. 39, no. 6, pp. 799–800, 2010.

[10] J. Shia, L. H. Tang, M. R. Weiser et al., "Is non small cell type high-grade neuroendocrine carcinoma of the tubular gastrointestinal tract a distinct disease entity?" *The American Journal of Surgical Pathology*, vol. 32, no. 5, pp. 719–731, 2008.

[11] J. Strosberg, A. Nasir, D. Coppola, M. Wick, and L. Kvols, "Correlation between grade and prognosis in metastatic gastroenteropancreatic neuroendocrine tumors," *Human Pathology*, vol. 40, no. 9, pp. 1262–1268, 2009.

[12] J. C. Yao, M. Hassan, A. Phan et al., "One hundred years after carcinoid: epidemiology of and prognostic factors for neuroendocrine tumors in 35,825 cases in the United States," *Journal of Clinical Oncology*, vol. 26, no. 18, pp. 3063–3072, 2008.

[13] A. Koumarianou, E. Chatzellis, G. Boutzios, N. Tsavaris, and G. Kaltsas, "Current concepts in the diagnosis and management of poorly differentiated gastrointestinal neuroendocrine carcinomas," *Endokrynologia Polska*, vol. 64, no. 1, pp. 60–72, 2013.

[14] C. M. Korse, J. M. G. Bonfrer, N. K. Aaronson et al., "Chromogranin A as an alternative to 5-hydroxyindoleacetic acid in the evaluation of symptoms during treatment of patients with neuroendocrine tumors," *Neuroendocrinology*, vol. 89, no. 3, pp. 296–301, 2009.

[15] P. Ferolla, A. Faggiano, G. Mansueto et al., "The biological characterization of neuroendocrine tumors: the role of neuroendocrine markers," *Journal of Endocrinological Investigation*, vol. 31, no. 3, pp. 277–286, 2008.

[16] B. Brenner, M. A. Shah, M. Gonen, D. S. Klimstra, J. Shia, and D. P. Kelsen, "Small-cell carcinoma of the gastrointestinal tract: a retrospective study of 64 cases," *British Journal of Cancer*, vol. 90, no. 9, pp. 1720–1726, 2004.

[17] J. Smith and D. Reidy-Lagunes, "The management of extrapulmonary poorly differentiated (high-grade) neuroendocrine carcinomas," *Seminars in Oncology*, vol. 40, no. 1, pp. 100–108, 2013.

[18] C. G. Moertel, L. K. Kvols, M. J. O'Connell, and J. Rubin, "Treatment of neuroendocrine carcinomas with combined etoposide and cisplatin. Evidence of major therapeutic activity in the anaplastic variants of these neoplasms," *Cancer*, vol. 68, no. 2, pp. 227–232, 1991.

[19] E. Mitry, E. Baudin, M. Ducreux et al., "Treatment of poorly differentiated neuroendocrine tumours with etoposide and cisplatin," *British Journal of Cancer*, vol. 81, no. 8, pp. 1351–1355, 1999.

Chinese Medicine Treatment for Afatinib-Induced Paronychia

Pei-Yuu Yang[1] and Chen-Jei Tai[1,2]

[1]*Department of Traditional Chinese Medicine, Taipei Medical University Hospital, Taipei 11031, Taiwan*
[2]*Department of OB/GYN, School of Medicine, College of Medicine, Taipei Medical University, Taipei 11031, Taiwan*

Correspondence should be addressed to Chen-Jei Tai; chenjtai@tmu.edu.tw

Academic Editor: Jeanine M. Buchanich

Afatinib (Gilotrif™) is widely used to treat patients with mutant activating epidermal growth factor receptor- (EGFR-) dependent lung adenocarcinoma; however, it has various adverse side effects. Here, we report a patient with afatinib-induced paronychia. After Chinese medicine treatment with the well-known anticancer Chinese herbs, Jen-Ren-Hwo-Minq-Saan, and decoction of Ban-Zhi-Lian *(Scutellaria barbata)* with Bai-Hua-She-She-Cao (*Hedyotis diffusa* Willd), patient's condition was significantly improved. This shows that these Chinese medicines can not only be used in cancer treatment but also be used in the afatinib-induced paronychia.

1. Introduction

Lung cancer is one of the most commonly diagnosed cancers and is the leading cause of cancer deaths around the world. Non-small-cell lung cancer (NSCLC) accounts for about 80% of all lung cancers and is often diagnosed at the late stage [1]. NSCLC comprises non-squamous-cell carcinoma (i.e., adenocarcinoma, large-cell carcinoma, and other cell types) and squamous cell carcinoma [1]. Some patients with lung adenocarcinoma have common activating epidermal growth factor receptor (EGFR) mutations: deletions in exon 19 and exon 21 L858R substitution mutations [2]. Thus, targeting EGFR has become an important strategy in the treatment of NSCLC. Specifically, oral afatinib (Gilotrif) is approved for the first-line treatment for patients who have metastatic NSCLC with EGFR exon 19 deletions or exon 21 (L858R) substitution mutations as detected by an FDA-approved test. The recommended dosage of afatinib is 40 mg once daily; treatment should be continued until disease progression or until afatinib is no longer tolerated [3]. Adverse events are generally manageable with dose reductions and delays. Among afatinib recipients, the most common treatment-related adverse events (all grades, incidence of >10%) included diarrhea (95.2% of patients), rash/acne (89.1%), stomatitis/mucositis (72.1%), paronychia (56.8%), dry skin (29.3%), decreased appetite (20.5%), pruritus (18.8%), nausea (17.9%), fatigue (17.5%), vomiting (17.0%), epistaxis (13.1%), and cheilitis (12.2%) [4]. Many people interrupt their therapies because of the seriously adverse side effects. Therefore, reducing the adverse side effects will greatly improve patients' outcome. This study reports that Chinese medicine can cure paronychia induced by afatinib.

2. Case Report

A 42-year-old female was diagnosed with adenocarcinoma in her lower and middle lobes of her right lung and bone, liver, and brain metastasis in 2015/8. She started taking afatinib from 2015/8/18. Then paronychia, oral ulcer, and diarrhea symptoms appeared.

We can see paronychia on both of her hands and left foot in the photos in 2015/9. From the pictures she took, we can see paronychia on the lateral side of the middle and ring finger of her left, both sides of the ring finger of her right, ulcers, and hypertrophic granulation tissue on the lateral side of the first and middle toes of her left foot (Figure 1).

The patient came to Chinese Medicine Clinics on 2015/10/1. Her chief complaint was paronychia with pain and tissue fluid exudation. We prescribed to her concentrated scientific herbal medicine of Jen-Ren-Hwo-Minq-Saan and Chinese herb decoction of Ban-Zhi-Lian with Bai-Hua-She-She-Cao. The dosage of concentrated scientific herbal

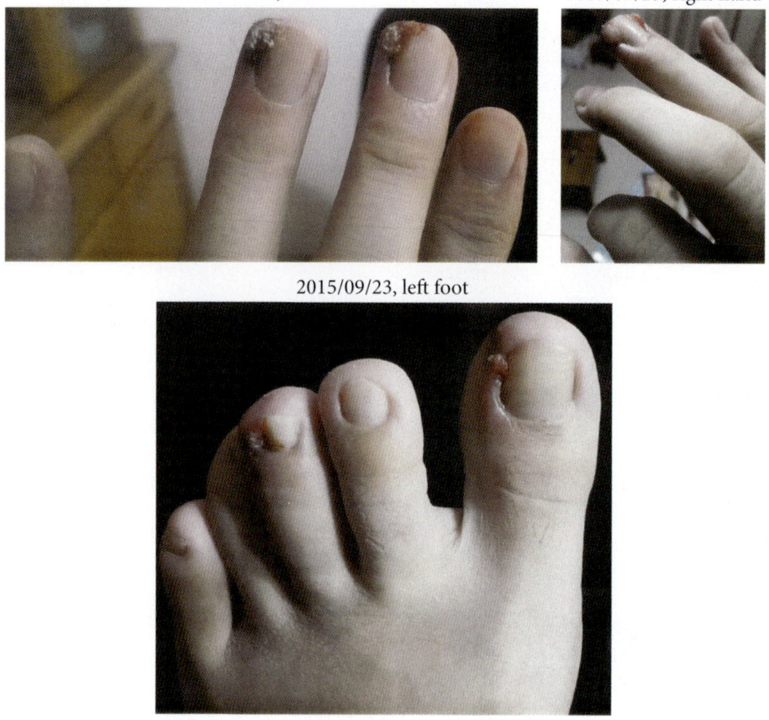

FIGURE 1

medicine, Jen-Ren-Hwo-Ming-Sann, was 6 grams per day in 3 divided doses taken after each meal. Besides, the dosage of crude drugs in each pack of decoction of Ban-Zhi-Liagn with Bai-Hua-She-She-Cao was 9.375 grams each. The patient had to take three packs every day. She took all these medicine above during the therapy.

To monitor whether the Chinese medicines affect the afatinib treatment, a blood test was issued. Her blood test report on 2015/10/19 was as follows: CEA: 134, WBC: 6520, GOT: 28, and GPT: 24.

The patient came back to clinic on 2015/10/22 with the pictures she took on 2015/10/3, when she had taken the medicine for 3 days (Figure 2).

We could observe that the granulation tissue almost disappeared and ulcer had improved, although the wound had not healed yet. Therefore, she continued taking the concentration scientific herbal medicine of Jen-Ren-Hwo-Minq-Saan and decoction of Ban-Zhi-Lian and Bai-Hua-She-She-Cao. The condition of the paronychia was recorded on 2015/10/22 and is shown in Figure 3.

We can find that the wounds on the left foot also continue improving with the pictures taken by patient herself in 2015/11/4 (Figure 4).

The wounds on both hands were almost cured in the pictures in 2015/12/10 (Figure 5). We advised her to continue the treatment.

The pictures showed that paronychia had been completely cured in 2016/1/7 (Figure 6). And her blood test report on 2016/1/18 was as follows: CEA: 124.4, WBC: 5910, and GOT: 17.

After the treatment of paronychia, she continued taking these medicines for controlling the tumor cells, and the paronychia never returns.

3. Discussion

The most tormenting side effect of afatinib for this patient is paronychia. From Figures 1–6, we can easily observe the efficacy of the Chinese medicine treatments. After the treatment, paronychia had almost been cured in two months. Note that the reduction of CEA showed that the Chinese medicine did not influence the effect of afatinib. This patient did not take any antibiotics or use topical medication to deal with paronychia during the treatment of traditional Chinese medicine. Because the patient keeps taking afatinib, we will not discontinue her Chinese medicine treatment even though her paronychia was cured. Therefore, we do not know whether the paronychia will recur after stopping taking Chinese medicine, but it is quite possible.

Zhen Ren Huo Ming Yin, also called Xian Fang Huo Ming Yin, is a traditional Chinese herbal complex medicine. It was often used to treat skin illness, such as skin ulcers, sores, and wounds. Nowadays, researches have shown the efficacy of Zhen Ren Huo Ming Yin on ulcerative colitis [5] and fibrocystic disease of the breast [6].

Bai-Hua-She-She-Cao, *Hedyotis diffusa* Willd, is a well-known Chinese herb. It has neuroprotective constituents [7] and antitumor activity [8]. *Hedyotis diffusa* has been proved to inhibit tumor angiogenesis [9] and fight against HepG2 carcinoma cells mediated via apoptosis [10]. *Hedyotis diffusa*

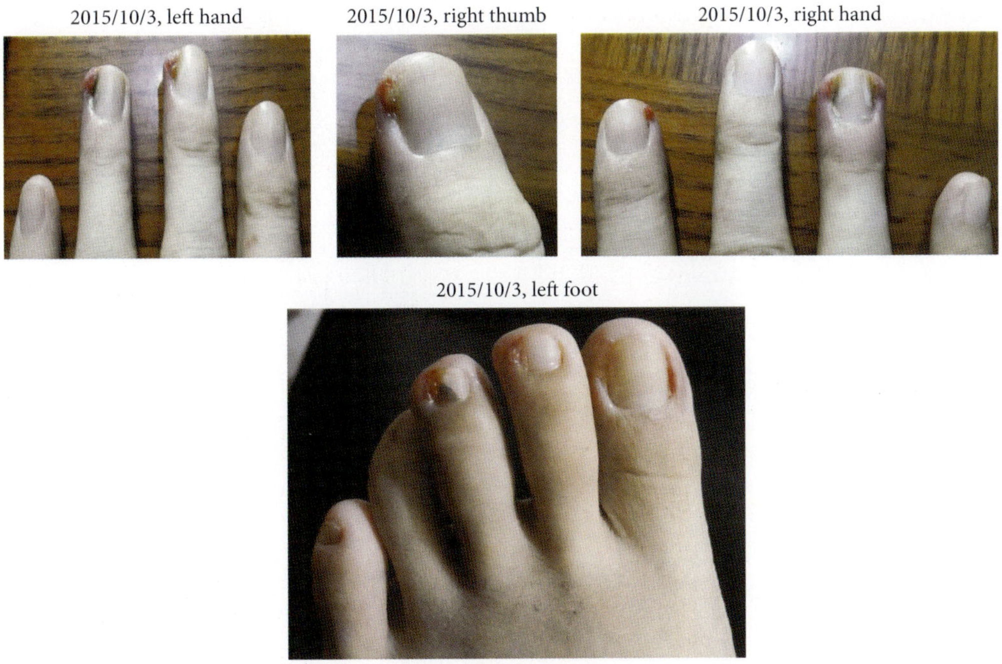

Figure 2

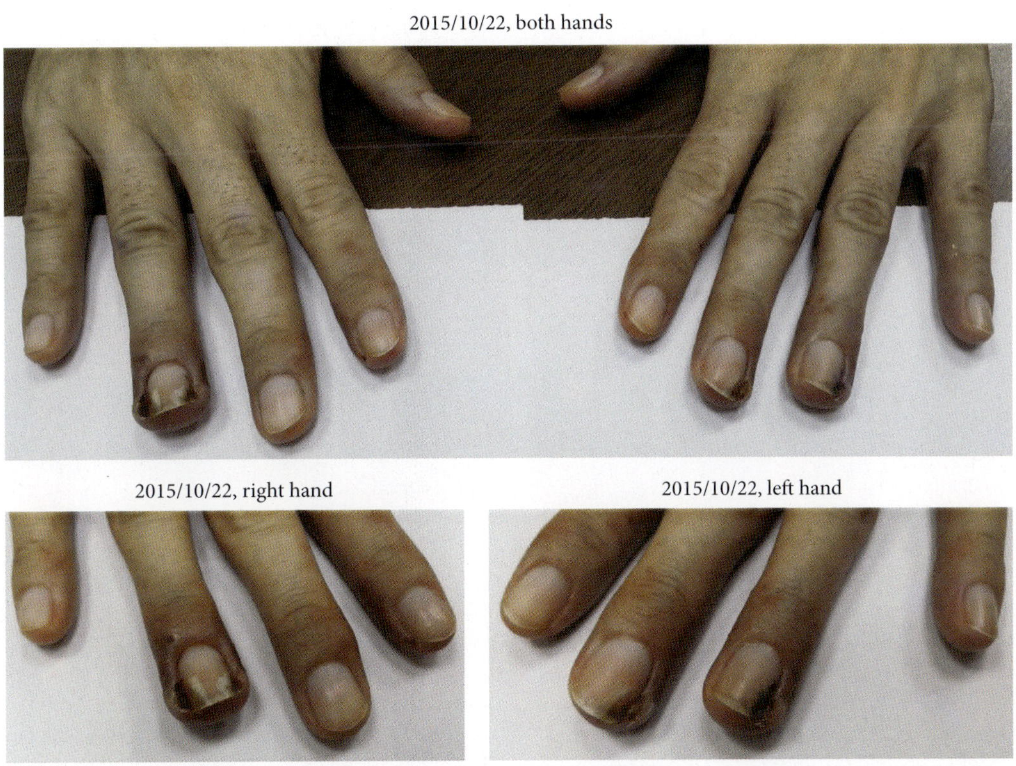

Figure 3

extract can inactivate human colorectal cancer cells [11] and breast cancer cells [12].

Ban-Zhi-Lian, *Scutellaria barbata*, is a traditional Chinese herbal medicine originated from southern China and is widely used as an anti-inflammatory and diuretic herb. Several studies have indicated that extracts of *Scutellaria barbata* have growth inhibition effects on a number of human cancers. Treatment of lung cancer, digestive system cancers, hepatoma, breast cancer, and chorioepithelioma by *Scutellaria barbata* extracts was reported [13].

In addition, many papers show the efficacy of *Hedyotis diffusa* plus *Scutellaria barbata* on multiple types of cancers.

2015/11/4, left foot

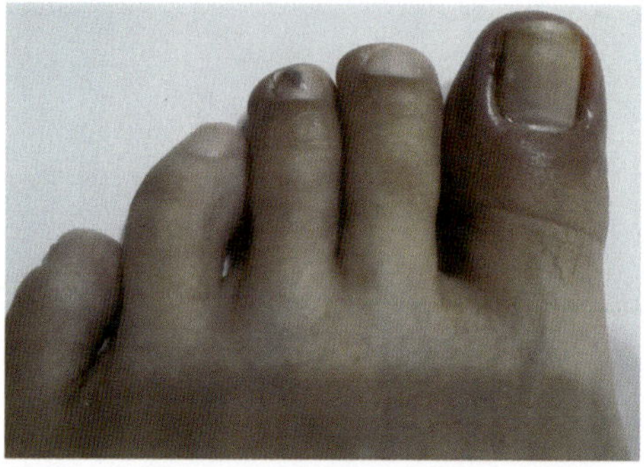

Figure 4

2015/12/10, both hands

2015/12/10, right hand

2015/12/10, left hand

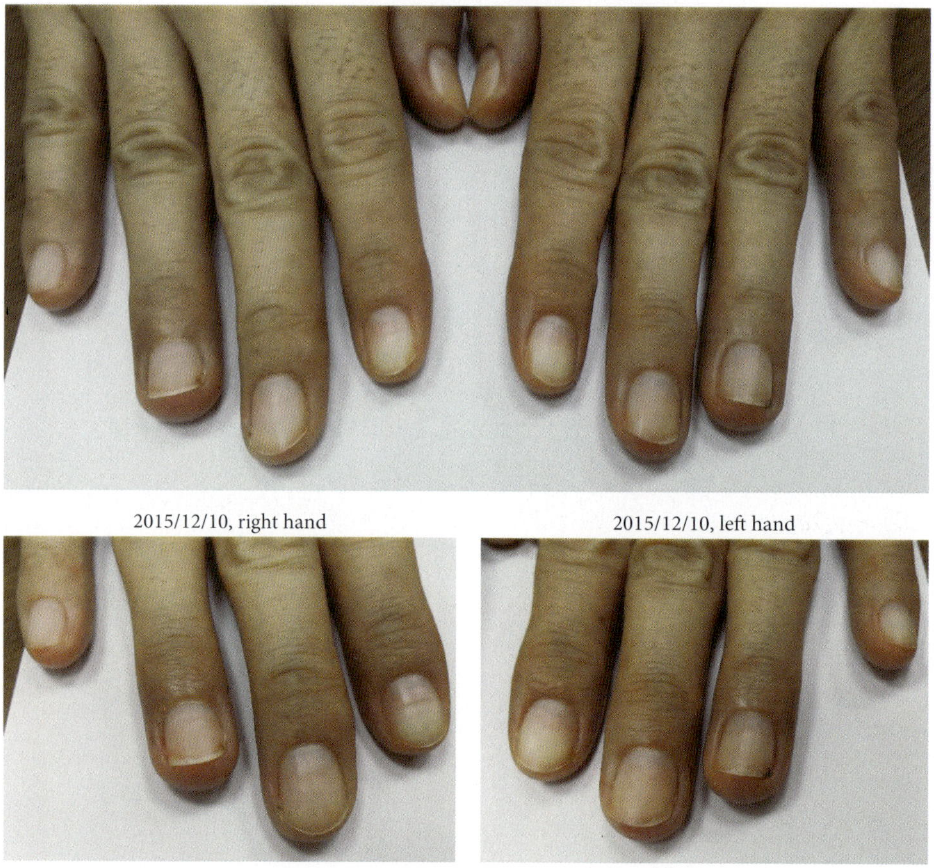

Figure 5

Hedyotis diffusa plus *Scutellaria barbata* can induce apoptosis in bladder cancer cells [14] and has been used for postsurgery colon cancer patients in Taiwan [15]. This kind of combined remedy is the core treatment for breast cancer patients in Chinese medicine [16].

4. Conclusion

The Chinese medicines that were used to treat paronychia in this report are well-known anticancer drugs. However, the efficacy for these anticancer drugs to treat paronychia induced by the targeted therapy, afatinib, was never reported to our knowledge. With the ability to cure afatinib-induced paronychia, we are confident that, with the combination of Jen-Ren-Hwo-Minq-Saan and decoction of Ban-Zhi-Lian with Bai-Hua-She-She-Cao, we can relieve the patients from severe side effect and reduce the rate for patients from dropping the afatinib treatment. Paronychia was almost completely recovered in two months in this case, but more cases are required to realize how long in average should the Chinese medicine be prescribed for paronychia sufferers.

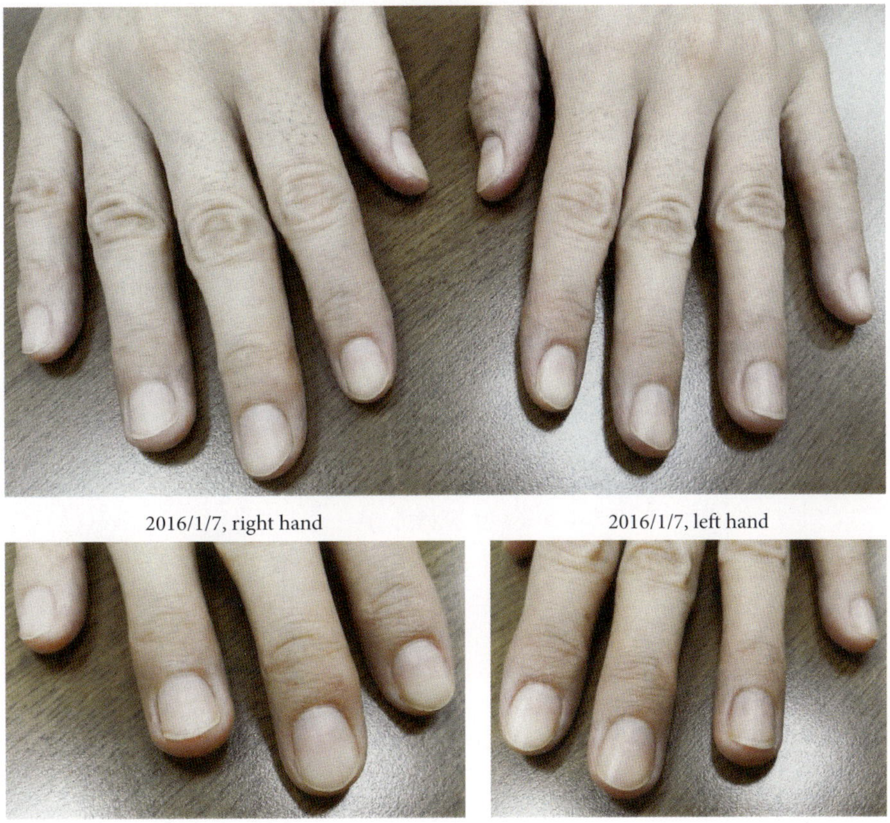

FIGURE 6

References

[1] V. Hirsh, "Afatinib (BIBW 2992) development in non-small-cell lung cancer," *Future Oncology*, vol. 7, no. 7, pp. 817–825, 2011.

[2] B.-C. Liao, C.-C. Lin, and J. C.-H. Yang, "First-line management of EGFR-mutated advanced lung adenocarcinoma: Recent developments," *Drugs*, vol. 73, no. 4, pp. 357–369, 2013.

[3] Boehringer Ingelheim Pharmaceuticals Inc. Gilotrif™ (afatinib) tablets, for oral use: US prescribing information. 2013.

[4] L. V. Sequist, J. C.-H. Yang, N. Yamamoto et al., "Phase III study of afatinib or cisplatin plus pemetrexed in patients with metastatic lung adenocarcinoma with EGFR mutations," *Journal of Clinical Oncology*, vol. 31, no. 27, pp. 3327–3334, 2013.

[5] L. Cai, L. Yun-mei, and W. Shu-qin, "Research status of traditional Chinese medicine treatment of ulcerative colitis," *Heilongjiang Medical Journal*, vol. 5, p. 67, 2015.

[6] G. Shao-bo, "Song Ai-li, Modified Xian Fang Huo Ming Yin in treatment of cyclomatopathy," *Journal of Liaoning University of Traditional Chinese Medicine*, vol. 10, no. 10, pp. 83-84, 2008.

[7] Y. Kim, E. J. Park, J. Kim, Y.-B. Kim, S. R. Kim, and Y. C. Kim, "Neuroprotective constituents from Hedyotis diffusa," *Journal of Natural Products*, vol. 64, no. 1, pp. 75–78, 2001.

[8] H.-Z. Lee, D.-T. Bau, C.-L. Kuo, R.-Y. Tsai, Y.-C. Chen, and Y.-H. Chang, "Clarification of the phenotypic characteristics and antitumor activity of hedyotis diffusa," *American Journal of Chinese Medicine*, vol. 39, no. 1, pp. 201–213, 2011.

[9] J. Lin, L. Wei, W. Xu, Z. Hong, X. Liu, and J. Peng, "Effect of Hedyotis Diffusa Willd extract on tumor angiogenesis," *Molecular Medicine Reports*, vol. 4, no. 6, pp. 1283–1288, 2011.

[10] Y.-L. Li, J. Zhang, D. Min, Z. Hongyan, N. Lin, and Q.-S. Li, "Anticancer effects of 1,3-dihydroxy-2-methylanthraquinone and the ethyl acetate fraction of hedyotis diffusa willd against HepG2 carcinoma cells mediated via apoptosis," *PLoS ONE*, vol. 11, no. 4, Article ID e0151502, 2016.

[11] J. M. Lin, Q. Y. Li, H. W. Chen, H. Lin, Z. J. Lai, and J. Peng, "*Hedyotis diffusa* willd. extract suppresses proliferation and induces apoptosis via IL-6-inducible STAT3 pathway inactivation in human colorectal cancer cells," *Oncology Letters*, vol. 9, no. 4, pp. 1962–1970, 2015.

[12] Z. Liu, M. Liu, and J. Li, "Methylanthraquinone from *Hedyotis diffusa* WILLD induces Ca^{2+}-mediated apoptosis in human breast cancer cells," *Toxicology in Vitro*, vol. 24, no. 1, pp. 142–147, 2010.

[13] X. Yin, J. Zhou, Y. Zhang, D. Xing, and C. Jie, "Anticancer activity and mechanism of Scutellaria barbata extract on human lung cancer cell line A549," *Life Sciences*, vol. 75, no. 18, pp. 2233–2244, 2004.

[14] L.-T. Pan, Y. Sheung, W.-P. Guo, Z.-B. Rong, and Z.-M. Cai, "Hedyotis diffusa plus scutellaria barbata induce bladder cancer cell apoptosis by inhibiting akt signaling pathway through downregulating miR-155 expression," *Evidence-based Complementary and Alternative Medicine*, vol. 2016, Article ID 9174903, 10 pages, 2016.

[15] T. Chao, P. Fu, C. Chang, S. Chang, F. Chiahung Mao, and C. Lin, "Prescription patterns of Chinese herbal products for post-surgery colon cancer patients in Taiwan," *Journal of Ethnopharmacology*, vol. 155, no. 1, pp. 702–708, 2014.

[16] Y.-C. Yeh, H.-Y. Chen, S.-H. Yang, Y.-H. Lin, J.-H. Chiu, and J.-L. Chen, "Hedyotis diffusa combined with scutellaria barbata are the core treatment of Chinese herbal medicine used for breast cancer patients: a population-based study," *Evidence-Based Complementary and Alternative Medicine*, vol. 2014, Article ID 202378, 9 pages, 2014.

A Case of Hyperammonemia Associated with High Dihydropyrimidine Dehydrogenase Activity

Keiki Nagaharu,[1] Kenji Ikemura,[2] Yoshiki Yamashita,[3] Hiroyasu Oda,[3] Mikiya Ishihara,[3] Yumiko Sugawara,[3] Satoshi Tamaru,[3] Toshiro Mizuno,[3] and Naoyuki Katayama[3]

[1]*Department of Hematology and Oncology, Suzuka General Hospital, Yamanohana, Yasuzuka, Suzuka, Mie Prefecture 1275-53, Japan*
[2]*Department of Pharmacy, Mie University Hospital, Edobashi 2-174, Tsu, Mie Prefecture 514-8507, Japan*
[3]*Department of Hematology and Oncology, Mie University Graduate School of Medicine, Edobashi 2-174, Tsu, Mie Prefecture 514-8507, Japan*

Correspondence should be addressed to Keiki Nagaharu; keiki.nagaharu@gmail.com

Academic Editor: Raffaele Palmirotta

Over the past decades, 5-Fluorouracil (5-FU) has been widely used to treat several types of carcinoma, including esophageal squamous cell carcinoma. In addition to its common side effects, including diarrhea, mucositis, neutropenia, and anemia, 5-FU treatment has also been reported to cause hyperammonemia. However, the exact mechanism responsible for 5-FU-induced hyperammonemia remains unknown. We encountered an esophageal carcinoma patient who developed hyperammonemia when receiving 5-FU-containing chemotherapy but did not exhibit any of the other common adverse effects of 5-FU treatment. At the onset of hyperammonemia, laboratory tests revealed high dihydropyrimidine dehydrogenase (DPD) activity and rapid 5-FU clearance. Our findings suggested that 5-FU hypermetabolism may be one of the key mechanisms responsible for hyperammonemia during 5-FU treatment.

1. Introduction

In 1957, Heidelberger et al. reported the use of 5-FU as a new antitumoral drug [1], and at present, 5-FU is one of the most commonly used anticancer drugs around the world. A combination of cisplatin and 5-FU is often used for first-line chemotherapy in unresectable cases of advanced esophageal carcinoma. As is the case for other anticancer drugs, the most common side effects of 5-FU, such as diarrhea, mucositis, neutropenia, and anemia, are due to its effects on the bone marrow and gastrointestinal epithelium. These common adverse effects are observed in more than half of the patients treated with 5-FU-containing regimens [2]. On the other hand, the prevalence of 5-FU-induced hyperammonemia has been reported to range within 5.7%–7.0% [3–5]. The exact mechanism responsible for 5-FU-induced hyperammonemia remains unknown. Herein, we report a patient who developed recurrent hyperammonemia.

2. Case Report

A 60-year-old man presented with a 1-month history of progressively worsening discomfort during swallowing. His medical history included treated gastric cancer (5 years earlier) and emphysema. The patient reported that he had smoked approximately 20 cigarettes per day since the age of 20. Laboratory tests did not detect hepatic disorders or renal problems. Upper gastrointestinal endoscopy revealed an ulcerative lesion with elevated distinct borders in the lower esophagus, and endoscopic ultrasound detected serosal invasion. The lesion was diagnosed as a squamous cell carcinoma from a biopsy. A positron emission tomography (PET) examination confirmed lung metastasis. As a result, the patient was clinically staged as cT3N1M1 and was treated with 5-FU and cisplatin. However, his obstructive swallowing problems continued to worsen. We next administered concurrent radiotherapy as a palliative treatment. The treatment regimen (FP regimen) consisted of 5-FU at a dose of

Table 1: Laboratory findings.

	Day of onset	The following day	[Normal range]
[Peripheral blood]			
WBC	8080/μL	5180/μL	3500–9000/μL
RBC	$382 \times 10^4/\mu L$	$414 \times 10^4/\mu L$	$376–500 \times 10^4/\mu L$
Hb	15.3 g/dL	12.9 g/dL	11.3–15.2 g/dL
Ht	33.3%	37.0%	33.4–44.9%
MCV	87.2 fL	89.4 fL	82.7–101 fL
Plt	$26.3 \times 10^4/\mu L$	$25.6 \times 10^4/\mu L$	$13.0–36.9 \times 10^4/\mu L$
[Coagulation test]			
APTT	31.0 sec		25.0–45.0 sec
PT	14.2 sec		13.5–15.0 sec
D-dimer	0.66 μg/mL		<0.50 μg/mL
[Biochemistry]			
TP	6.2 g/dL	5.6 g/dL	6.5–8.5 g/dL
Alb	3.4 g/dL	3.4 g/dL	4.1–5.3 g/dL
AST	20 IU/L	20 IU/L	10–35 IU/L
ALT	25 IU/L	23 IU/L	10–35 IU/L
LDH	182 IU/L	155 IU/L	110–225 IU/L
γ-GTP		50 IU/L	8–60 IU/L
T-Bil	0.6 mg/dL	0.60 mg/dL	0.2–1.3 mg/dL
Glu	101 mg/dL		80–120 mg/dL
BUN	34 mg/dL	31 mg/dL	9.6–22.0 mg/dL
Cre	0.95 mg/dL	1.09 mg/dL	<1.20 mg/dL
Na	129 mEq/L	136 mEq/L	138–145 mEq/L
K	2.6 mEq/L	3.1 mEq/L	3.4–4.7 mEq/L
Cl	93 mEq/L	97 mEq/L	99–108 mEq/L
CRP	0.47 mg/dL	0.44 mg/dL	<0.30 mg/dL
NH^3	131 μg/dL	44 μg/dL	<18 μg/dL
5-FU concentration	13 ng/mL	<10 ng/mL	600 ng/mL (steady state)

Laboratory findings revealed hyperammonemia and mild hyponatremia. Serum concentration of 5-FU was low.

800 mg/m^2 on days 1–5 and cisplatin at a dose of 80 mg/m^2 on day 1 and was repeated every 28 days. The patient did not exhibit specific adverse effects during the first course of treatment. After the completion of that, a second course of the same regimen was started. However, the patient fell unconscious 72 hours after the initiation of treatment.

On physical examination, he was unconscious (Glasgow Coma Scale: E1V3M5) and afebrile and had a pulse rate of 69 bpm and a blood pressure of 111/61 mmHg. There were no signs of mucositis. A neurological examination did not detect paralysis or abnormal reflexes. The patient's laboratory data revealed hyperammonemia, mild hyponatremia, and a high blood urea nitrogen (BUN) level. Other findings are shown in Table 1. Radiological assessments including computed tomography (CT) and magnetic resonance imaging (MRI) scans of the patient's head did not detect any apparent cause of the patient's condition. On the following day, his condition normalized with only normal saline hydration, and he did not exhibit sequelae. We subsequently diagnosed the patient with 5-FU-related hyperammonemia.

Table 2: Urinary analysis of dihydrouracil and uracil.

	Dihydrouracil	Uracil	Ratio
Patient's value	5.325 μg/mL	0.495 μg/mL	10.75
Normal range [6]	1.7–13.1 μg/mL	4–30 μg/mL	0.3–0.77

Urinary DHU/U was much higher than normal. These findings supported the high activity of dihydropyrimidine dehydrogenase.

At the onset of hyperammonemia, the patient's serum 5-FU concentration during the unconscious state was significantly lower (13 ng/mL) than the normal range (500–600 ng/mL). In 5-FU metabolism, approximately 80% of infused 5-FU is degraded by DPD, the initial and rate-limiting enzyme in the catabolism of pyrimidine bases, and this process produces ammonia as the end product. Due to the rapid clearance of 5-FU, we evaluated the patient's DPD activity using the urinary dihydrouracil to uracil ratio (DHU/U). Table 2 shows the patient's DPD activity and a high DHU/U ratio, which indicated that his 5-FU metabolism had not been suppressed.

We concluded that continuing with the FP regimen would be harmful to the patient. He was subsequently treated with taxane-based treatment, which resulted in PD. He died approximately six months after being diagnosed due to cancer progression.

3. Discussion

Our patient developed hyperammonemia without other adverse effects. Laboratory examination revealed a high DHU/U ratio. Although urinary DHU/U is an indirect method to assess DPD activity, his high DPD activity was supported by his undetectably low serum 5-FU concentration and the absence of most of the common adverse effects of 5-FU treatment (including diarrhea, mucositis, neutropenia, and anemia). These findings suggested that rapid metabolism of 5-FU may cause faster than normal accumulation of ammonia.

Previous studies have investigated the relationship between DPD activity and 5-FU toxicity [7–11]. Clinically severe 5-FU toxicity was reported in a family with DPD deficiency [12]. Moreover, relatively low DPD activity was reported to be a risk factor for severe cytotoxic adverse effects [7]. On the other hand, Kim et al. described a case of hyperammonemia with high DPD synthesis, similar to our case [13]. Although the etiology for acquisition of high DPD is unknown, Li et al. demonstrated that exposure to 5-FU causes resistance to 5-FU, with upregulation of DPD activity, using a human colorectal carcinoma xenograft nude mouse model [14]. In the present and previous cases, the first administration of 5-FU may have induced upregulation of DPD activity.

There are some limitations in our hypothesis. First, we were unable to assess the actual DPD activity in the liver tissue. Because it was reported that hepatic DPD activity is correlated with the urinary DHU/U ratio, we indirectly analyzed the patient's DPD activity using the urinary DHU/U ratio, as was performed in a previous study [6]. Although urine and salivary DHU/U ratios were reported to be good predictors of the adverse effect of 5-FU [7, 15], further investigation is required to establish a method for precise DPD evaluation. Second, the DPD activity before treatment was not evaluated. Thus, we were unable to identify whether the high DPD of our case was congenital or acquired. As mentioned above, the absence of hyperammonemia during his first course suggested acquired high DPD. However, previous reports also performed the same regimen without incidence of hyperammonemia [13]. This suggests that other factors may be required for development of hyperammonemia. Third, we did not evaluate genetic analysis of DPD and other enzymes in our case. Kim et al. reported genetic mutations of thymidylate synthetase which is the main target enzyme of 5-FU in their hyperammonemia cases [16]. Not only catabolic enzymes but also the target of 5-FU may play a role in hyperammonemia.

In conclusion, the present case suggested that high DPD activity may be a trigger of hyperammonemia. While this report suggested a possible mechanism for such hyperammonemia, the exact mechanism remains unknown, and further investigation on the association between hyperammonemia and DPD activity is warranted.

Abbreviation

5-FU:	5-Fluorouracil
DPD:	Dihydropyrimidine dehydrogenase
CT:	Computed tomography
BUN:	Blood urea nitrogen
MRI:	Magnetic resonance imaging
DHU/U:	Dihydrouracil to uracil ratio.

Authors' Contribution

Keiki Nagaharu participated in the treatment of the patient in this case report and drafted the paper. Kenji Ikemura assisted in the examination of catabolites. Yoshiki Yamashita participated in the treatment of the patient. Hiroyasu Oda, Mikiya Ishihara, Yumiko Sugawara, and Satoshi Tamaru participated in the planning of treatment. Toshiro Mizuno and Naoyuki Katayama supervised and assisted in drafting the paper. All authors read and approved the final paper.

Acknowledgment

The authors thank their patient's family for allowing them to write about the case for the benefit of the future patients.

References

[1] C. Heidelberger, N. K. Chaudhuri, P. Danneberg et al., "Fluorinated pyrimidines, a new class of tumour-inhibitory compounds," *Nature*, vol. 179, no. 4561, pp. 663–666, 1957.

[2] K. Tsuji, H. Yasui, Y. Onozawa et al., "Modified folfox-6 therapy for heavily pretreated advanced gastric cancer refractory to fluorouracil, irinotecan, cisplatin and taxanes: a retrospective study," *Japanese Journal of Clinical Oncology*, vol. 42, no. 8, pp. 686–690, 2012.

[3] C.-C. Liaw, S.-J. Liaw, C.-H. Wang, M.-C. Chiu, and J.-S. Huang, "Transient hyperammonemia related to chemotherapy with continuous infusion of high-dose 5-fluorouracil," *Anti-Cancer Drugs*, vol. 4, no. 3, pp. 311–315, 1993.

[4] K. H. Yeh and A. L. Cheng, "High-dose 5-fluorouracil infusional therapy is associated with hyperammonaemia, lactic acidosis and encephalopathy," *British Journal of Cancer*, vol. 75, no. 3, pp. 464–465, 1997.

[5] M. Nobuhiro, G. Takashi, M. Takanori et al., "Risk factors for hyperammonemia during mFOLFOX6 treatment," *Gan To Kagaku Ryoho*, vol. 40, no. 4, pp. 483–487, 2013.

[6] R. W. Sparidans, T. M. Bosch, M. Jörger, J. H. M. Schellens, and J. H. Beijnen, "Liquid chromatography–tandem mass spectrometric assay for the analysis of uracil, 5,6-dihydrouracil and β-ureidopropionic acid in urine for the measurement of

the activities of the pyrimidine catabolic enzymes," *Journal of Chromatography B: Analytical Technologies in the Biomedical and Life Sciences*, vol. 839, no. 1-2, pp. 45–53, 2006.

[7] A. B. P. van Kuilenburg, J. Haasjes, D. J. Richel et al., "Clinical implications of dihydropyrimidine dehydrogenase (DPD) deficiency in patients with severe 5-fluorouracil-associated toxicity: identification of new mutations in the DPD gene," *Clinical Cancer Research*, vol. 6, no. 12, pp. 4705–4712, 2000.

[8] Y. Wettergren, G. Carlsson, E. Odin, and B. Gustavsson, "Pretherapeutic uracil and dihydrouracil levels of colorectal cancer patients are associated with sex and toxic side effects during adjuvant 5-fluorouracil-based chemotherapy," *Cancer*, vol. 118, no. 11, pp. 2935–2943, 2012.

[9] M. Gamelin, M. Boisdron-Celle, V. Guérin-Meyer et al., "Correlation between uracil and dihydrouracil plasma ratio, fluorouracil (5-FU) pharmacokinetic parameters, and tolerance in patients with advanced colorectal cancer: a potential interest for predicting 5-FU toxicity and determining optimal 5-FU dosage," *Journal of Clinical Oncology*, vol. 17, no. 4, pp. 1105–1110, 1999.

[10] Y. Nakayama, K. Matsumoto, Y. Inoue et al., "Correlation between the urinary dihydrouracil-uracil ratio and the 5-FU plasma concentration in patients treated with oral 5-FU analogs," *Anticancer Research*, vol. 26, no. 5, pp. 3983–3988, 2006.

[11] M. H. Kristensen, P. Pedersen, and J. Mejer, "The value of dihydrouracil/uracil plasma ratios in predicting 5-fluorouracil-related toxicity in colorectal cancer patients," *Journal of International Medical Research*, vol. 38, no. 4, pp. 1313–1323, 2010.

[12] B. E. Harris, J. T. Carpenter, and R. B. Diasio, "Severe 5-fluorouracil toxicity secondary to dihydropyrimidine dehydrogenase deficiency. A potentially more common pharmacogenetic syndrome," *Cancer*, vol. 68, no. 3, pp. 499–501, 1991.

[13] Y.-A. Kim, H. C. Chung, H. J. Choi, S. Y. Rha, J. S. Seong, and H.-C. Jeung, "Intermediate dose 5-fluorouracil-induced encephalopathy," *Japanese Journal of Clinical Oncology*, vol. 36, no. 1, pp. 55–59, 2006.

[14] L.-H. Li, H. Dong, F. Zhao et al., "The upregulation of dihydropyrimidine dehydrogenase in liver is involved in acquired resistance to 5-fluorouracil," *European Journal of Cancer*, vol. 49, no. 7, pp. 1752–1760, 2013.

[15] G. Carlsson, E. Odin, B. Gustavsson, and Y. Wettergren, "Pretherapeutic uracil and dihydrouracil levels in saliva of colorectal cancer patients are associated with toxicity during adjuvant 5-fluorouracil-based chemotherapy," *Cancer Chemotherapy and Pharmacology*, vol. 74, no. 4, pp. 757–763, 2014.

[16] S.-R. Kim, C.-H. Park, S. Park, J.-O. Park, J. Lee, and S.-Y. Lee, "Genetic polymorphisms associated with 5-fluorouracil-induced neurotoxicity," *Chemotherapy*, vol. 56, no. 4, pp. 313–317, 2010.

Complete Response after Treatment with Neoadjuvant Chemoradiation with Prolonged Chemotherapy for Locally Advanced, Unresectable Adenocarcinoma of the Pancreas

Tiffany A. Pompa,[1] William F. Morano,[2] Chetan Jeurkar,[1] Hui Li,[3] Suganthi Soundararajan,[3] Jaganmohan Poli,[4] Wilbur B. Bowne,[2] and Michael Styler[1]

[1]*Department of Medicine, Division of Hematology/Oncology, Drexel University College of Medicine, Philadelphia, PA 19102, USA*
[2]*Department of Surgery, Division of Surgical Oncology, Drexel University College of Medicine, Philadelphia, PA 19102, USA*
[3]*Department of Pathology & Laboratory Medicine, Drexel University College of Medicine, Philadelphia, PA 19102, USA*
[4]*Department of Radiation Oncology, Drexel University College of Medicine, Philadelphia, PA 19102, USA*

Correspondence should be addressed to Wilbur B. Bowne; wilbur.bowne@drexelmed.edu

Academic Editor: Francesco A. Mauri

Surgery is the only chance for cure in pancreatic ductal adenocarcinoma. In unresectable, locally advanced pancreatic cancer (LAPC), the National Comprehensive Cancer Network (NCCN) suggests chemotherapy and consideration for radiation in cases of unresectable LAPC. Here we present a rare case of unresectable LAPC with a complete histopathological response after chemoradiation followed by surgical resection. A 54-year-old female presented to our clinic in December 2013 with complaints of abdominal pain and 30-pound weight loss. An MRI demonstrated a mass in the pancreatic body measuring 6.2×3.2 cm; biopsy revealed proven ductal adenocarcinoma. Due to splenic vein/artery and contiguous celiac artery encasement, she was deemed surgically unresectable. She was started on FOLFIRINOX therapy (three cycles), intensity modulated radiation to a dose of 54 Gy in 30 fractions concurrent with capecitabine, followed by FOLFIRI, and finally XELIRI. After 8 cycles of ongoing XELIRI completed in March 2015, restaging showed a remarkable decrease in tumor size, along with PET-CT revealing no FDG-avid uptake. She was reevaluated by surgery and taken for definitive resection. Histopathological evaluation demonstrated a complete R0 resection and no residual tumor. Based on this patient and literature review, this strategy demonstrates potential efficacy of neoadjuvant chemoradiation with prolonged chemotherapy, followed by surgery, which may improve outcomes in patients deemed previously unresectable.

1. Introduction

Pancreatic cancer is the fourth leading cause of cancer death in the United States with pancreatic ductal adenocarcinoma (PDAC), accounting for nearly 90% of the cases [1]. Surgery offers the best chance for cure with prolonged survival, yet only 15–20% of patients present as candidates for resection at diagnosis [2, 3]. Nonmetastatic, locally advanced, pancreatic cancer (LAPC) is observed in about 40% of patients upon presentation thus posing a difficult challenge for the oncologist.

The most important aspect after diagnosis of PDAC is determining resectability of the tumor. Dedicated radiographic imaging of PDAC serves as a window for an experienced radiologist and pancreatic surgeon to determine resectability. The recommended imaging modality for visualization of a pancreatic tumor and surrounding structures is multidetector computed tomography (MDCT) which uses thin-sliced, incremental vascular phases and parenchymal contrast to assess advanced disease [4]. These images are best obtained prior to interventions such as biopsy or stent placement, as these can limit accuracy of interpretation [5].

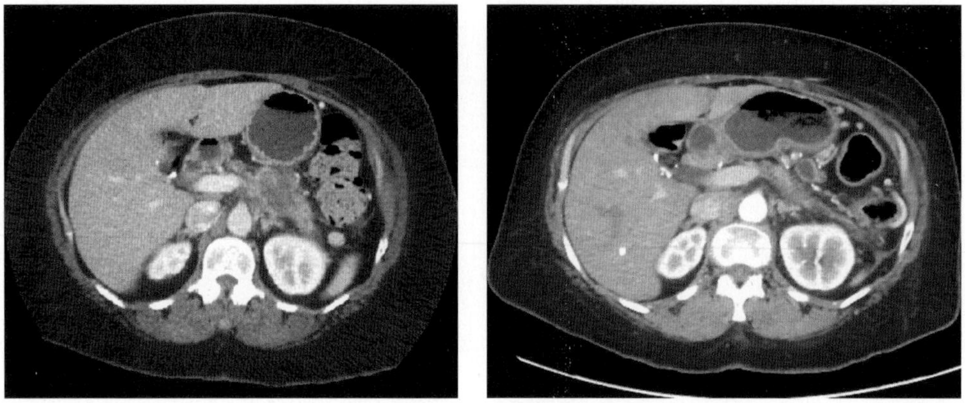

(a) (b)

Figure 1: (a) Axial CT demonstrating large mass in body/tail of pancreas before neoadjuvant therapy. (b) Axial CT demonstrating tumor response after neoadjuvant therapy.

Magnetic resonance imaging may be used to further define local and distant extent of disease.

As per the National Comprehensive Cancer Network (NCCN) guidelines, presentation of PDAC is divided into resectable, borderline resectable, and unresectable (LAPC and metastatic) disease, with distinctions for pancreatic anatomy, as well as venous and arterial involvement [6, 7]. Traditionally, the goals of care for patients with unresectable disease have been to extend survival and limit symptomatology with palliative intent using chemotherapy and/or radiation. More recently, focus has shifted toward the use of chemoradiation to downstage borderline resectable disease, allowing for resection [8–10].

A complete pathological response describes the presence of neoplastic tissue without viable invasive cancer cells within the specimen [11]. In pancreatic cancer, a complete pathologic response is associated with improved survival, yet a complete pathologic response following neoadjuvant therapy in LAPC is rarely reported [11, 12]. We present a case of a patient with a locally advanced, initially unresectable PDAC of the body and tail, who underwent neoadjuvant chemoradiation, with prolonged chemotherapy, followed by R0 radical resection that included subtotal pancreatectomy, splenectomy, and left adrenalectomy with no residual tumor identified in the pathologic specimen.

2. Case Report

A 54-year-old female presented in December 2013 with abdominal pain and 30-pound weight loss. A pancreatic mass was identified on routine cross-sectional imaging. CT with pancreatic protocol revealed an ill-defined soft tissue density in the region of the pancreatic body with proximal pancreatic ductal dilation central necrosis and obliteration of the splenic vein and encasement of the splenic and celiac arteries (Figure 1(a)). An MRI confirmed a soft tissue mass in the body of the pancreas, measuring 6.2 × 3.2 cm. An endoscopic ultrasound and fine-needle aspiration of the mass revealed PDAC and confirmed vascular encasement. Her initial CA 19-9 was elevated at 531. She was then evaluated by the surgical oncology service that determined the lesion was unresectable due to locally advanced extension of tumor with vascular involvement.

The patient had an optimal ECOG performance status despite her significant weight loss. She began neoadjuvant chemotherapy with three cycles of FOLFIRINOX (5-FU, leucovorin, irinotecan, and oxaliplatin) followed by concurrent intensity modulated radiation therapy (IMRT) to a dose of 54 Gy in 30 fractions (Figure 2) and capecitabine, which was tolerated well, except for development of mild peripheral neuropathy [13]. A repeat CT scan of the abdomen in July 2014, approximately 6 weeks after completing concurrent chemotherapy and radiation, showed a reduction in the size of her tumor to 3.7×2.7×3.9 cm, although there was persistent encasement of the celiac and splenic arteries.

Chemotherapy with FOLFIRI (5-FU, leucovorin and irinotecan) was started in July 2014 [14]. However, to obviate the need for central venous catheter placement, this regimen was later switched to XELIRI (capecitabine and irinotecan) beginning with cycle two [15]. Repeat CT imaging of the abdomen in December 2014, after her fifth cycle of XELIRI, revealed mild decrease in the size of the pancreatic mass but persistent peripancreatic soft tissue involvement and encasement of the celiac and splenic arteries.

We performed a restaging PET-CT in January 2015, eight months after initiation of therapy, which showed no FDG-avid uptake in the pancreas or the surrounding structures (Figure 3). Minimal stranding in the peripancreatic tissue was believed to be treatment-related fibrosis replacing tumor. She received a total of eight cycles of XELIRI, completed in March 2015. At that time, repeat CT imaging showed decrease in the size of her mass and persistent splenic artery encasement but minimal involvement of the celiac artery and findings consistent with possible radiation-induced fibrosis (Figure 1(b)). Additionally, at that time, her CA 19-9 was normal (14 U/mL).

Given the negative FDG-avid uptake on PET-CT and significantly improved CT, the patient was considered for surgical resection. After discussion at our multidisciplinary tumor conference, she was taken for radical antegrade

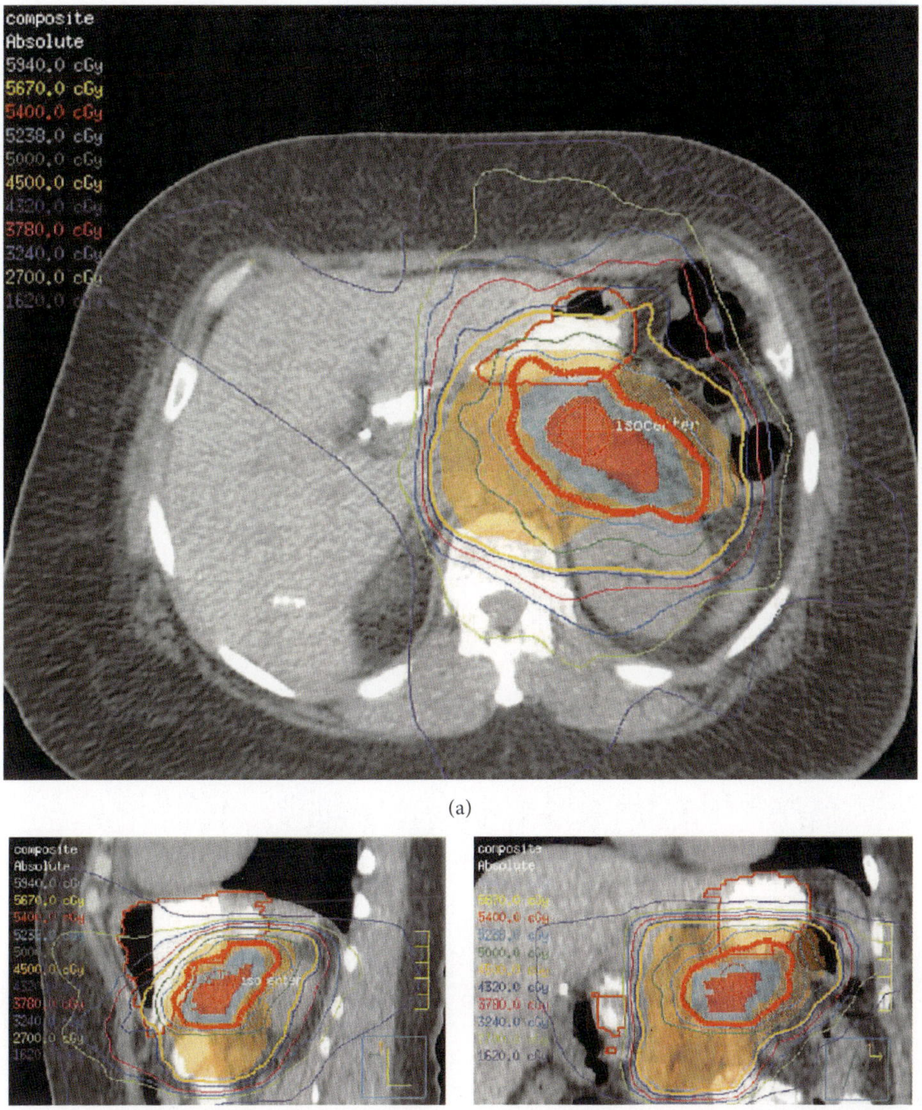

(a)

(b) (c)

FIGURE 2: Axial, sagittal, and coronal isodose distribution of IMRT plan to 54 Gy in 30 fractions.

modular pancreatosplenectomy in April 2015 [16, 17]. Initially, a diagnostic laparoscopy was performed, which did not demonstrate evidence of disseminated or peritoneal metastasis. The procedure continued with a left subcostal incision, which was extended to the right side. After reflection of the stomach superiorly and transverse colon inferiorly, a large degree of dense-appearing fibrosis was found obscuring the ventral surface of the pancreas with anterior and posterior extension to the spleen and left adrenal gland, respectively. The posterior surface of the stomach did not show any involvement. The body and tail of the pancreas and spleen were subsequently resected en bloc with Gerota's fascia and left adrenal gland. The celiac artery was skeletonized and appeared to have no residual disease. The procedure continued to conclusion without complications and with approximate estimated blood loss of 500 mL. Her postoperative course was complicated by pneumonia. The patient was discharged home on postoperative day 16. During the immediate 60-day postoperative period, there was no surgery-related morbidity. Histopathological analysis revealed an R0 resection with no residual tumor, but extensive fibrosis was found throughout the surgical specimen to the margins (Figures 4 and 5). The ten lymph nodes evaluated were negative. Ten months following resection, a small focus of local disease recurrence was detected on PET-CT and confirmed by fine-needle aspiration. The patient was subsequently treated with proton radiation therapy at an outside hospital and followed for three months until death from a treatment-related complication.

3. Discussion

The goals of treatment for patients with LAPC are predominantly palliation and extending survival. Patients with

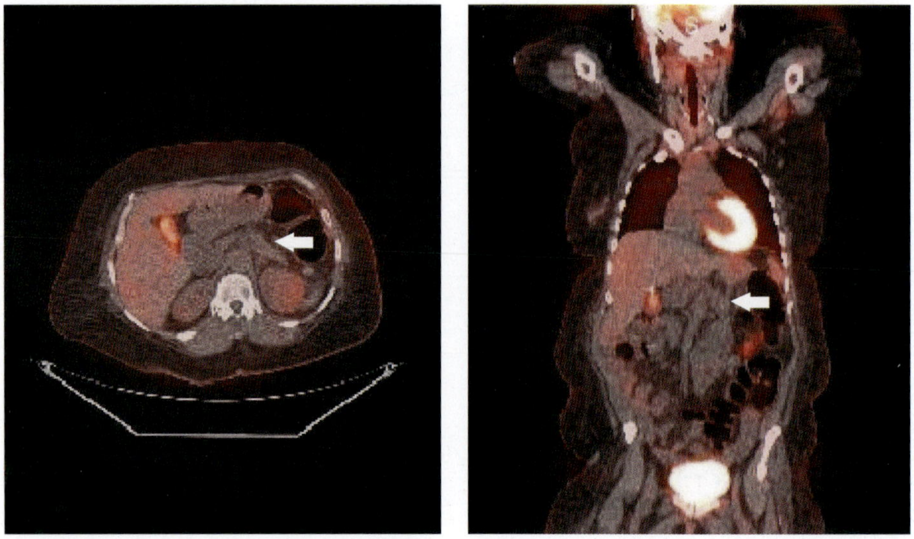

(a) (b)

Figure 3: PET-CT ((a) axial, (b) coronal) images showing lack of FDG-avid uptake in pancreas after neoadjuvant chemoradiation.

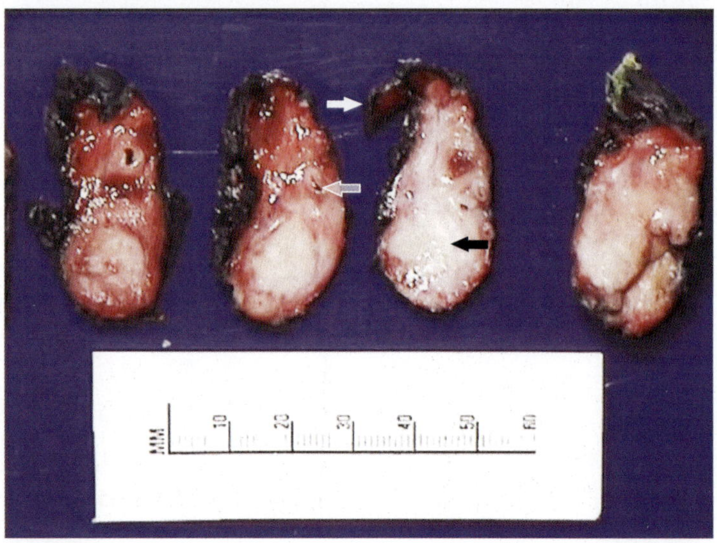

Figure 4: Cross sections of gross pathologic specimen. Black arrow points to fibrosis within the body of the resected pancreas. White arrow points to resected adrenal gland. Translucent arrow denotes the splenic artery encased in fibrosis.

borderline disease may benefit from neoadjuvant chemoradiation, increasing the potential for operative resection. This neoadjuvant treatment paradigm was originally described in a case series of patients with borderline disease from Varadhachary et al. in 2006 [18]. Evans et al. later published an expert consensus statement in 2009, which recommended an aggressive approach for this patient population, in collaboration with medical and radiation oncologists [19]. A similar strategy may prove applicable for unresectable LAPC.

In 2013, Heinemann et al. reported an overall resection rate after neoadjuvant therapy in LAPC of 33%, 79% of which had negative resection margins. Patients that remained unresectable had recorded median survival of 10.2 months, while the 33% of patients that underwent resection had a median overall survival of 20.5 months [6]. In this report, up to one-third of patients with initially unresectable LAPC became resectable after neoadjuvant therapy with chemotherapy, radiotherapy, or a combination of the two [6]. Importantly, if R0 resection could be achieved, overall survival was similar to those with primary resectable disease [6, 20].

Current treatment approaches for unresectable LAPC involve chemotherapy and/or radiation [9]. Treatment goals include controlling the spread of tumor, reducing metastatic potential, and downstaging of tumor status to allow for possible surgical resection. Chemotherapeutic regimens in LAPC are extrapolated from their use in metastatic disease. The Accord 11 trial demonstrated FOLFIRINOX to be superior to single agent gemcitabine in patients with

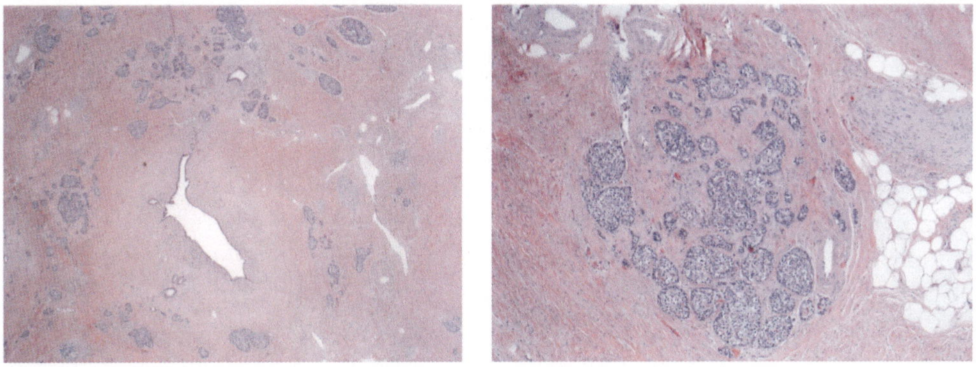

(a) (b)

FIGURE 5: (a) H&E sections demonstrating pancreatic tissue with dense fibrosis, residual ducts, and islet cells. No evidence of residual carcinoma. (b) Cluster of islets of Langerhans within the fibrotic tissue.

metastatic disease. This study showed that a combination of 5-fluorouracil, irinotecan, and oxaliplatin (FOLFIRINOX) produced increased response rates, progression-free survival, and overall survival (6.8 versus 11.1 months, $p < 0.001$) compared to standard monotherapy with gemcitabine [13]. Based on this response rate, FOLFIRINOX followed by radiation became the rational treatment option as neoadjuvant therapy in these patients, like ours, with unresectable LAPC. Hosein et al. subsequently reported an R0 resection rate of 44% in patients who received FOLFIRINOX as neoadjuvant therapy [21]. Moreover, a recent observational study including 101 patients with locally advanced, unresectable disease treated with FOLFIRINOX as induction therapy showed that 29% of patients had a reduction in tumor size of and half of those patients underwent resection with 55% undergoing an R0 resection [10].

Radiographic criteria to determine response to neoadjuvant therapy remain equivocal for borderline and more so for LAPC [22]. In our patient, evaluation of treatment efficacy was determined by RECIST Criteria with a CT dedicated pancreatic protocol. PET-CT imaging was also used to measure associated metabolic, tumor-related activity, which was not detected [23]. In monitoring treatment efficacy, Picchio et al. found that PET-CT can detect a metabolic response to treatment not identified by CT, while Chang et al. found PET-CT scanning to be a more effective method for evaluating tumor response than conventional CT scanning [24, 25]. There have also been noted instances where patients were spared unnecessary pancreaticoduodenectomy after "occult" metastases were revealed on PET imaging [24]. Nevertheless, the role of PET-CT in diagnosis and treatment response for PDAC remains controversial. NCCN currently recommends not to substitute a PET-CT for high quality standard CT evaluation in any stage of pancreatic cancer [7].

Challenges for evaluating response to neoadjuvant therapy include radiographic underestimation of treatment-related effects, such as peripancreatic inflammation and fibrosis [26]. Ferrone et al. recently published the largest study of LAPC patients who underwent neoadjuvant treatment and surgical resection. This study concluded that, after neoadjuvant FOLFIRINOX and RT (in most patients), imaging no longer accurately predicted patients for resectability. Among 40 patients undergoing resection, 19 were deemed unresectable by imaging, yet there was a 92% R0 resection rate. This study used surgical exploration with biopsies prior to proceeding to resection [8].

Neoadjuvant therapy-induced fibrosis often masquerades as residual, posttreatment tumor. Sasson et al. performed a retrospective review of 116 patients who underwent resection for PDAC following neoadjuvant therapy, demonstrating 56% mean fibrosis level in surgical specimens. Patients that received neoadjuvant therapy, as well as those with negative margins and lymph nodes, had higher levels of fibrosis than those patients with no preoperative treatment. Patients undergoing neoadjuvant therapy had higher pathological curative resection rates and median survival (23 mo versus 16 mo) [27, 28]. As recently shown, patients who undergo a prolonged time interval after neoadjuvant chemoradiation with ongoing chemotherapy are more likely to have an improved pathological response at time of surgical resection, which is associated with improved median overall survival; an apparent benefit observed in this case report (30-month survival) [29].

The use of combined neoadjuvant treatment with chemotherapy and/or radiation increases median survival for patients with locally advanced cancers to approximately 9 to 13 months but rarely results in long-term survival [30]. Despite this, the percentage of approximately 17,000 new LAPC cases diagnosed each year, considered for neoadjuvant therapy, and followed by resection in the United States remains small [6]. Reasons for this include indeterminate resectability of vascular involvement, patient comorbidities, oncology/community bias, and insufficient surgical expertise. The NCCN guidelines now recommend that patients with unresectable LAPC that demonstrate a significant response to therapy be considered for resection [7].

4. Conclusion

In our patient after neoadjuvant chemoradiation, with prolonged time interval and ongoing chemotherapy, a notable change in disease-status on imaging and normalization of surrogate tumor markers warranted an aggressive approach to therapy. A complete pathological response was determined, in this patient, after resection. With recent advances in neoadjuvant therapies (e.g., FOLFIRINOX, IMRT) and comprehensive multidisciplinary approach, more patients with unresectable LAPC may become candidates for curative resection. Pancreatic cancer is projected to become the second leading cause of cancer death in the US by 2030; treatment strategies to increase resectability are clearly needed [31]. This approach should be considered in carefully selected patients and validated by future studies in this patient population.

Consent

Written informed consent was obtained from the patient for publication of this case report and any accompanying images.

References

[1] M. Carpelan-Holmström, S. Nordling, E. Pukkala et al., "Does anyone survive pancreatic ductal adenocarcinoma? A nationwide study re-evaluating the data of the Finnish Cancer Registry," *Gut*, vol. 54, no. 3, pp. 385–387, 2005.

[2] C. R. Ferrone, M. F. Brennan, M. Gonen et al., "Pancreatic adenocarcinoma: the actual 5-year survivors," *Journal of Gastrointestinal Surgery*, vol. 12, no. 4, pp. 701–706, 2008.

[3] E. M. O'Reilly, "Pancreatic adenocarcinoma: new strategies for success," *Gastrointestinal Cancer Research*, vol. 3, no. 2, supplement 1, pp. S11–S15, 2009.

[4] D. B. Evans, "Resectable pancreatic cancer: the role for neoadjuvant/preoperative therapy," *HPB*, vol. 8, no. 5, pp. 365–368, 2006.

[5] W. Small Jr., J. Berlin, G. M. Freedman et al., "Full-dose gemcitabine with concurrent radiation therapy in patients with nonmetastatic pancreatic cancer: a multicenter phase II trial," *Journal of Clinical Oncology*, vol. 26, no. 6, pp. 942–947, 2008.

[6] V. Heinemann, M. Haas, and S. Boeck, "Neoadjuvant treatment of borderline resectable and non-resectable pancreatic cancer," *Annals of Oncology*, vol. 24, no. 10, pp. 2484–2492, 2013.

[7] Network NCC, "Pancreatic Adenocarcinoma (Version 2.2016)," 2016, https://www.nccn.org/professionals/physician_gls/PDF/pancreatic.pdf.

[8] C. R. Ferrone, G. Marchegiani, T. S. Hong et al., "Radiological and surgical implications of neoadjuvant treatment with FOLFIRINOX for locally advanced and borderline resectable pancreatic cancer," *Annals of Surgery*, vol. 261, no. 1, pp. 12–17, 2015.

[9] S. Tsai, K. K. Christians, P. S. Ritch et al., "Multimodality therapy in patients with borderline resectable or locally advanced pancreatic cancer: importance of locoregional therapies for a systemic disease," *Journal of Oncology Practice*, vol. 12, no. 10, pp. 915–923, 2016.

[10] E. Sadot, A. Doussot, E. M. O'Reilly et al., "FOLFIRINOX induction therapy for stage 3 pancreatic adenocarcinoma," *Annals of Surgical Oncology*, vol. 22, no. 11, pp. 3512–3521, 2015.

[11] S. Lorenzen, P. Thuss-Patience, S. E. Al-Batran et al., "Impact of pathologic complete response on disease-free survival in patients with esophagogastric adenocarcinoma receiving preoperative docetaxel-based chemotherapy," *Annals of Oncology*, vol. 24, no. 8, pp. 2068–2073, 2013.

[12] Q. Zhao, A. Rashid, Y. Gong et al., "Pathologic complete response to neoadjuvant therapy in patients with pancreatic ductal adenocarcinoma is associated with a better prognosis," *Annals of Diagnostic Pathology*, vol. 16, no. 1, pp. 29–37, 2012.

[13] T. Conroy, F. Desseigne, M. Ychou et al., "FOLFIRINOX versus gemcitabine for metastatic pancreatic cancer," *The New England Journal of Medicine*, vol. 364, no. 19, pp. 1817–1825, 2011.

[14] C. Yoo, J. Y. Hwang, J.-E. Kim et al., "A randomised phase II study of modified FOLFIRI.3 vs modified FOLFOX as second-line therapy in patients with gemcitabine-refractory advanced pancreatic cancer," *British Journal of Cancer*, vol. 101, no. 10, pp. 1658–1663, 2009.

[15] S. Cereda, M. Reni, A. Rognone et al., "XELIRI or FOLFIRI as salvage therapy in advanced pancreatic cancer," *Anticancer Research*, vol. 30, no. 11, pp. 4785–4790, 2010.

[16] S. M. Strasberg, J. A. Drebin, and D. Linehan, "Radical antegrade modular pancreatosplenectomy," *Surgery*, vol. 133, no. 5, pp. 521–527, 2003.

[17] J. G. Grossman, R. C. Fields, W. G. Hawkins, and S. M. Strasberg, "Single institution results of radical antegrade modular pancreatosplenectomy for adenocarcinoma of the body and tail of pancreas in 78 patients," *Journal of Hepato-Biliary-Pancreatic Sciences*, vol. 23, no. 7, pp. 432–441, 2016.

[18] G. R. Varadhachary, E. P. Tamm, J. L. Abbruzzese et al., "Borderline resectable pancreatic cancer: definitions, management, and role of preoperative therapy," *Annals of Surgical Oncology*, vol. 13, no. 8, pp. 1035–1046, 2006.

[19] D. B. Evans, M. B. Farnell, K. D. Lillemoe, C. Vollmer Jr., S. M. Strasberg, and R. D. Schulick, "Surgical treatment of resectable and borderline resectable pancreas cancer: expert consensus statement," *Annals of Surgical Oncology*, vol. 16, no. 7, pp. 1736–1744, 2009.

[20] S. Gillen, T. Schuster, C. M. Z. Büschenfelde, H. Friess, and J. Kleeff, "Preoperative/neoadjuvant therapy in pancreatic cancer: a systematic review and meta-analysis of response and resection percentages," *PLoS Medicine*, vol. 7, no. 4, Article ID e1000267, 2010.

[21] P. J. Hosein, J. Macintyre, C. Kawamura et al., "A retrospective study of neoadjuvant FOLFIRINOX in unresectable or borderline-resectable locally advanced pancreatic adenocarcinoma," *BMC Cancer*, vol. 12, article 199, 2012.

[22] M. H. G. Katz, J. B. Fleming, P. Bhosale et al., "Response of borderline resectable pancreatic cancer to neoadjuvant therapy is not reflected by radiographic indicators," *Cancer*, vol. 118, no. 23, pp. 5749–5756, 2012.

[23] E. A. Eisenhauer, P. Therasse, J. Bogaerts et al., "New response evaluation criteria in solid tumours: revised RECIST guideline (version 1.1)," *European Journal of Cancer*, vol. 45, no. 2, pp. 228–247, 2009.

[24] M. Picchio, E. Giovannini, P. Passoni et al., "Role of PET/CT in the clinical management of locally advanced pancreatic cancer," *Tumori*, vol. 98, no. 5, pp. 643–651, 2012.

[25] S. T. Chang, K. A. Goodman, G. P. Yang, and A. C. Koong, "Stereotactic body radiotherapy for unresectable pancreatic cancer," *Frontiers of Radiation Therapy and Oncology*, vol. 40, pp. 386–394, 2007.

[26] Z. Li, H. Shang, X. Zhang, H. Zhang, J. Bao, and C. Hao, "Surgical treatment for locally advanced pancreatic cancer localized in the pancreatic body and tail (Report of 11 cases)," *International Journal of Clinical and Experimental Medicine*, vol. 8, no. 3, pp. 4676–4681, 2015.

[27] A. R. Sasson, R. W. Wetherington, J. P. Hoffman et al., "Neoadjuvant chemoradiotherapy for adenocarcinoma of the pancreas: analysis of histopathology and outcome," *International Journal of Gastrointestinal Cancer*, vol. 34, no. 2-3, pp. 121–127, 2004.

[28] J.-L. Lee, S. C. Kim, J.-H. Kim et al., "Prospective efficacy and safety study of neoadjuvant gemcitabine with capecitabine combination chemotherapy for borderline-resectable or unresectable locally advanced pancreatic adenocarcinoma," *Surgery*, vol. 152, no. 5, pp. 851–862, 2012.

[29] K. T. Chen, K. Devarajan, B. N. Milestone et al., "Neoadjuvant chemoradiation and duration of chemotherapy before surgical resection for pancreatic cancer: does time interval between radiotherapy and surgery matter?" *Annals of Surgical Oncology*, vol. 21, no. 2, pp. 662–669, 2014.

[30] B. G. Czito, C. G. Willett, J. W. Clark, and C. F. Del Castillo, "Current perspectives on locally advanced pancreatic cancer," *Oncology*, vol. 14, no. 11, pp. 1535–1545, 2000.

[31] L. Rahib, B. D. Smith, R. Aizenberg, A. B. Rosenzweig, J. M. Fleshman, and L. M. Matrisian, "Projecting cancer incidence and deaths to 2030: the unexpected burden of thyroid, liver, and pancreas cancers in the united states," *Cancer Research*, vol. 74, no. 11, pp. 2913–2921, 2014.

Synchronous Diagnosis of Multiple Myeloma, Breast Cancer, and Monoclonal B-Cell Lymphocytosis on Initial Presentation

A. Vennepureddy,[1] V. Motilal Nehru,[1] Y. Liu,[2] F. Mohammad,[3] and J. P. Atallah[3]

[1] *Department of Internal Medicine, Staten Island University Hospital, 475 Seaview Avenue, Staten Island, NY 10305, USA*
[2] *Department of Pathology, Staten Island University Hospital, 475 Seaview Avenue, Staten Island, NY 10305, USA*
[3] *Division of Hematology and Oncology, Staten Island University Hospital, 475 Seaview Avenue, Staten Island, NY 10305, USA*

Correspondence should be addressed to A. Vennepureddy; avenn4@gmail.com

Academic Editor: Su Ming Tan

The cooccurrence of more than one oncologic illness in a patient can present a diagnostic challenge. Here we report an unusual case of concomitant existence of multiple myeloma, breast cancer, and monoclonal B-cell lymphocytosis on initial presentation. The challenge was to accurately diagnose each disease and stage in order to maximize the therapeutic regimen to achieve cure/remission. Successful management of the patient and increased life expectancy can be achieved by multidisciplinary management and patient-oriented approach in multiple primary malignant synchronous tumors.

1. Introduction

Multiple primary malignant tumors (MPMTs) are rarely observed in clinical practice; however, certain fundamental factors for the potential etiology have been described in the literature, including the environment and behavior (tobacco, occupation, pollution, and ultraviolet light), genetic predisposition (Li-Fraumeni or Beckwith-Wiedemann syndromes), previous medical treatment (radiotherapy or chemotherapy), and complex interaction between all these factors [1]. The association between varying cancer types can be classified into two categories, which are dependent on the timing of their discovery. An American review stated that the tumors are synchronous when the cancers occur at the same time or within 2 months of each other, whereas metachronous tumors occur when the cancers follow in sequence more than 2 months apart [2]. The majority of MPMTs that occur in multiple organs are metachronous, while the presence of synchronous lesions is less common, and in accordance with the behavior of malignancy lesions, these tumors are more frequent with aging.

This distinction implies important diagnostic and therapeutic challenges. From a diagnostic point of view the different patterns of MPMs should be considered. Therapeutically, a multidisciplinary and patient-oriented approach should be considered.

2. Case Report

A 77-year-old female with history of hypertension, diabetes mellitus type II, dyslipidemia, and chronic kidney disease stage II presented to our hospital after a fall initially suspected to be secondary to mechanical factors without any loss of consciousness. Her lab tests on admission were found to be as follows: hemoglobin of 10.8 g/dL (baseline was 12.5 g/dL) with red blood cell indices within normal limits, white blood cell count of 9.8×10^9 cells/L with absolute lymphocyte count of 1.4×10^9 cells/L, absolute granulocyte count of 7.8×10^9 cells/L, and normal platelets. Her serum creatinine was 2.01 (baseline was 1.03) with a GFR of 29 and normal serum electrolytes. The patient's initial trauma workup and physical exam revealed a palpable mass in the upper outer quadrant of the left breast and multiple lytic lesions on C2 and C5 vertebral bodies and T2 spinous process on the computerized tomography (CT) scan. Subsequent magnetic

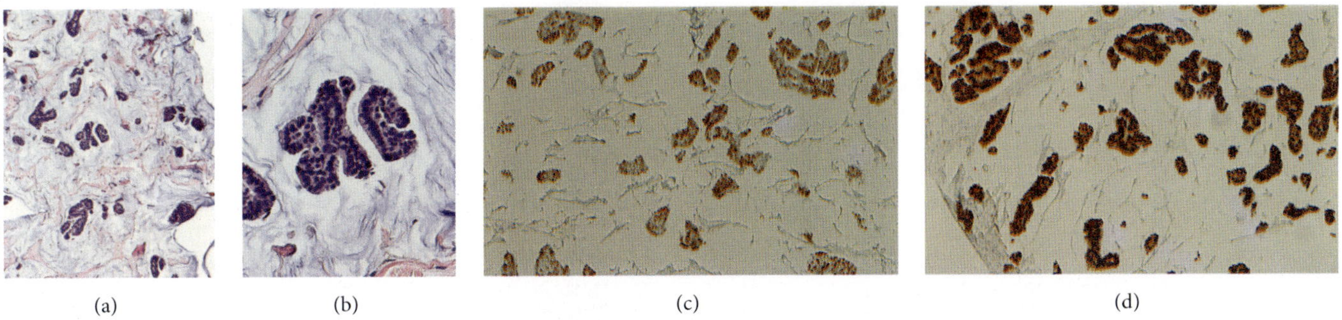

FIGURE 1: Colloid carcinoma of the breast. This invasive ducal carcinoma exhibits dominant mucin production and tumor cells are arranged in clusters and nests, floating in pools of extracellular mucin (a). Tumor cells are uniform in size and shape with hyperchromatic nuclei without prominent nucleoli and mitosis (b). PR (c) and ER (d) are positive in tumor cells. [(a) H&E, ×100; (b) H&E, ×400; (c) IHC, ×100; (d) IHC, ×100.]

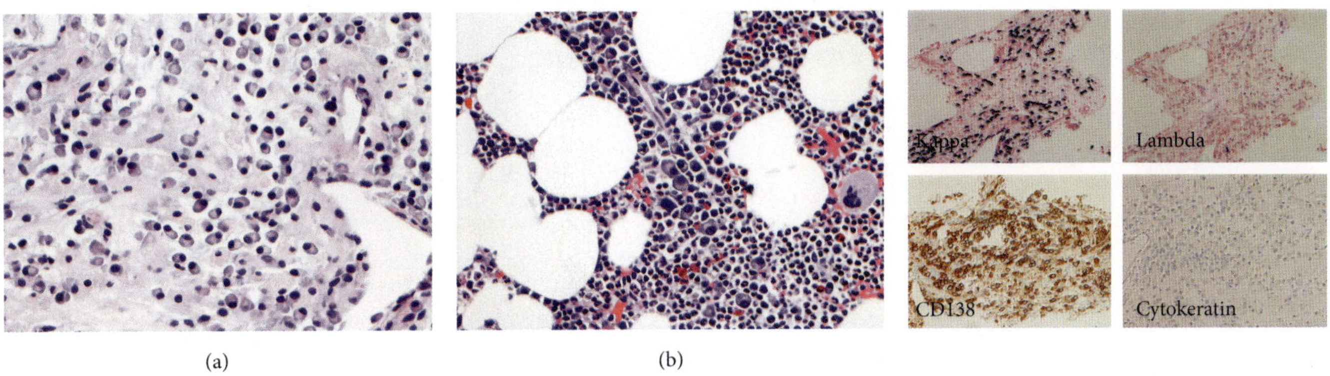

FIGURE 2: Photomicrographs from femur bone biopsy (a) and bone marrow clot preparation (b) showing a monomorphic population of plasma cells intermixed with few small lymphocytes and other hematopoietic cells in the bone marrow. The plasma cells show mature cytological features with strong CD138 reactivity and restriction for kappa light chain. No morphologic evidence of carcinoma is identified in both specimens and staining with cytokeratin marker is negative. [(a) H&E, ×100; (b) H&E, ×400.]

resonance imaging (MRI) noncontrast of the brain and cervical spine exhibited multiple focal lesions of the calvarium, clivus, C2 and C5 vertebral bodies, and T1 spinous process and cord compression of C3-C4, C4-C5, C5-C6, and C6-C7 suggestive of metastatic disease. The patient was started on dexamethasone while undergoing malignancy workup. She then underwent a nuclear medicine bone scan of the whole body which showed multiple bony abnormalities in the left femoral shaft, left acetabulum, L1, L2, and multiple bilateral ribs consistent with metastatic disease.

The patient's mammogram and left breast ultrasound showed a 7.5 × 3.7 × 7.8 cm heterogeneous irregularly shaped mass at the 2:00 position, 15 cm from the nipple on the upper outer quadrant of the left breast. Subsequent biopsy of the mass revealed an invasive well differentiated ductal carcinoma with mucinous features (colloid carcinoma) (Figure 1). The breast cancer proved to be triple positive for estrogen, progesterone receptors, and HER2 via immunohistochemistry and fluorescence in situ hybridization testing. The lytic lesions on bone scan were initially suspected to be of metastatic breast cancer.

The combination of acute kidney injury, normocytic normochromic anemia, and multiple bony lesions was suspected of being multiple myeloma (MM) and its workup was done by serum and urine electrophoresis, serum and urine immunofixation, and free light chain ratio. The results revealed abnormal IgA kappa monoclonal protein with elevated free light chain ratio. The patient's subsequent bone marrow biopsy confirmed the diagnosis of MM but also revealed a minute monoclonal B-cell population with typical chronic lymphocytic leukemia (CLL)/small lymphocytic lymphoma (SLL) phenotype confirmed via flow cytometry (Figure 2).

The patient improved significantly with the supportive treatment and was discharged from the hospital with outpatient follow-up. The patient was then started on REVLIMID and Decadron for MM and pertuzumab, trastuzumab, and letrozole for invasive ductal carcinoma of the breast. She underwent positron emission tomography (PET-CT) as part of the initial treatment workup as well as for determining the appropriate site for bone biopsy to differentiate between metastatic breast cancer and MM as MM lesions usually do not light up on the bone scan. The PET-CT revealed a fluorodeoxyglucose (FDG) avid 4.3 × 5.1 cm partially calcified left breast mass (SUV 3.2) as well as increased uptake (SUV 4.3) in the 5.3 × 4.3 cm lytic lesion of the right distal femur. The right femur and left pubic bone were biopsied which showed only monomorphic population of plasmacytoid cells consistent with plasma cell neoplasm with no evidence of metastatic breast cancer (Figure 2).

The patient is currently continuing the neoadjuvant chemotherapy with pertuzumab, trastuzumab, and letrozole while awaiting surgical evaluation for the triple positive localized left breast cancer and REVLIMID and Decadron for symptomatic multiple myeloma. She is also being monitored for the progression of the CLL/SLL clone.

Synchronous diagnosis of two different primaries is very important as the management of these coexisting malignancies is different. In our case report, we initially thought the lytic lesions could be from metastatic breast cancer which in turn proved to be pure myelomatous involvement of bone and no signs of metastases from breast cancer which changed the management and made the patient undergo mastectomy. This patient should also be monitored for any evidence of development of CLL as we found monoclonal B-cell population with typical CLL/SLL phenotypic picture on flow cytometry of bone marrow biopsy.

3. Discussion

Primary soft tissue extramedullary plasmacytoma is uncommon and is defined as a malignant tumor of plasma cells arising in the soft tissue in the absence of bone involvement. It can occur in any organ as a solitary form of plasma cell neoplasm [3]. Breast plasmacytoma is one of the major differential diagnoses in synchronous diagnosis of breast cancer and multiple myeloma as plasmacytomas may mimic breast cancer in some cases, especially when axillary lymph nodes are involved. Few case reports have been published in the literature where breast plasmacytomas can occur either as a solitary lesion without evidence of systemic disease [4–7] or concurrently with multiple myeloma [8–11] or as a sign of relapse in patients with known history of myeloma [12–15].

To the best of our knowledge, few case reports have been described in the literature with synchronous diagnosis of multiple myeloma and breast cancer. Cao et al. reported a case of breast tumor where infiltrating ductal carcinoma of the breast and breast plasmacytoma occurred which was coexistent in the breast tumor on initial presentation and the patient got successfully treated with chemotherapy for breast cancer and radiotherapy for plasmacytoma [16]. Khalbuss et al. reported a case of synchronous diagnosis of multiple myeloma and breast cancer with plasmacytoid morphology on initial presentation [17]. This case illustrated the deceptive cytomorphologic similarities between an epithelial malignancy and a hematopoietic malignancy. Since myeloma plasma cells vary from mature forms to pleomorphic, anaplastic plasma cells, they can easily mimic the cytomorphology of adenocarcinoma and vice versa. The distinction may be challenging by cytomorphology alone [17]. Kherfani et al. reported a case of spinal cord compression from concurrent multiple myeloma and metastatic breast cancer in the same vertebra [18]. Al-Said Ali et al. reported synchronous diagnosis of multiple myeloma and breast cancer on initial presentation similar to our case in 2009 [19].

4. Conclusion

In summary, here we presented a case of synchronous diagnosis of MM, breast cancer, and monoclonal B-cell lymphocytosis on initial presentation. The diagnosis of dual malignancy in a patient at the time of the first presentation is rare. We initially suspected the lytic lesions on bone scan could be from metastatic breast cancer but were found out to be only localized breast cancer with pure myelomatous involvement of bony lesions. This made the patient undergo mastectomy along with continuation of neoadjuvant chemotherapy. The patient also needs to be monitored for any development of CLL from monoclonal B-cell lymphocytosis. Recognizing both malignancies at the time of presentation and before initiation of treatment is crucial since the management of these coexisting malignancies is different.

In conclusion, successful patient's management and increased life expectancy can be achieved by multidisciplinary management and patient-oriented approach in multiple primary malignant synchronous tumors.

Disclosure

The authors stipulate that all persons listed as authors have contributed to preparing of the manuscript and that no person or persons other than the authors listed have contributed significantly in its preparation.

References

[1] F. Rabbani, G. Grimaldi, and P. Russo, "Multiple primary malignancies in renal cell carcinoma," *Journal of Urology*, vol. 160, no. 4, pp. 1255–1259, 1998.

[2] H. L. Howe, "A review of the definition for multiple primary cancers in the united states," in *Workshop Proceedings From December 4–6, 2002*, North American Association of Central Cancer Registries, Princeton, NJ, USA, May 2003.

[3] C. Van Nieuwkoop, R. W. M. Giard, H. F. Veen, and A. Dees, "Extramedullary plasmacytoma of the breast simulating breast cancer," *Netherlands Journal of Medicine*, vol. 58, no. 4, pp. 174–176, 2001.

[4] C. W. Cutler, "Plasma-cell tumor of the breast with metastases," *Annals of Surgery*, vol. 100, no. 2, pp. 392–394, 1934.

[5] J. Innes and J. Newall, "Myelomatosis," *The Lancet*, vol. 277, no. 7171, pp. 239–245, 1961.

[6] N. S. F. Proctor, J. J. Rippey, G. Shulman, and C. Cohen, "Extramedullary plasmacytoma of the breast," *Journal of Pathology*, vol. 116, no. 2, pp. 97–100, 1975.

[7] T. J. Bloomberg, J. P. Glees, and J. E. Williams, "Bilateral breast lumps: an unusual feature of extramedullary plasmacytoma," *British Journal of Radiology*, vol. 53, no. 629, pp. 498–501, 1980.

[8] B. Rosenberg, J. N. Attie, and H. L. Mandelbaum, "Breast tumor as the presenting sign of multiple myeloma," *The New England Journal of Medicine*, vol. 269, pp. 359–361, 1963.

[9] K. Maeda, C. M. Abesamis, L. M. Kuhn, and B. H. Hyun, "Multiple myeloma in childhood: report of a case with breast tumors as a presenting manifestation," *American Journal of Clinical Pathology*, vol. 60, no. 4, pp. 552–558, 1973.

[10] W. B. Bassett and R. B. Weiss, "Plasmacytomas of the breast: an unusual manifestation of multiple myeloma," *Southern Medical Journal*, vol. 72, no. 11, pp. 1492–1494, 1979.

[11] A. Ben-Yehuda, D. Steiner-Saltz, E. Libson, and A. Polliack, "Plasmacytoma of the breast—unusual initial presentation of myeloma: report of two cases and review of the literature," *Blut*, vol. 58, no. 3, pp. 169–170, 1989.

[12] I. L. Craft, "The late appearance of extramedullary lesions in myelomatosis," *British Journal of Cancer*, vol. 21, no. 3, pp. 501–504, 1967.

[13] A. Mangalik and P. K. Gupta, "Soft tissue involvement in plasmacytoma and multiple myeloma: a report of seven cases," *Indian Journal of Pathology and Microbiology*, vol. 17, no. 1, pp. 45–51, 1974.

[14] J. S. Ross, T. M. King, J. I. Spector, H. Zimbler, and R. M. Basile, "Plasmacytoma of the breast. An unusual case of recurrent myeloma," *Archives of Internal Medicine*, vol. 147, no. 10, pp. 1838–1840, 1987.

[15] C. Lombardi, A. Calvi, E. Bonera, A. Savio, and E. Savio, "Bilateral breast involvement in a 71-year-old white man with lambda light chain disease. Regression after a new chemotherapy combination. A case report," *Tumori*, vol. 78, no. 1, pp. 35–36, 1992.

[16] S. Cao, H.-G. Kang, Y.-X. Liu, and X.-B. Ren, "Synchronous infiltrating ductal carcinoma and primary extramedullary plasmacytoma of the breast," *World Journal of Surgical Oncology*, vol. 7, article 43, 2009.

[17] W. E. Khalbuss, G. Fischer, M. Ahmad, and B. Villas, "Synchronous presentation of breast carcinoma with plasmacytoid cytomorphology and multiple myeloma," *Breast Journal*, vol. 12, no. 2, pp. 165–167, 2006.

[18] A. Kherfani, K. Amri, M. Hachem, L. Abid, M. Bouaziz, and M. Mestiri, "An association of vertebral breast cancer metastasis and multiple myeloma, revealed by a spinal cord compression," *Pan African Medical Journal*, vol. 19, article 168, 2014.

[19] A. Al-Said Ali, I. Al-Bader, F. Al-Ali, A. H. Elgazzar, and S. Fayez, "Breast cancer and multiple myeloma at initial presentation," *Breast Journal*, vol. 15, no. 1, pp. 103–105, 2009.

Paclitaxel Induced MDS and AML: A Case Report

Udit Bhaskar Bhatnagar,[1] Daulath Singh,[1] Alexy Glazyrin,[2] and Jill Moormeier[3]

[1] *Internal Medicine, University of Missouri-Kansas City School of Medicine, 2301 Holmes Street, Kansas City, MO 64108, USA*
[2] *Department of Pathology, University of Missouri-Kansas City School of Medicine, 2301 Holmes Street, Kansas City, MO 64108, USA*
[3] *Department of Medicine, Hematology/Oncology, University of Missouri-Kansas City School of Medicine, 2301 Holmes Street, Kansas City, MO 64108, USA*

Correspondence should be addressed to Udit Bhaskar Bhatnagar; bhatnagaru@umkc.edu

Academic Editor: Yoshihito Yokoyama

Therapy related acute myelogenous leukemia (AML) and myelodysplastic syndromes (MDS) have been classically linked to alkylating agents and topoisomerase inhibitors. They constitute about 1% of all AMLs. There is less evidence on association of taxanes (paclitaxel and docetaxel) with these myeloid neoplasms. We present a case of paclitaxel therapy related acute myelogenous leukemia after treatment of endometrial cancer with a regimen containing paclitaxel and carboplatin. A 63-year-old female underwent surgery followed by a total of 6 cycles of chemotherapy with carboplatin and paclitaxel. Six months after last cycle of chemotherapy, she was diagnosed with myelodysplastic syndrome with refractory anemia and excess blasts. Six weeks later, she had worsening anemia and thrombocytopenia which prompted a bone marrow biopsy which revealed acute myelomonocytic leukemia. A thorough literature review revealed 12 other case reports where taxanes have been implicated in the development of therapy related myeloid neoplasm. Based on the timeline of events in our patient, paclitaxel is the likely culprit in the pathogenesis of this myeloid neoplasm. This rare but significantly grave adverse effect should be kept in consideration when deciding on treatment options for gynecological malignancies.

1. Introduction

Advancements in the treatment of gynecologic cancers with newer chemoradiotherapies have significantly improved the mortality and life expectancy of patients with these cancers. But with increased use of these chemotherapeutic agents, prescribers should be mindful of the potential long term side effects of these agents. One of the most serious complications of chemotherapeutic agents is dysplasia and malignancy.

Therapy related AML (t-AML) makes up about 10% of AML and has been studied and well documented in association with alkylating agents and topoisomerase inhibitors [1]. It usually involves a rapidly progressive disease, complex karyotype abnormalities, and poor prognosis with lesser response to treatment than archetypal AMLs.

Taxanes are the cornerstone of management of gynecological malignancies but recent data has linked them to cases of therapy related AML and MDS.

2. Case Presentation

We report a case of a 63-year-old Caucasian female found to have high grade endometrial carcinoma while undergoing evaluation for postmenopausal bleeding. The initial suspicion was from an abnormal pap smear done 3 years ago showing possible adenocarcinoma cells. Endometrial biopsy was done and showed high grade endometrial adenocarcinoma with serous features. The patient underwent surgical staging 4 months later with total abdominal hysterectomy, bilateral salpingo-oophorectomy, pelvic lymphadenectomy, and omentectomy. Out of the total 21 resected lymph nodes, one was involved with cancer and the carcinoma was staged at T3aN1M0, Stage 3.

Following surgical staging and tumor resection, the patient underwent chemotherapy with three cycles of carboplatin and paclitaxel at 21-day intervals, followed by pelvic radiotherapy (planned total dose 5040 cGy), and finally three

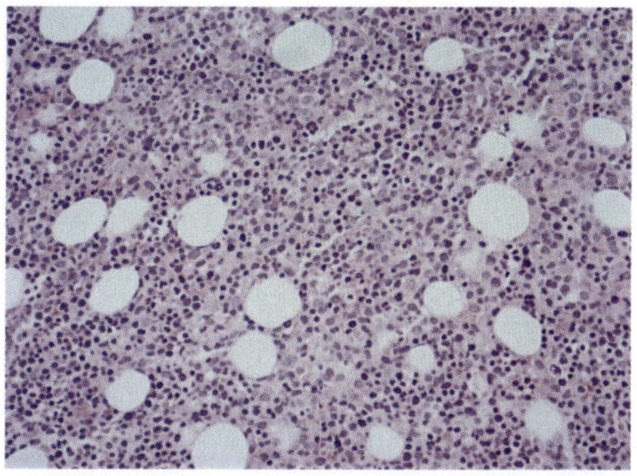

FIGURE 1: Bone marrow aspiration cytology (H&E stain, magnification 400x) shows hypercellular bone marrow with proliferating blasts replacing most of the normal bone marrow.

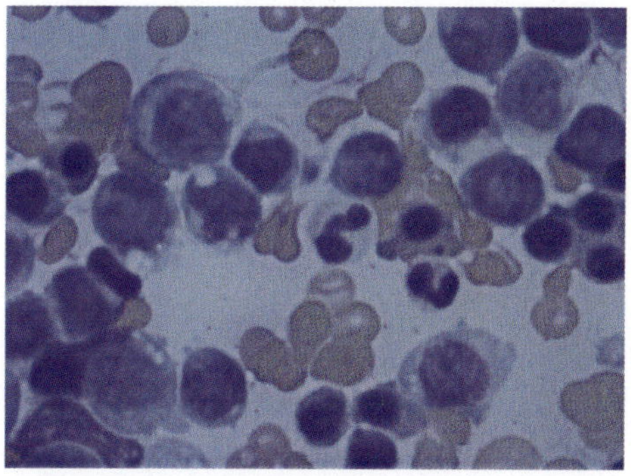

FIGURE 2: Bone marrow aspiration cytology (W&G stain, magnification 1000x) shows medium to large blast cells replacing normal bone marrow cellularity. Dysplastic granules and occasional vacuoles are observed.

additional cycles of carboplatin and paclitaxel. Initial doses of carboplatin were targeted at 750 mg/cycle (AUC = 6) and paclitaxel at 175 mg/m^2. Because of extended duration radiation related Grade 3 colitis, radiation therapy was stopped after receipt of 1980 cGy. Patient then underwent 3 more cycles (cycles 4–6) of chemotherapy with carboplatin and paclitaxel. The total cumulative dose of paclitaxel was 1511 mg and that of carboplatin was 4312 mg.

Prior to beginning chemotherapy, the patient had normal blood counts except for a mild iron deficiency anemia (hemoglobin 11.2 gm/dL, white blood cell count 7200/mm^3, and platelets 168,000/mm^3). Her platelet count after completion of radiation therapy was 120,000–140,000/mm^3, with mild anemia and a normal white blood cell count. After receiving the sixth and final dose of chemotherapy, her platelet count fell to 80,000/mm^3 and did not recover.

Six months after last cycle of chemotherapy, patient was hospitalized thrice over a period of two months with high grade fevers. She had worsening anemia and thrombocytopenia during this period which prompted a bone marrow biopsy. This revealed a hypercellular marrow with overall 5% myeloblasts with megaloblastic changes in the red cells and myeloid series and normal appearing megakaryocytes (Figures 1–3). The peripheral blood showed marked anisocytosis with moderate normocytic normochromic anemia and left shifted myeloid series and thrombocytopenia (Figure 4). The findings were consistent with treatment related myelodysplastic syndrome with refractory anemia and excess blasts. Karyotyping revealed abnormal female karyotype: 45,XX,add(3)(p13),del(3)(q23q25),−5, add(5)(q13),add(7)(q11.2),der(17)t(5,17)(q15;q25).

Within six weeks of the diagnosis of myelodysplasia, she had progressed to acute leukemia. Initial lab work revealed leukocytosis up to 76000 with 22% blasts; anemia with Hb 6.4 g/dL; and thrombocytopenia with counts of 15,000/mm^3. She was given a provisional diagnosis of therapy related AML. A bone marrow biopsy revealed hypercellular marrow with 29% of cells blasts. The blasts exhibited both myeloid and monocytic features and a diagnosis of acute myelomonocytic leukemia (AML; FAB classification: M4) was made. Peripheral smear also showed persistent leukocytosis with blasts >27% along with anemia and thrombocytopenia which eventually required transfusions.

Patient was offered treatment options including chemotherapy for AML and then possible stem cell transplant but decided not to pursue chemotherapy and opted for supportive treatment. She died a week later due to pneumonia and respiratory failure.

3. Discussion

Therapy related myeloid neoplasm (t-MN) is the term recently proposed by the World Health Organization to cover the spectrum of malignant disorders that were previously described as therapy related myelodysplastic syndromes (t-MDSs) or acute myeloid leukemia (t-AML).

Several chemotherapeutic regimens have been implicated in causing therapy related myeloid neoplasms. The most common of these agents are alkylating agents like cyclophosphamide, nitrosourea, or melphalan and topoisomerase inhibitors such as etoposide, daunorubicin, and doxorubicin. The latency period between first exposure to a cytotoxic agent and the development of therapy related myeloid neoplasms (t-MN) usually ranges from one to 10 years. This latency period and predominant cytogenetics observed often vary according to the chemotherapeutic agent used.

t-MNs after exposure to alkylating agents typically present after a latency period of approximately five to seven years [2]. Two-thirds of these patients are first recognized by evidence of myelodysplasia (usually trilineage dysplasia), marrow failure, and pancytopenia. The chromosomal abnormalities seen in these t-MNs often involve complex abnormalities and monosomies such as −5 or −7 that have been associated with unfavorable risk [3]. Combination of radiotherapy and chemotherapy was further shown to have increased risk of t-AML in some studies [4].

t-MNs that develop after the use of topoisomerase II inhibitors have a considerably shorter latency period of one to three years and most often present with overt leukemia and rarely with MDS or MDS/MPN [5]. The cytogenetic alterations typically apparent in these t-MNs often involve

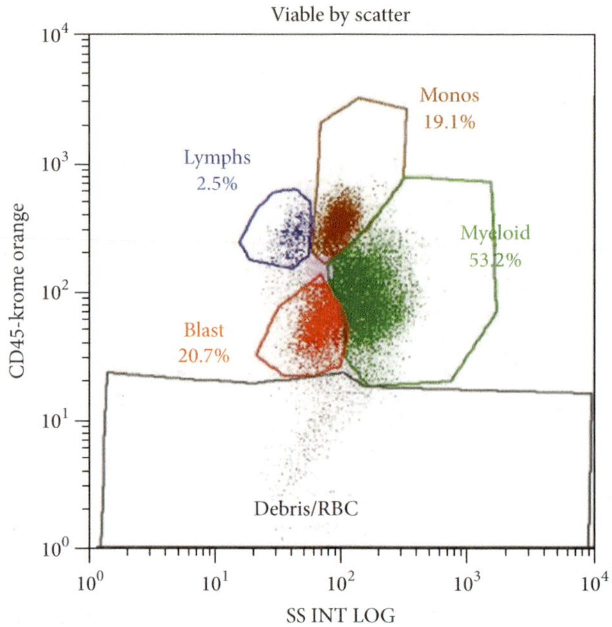

FIGURE 3: Bone marrow aspirate flow cytometry showing increased number of blasts and left shifted granulopoiesis.

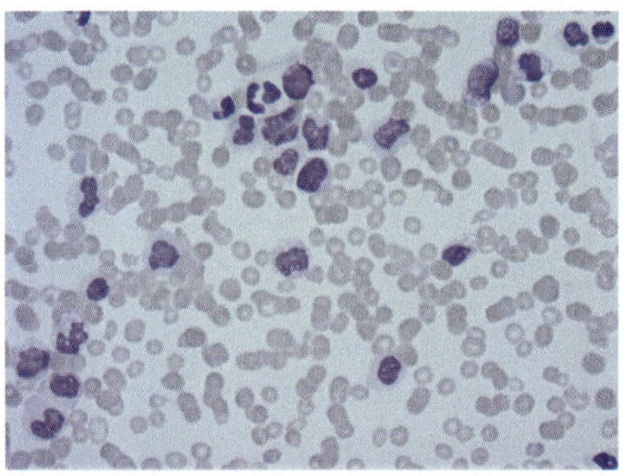

FIGURE 4: Peripheral blood smear: (W&G stain) show circulating blasts, dysplastic neutrophils, and nucleated red blood cells.

11q23 abnormalities, such as t(9;11), or 21q22 abnormalities, such as t(8;21) or t(3;21) [6].

The platinum containing derivatives like carboplatin and cisplatin also have some leukemogenic potential. In a case control study by Travis et al., platinum containing agents were associated with an increased risk of *t*-MDS/*t*-AML [7]. Most of the cases seen in our literature review were treated concomitantly with taxanes (paclitaxel) and carboplatin. However, as reported in the study by Travis et al., carboplatin related t-AML have a higher latency period, averaging at 4 years (the minimum latency being 1.3 years in the report), which was not the case with our patient, making the platinum agent a less likely culprit.

Review of the English language literature revealed 12 other similar case reports where taxanes had been implicated in development of therapy related myelogenous leukemia (Table 1) [8–17]. Of these, mean time of onset of disease from beginning of chemotherapy and diagnosis of leukemia was about 8.75 months. The total dosage of paclitaxel used was specified clearly in 8 studies. Among these studies, the total mean dosage of paclitaxel used was 1342.5 mg which is the usual dose for gynecological malignancies, 175 mg/m^2 [18, 19]. The malignant potential thus does not seem to be related to the dose of paclitaxel but rather to an idiosyncratic response to the treatment. It is unclear why taxanes lead to therapy related AML but treatment specific DNA damage is likely to be important in the pathogenesis [20]. Five of the nine cases which report the AML subtype revealed a M4 AML subtype (FAB classification). On review of the cytogenetics, there was no specific chromosomal abnormality that was common to the cases but almost all cases had a multitude of cytogenetic abnormalities which, not surprisingly, points to the poor prognosis seen in these cases. Larson, RA, in a recent review noted that it is the cytogenetics, and not merely prior exposures, which are the strongest predictors for outcome for these treatment related AMLs [21].

As seen in the literature review, the myelodysplastic syndromes and myelogenous malignancies associated with these agents are characterized by multiple cytogenetic abnormalities and typically have a very poor prognosis. Of the four patients who received treatment for secondary leukemia, two died within a year, one died 13 months later due to progression of the primary tumor, and one survived. Of the patients who did not receive treatment, the average survival was 7.5 months. In all of the reviewed cases, only two cases had gone into remission: the first described by Christodoulou et al. was detected early in the MDS stage and was treated two months after diagnosis with bone marrow transplantation [15] and the second case described by Seymour et al. had progressed to AML M4 subtype and had leptomeningeal leukemic infiltrate but was treated with intensified cytarabine therapy leading to remission [16]. However, due to the rarity

TABLE 1: Case reports of taxane chemotherapy related myelogenous leukemias.

Author	Year	Age	Primary tumor	Docetaxel	Paclitaxel (total dose in mg)	Carboplatin (total dose in mg)	Karyotype	Latency of leukemia (period from initial treatment to onset of AML)	MDS	AML	Prognostic: time from Dx of AML to death
Ishikawa et al. [8]	2014	65	Ovarian cancer		1968	6480	45,XX,der(6)t(6:17)(p23;q21)inv(6)(p23q13),17, add(19)(p13)[4]/44,sl-5[10]/46,XX[5]	3 years 10 months	MDS-RCMD	—	15 m
Vanajakshi et al. [9]	2014	69	Ovarian cancer		1200	2700	53XX; trisomies 8, 12, 16, 18, 19, and +2mar JAK2V617F; 5q31 and 7q31 deletions	33 months	MDS-U	M4	1 m of AML
See et al. [10]	2006	54	Ovarian cancer		1710	6820	Abnormal karyotype with multiple complex abnormalities, including 45XX t(1,5)(q25;q35),del(4)(q21q26),ins(7)(p15;?),del(12)(p12),213,217,217, add(19)(p13.3), add(22)(q13),12mar in 11 metaphases and 43–45,XX,t(1;5)(q25;q35),del(4)(q21q26),ins(7)(p15;?) del(12)(p12),213,217,217,add(19)(p13.3), add(22)(q13),1224mar in 8 metaphases were identified at diagnosis of erythroleukemia	36 months	—	M6	10 m after dx of AML
Yeasmin et al. [11]	2008	73	Ovarian cancer		2085	1910	46,XX,der(5,19)(p10:q10),−6,del(7)(q?), add(12)(p11.2),−13,−17,+19	24 months	MDS-RAEB	M7	2 m
Kim et al. [12]	2006	64	NSCLC		525	1123	NR	27 months	MDS-CMML		9 m
Gupta et al. [13]	2014	64	Breast cancer		(Dose not specified)		46,XX,t(8;16)(p11.2;p13.3),der(22)t(1;22)(q21;q13)	2 years		M4	1 m
Melichar et al. [14]	2012	54	Ovarian and breast cancer		(Dose not specified)	Cisplatin equivalents 3798 mg	NR	5 years	MDS-RAEB	—	3 m
Melichar et al. [14]	2012	66	Ovarian cancer		31 cycles × 175 mg/m^2	Cisplatin equivalents 4050 mg	NR	43 months		Unclassified	1 m
Christodoulou et al. [15]	2004	21	Mixed germ cell tumor (seminoma)		1000		47,XY,i(5)(p10),del(12)(p11),+i(12)(p10) [18]	10 months	MDS (RARS)	—	Survived
Seymour et al. [16]	1999	59	Ovarian cancer		1800	3600	NR	22 months		M4	Survived
Seymour et al. [16]	1999	54-55	Neuroendocrine cancer of ovary		450	750	NR	8 months		M4	10 weeks
Griesinger et al. [17]	2004	74	NSCLC stage IIIB	4 cycles × 100 mg/m^2		4800	NR	40 months	MDS-RA	M2	40 m
Current	2014	63	Endometrial cancer		1511	4312	45,XX,add(3)(p13),del(3)(q23q25),−5,add(5)(q13), add(7)(q11.2),der(17)t(5,17)(q15;q25)	7.5 months	MDS-RAEB	M4	2 weeks

of this adverse event, our review was limited by the paucity of similar case reports. Given that taxanes are commonly used in gynecological cancers, this rare but significant risk of myeloid neoplasms secondary to these agents should be taken into account while discussing and deciding on treatment options.

Abbreviations

MDS: Myelodysplastic syndrome
AML: Acute myelogenous leukemia
t-AML: Therapy related acute myelogenous leukemia
t-MN: Therapy related myeloid neoplasm
cGY: Centigrays.

References

[1] D. J. Park and H. P. Koeffler, "Therapy-related myelodysplastic syndromes," *Seminars in Hematology*, vol. 33, no. 3, pp. 256–273, 1996.

[2] W. Kern, T. Haferlach, S. Schnittger, W. Hiddemann, and C. Schoch, "Prognosis in therapy-related acute myeloid leukemia and impact of karyotype," *Journal of Clinical Oncology*, vol. 22, no. 12, pp. 2510–2511, 2004.

[3] H. M. Kantarjian, M. J. Keating, R. S. Walters et al., "Therapy-related leukemia and myelodysplastic syndrome: clinical, cytogenetic, and prognostic features," *Journal of Clinical Oncology*, vol. 4, no. 12, pp. 1748–1757, 1986.

[4] G. Chaplain, C. Milan, C. Sgro, P.-M. Carli, and C. Bonithon-Kopp, "Increased risk of acute leukemia after adjuvant chemotherapy for breast cancer: a population-based study," *Journal of Clinical Oncology*, vol. 18, no. 15, pp. 2836–2842, 2000.

[5] M. J. Ratain and J. D. Rowley, "Therapy-related acute myeloid leukemia secondary to inhibitors of topoisomerase II: from the bedside to the target genes," *Annals of Oncology*, vol. 3, supplement 2, pp. S107–S111, 1992.

[6] J. Pedersen-Bjergaard, "Insights into leukemogenesis from therapy-related leukemia," *The New England Journal of Medicine*, vol. 352, no. 15, pp. 1591–1594, 2005.

[7] L. B. Travis, E. J. Holowaty, K. Bergfeldt et al., "Risk of leukemia after platinum-based chemotherapy for ovarian cancer," *The New England Journal of Medicine*, vol. 340, no. 5, pp. 351–357, 1999.

[8] M. Ishikawa, K. Nakayama, M. T. Rahman et al., "Therapy-related myelodysplastic syndrome and acute myeloid leukemia following chemotherapy (paclitaxel and carboplatin) and radiation therapy in ovarian cancer: a case report," *European Journal of Gynaecological Oncology*, vol. 35, no. 4, pp. 443–448, 2014.

[9] S. Vanajakshi, S. V. S. S. Prasad, S. S. Amina, E. Kavitha, K. Iravathy Goud, and K. Kshitija, "Therapy related myelodysplasia/myeloproliferative neoplasia-unclassified with acute leukemic transformation following Paclitaxel and Carboplatin based chemotherapy in an ovarian cancer patient," *Indian Journal of Hematology and Blood Transfusion*, vol. 30, supplement 1, pp. 258–263, 2014.

[10] H. T. See, D. A. Thomas, C. Bueso-Ramos, and J. Kavanagh, "Secondary leukemia after treatment with paclitaxel and carboplatin in a patient with recurrent ovarian cancer," *International Journal of Gynecological Cancer*, vol. 16, supplement 1, pp. 236–240, 2006.

[11] S. Yeasmin, K. Nakayama, M. Ishibashi et al., "Therapy-related myelodysplasia and acute myeloid leukemia following paclitaxel- and carboplatin-based chemotherapy in an ovarian cancer patient: a case report and literature review," *International Journal of Gynecological Cancer*, vol. 18, no. 6, pp. 1371–1376, 2008.

[12] K. B. Kim, S. Fader, C. S. Hwang, and F. R. Khuri, "Chronic myelomonocytic leukaemia after platinum-based therapy for non-small cell lung cancer: case report and review of the literature," *Journal of Clinical Pharmacy and Therapeutics*, vol. 31, no. 4, pp. 401–406, 2006.

[13] A. Gupta, M. M. Patnaik, and H. V. Naina, "*MYST3/CREBBP* rearranged acute myeloid leukemia after adjuvant chemotherapy for breast cancer," *Case Reports in Oncological Medicine*, vol. 2014, Article ID 361748, 3 pages, 2014.

[14] B. Melichar, J. Laco, P. Fridrichov, M. Imkovia, T. Papajk, and L. Foretov, "Therapy-related myeloid neoplasms in epithelial ovarian cancer patients carrying BRCA1 mutation: report of two cases," *Acta Oncologica*, vol. 51, no. 1, pp. 136–138, 2012.

[15] J. Christodoulou, C. Schoch, S. Schnittger, and T. Haferlach, "Myelodysplastic syndrome (RARS) with +i(12p) abnormality in a patient 10 months after diagnosis and successful treatment of a mediastinal germ cell tumor (MGCT)," *Annals of Hematology*, vol. 83, no. 6, pp. 386–389, 2004.

[16] J. F. Seymour, S. K. Juneja, L. J. Campbell, P. H. Ellims, E. H. Estey, and H. M. Prince, "Secondary acute myeloid leukemia with inv(16): report of two cases following paclitaxel-containing chemotherapy and review of the role of intensified ara-C therapy," *Leukemia*, vol. 13, no. 11, pp. 1735–1740, 1999.

[17] F. Griesinger, M. Metz, L. Trümper, T. Schulz, and D. Haase, "Secondary leukaemia after cure for locally advanced NSCLC: alkylating type secondary leukaemia after induction therapy with docetaxel and carboplatin for NSCLC IIIB," *Lung Cancer*, vol. 44, no. 2, pp. 261–265, 2004.

[18] T. Arimoto, S. Nakagawa, T. Yasugi et al., "Treatment with paclitaxel plus carboplatin, alone or with irradiation, of advanced or recurrent endometrial carcinoma," *Gynecologic Oncology*, vol. 104, no. 1, pp. 32–35, 2007.

[19] C. M. Michener, G. Peterson, B. Kulp, K. D. Webster, and M. Markman, "Carboplatin plus paclitaxel in the treatment of advanced or recurrent endometrial carcinoma," *Journal of Cancer Research and Clinical Oncology*, vol. 131, no. 9, pp. 581–584, 2005.

[20] R. E. Smith, "Risk for the development of treatment-related acute myelocytic leukemia and myelodysplastic syndrome among patients with breast cancer: review of the literature and the National Surgical Adjuvant Breast and Bowel Project experience," *Clinical Breast Cancer*, vol. 4, no. 4, pp. 273–279, 2003.

[21] R. A. Larson, "Cytogenetics, not just previous therapy, determines the course of therapy-related myeloid neoplasms," *Journal of Clinical Oncology*, vol. 30, no. 19, pp. 2300–2302, 2012.

Two Cases of Heavy Chain MGUS

Jan Van Keer,[1] Björn Meijers,[1,2] Michel Delforge,[3,4] Gregor Verhoef,[3,5] and Koen Poesen[6,7]

[1]*Nephrology, Dialysis and Renal Transplantation, University Hospitals Leuven, 3000 Leuven, Belgium*
[2]*Laboratory of Nephrology, Department of Microbiology and Immunology, KU Leuven, 3000 Leuven, Belgium*
[3]*Hematology, University Hospitals Leuven, 3000 Leuven, Belgium*
[4]*Laboratory for Stem Cell Biology and Embryology, Department of Development and Regeneration, KU Leuven, 3000 Leuven, Belgium*
[5]*Laboratory for Experimental Hematology, Department of Oncology, KU Leuven, 3000 Leuven, Belgium*
[6]*Laboratory Medicine, University Hospitals Leuven, 3000 Leuven, Belgium*
[7]*Laboratory for Molecular Neurobiomarker Research, Department of Neurosciences, KU Leuven, 3000 Leuven, Belgium*

Correspondence should be addressed to Koen Poesen; koen.poesen@uzleuven.be

Academic Editor: Josep M. Ribera

Heavy chain diseases are rare variants of B-cell lymphomas that produce one of three classes of immunoglobulin heavy chains, without corresponding light chains. We describe two patients with asymptomatic heavy chain monoclonal gammopathy. The first patient is a 51-year-old woman with alpha paraprotein on serum immunofixation. The second case is a 46-year-old woman with gamma paraprotein on urine immunofixation. Neither patient had corresponding monoclonal light chains. Workup for multiple myeloma and lymphoma was negative in both patients. These two cases illustrate that heavy chain monoclonal gammopathy can exist in the absence of clinically apparent malignancy. Only a few reports of "heavy chain MGUS" have been described before. In the absence of specialized guidelines, we suggest a similar follow-up as for MGUS, while taking into account the higher probability of progression to lymphoma than to myeloma.

1. Introduction

Heavy chain diseases are characterized by the presence of monoclonal heavy chains without light chains in serum and/or urine [1]. They are rare variants of B-cell lymphomas that produce one of three classes of immunoglobulin heavy chains: alpha, gamma, or mu [2–4]. The clinical manifestations vary with the heavy chain isotype and range from an asymptomatic presentation to aggressive lymphoma [5]. In this report, we describe two patients with asymptomatic heavy chain monoclonal gammopathy, who meet the criteria of "monoclonal gammopathy of undetermined significance" (MGUS) [6].

2. Case 1

A 51-year-old woman with a past medical history of depression and dyslipidemia was referred by her general practitioner to the hematology consultation. During the workup of myalgia after start of rosuvastatin therapy, an abnormal serum protein electrophoresis was discovered. At the time of referral, rosuvastatin was stopped and myalgia had disappeared. The patient was asymptomatic. Her only medication consisted of risperidone 1 mg. She never smoked. Physical findings were normal. Laboratory findings included hemoglobin of 14.0 g/dL, total leukocyte count of 8.4×10^9/L with normal differential count, and platelets of 360×10^9/L. Serum creatinine was 0.62 mg/dL (eGFR > 90 mL/min/1.73 m^2) and blood urea nitrogen 10 mg/dL. Calcium level was normal. Liver function, lactate dehydrogenase, creatine kinase, and coagulation tests were within normal limits. C-reactive protein was 1.6 mg/L (reference value < 5 mg/L).

Serum protein electrophoresis showed a monoclonal spike of 8.9 g/L in the beta-fraction (see Figure 1). Immunofixation revealed an alpha paraprotein, without corresponding monoclonal kappa or lambda chains. 24-hour urine collection contained 0.11 g of protein, without monoclonal spike. Serum total IgA level was 7.20 g/L.

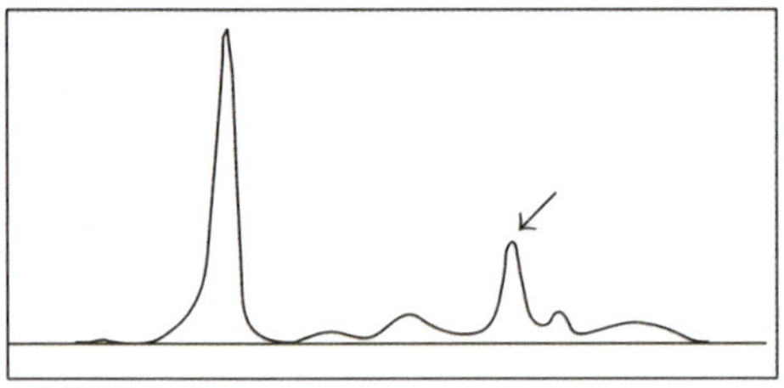

(a)

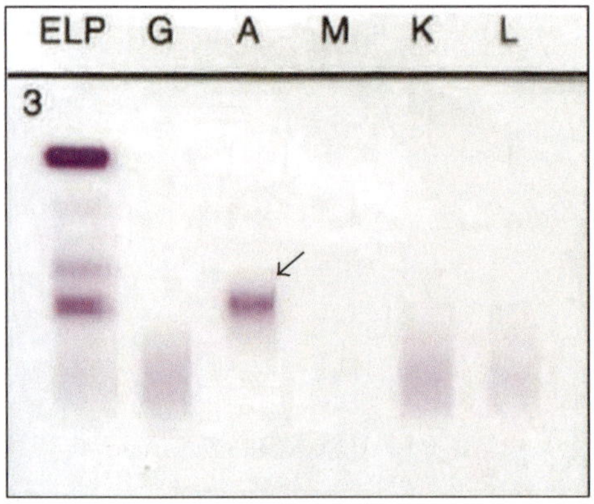

(b)

FIGURE 1: (a) Serum protein electrophoresis showing monoclonal spike in the beta-fraction (arrow). (b) Serum immunofixation showing presence of alpha paraprotein (arrow), without corresponding kappa or lambda light chains.

TABLE 1: Evolution of total IgA and estimated monoclonal spike during 8 years of follow-up.

Time (y)	IgA (g/L)	Estimated monoclonal spike (g/L)
0	7.20	8.9
1	6.72	NA
2	7.08	NA
3	8.18	9.1
4	8.63	NA
5	7.72	NA
6	NA	NA
7	NA	NA
8	9.53	10.9

Bone marrow was normocellular with trilineage hematopoiesis and normal percentage of plasma and lymphoid cells. X-ray metastatic bone survey was negative. Chest X-ray and abdominal ultrasound showed no lymphadenopathy or organomegaly. Upper gastrointestinal endoscopy excluded MALT lymphoma. During 8 years of follow-up, the patient developed hypertension and type 2 diabetes; otherwise she remained asymptomatic. Kidney function remained stable. Serum monoclonal spike rose from 8.9 to 10.9 g/L and total IgA from 7.20 to 9.53 g/L (see Table 1). Urine electrophoresis stayed negative.

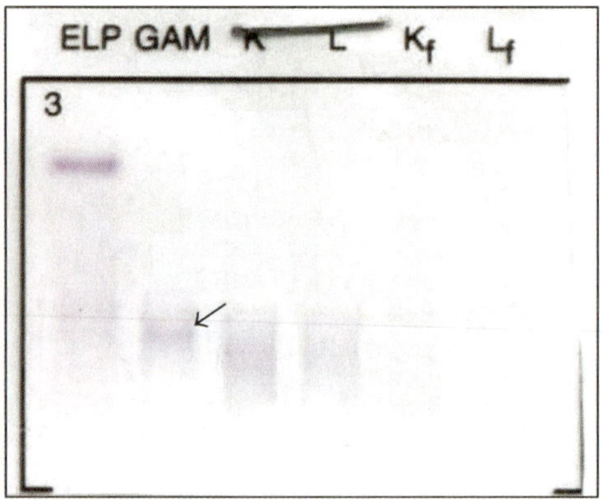

FIGURE 2: Urinary immunofixation shows a gamma paraprotein (arrow), without corresponding monoclonal light chains.

In conclusion, we describe an asymptomatic patient with an incidental finding of monoclonal gammopathy, corresponding to alpha heavy chains without monoclonal light chains. As workup for lymphoma, myeloma, and monoclonal gammopathy related end organ damage was negative, we diagnosed a heavy chain monoclonal gammopathy of undetermined significance (MGUS). During 8 years of follow-up, serum monoclonal spike was relatively stable and urine electrophoresis remained negative.

3. Case 2

A 46-year-old woman was referred to the nephrology consultation for the investigation of chronic kidney disease, with serum creatinine of 1.72 mg/dL (eGFR: 35 mL/min/1.73 m^2) and blood urea nitrogen of 66 mg/dL. The patient's medical history included squamous cell carcinoma of the right ovary, for which she had undergone extensive surgery (total pelvic exenteration with colostomy and Bricker diversion, sigmoid resection, and partial enterectomy), chemotherapy (cisplatinum, 5-fluorouracil, and mitomycin C, followed by carboplatin, etoposide, ifosfamide, and paclitaxel), and pelvic radiotherapy. The remainder of her past medical history was remarkable for hypertension, anemia of chronic kidney disease, and short bowel syndrome after the aforementioned surgery, for which she was treated with total parenteral nutrition. Her medication included darbepoetin alfa 60 μg per 2 weeks, ramipril 5 mg, barnidipine 10 mg, sodium bicarbonate 4 g daily, and an estradiol patch. She never smoked. Blood pressure was well controlled.

Serum and urine protein electrophoresis and immunofixation were ordered in the workup of chronic kidney disease. Immunofixation of the 25-fold concentrated 24-hour urine collection showed the presence of a weak monoclonal band typed as gamma heavy chain, without monoclonal kappa or lambda immunoglobulin light chains (see Figure 2). Serum electrophoresis and immunofixation were normal. Total IgG, IgA, and IgM values were 14.40 g/L, 2.73 g/L, and 0.78 g/L, respectively. Serum free light chains were elevated in accordance with the degree of renal insufficiency: 35.00 mg/L for kappa and 35.80 mg/L for lambda light chains, with a normal kappa/lambda ratio (0.98).

Hemogram showed a hemoglobin of 11.2 g/dL, total leukocyte count of 5.14 × 10^9/L with a normal differential count, and platelets of 125 × 10^9/L. Peripheral blood smear showed no abnormal lymphocyte population. Liver function, coagulation tests, lipid profile, and fasting and postprandial blood sugars were within normal limits. C-reactive protein was 1.9 mg/L (reference value, < 5 mg/L). Urine sediment showed sterile pyuria and microscopic hematuria (48/μL), a normal finding given the Bricker urinary diversion. Proteinuria on a 24-hour urine collection was 0.23 g.

Bone marrow biopsy showed normal presence of all cell lines with a mild elevation of plasma cells (3.7%), without an atypical morphology. Whole body computed tomography (CT) with 18-fluorodeoxyglucose (FDG) positron emission tomography (PET) showed no evidence of lymphoma. Ultrasound examination revealed relatively small kidneys (left: 99 mm, right: 94 mm) with bilateral significant dilatation of the pyelocaliceal system. Kidney biopsy showed extensive chronic destruction of renal parenchyma in a zonal pattern. All these findings are suggestive of reflux nephropathy. There was no evidence of cast nephropathy, amyloidosis, or heavy or light chain deposition disease on renal biopsy.

In conclusion, we describe a patient with chronic kidney disease due to reflux nephropathy after Bricker urinary diversion, whose urine immunofixation showed presence of monoclonal gamma heavy chains. Workup for lymphoma and myeloma was negative; kidney biopsy showed no monoclonal gammopathy related pathology. Since only one year of follow-up is available, early stage Franklin's disease cannot be entirely excluded. No specific treatment was started. During one year of follow-up the clinical situation remained unchanged.

4. Discussion

Heavy chain diseases are B-cell lymphoproliferative disorders that are characterized by the production of monoclonal immunoglobulins consisting of heavy chains without associated light chains [1]. The diagnosis is established by demonstration of alpha, gamma, or mu paraprotein on serum and/or urine protein electrophoresis and immunofixation, without corresponding monoclonal kappa or lambda chains. One should be aware that differing sensitivity of heavy and light chain reagents could potentially cause false negative results of light chain immunofixation. This would incorrectly suggest the diagnosis of heavy chain disease in a case of a regular, intact monoclonal gammopathy.

Alpha, gamma, and mu heavy chain diseases have been described [2–4]. Of these, alpha heavy chain disease (Seligmann's disease) is the most common. It was first described in 1968 by Seligmann et al. [7], hence its eponym. Approximately 175 cases have been described. The patients typically present with chronic diarrhea, malabsorption, and weight loss. Some patients develop extensive mesenteric adenopathy [2]. Alpha heavy chain disease is also known as immunoproliferative small intestinal disease. It is a form of MALT lymphoma and is associated with poor sanitation and *Campylobacter jejuni* infection [8]. Some cases may respond to treatment with antibiotics. Therefore an endoscopic and microbiologic study of the digestive tract is indicated in the workup of alpha heavy chain disease.

Gamma heavy chain disease is intermediate in frequency. It is also called Franklin's disease [9], after the author of the first report in 1964. Since then, approximately 130 cases have been described in the literature. The classical presentation is one with generalized lymphadenopathy, splenomegaly, and anemia [10]. The most distinctive symptom is palatal edema resulting from enlargement of nodes in Waldeyer's ring, sometimes leading to respiratory compromise [2]. Gamma heavy chain disease is associated with autoimmune disease in almost one-third of cases: rheumatoid arthritis is most common; other associated diseases include autoimmune hemolytic anemia and idiopathic thrombocytopenic purpura [1].

Mu heavy chain disease is the least common of the heavy chain diseases. Less than 30 cases have been reported. Its clinical features resemble chronic lymphocytic leukemia. Vacuolated lymphocytes in the bone marrow are characteristic [11]. Unlike alpha and gamma heavy chain diseases, mu heavy chain disease can be associated with increased free light chain excretion as some tumor cells seem to have a defect in the assembly of both light and heavy chains.

We described two cases (one alpha and one gamma) of heavy chain monoclonal gammopathy who were asymptomatic. Based the low value of the monoclonal spike (<30 g/L) and bone marrow monoclonal plasma cells (<10%), absence of end organ damage, and clinical or radiographic evidence of lymphoma, these cases met the criteria for monoclonal gammopathy of undetermined significance (MGUS) [6].

Only a few reports of "heavy chain MGUS" have been described previously [1, 11–15]. There are no established guidelines for follow-up. We propose the same follow-up as for normal MGUS. However, unlike normal MGUS, there are no validated risk factors for progression that could guide intensity of follow-up. Note that most heavy chain diseases are lymphoproliferative disorders. Therefore, heavy chain MGUS is more likely to progress to lymphoma than to myeloma. Follow-up should focus on assessment of lymphadenopathy and organomegaly. This can be done by regular physical examination in most cases and imaging on indication. Follow-up should include measurement of serum and urinary M-protein, complete blood count, creatinine, and electrolytes. M-protein level can be determined semiquantitatively by protein electrophoresis and immunofixation. At this moment, there are no commercially available quantitative techniques to measure monoclonal free heavy chains.

5. Conclusion

Heavy chain diseases are rare variants of B-cell lymphomas characterized by the presence of monoclonal heavy chains, alpha, gamma, or mu, without corresponding light chains. Clinical presentation is diverse. We describe two asymptomatic cases that meet the criteria of MGUS. This report demonstrates that heavy chain monoclonal gammopathy can exist in the absence of clinically apparent malignancy, similar to other forms of MGUS. In the absence of specialized guidelines, we suggest a similar follow-up as for MGUS, while taking into account the higher probability of progression to lymphoma than to myeloma.

Consent

Written informed consent was obtained from both patients for publication of this case report.

References

[1] D. L. Wahner-Roedler, T. E. Witzig, L. L. Loehrer, and R. A. Kyle, "γ-Heavy chain disease: review of 23 cases," *Medicine*, vol. 82, no. 4, pp. 236–250, 2003.

[2] N. C. Munshi, L. Longo Dan, and C. Anderson Kenneth, "Plasma cell disorders," in *Harrison's Principles of Internal Medicine*, A. S. Fauci, E. Braunwald, D. L. Kasper et al., Eds., chapter 106, McGraw-Hill, 17th edition, 2008, http://www.accessmedicine.com/content.aspx.

[3] T. M. Grogan, B. Van Camp, R. A. Kyle, H. K. Müller-Hermelink, and N. L. Harris, "Pathology and genetics of tumors of haemato-poietc and lymphoid tissues," in *World Health Organization Classification of Tumors (WHO): Plasma Cell Neoplasm*, pp. 75–107, World Health Organization, Geneva, Switzerland, 2001.

[4] J.-P. Fermand, J.-C. Brouet, F. Danon, and M. Seligmann, "Gamma heavy chain 'disease': heterogeneity of the clinicopathologic features report of 16 cases and review of the literature," *Medicine*, vol. 68, no. 6, pp. 321–335, 1989.

[5] S. Bieliauskas, R. R. Tubbs, C. M. Bacon et al., "Gamma heavy-chain disease: defining the spectrum of associated lymphoproliferative disorders through analysis of 13 cases," *The American Journal of Surgical Pathology*, vol. 36, no. 4, pp. 534–543, 2012.

[6] The International Myeloma Working Group, "Criteria for the classification of monoclonal gammopathies, multiple myeloma and related disorders: a report of the International Myeloma Working Group," *British Journal of Haematology*, vol. 121, no. 5, pp. 749–757, 2003.

[7] M. Seligmann, F. Danon, D. Hurez, E. Mihaesco, and J. L. Preud'Homme, "Alpha-chain disease: a new immunoglobulin abnormality," *Science*, vol. 162, no. 3860, pp. 1396–1397, 1968.

[8] M. Lecuit, E. Abachin, A. Martin et al., "Immunoproliferative small intestinal disease associated with campylobacter jejuni," *The New England Journal of Medicine*, vol. 350, no. 3, pp. 239–248, 2004.

[9] E. C. Franklin, "Structural studies of human 7S y-globulin (G immunoglobulin). Further observations of a naturally occurring protein related to the crystallizable (fast) fragment," *The Journal of Experimental Medicine*, vol. 120, no. 5, pp. 691–709, 1964.

[10] N. C. Munshi, S. Digumarthy, and A. Rahemtullah, "Case 13-2008: a 46-year-old man with rheumatoid arthritis and lymphadenopathy," *The New England Journal of Medicine*, vol. 358, no. 17, pp. 1780–1848, 2008.

[11] D. L. Wahner-Roedler and R. A. Kyle, "μ-Heavy chain disease: presentation as a benign monoclonal gammopathy," *American Journal of Hematology*, vol. 40, no. 1, pp. 56–60, 1992.

[12] L. M. Galanti, C. Doyen, C. V. Maelen et al., "Biological diagnosis of a gamma-1-heavy chain disease in an asymptomatic patient," *European Journal of Haematology*, vol. 54, no. 3, pp. 202–204, 1995.

[13] J. W. Lenders, R. S. Holdrinet, C. T. Nguyen, and R. De Waal, "A case of gamma-heavy chain monoclonal gammopathy of undetermined significance," *The Netherlands Journal of Medicine*, vol. 27, no. 10, pp. 412–416, 1984.

[14] J. Westin, R. Eyrich, E. Falsen et al., "Gamma heavy chain disease. Reports of three patients," *Acta Medica Scandinavica*, vol. 192, no. 4, pp. 281–292, 1972.

[15] M. Seligmann, "Heavy chain diseases," *La Revue du Praticien*, vol. 43, no. 3, pp. 317–320, 1993.

50

Laparoscopic Resection of Recurrence from Hepatocellular Carcinoma after Liver Transplantation: Case Reports

Mushegh A. Sahakyan,[1,2,3] Airazat M. Kazaryan,[1,4] Ewa Pomianowska,[5] Andreas Abildgaard,[6] Pål-Dag Line,[7] Bjørn Atle Bjørnbeth,[5] Bjørn Edwin,[1,2,5] and Bård Ingvald Røsok[5]

[1] *The Intervention Centre, Oslo University Hospital, Rikshospitalet, 0027 Oslo, Norway*
[2] *Institute of Clinical Research, Medical Faculty, University of Oslo, 0318 Oslo, Norway*
[3] *Department of Surgery No. 1, Yerevan State Medical University after M. Heratsi, 0025 Yerevan, Armenia*
[4] *Department of Gastrointestinal Surgery, Akershus University Hospital, 1478 Lørenskog, Norway*
[5] *Department of HPB Surgery, Oslo University Hospital, Rikshospitalet, 0407 Oslo, Norway*
[6] *Department of Radiology, Oslo University Hospital, Rikshospitalet, 0027 Oslo, Norway*
[7] *Department of Transplantation Medicine, Oslo University Hospital, Rikshospitalet, 0424 Oslo, Norway*

Correspondence should be addressed to Mushegh A. Sahakyan; sahakyan.mushegh@gmail.com

Academic Editor: Constantine Gennatas

Background. Recurrence of hepatocellular carcinoma (HCC) after liver transplantation (LT) indicates a poor prognosis. Surgery is considered the only curative option for selected patients with HCC recurrence following LT. Traditionally, the preference is given to the open approach. *Methods.* In this report, we present two cases of laparoscopic resections (LR) for recurrent HCC after LT, performed at Oslo University Hospital, Rikshospitalet. *Results.* Both procedures were executed without intraoperative and postoperative adverse events. Whereas one of the patients had a recurrence one year after LR, the other patient did not have any sign of disease during 3-year follow-up. *Conclusions.* We argue that, in selected cases, patients with HCC recurrence following LT may benefit from LR due to its limited tissue trauma and timely start of subsequent treatment if curative resection cannot be obtained. In patients with relatively favorable prognosis, LR facilitates postoperative recovery course and avoids unnecessary laparotomy.

1. Introduction

Hepatocellular carcinoma (HCC) is the fifth most common cancer and the second leading cause of cancer related death in the world with more than a half million new cases annually [1, 2].

The key aspect in successful treatment of HCC is linked to proper preoperative staging. The most widely adopted staging system is the Barcelona Clinic Liver Cancer (BCLC) system, based on tumor stage, severity of liver disease, and performance status of the patients to different therapeutic alternatives. According to BCLC recommendations, the patients with early HCC are suitable candidates for radical treatment (i.e., resection, liver transplantation, or radio frequency ablation). Among these approaches, liver transplantation (LT) seems to be an attractive therapeutic option, particularly in patients with significant liver parenchymal disease (Child-Pugh B and C), as it has the potential to cure both the tumor and underlying liver disease [3].

However LT is often limited to early stages of disease in order to ensure outcomes that are comparable to those of liver transplantation for noncancer related indications. Selection criteria, such as Milan (a single tumor ≤ 5 cm or ≤ 3 tumors ≤ 3 cm without signs of macrovascular invasion), UCSF (a single tumor ≤ 6.5 cm, or ≤ 3 tumors with the largest being ≤ 4.5 cm, and a total tumor burden of ≤ 8 cm), and up-to-seven

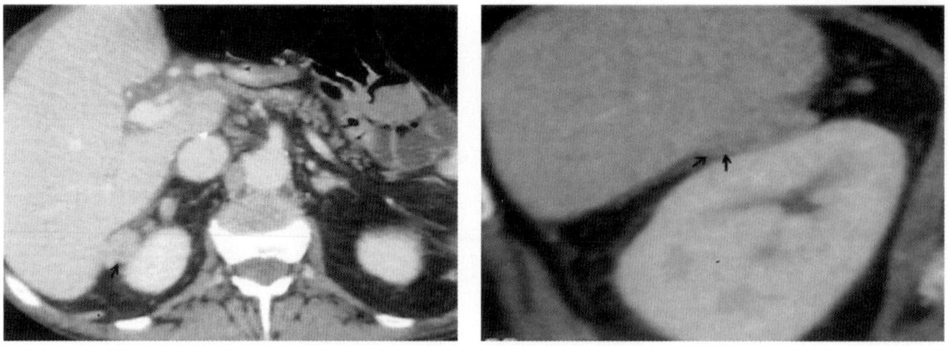

FIGURE 1: CT with intravenous contrast. Extrahepatic lesion between liver segment 6 and right kidney, largest diameter 2 cm.

(the sum of the number of nodules and of the diameter of the largest tumor (in cm) not exceeding seven, in absence of macrovascular invasion and extrahepatic spread), have been introduced up to date [4–8].

At the same time, recurrence of HCC after LT still occurs and is to a large extent related to tumor stage. Relapse after transplantation is usually associated with poor prognosis, since in most cases it must be considered as a sign of systemic disease. Extrahepatic lesions, present in majority of these patients, are not amenable to curative treatment, thereby being considered for palliative therapy only. However, the efficacy of the latter remains unsatisfactory [9]. Several authors emphasized the curative role of surgery for HCC recurrences, indicating that longer time interval between LT and the recurrence and feasibility of resection are associated with improved survival [10–12].

Today, laparoscopic surgery is comparable to open technique for primary resection in a large fraction of patients with HCC [13]. However, in terms of tumor recurrences, a conventional open technique is usually preferred, perhaps considering the fact that patients had previously undergone major surgical procedure. In our review of current literature, we are not aware of any report concerning laparoscopic approach for HCC recurrence after LT. Herein we report on two cases of recurrences following LT that were treated by laparoscopic resections at our institution.

2. Materials and Methods

Hospital records review revealed that 89 patients with HCC on final pathology underwent LT at Oslo University Hospital, Rikshospitalet, from 2004 to 2014. Eighteen of these patients (20.2%) had recurrence during follow-up. Of these, two with locoregional isolated recurrences and performance status of 0 according to Eastern Cooperative Oncology Group (ECOG) scale were considered eligible for curative resection. Laparoscopic approach was applied.

3. Results

3.1. Case 1. A 62-year-old male underwent LT for multifocal HCC, combined with hepatitis C related cirrhosis. According to preoperative CT scan images, a massive lesion with greatest extent over 8 cm was found in the right lobe and 2-3 small lesions were found in segment 2. AFP level was elevated at 278 ng/mL. Histological examination of the explanted liver revealed disseminated HCC with numerous nodules in all segments and widespread vessel infiltration. In the posttransplant period the patient received immunosuppressive therapy with tacrolimus, prednisolone, and mycophenolate mofetil (MMF).

Nine months after LT a routine CT scan revealed an extrahepatic, 2 cm lesion adjacent to segment 6 (Figure 1). Ultrasound guided biopsy verified HCC. The case was determined suitable for laparoscopic resection.

Pneumoperitoneum was established through an open approach via right pararectal region, supplemented by three trocars: a 12 mm through the scar from previous incision and two 5 mm in the right flank. After complete mobilization of the right lobe, the tumor was found retroperitoneally between the right kidney and adrenal gland. Intraoperative ultrasound was carried out to determine the borders of the tumor. Despite close relation with renal capsule, no signs of infiltration to the kidney were revealed. Division of Gerota's fascia and exposing the upper part of the kidney allowed mobilization of the tumor laterally and cranially, separating it from the renal capsule. No evidence of infiltration to adjacent structures was found and the tumor was removed. No significant bleeding occurred during the surgery and the operation time was 131 min.

Histological findings confirmed the presence of two (40 mm and 12 mm) extrahepatic recurrences from HCC. The postoperative course was uneventful.

Surveillance for the first 8 months revealed no signs of disease recurrence, but one year after the reresection, metastases in liver, lungs, and adrenal gland were detected. Subsequent therapy with sorafenib was considered as the only possible active treatment.

3.2. Case 2. HCC was diagnosed in a 57-year-old male with hepatitis C and cirrhosis. A 3 cm tumor, located in segment 5, and two small hypervascular lesions, suggestive of HCC, were discovered by CT scan. The AFP level was significantly elevated (>20.000).

The patient was assessed and accepted as a liver recipient and LT was performed. The postoperative course was uneventful and the patient received immunosuppression with tacrolimus, prednisolone, and MMF.

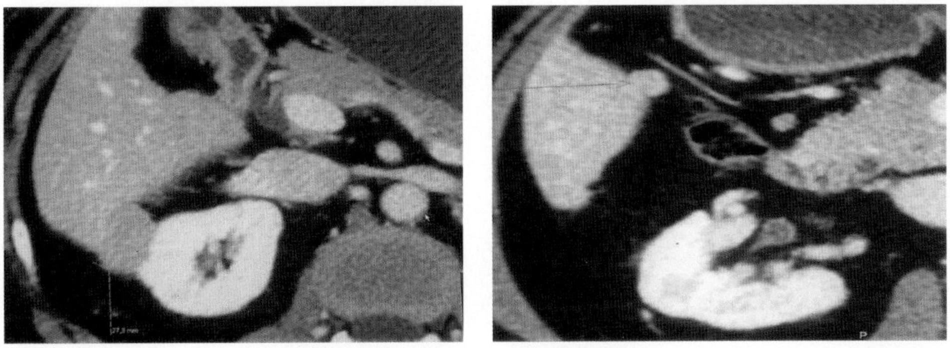

(a) (b)

FIGURE 2: CT with intravenous contrast. Two lesions detected. First lesion adjacent to lateral part of right kidney, largest diameter 2.7 cm (a). Second lesion close to duodenum, largest diameter 1.4 cm (b).

An abdominal CT scan, 6 years after LT, detected two intrahepatic lesions. The larger one, measuring 2.7 cm, was located laterally in segment 6, close to the right kidney (Figure 2(a)). The second lesion of 1.4 cm was located between the segments 5 and 6, adjacent to the wall of duodenum (Figure 2(b)).

The laparoscopic approach was chosen for reresection. Pneumoperitoneum was obtained through an open access technique via umbilicus. Adhesiolysis was carried out. Afterwards, one 12 mm trocar was placed high in the midline, followed by two 5 mm trocars in the right pararectal area and more laterally. Mobilizing the right lobe of the liver, the lateral tumor was found to infiltrate into Gerota's fascia. Using LigaSure (Valleylab/Covidien, Boulder, CO, USA) device, the tumor was completely mobilized and separated from the fascia. Finally, both of the tumors were removed by wedge resection of the liver. Operative time was 127 min with only minor intraoperative blood loss observed.

A pathological examination revealed 32 mm and 18 mm measuring moderately differentiated HCC with trabecular pattern. The postoperative course was uneventful. During further surveillance for more than 3 years, no signs of disease recurrence have been observed.

4. Discussion

LT is associated with significantly higher 5-year overall and disease-free survival rates, compared to LR (65.7% versus 43.8%; $P = 0.005$ and 85.3% versus 22.7%; $P < 0.001$, resp.); hence it should be considered in patients with liver disease and cirrhosis within the various transplantation criteria [14, 15]. Unlike resection, LT is also an ultimate solution for treatment of HCC and underlying cirrhosis [16]. Up to 83% 5-year recurrence-free survival rates have been reported after LT for HCC, which is comparable to LT for nonmalignant disease [17].

Unfortunately, even the utilization of criteria for LT does not prevent tumor recurrence. According to Welker and coworkers [10], the recurrence rates following LT vary between 15% and 20%. The latter was assumed to be dependent from patient selection criteria for initial LT. In another paper by Sotiropoulos and colleagues [18] a 12.6% recurrence rate was found among the patients within the Milan criteria.

Numerous retrospective analyses have been performed to estimate the factors leading to the recurrence and eventual poor outcome. Parameters such as vascular invasion, poor differentiation, tumor size >5 cm, number of lesions, HCC exceeding the Milan criteria, and elevated pretransplant AFP levels have been reported to have significant impact on the rate of posttransplant recurrences [18–20].

The limitations of therapeutic options for recurrent HCC after LT lead to an absence of established treatment strategies [18, 21]. A major contraindication for reresection is the presence of extrahepatic recurrences that have been described in 10–43% of patients. These are typically located in lungs, bones, abdominal lymph nodes, and adrenal glands [22]. Nevertheless, even though disseminated disease commonly precludes curative treatment, patients with limited intra- or extrahepatic lesions may still benefit from local treatment, including surgical resection [17]. Roayaie et al. [12] reported that recurrent disease should be treated by surgery whenever possible, since it was independently associated with prolonged survival of 47% at 5 years. Hwang et al. [23] recommended performing pulmonary metastasectomy for resectable HCC metastases in lungs following LT, as it may provide a chance of long-term survival in a substantial proportion of patients. According to recent clinical studies, resection of both intra- and/or extrahepatic lesions in a selected group of patients can be associated with an improved overall 5-year survival ranging from 27 to 88% [22, 24–26]. Furthermore, the authors conclude that even noncurative surgery seems to prolong survival [18]. Reportedly, resection rates for recurrent HCC may vary from 31 to 43% among different centers [19]. However, the studies are limited by retrospective design and a small series of cases, reported so far (Table 1).

Another available surgical option seems to be retransplantation. Nevertheless, the attempts are currently made to salvage graft rather than performing retransplantation, because of the organ shortage. Hence, although the resections are relatively rare, they are associated with favorable outcome

TABLE 1: Recurrence and resection rates following liver transplantation.

Authors	Year of publication	Liver transplantations	Total number of recurrences	Resections for recurrent HCC
Pfeiffenberger et al. [29]	2013	136	18	3 (16.6%)
Hwang et al. [23]	2012	587	43	23*
Chok et al. [16]	2011	139	24	17 (70.8%)
Pfiffer et al. [24]	2011	139	24	7 (29.1%)
Kornberg et al. [17]	2010	60	16	7 (44%)
Shin et al. [30]	2010	138	28	4 (14.3%)
Valdivieso et al. [19]	2010	182	23	11 (47.8%)
Taketomi et al. [25]	2010	101	17	9 (52.9%)
Roayaie et al. [12]	2004	311	57	15 (32%)
Schlitt et al. [11]	1999	69	39	15 (38%)
Regalia et al. [26]	1998	132	21	7 (32%)

*Hwang et al. reported on 43 HCC cases with pulmonary recurrences after LT. 23 patients underwent resections.

in selected patients and avoid retransplantation in most of the cases [27].

There has been a considerable development in laparoscopic liver surgery during the last decade and it is now generally accepted that laparoscopic resection offers advantages, compared to the open approach in terms of severity of complications, 30-day readmission rate, length of hospital stay, and blood loss [28]. However, no reports in the literature concerning laparoscopic resections for recurrent HCC after LT have been observed to date.

In this report we present two cases that may suggest that laparoscopic resection is a feasible and safe procedure in selected patients with recurrent HCC following LT. Since these patients often have a dismal prognosis, emphasis should be on minimizing surgical risk and trauma when choosing therapeutic options for treatment of recurrence. In this context laparoscopy seems to be a rational approach that may be well suited in selected patients. The disparity in long-term outcome in two patients can probably be related to the difference between the risk factors for recurrence. While the first patient exceeded all morphological criteria systems, the second patient fulfilled each of them (BCLC, Milan, UGSF, and "up-to-seven"). On the other hand, the occurrence of so-called "de novo" cancer cannot be excluded in Case 2, considering the fact that the lesions developed 6 years after LT.

In the light of the limited role of medical therapy in palliative treatment of recurrent HCC, patients with poor prognosis and limited survival prospects can benefit from laparoscopy due to shortened recovery period. In case of indications for subsequent therapy, laparoscopy may avoid potential delay in treatment, caused by open surgery. Conversely, the patients with favorable prognosis may also benefit from the fast recovery course, provided by laparoscopy. Extensive experience in the field of laparoscopic surgery coupled with the evaluation of therapeutic options will establish the new surgical guidelines in treatment of resectable recurrent HCC after LT.

References

[1] S. Bhoori and V. Mazzaferro, "Current challenges in liver transplantation for hepatocellular carcinoma," *Best Practice & Research Clinical Gastroenterology*, vol. 28, no. 5, pp. 867–879, 2014.

[2] F. Pons, M. Varela, and J. M. Llovet, "Staging systems in hepatocellular carcinoma," *HPB*, vol. 7, no. 1, pp. 35–41, 2005.

[3] P.-A. Clavien, M. Lesurtel, P. M. Bossuyt, G. J. Gores, B. Langer, and A. Perrier, "Recommendations for liver transplantation for hepatocellular carcinoma: an international consensus conference report," *The Lancet Oncology*, vol. 13, no. 1, pp. e11–e22, 2012.

[4] V. Mazzaferro, E. Regalia, R. Doci et al., "Liver transplantation for the treatment of small hepatocellular carcinomas in patients with cirrhosis," *The New England Journal of Medicine*, vol. 334, no. 11, pp. 693–699, 1996.

[5] F. Y. Yao, L. Ferrell, N. M. Bass et al., "Liver transplantation for hepatocellular carcinoma: expansion of the tumor size limits does not adversely impact survival," *Hepatology*, vol. 33, no. 6, pp. 1394–1403, 2001.

[6] V. Mazzaferro, J. M. Llovet, R. Miceli et al., "Predicting survival after liver transplantation in patients with hepatocellular carcinoma beyond the Milan criteria: a retrospective, exploratory analysis," *The Lancet Oncology*, vol. 10, no. 1, pp. 35–43, 2009.

[7] D. A. Kooby, V. Egnatashvili, M. Graiser et al., "Changing management and outcome of hepatocellular carcinoma: evaluation of 501 patients treated at a single comprehensive center," *Journal of Surgical Oncology*, vol. 98, no. 2, pp. 81–88, 2008.

[8] K. V. Menon, A. R. Hakeem, and N. D. Heaton, "Review article: liver transplantation for hepatocellular carcinoma—a critical appraisal of the current worldwide listing criteria," *Alimentary Pharmacology and Therapeutics*, vol. 40, no. 8, pp. 893–902, 2014.

[9] J.-O. Lee, D.-Y. Kim, J. H. Lim et al., "Palliative chemotherapy for patients with recurrent hepatocellular carcinoma after liver transplantation," *Journal of Gastroenterology and Hepatology*, vol. 24, no. 5, pp. 800–805, 2009.

[10] M.-W. Welker, W.-O. Bechstein, S. Zeuzem, and J. Trojan, "Recurrent hepatocellular carcinoma after liver transplantation—an emerging clinical challenge," *Transplant International*, vol. 26, no. 2, pp. 109–118, 2013.

[11] H. J. Schlitt, M. Neipp, A. Weimann et al., "Recurrence patterns of hepatocellular and fibrolamellar carcinoma after liver transplantation," *Journal of Clinical Oncology*, vol. 17, no. 1, pp. 324–331, 1999.

[12] S. Roayaie, J. D. Schwartz, M. W. Sung et al., "Recurrence of hepatocellular carcinoma after liver transplant: patterns and prognosis," *Liver Transplantation*, vol. 10, no. 4, pp. 534–540, 2004.

[13] T. Kamiyama, M. Tahara, K. Nakanishi et al., "Long-term outcome of laparoscopic hepatectomy in patients with hepatocellular carcinoma," *Hepatogastroenterology*, vol. 61, no. 130, pp. 405–409, 2014.

[14] M. H. Squires III, S. I. Hanish, S. B. Fisher et al., "Transplant versus resection for the management of hepatocellular carcinoma meeting Milan Criteria in the MELD exception era at a single institution in a UNOS region with short wait times," *Journal of Surgical Oncology*, vol. 109, no. 6, pp. 533–541, 2014.

[15] R. J. Wong, J. Wantuck, A. Valenzuela et al., "Primary surgical resection versus liver transplantation for transplant-eligible hepatocellular carcinoma patients," *Digestive Diseases and Sciences*, vol. 59, no. 1, pp. 183–191, 2014.

[16] K. S. H. Chok, S. C. Chan, T. T. Cheung, A. C. Y. Chan, S. T. Fan, and C. M. Lo, "Late recurrence of hepatocellular carcinoma after liver transplantation," *World Journal of Surgery*, vol. 35, no. 9, pp. 2058–2062, 2011.

[17] A. Kornberg, B. Küpper, A. Tannapfel et al., "Long-term survival after recurrent hepatocellular carcinoma in liver transplant patients: clinical patterns and outcome variables," *European Journal of Surgical Oncology*, vol. 36, no. 3, pp. 275–280, 2010.

[18] G. C. Sotiropoulos, E. P. Molmenti, C. Lösch, S. Beckebaum, C. E. Broelsch, and H. Lang, "Meta-analysis of tumor recurrence after liver transplantation for hepatocellular carcinoma based on 1,198 cases," *European Journal of Medical Research*, vol. 12, no. 10, pp. 527–534, 2007.

[19] A. Valdivieso, J. Bustamante, M. Gastaca et al., "Management of hepatocellular carcinoma recurrence after liver transplantation," *Transplantation Proceedings*, vol. 42, no. 2, pp. 660–662, 2010.

[20] M. Abdel-Wahab, A. M. Sultan, O. M. Fathy et al., "Factors affecting recurrence and survival after living donor liver transplantation for hepatocellular carcinoma," *Hepato-Gastroenterology*, vol. 60, no. 128, pp. 1847–1853, 2013.

[21] H. R. Kim, S. H. Cheon, S. Y. Rha et al., "Treatment of recurrent hepatocellular carcinoma after liver transplantation," *Asia-Pacific Journal of Clinical Oncology*, vol. 7, no. 3, pp. 258–269, 2011.

[22] P. J. Kneuertz, D. P. Cosgrove, A. M. Cameron et al., "Multidisciplinary management of recurrent hepatocellular carcinoma following liver transplantation," *Journal of Gastrointestinal Surgery*, vol. 16, no. 4, pp. 874–881, 2012.

[23] S. Hwang, Y.-H. Kim, D. K. Kim et al., "Resection of pulmonary metastases from hepatocellular carcinoma following liver transplantation," *World Journal of Surgery*, vol. 36, no. 7, pp. 1592–1602, 2012.

[24] T. E. F. Pfiffer, D. Seehofer, A. Nicolaou, R. Neuhaus, H. Riess, and R. U. Trappe, "Recurrent hepatocellular carcinoma in liver transplant recipients: parameters affecting time to recurrence, treatment options and survival in the sorafenib era," *Tumori*, vol. 97, no. 4, pp. 436–441, 2011.

[25] A. Taketomi, T. Fukuhara, K. Morita et al., "Improved results of a surgical resection for the recurrence of hepatocellular carcinoma after living donor liver transplantation," *Annals of Surgical Oncology*, vol. 17, no. 9, pp. 2283–2289, 2010.

[26] E. Regalia, L. R. Fassati, U. Valente et al., "Pattern and management of recurrent hepatocellular carcinoma after liver transplantation," *Journal of Hepato-Biliary-Pancreatic Surgery*, vol. 5, no. 1, pp. 29–34, 1998.

[27] G. Marangoni, W. Faraj, H. Sethi, M. Rela, P. Muiesan, and N. Heaton, "Liver resection in liver transplant recipients," *Hepatobiliary and Pancreatic Diseases International*, vol. 7, no. 6, pp. 590–594, 2008.

[28] J. J. Lee, J. B. Conneely, R. L. Smoot et al., "Laparoscopic versus open liver resection for hepatocellular carcinoma at a North-American Centre: a 2-to-1 matched pair analysis," *HPB*, vol. 17, no. 4, pp. 304–310, 2015.

[29] J. Pfeiffenberger, R. Koschny, K. Hoffmann et al., "Sorafenib treatment is save and may affect survival of recurrent hepatocellular carcinoma after liver transplantation," *Langenbeck's Archives of Surgery*, vol. 398, no. 8, pp. 1123–1128, 2013.

[30] W. Y. Shin, K.-S. Suh, H. W. Lee et al., "Prognostic factors affecting survival after recurrence in adult living donor liver transplantation for hepatocellular carcinoma," *Liver Transplantation*, vol. 16, no. 5, pp. 678–684, 2010.

51

A Rare Case of Primary Anterior Mediastinal Yolk Sac Tumor in an Elderly Adult Male

Sammy G. Nakhla[1] **and Srinath Sundararajan**[2]

[1]*Department of Medicine, Southern Arizona VA Health Care System, Tucson, AZ 85723, USA*
[2]*Department of Hematology/Oncology, University of Arizona Cancer Center, Tucson, AZ 85724, USA*

Correspondence should be addressed to Sammy G. Nakhla; sammy.nakhla@va.gov

Academic Editor: Didier Frappaz

Mediastinal germ cell tumors are extragonadal germ cell tumors (EGGCTs) commonly seen in children and young adults. They are more common in men. Clinically they are classified as teratomas, seminomas, and nonseminomatous germ cell tumors. Primary mediastinal yolk sac neoplasm is an extremely rare tumor. We present here a very rare case of primary yolk sac tumor of the anterior mediastinum in a 73-year-old male. Mediastinal germ cell tumors have a worse prognosis than gonadal germ cell tumors. Chemotherapy followed by adjuvant surgery improves overall response in EGGCTs. However, comorbidities can render treatment with chemotherapy and surgery challenging in elderly patients.

1. Introduction

Yolk sac tumor is a subtype of germ cell tumor that is highly malignant. In addition to presenting in ovaries and testes, the tumor has been detected at several extragonadal sites such as the retroperitoneum, sacrococcygeal region, pineal gland, and the anterior mediastinum [1]. Primary yolk sac tumor (YST) of the anterior mediastinum is rare and has a grave prognosis. Often patients present with advanced stage tumors that are bulky and unresectable [2]. Like other germ cell tumors (GCTs), YST is predominantly a disease of young adults and the average age at diagnosis is 18 years [1]. However, a few cases of gonadal and extragonadal germ cell tumors have been reported in elderly patients as well [3–6]. We present a very rare case of an elderly 73-year-old male with primary yolk sac tumor of the mediastinum.

2. Case Report

A 73-year-old Caucasian male with past medical history of chronic lymphocytic leukemia, atrial fibrillation, and dyslipidemia presented to the emergency department with complaints of worsening dyspnea on exertion for approximately three to four days and occasional night sweat. He did not have fever, chills, night sweat, cough, sputum production, sick contacts, or recent travel. His physical examination was unrevealing except for right mid posterior egophony and decreased breath sounds in the right lung base. His labs revealed a leukocytosis of 15×10^3 cells/uL with 70% lymphocytes and smudge cells present consistent with his prior CLL. Patient's chest X-ray revealed a large right unilateral pleural effusion with loculation. A computerized tomography (CT) scans of his chest, abdomen, and pelvis revealed a large mass/conglomerate lymphadenopathy measuring 6.6 cm × 14.5 cm × 7 cm in the anterior inferior mediastinum extending to involve the anterior right hemithorax, along the pleural surface, associated with a very large right-sided pleural effusion, causing partial collapse of the right inferior and middle lobes (Figures 1 and 2).

The patient was worked up for an anterior mediastinal mass. Tests for alpha-fetoprotein (AFP), LDH, beta-human chorionic gonadotropin (B-HCG), thyroid-stimulating hormone, and cortisol were requested. AFP was elevated at 5,610 IU/ML, serum beta-HCG < 2.0 mIU/mL, TSH was at 2.11 mIU/L, and LDH was 903 U/L. Ultrasound examination of the scrotum was done as well, results of which were negative. Fine needle aspiration of the mediastinal

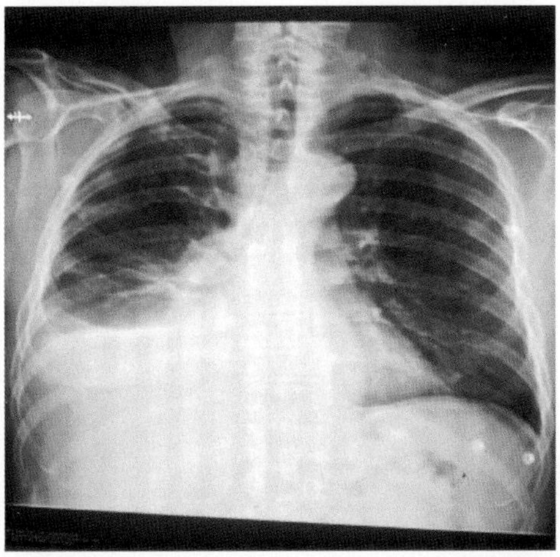

FIGURE 1: Chest X-ray of 73-year-old male revealing large right unilateral pleural effusion.

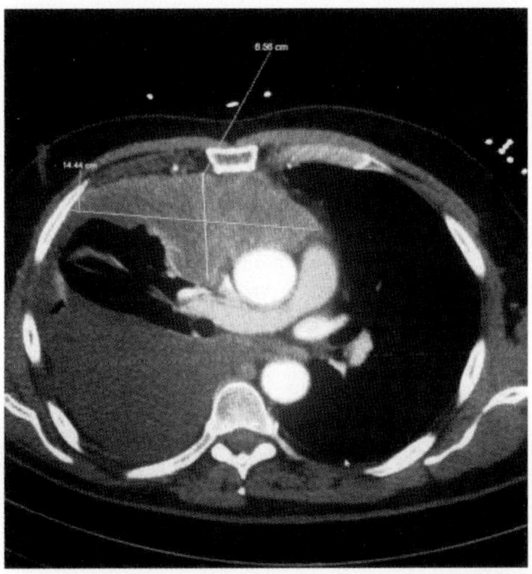

FIGURE 2: Computerized tomography (CT) scans of chest revealed a large mass/conglomerate lymphadenopathy measuring 6.6 cm × 14.5 cm × 7 cm in the anterior inferior mediastinum extending to involve the anterior right hemithorax, along the pleural surface, associated with a very large right-sided pleural effusion, causing partial collapse of the right inferior and middle lobes.

mass revealed abundant tumor cells that were pleomorphic with reticular growth pattern (Figures 3(a), 3(b), and 3(c)). Immunohistochemistry showed focal reactivity with AFP and CDX2 and focal weak reactivity with TTF-1. The tumor cells were nonreactive with CK7, CK20, Napsin A, p63, calretinin, CK5/6, D2-40, CD31, PSA, PSAP, synaptophysin, chromogranin, CD56, hepar, CD45, CD5, CD10, and CD30. Based on the light microscopy morphology and immune-phenotype, final diagnosis of a yolk sac tumor, pleomorphic variant was made. Considering the negative ultrasound of the scrotum, patient was diagnosed to have an extragonadal or primary anterior mediastinal yolk sac tumor (YST). Patient was referred to oncology and had a PleurX chest catheter placed for drainage of right-sided effusion prior to discharge.

Patient was readmitted within a few days with worsening shortness of breath and new segmental pulmonary embolism. He was started on anticoagulation and was treated as inpatient with chemotherapy. The patient was treated with VIP regimen comprising of etoposide (Vepesid) at 80 mg/m^2, ifosfamide at 1200 mg/m^2 (with mesna 120 mg/m^2), and cisplatin 20 mg/m^2 on days 1–5. Granulocyte colony stimulating factor was started prophylactically starting day 7. His postchemotherapy course was complicated by pancytopenia, hemothorax, sepsis, and multiorgan failure. Due to continued decline of his overall health status despite aggressive supportive measures, patient's family resorted to comfort care measures and all life support measures were withdrawn.

3. Discussion

Germ cell tumors (GCTs) mostly occur in the gonads. Extragonadal germ cell tumors (ECGCTs) are rare and most can arise in the pineal gland, retroperitoneum, and the mediastinum [7]. EGGCTs have been speculated to develop from primordial germ cell remnants that fail to migrate to gonadal ridge during embryogenesis [2]. Hence, the locations of development of EGGCT fall along the migration pathway of the primordial germ cells to gonadal ridge. The mediastinum is the most common site of EGGCTs [8]. Malignant GCT in the mediastinum accounts for 1–6% of all mediastinal tumors [9]. Primary extragonadal GCTs, especially primary mediastinal tumors, are considered to have poor prognosis [10].

GCTs are histologically categorized into teratomas, teratocarcinomas, seminomas, and nonseminomatous carcinoma, including choriocarcinoma, embryonal carcinoma, yolk sac carcinoma, and mixed type carcinoma [1]. Greater than 90% of malignant extragonadal tumors of the mediastinum occur in men. In a retrospective study by Sakurai et al. with 48 patients, the median age at presentation of extragonadal GCT was 28.8 years [11].

Yolk sac tumors (YSTs) can occur in both men and women, usually arising from germ cells in testes and ovaries, respectively. Pure YST tumors are usually found in young children and mixed germ cell tumors with YST are found in adults [1]. Yolk sac tumors, similar to other nonseminomatous germ tumors, can be associated with hematologic Klinefelter's syndrome (up to 20%) and other hematological malignancies such as acute leukemia and myelodysplastic syndrome [12]. In an international study by Bokemeyer et al. with 381 mediastinal GCTs, the most common symptoms on presentation were dyspnea (25%), chest pain (23%), cough (17%), fever (13%), night sweat, or weight loss (11%). Night sweat, fatigue, hemoptysis, and symptoms of superior vena cava compression were seen in <10% of patients with mediastinal GCT [7].

Histologically, extragonadal GCTs and mediastinal GCTs have many similarities. Microcystic/reticular pattern is the most common histological presentation [13]. Schiller-Duval bodies are pathognomonic and are helpful for identification. Yolk sac tumors immunohistochemical testing is positive for AFP, glypican-3, SALL4, and placental alkaline phosphatase.

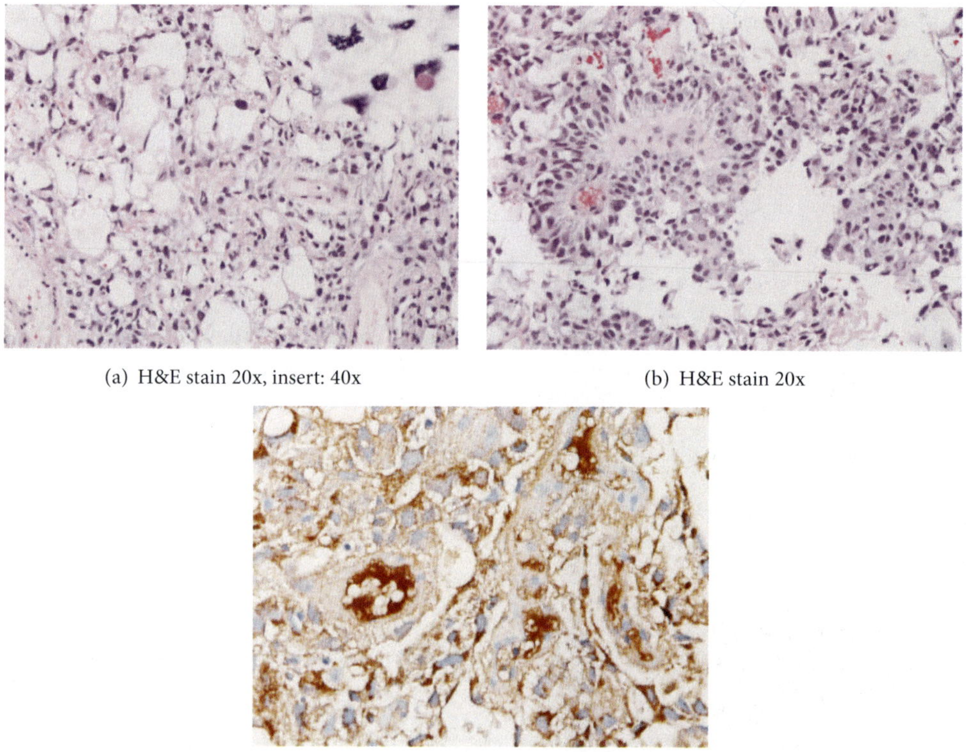

(a) H&E stain 20x, insert: 40x

(b) H&E stain 20x

(c) AFP immunostaining, 40x

FIGURE 3: The fine needle aspiration/core biopsy revealed abundant tumor cells that were pleomorphic with reticular growth pattern. The tumor showed focal reactivity with AFP and CDX2 and focal weak reactivity with TTF-1 and is nonreactive with CK7, CK20, Napsin A, p63, calretinin, CK5/6, D2-40, CD31, PSA, PSAP, synaptophysin, chromogranin, CD56, hepar, CD45, CD5, CD10, and CD30.

In a study by Moran et al. with 38 YST patients, the most common pattern observed was the reticular type, characterized by strands and cords of cells embedded in a myxoid or edematous stroma [12]. Yolk sac tumors secrete substances such as AFP, B-hCG, and cytokeratin (CEA), which can be measured in the serum [10]. Although extragonadal GCTs and mediastinal GCTs have similar histologic feature, they are clinically and biologically distinct from their testicular counterparts [11].

The treatment regimens of extragonadal and gonadal YSTs are similar since they share histological patterns. Extragonadal nonseminomatous germ cell tumors have considerably poorer prognosis. Chemotherapeutic schemes based on cisplatin have shown significant results with up to 50% of patients achieving long-term survival [14, 15]. Bleomycin-Etoposide-Cisplatin (BEP) therapy or etoposide (Vepesid), ifosfamide, and cisplatin (VIP), at least 4 cycles, are widely accepted chemotherapy regimens [16, 17]. VIP regimen may be preferred over BEP since patients with mediastinal GCTs might need postchemotherapy thoracotomy for removal of residual tumor and bleomycin induced pulmonary toxicities can be potentiated by surgery.

Surgical resection as the primary treatment modality is not recommended in mediastinal GCTs because of the likelihood of early metastasis [11]. However, there is a definite role for postchemotherapy adjuvant surgery to remove residual lesions and a rising serum tumor marker after completion of chemotherapy is not considered as a contraindication for surgery [18, 19]. Complete resolution of serum AFP marker occurs in less than 5% of patients [20]. Survival rates have increased in patients who have decrease in serum of AFP after chemotherapy and in cases with residual tumor surgical excision [21]. According to the International Germ Cell Collaborative Group, prognosis is considered poor (5-year survival rate of 48%), if only one of three following criteria is met: primary mediastinal locations of the NSGCT, the nonpulmonary visceral metastases, and an AFP level greater than 10,000 IU/mL [22].

Elderly patients with germ cell tumor generally have worse clinical outcomes compared to younger patients. A Surveillance, Epidemiology, and End Results (SEER) database analysis with 12,811 patients compared the outcomes of testicular cancers in young adults (age $<$ 50) versus older adults (age $>$ 50 years) [23]. In this study, survival from both localized and metastatic NSGCT was noted to be much better in younger patients compared to elderly (76.9% versus 57.0%). Another study that evaluated the clinic-pathological features and tolerance of platinum based chemotherapy of 50 older adults (age $>$ 50) treated for testicular germ cell tumor noted that 30 of 50 (60%) patients had significant dose delays or could not complete their planned chemotherapy course and a majority of patients required regimen change [6]. Neutropenic fever was noted in 44% of patients overall and in 12% of patients despite prophylactic G-CSF. Our patient had overall poor prognosis due to multiple reasons such as his age, tumor location, and tumor bulk.

4. Conclusion

Extragonadal and mediastinal GCTs are diseases of childhood or early adulthood. It rarely appears after the age of 30 years. Primary mediastinal yolk sac neoplasm is a rare tumor. To the best of our knowledge, this is the first reported case of a primary yolk sac tumor of the mediastinum in an elderly 73-year-old male. High index of suspicion is needed to diagnose extragonadal GCTs in elderly patients. Diagnosis can be made with elevated AFP in conjunction with a supporting histopathology. Elderly patients with EGGCT have considerably worse outcome due to their functional status and comorbidities.

References

[1] A. Papaioannou, K. Porpodis, D. Spyratos, and K. Zarogoulidis, "Yolk sac tumour in the anterior mediastinum," *Pneumon*, vol. 26, no. 4, pp. 361–365, 2013.

[2] C. R. Nichols, "Mediastinal germ cell tumors," *Seminars in Thoracic and Cardiovascular Surgery*, vol. 4, no. 1, pp. 45–50, 1992.

[3] K. Fizazi, L. Pagliaro, A. Laplanche et al., "Personalised chemotherapy based on tumour marker decline in poor prognosis germ-cell tumours (GETUG 13): a phase 3, multicentre, randomised trial," *The Lancet Oncology*, vol. 15, no. 13, pp. 1442–1450, 2014.

[4] A. Necchi, P. Giannatempo, S. Lo Vullo et al., "A prognostic model including pre- and postsurgical variables to enhance risk stratification of primary mediastinal nonseminomatous germ cell tumors: the 27-year experience of a referral center," *Clinical Genitourinary Cancer*, vol. 13, no. 1, pp. 87.e1–93.e1, 2015.

[5] A. J. Rodney, N. M. Tannir, A. O. Siefker-Radtke et al., "Survival outcomes for men with mediastinal germ-cell tumors: the University of Texas M. D. Anderson Cancer Center experience," *Urologic Oncology: Seminars and Original Investigations*, vol. 30, no. 6, pp. 879–885, 2012.

[6] D. R. Feldman, M. H. Voss, E. P. Jacobsen et al., "Clinical features, presentation, and tolerance of platinum-based chemotherapy in germ cell tumor patients 50 years of age and older," *Cancer*, vol. 119, no. 14, pp. 2574–2581, 2013.

[7] C. Bokemeyer, C. R. Nichols, J.-P. Droz et al., "Extragonadal germ cell tumors of the mediastinum and retroperitoneum: results from an international analysis," *Journal of Clinical Oncology*, vol. 20, no. 7, pp. 1864–1873, 2002.

[8] G. L. Walsh, G. D. Taylor, J. C. Nesbitt, and R. J. Amato, "Intensive chemotherapy and radical resections for primary nonseminomatous mediastinal germ cell tumors," *Annals of Thoracic Surgery*, vol. 69, no. 2, pp. 337–344, 2000.

[9] E. M. Dulmet, P. Macchiarini, B. Suc, and J. M. Verley, "Germ cell tumors of the mediastinum. A 30-year experience," *Cancer*, vol. 72, no. 6, pp. 1894–1901, 1993.

[10] B. T. Ie Roux, S. Kallichurum, and D. M. Shama, "Mediastinal cysts and tumors," *Current Problems in Surgery*, vol. 21, no. 11, pp. 6–77, 1984.

[11] H. Sakurai, H. Asamura, K. Suzuki, S.-I. Watanabe, and R. Tsuchiya, "Management of primary malignant germ cell tumor of the mediastinum," *Japanese Journal of Clinical Oncology*, vol. 34, no. 7, pp. 386–392, 2004.

[12] C. A. Moran, S. Suster, and M. N. Koss, "Primary germ cell tumors of the mediastinum: III. Yolk sac tumor, embryonal carcinoma, choriocarcinoma, and combined nonteratomatous germ cell tumors of the mediastinum—a clinicopathologic and immunohistochemical study of 64 cases," *Cancer*, vol. 80, no. 4, pp. 699–707, 1997.

[13] M. B. Amin, J. K. McKenney, S. Tickoo et al., *Diagnostic Pathology. Genitourinary*, Lippincott Williams & Wilkins, 2010.

[14] M. Giannis, B. Aristotelis, K. Vassiliki et al., "Cisplatin-based chemotherapy for advanced seminoma: report of 52 cases treated in two institutions," *Journal of Cancer Research and Clinical Oncology*, vol. 135, no. 11, pp. 1495–1500, 2009.

[15] J. Heinzelbecker, M. Katzmarzik, C. Weiss, L. Trojan, and A. Haecker, "During twenty years of Cisplatin-based therapy the face of nonseminomatous testicular germ cell tumors is still changing: an evaluation of presentation, management, predictive factors and survival," *International Brazilian Journal of Urology*, vol. 39, no. 1, pp. 10–21, 2013.

[16] K. Fizazi, S. Culine, J. P. Droz et al., "Primary mediastinal nonseminomatous germ cell tumors: results of modern therapy including cisplatin-based chemotherapy," *Journal of Clinical Oncology*, vol. 16, no. 2, pp. 725–732, 1998.

[17] C. R. Nichols, P. J. Catalano, E. D. Crawford, N. J. Vogelzang, L. H. Einhorn, and P. J. Loehrer, "Randomized comparison of cisplatin and etoposide and either bleomycin or ifosfamide in treatment of advanced disseminated germ cell tumors: an Eastern Cooperative Oncology Group, Southwest Oncology Group, and cancer and leukemia group B study," *Journal of Clinical Oncology*, vol. 16, no. 4, pp. 1287–1293, 1998.

[18] S. M. Radaideh, V. C. Cook, K. A. Kesler, and L. H. Einhorn, "Outcome following resection for patients with primary mediastinal nonseminomatous germ-cell tumors and rising serum tumor markers post-chemotherapy," *Annals of Oncology*, vol. 21, no. 4, pp. 804–807, 2009.

[19] J. Vuky, M. Bains, J. Bacik et al., "Role of postchemotherapy adjunctive surgery in the management of patients with nonseminoma arising from the mediastinum," *Journal of Clinical Oncology*, vol. 19, no. 3, pp. 682–688, 2001.

[20] B. V. Duwe, D. H. Sterman, and A. I. Musani, "Tumors of the mediastinum," *Chest*, vol. 128, no. 4, pp. 2893–2909, 2005.

[21] C. H. Kang, Y. T. Kim, S.-H. Jheon, S.-W. Sung, and J. H. Kim, "Surgical treatment of malignant mediastinal nonseminomatous germ cell tumor," *Annals of Thoracic Surgery*, vol. 85, no. 2, pp. 379–384, 2008.

[22] "International Germ Cell Consensus Classification: a prognostic factor-based staging system for metastatic germ cell cancers. International Germ Cell Cancer Collaborative Group," *Journal of Clinical Oncology*, vol. 15, no. 2, pp. 594–603, 1997.

[23] J. R. Spermon, J. A. Witjes, and L. A. L. M. Kiemeney, "Difference in stage and morphology-adjusted survival between young and elderly patients with a testicular germ cell tumor," *Urology*, vol. 60, no. 5, pp. 889–893, 2002.

Plasmablastic Lymphoma Mimicking Acute Pancreatitis

Faisal Inayat,[1] Hafeez Ul Hassan Virk,[2] Ahmad R. Cheema,[2] and Muhammad Wasif Saif[3]

[1] *Department of Medicine, New York-Presbyterian Hospital, Weill Cornell Medical College, New York, NY 10065, USA*
[2] *Department of Medicine, Mount Sinai St. Luke's and Mount Sinai Roosevelt Hospitals, Icahn School of Medicine, New York, NY 10019, USA*
[3] *Department of Hematology/Oncology, Tufts Medical Center, Tufts University School of Medicine, Boston, MA 02111, USA*

Correspondence should be addressed to Faisal Inayat; faisalinayat@hotmail.com

Academic Editor: Josep M. Ribera

Background. Plasmablastic lymphoma (PBL) is a rare B-cell neoplasm. It predominantly occurs in the oral cavity of human immunodeficiency virus (HIV)-positive patients and exhibits a highly aggressive clinical behavior. *Case Presentation.* We describe an unusual case of a 37-year-old HIV-positive male who presented with acute pancreatitis secondary to multiple peripancreatic masses compressing the pancreas. Histopathological examination of the lesions showed diffuse and cohesive pattern of large B-cells resembling immunoblasts or plasmablasts. The neoplastic cells were positive for BOB1 and MUM1, partially positive for CD79a, and negative for CD20, CD56, CD138, CD3, CD5, AE1/AE3, and HHV8. Epstein-Barr virus-encoded RNA in situ hybridization was positive. These features were consistent with PBL. The patient was initiated on cyclophosphamide, doxorubicin, vincristine, and prednisone (CHOP) chemotherapy, demonstrating a striking response. *Conclusion.* To our research, this is the first report of PBL with the initial presentation of acute pancreatitis. The findings in this case suggest that PBL should be included in the differential diagnosis of pancreatic and peripancreatic tumors.

1. Introduction

Plasmablastic lymphoma (PBL) is a rare and an almost invariably fatal clinicopathologic entity that predominantly occurs in human immunodeficiency virus (HIV)-positive patients [1]. In HIV-negative patients, PBL has been associated with older age and underlying immunosuppression secondary to transplantation, lymphoproliferative disorders, or autoimmune diseases [2]. PBL demonstrates a strong predilection for oral cavity. However, clinical spectrum of PBL has been expanding since it was first described in 1997 as a distinct entity and a subtype of diffuse large B-cell lymphoma [1]. A number of case reports in HIV-negative and multiple case series in HIV-positive patients demonstrated numerous extra-oral locations for PBL [3–12]. However, we report this rare case of PBL initially presenting with acute pancreatitis-related epigastric pain. Our patient showed a dramatic response to cyclophosphamide, doxorubicin, vincristine, and prednisone (CHOP) chemotherapy achieving near complete resolution in three months. PBL poses a formidable diagnostic challenge owing to very low incidence and associated unique morphology. It reportedly has a rapid progression with dismal outcomes resulting in death in majority of the patients within 2 years from initial presentation [13, 14]. Standard chemotherapy protocol for treatment of PBL is nonexistent.

2. Case Presentation

A 37-year-old African-American male with past medical history of HIV (detected in 2001; transmitted by heterosexual intercourse; latest CD4 count 320 cells/mm^3 with undetectable viral load; compliant with highly active antiretroviral therapy (HAART); no opportunistic infections in past) and nephrolithiasis presented to emergency department of our hospital with progressively worsening epigastric pain and nausea for one week. Pain was constant and was rated severe and radiated to his back. The patient denied hematemesis, hematochezia, or diarrhea. However, he reported weight loss of 12 lbs in last 2 months but denied night sweats. There was no history of recent travel, sick contacts, or illicit drug use.

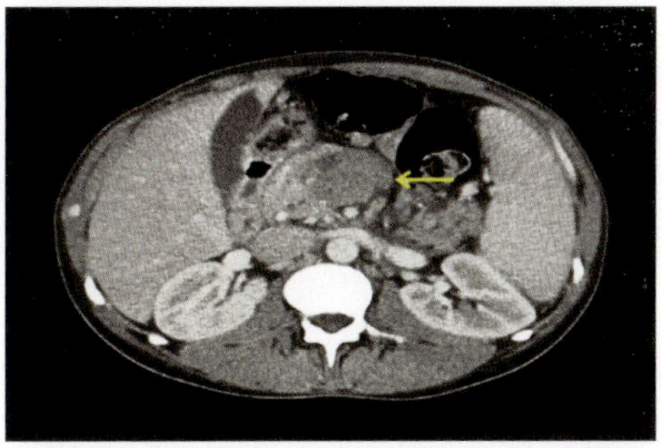

FIGURE 1: Contrast-enhanced computed tomography at the level of pancreas. Arrow demarcates multiple peripancreatic soft tissue masses to left of the uncinate process.

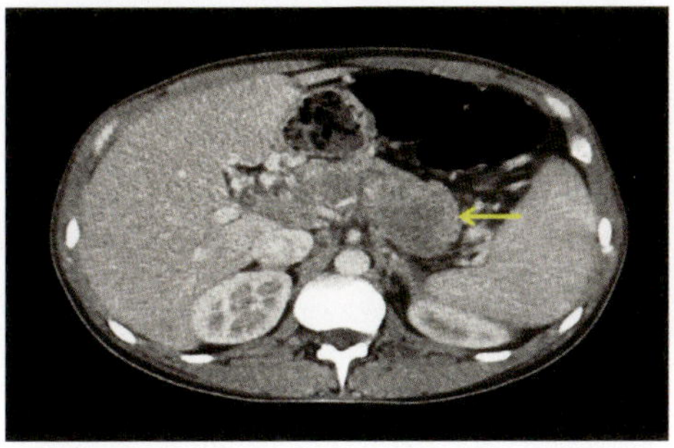

FIGURE 2: Contrast-enhanced computed tomography at the level of pancreas. Arrow demonstrates multiple peripancreatic soft tissue masses posterior to the pancreatic tail.

Vital signs were notable for tachycardia of 120 beats/minute and low-grade fever of 38.8°C. The physical examination revealed epigastric tenderness with no rebound. Initial laboratory evaluation showed elevated levels of lipase 629 IU/L (33–200), amylase 250 IU/L (30–110), lactate dehydrogenase (LDH) 936 IU/L (313–618), and C-reactive protein 3.6 mg/dL (0-1), with normal liver and renal function tests. White cell count was 3.8×10^9cells/L ($3.8–9.8 \times 10^9$), hemoglobin was 13.2 g/dL (13.5 to 17.5), and platelets were 139×10^9 cells/L ($150–450 \times 10^9$). Cardiac troponins came out negative with unchanged EKG. Preliminary diagnosis of acute pancreatitis was made. Subsequently, abdominal computed tomography (CT) demonstrated multiple, well-defined, peripancreatic, soft tissue masses to left of the uncinate process (Figure 1), posterior to the pancreatic tail, and near the hepatic hilum (Figure 2). The peripancreatic masses were found to be compressing the body of pancreas, causing acute pancreatitis in our patient. Furthermore, there was partial compression of the portal vein with multiple surrounding portal venous system collaterals.

Differential diagnoses included lymphoma, mycobacterium avium complex (MAC), disseminated fungal infection, and tuberculosis (TB). The case was discussed in the multidisciplinary tumor board. It was concluded that, due to the advanced disease, tissue diagnosis will be difficult employing surgery or interventional radiology. Thereafter, an uneventful endoscopic ultrasound (EUS)-guided fine-needle aspiration biopsy of one of the masses was performed, and preliminary pathology suggested lymphoma. Cancer antigen 19-9 (CA 19-9), carcinoembryonic antigen (CEA), alpha-fetoprotein (AFP), and serotonin levels were within normal limits. Sputum AFB culture and QuantiFERON-TB Gold (QFT) were negative ruling out TB. Fungal cultures and isolated bacterial cultures for MAC also came out negative. Total body scan showed subcentimeter bilateral mediastinal and axillary lymphadenopathy. Histopathology analysis revealed diffused infiltration of large B-cells with plasmablastic (cells with rounded nuclei, coarser chromatin, and smaller two to three nucleoli) and immunoblastic morphological features (cells with vesicular enlarged nuclei and single prominent nucleolus). A high proliferative index with frequent apoptosis and focal necrosis was demonstrated. Immunohistochemistry of the peripancreatic specimen revealed neoplastic cells positive for BOB1, MUM1, and EBER-ISH, partially positive for CD79a, and negative for CD20, CD56, CD138, CD3, CD5, AE1/AE3, and HHV8, most consistent with plasmablastic lymphoma. A bone marrow biopsy was performed for staging purposes. It revealed normocellular marrow with maturing trilineage hematopoiesis with no evidence of excess blasts or lymphoma. Furthermore, lumber puncture cytology was negative for malignant cells and CSF flow cytometry did not show any abnormal cells; based on these findings, the patient was deemed as stage III.

Subsequently, epigastric pain improved with oral opioids and other pancreatitis-related symptoms resolved with the symptomatic treatment. The patient was discharged from the hospital with oncology out-patient follow-up. Therein, he was initiated on cyclophosphamide, doxorubicin, vincristine, and prednisone (CHOP) therapy. Central nervous system prophylaxis was achieved by employing intrathecal chemotherapy. Filgrastim (G-CSF) was administered twenty-four hours after CHOP cycles and was continued daily for seven days. Our patient tolerated the treatment well, with no significant interactions with HAART for his HIV-infection, and achieved remission after six cycles of chemotherapy. Contrast-enhanced CT at the level of pancreas 3 months after initiation of CHOP treatment demonstrated near complete resolution of previously seen soft tissue masses (Figure 3). The patient has been disease-free for over a year now without any additional specific therapy.

3. Discussion

Plasmablastic lymphoma (PBL) is a distinct, diffuse large B-cell lymphoma, commonly associated with HIV-infection [1]. It accounts for 1.5% of all nodal non-Hodgkin's lymphomas and 2.6% of all AIDS-related neoplasms [2]. PBL typically involves oral sites in HIV-positive population [2]. However, newer reports demonstrated PBL in numerous extra-oral locations predominantly gastrointestinal tract, lymph nodes, skin, bone, genitourinary, nose, central nervous system, liver, and lung, with or without HIV-infection [3–12]. Previously, pancreas or peripancreatic tissue involvement has rarely been described. To the best of our knowledge, this is the first case of PBL with initial presentation of acute pancreatitis.

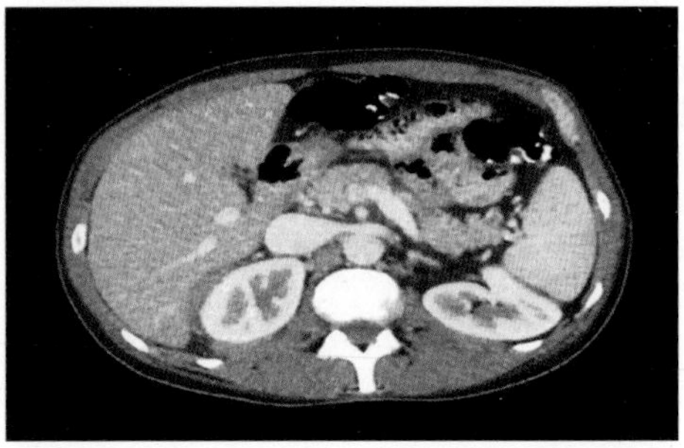

Figure 3: Contrast-enhanced computed tomography at the level of pancreas after 3 months of cyclophosphamide, doxorubicin, vincristine, and prednisone (CHOP) treatment demonstrating near complete resolution of previously seen soft tissue masses.

PBL is associated with Epstein-Barr virus (EBV) infection in over 75% of the HIV-positive cases [11]. Chronic EBV infection thrives in the environment generated by HIV and EBV inhibits apoptosis in B-cells by mechanisms related to EBV antigens, unlocking their malignant potential. Hence, it plays a significant role in the tumorigenesis in HIV-positive PBL patients [2, 11–14]. Apart from the role of EBV as an effective diagnostic marker, it has also been implicated in investigating potential EBV-directed PBL therapies and predicting treatment response and relapse in PBL cases [15–17].

PBL represents a diagnostic and therapeutic challenge for pathologists and clinicians alike, owing to scarcity of the available literature and indistinguishable tumor cells from plasmablastic myeloma [18]. It is a high-grade neoplasm with diffuse lymphoid infiltrates and cohesive growth pattern, having cytomorphologic features such as large B-immunoblasts with an immunophenotype of plasma cells [18]. PBL cells are immunohistologically positive for CD79a, IRF-4/MUM-1, BLIMP-1, CD38, and CD138; negative for B-cell markers CD19, CD20, and PAX-5 and some cases express T-cell marker CD2 or CD4 [19]. Immunohistochemistry with antibody MIB-1 revealed that most or all neoplastic cells are positive for Ki-67 and negative for HHV8. 50% of the PBL cases express an *MYC* translocation indicatingpoor prognosis [20]. EBV-encoded RNA in situ hybridization (EBER-ISH) is a very sensitive modality that is usually implicated in HIV-positive PBL patients with oral locations [21]. In our case, tumor cells were positive for BOB1, MUM1, and EBER-ISH, partially positive for CD79a, and negative for CD20, CD56, CD138, CD3, CD5, AE1/AE3, and HHV8, which was most consistent with plasmablastic lymphoma. Therefore, clinicians and pathologists should have this location in mind for plasmablastic lymphoma.

Clinically, PBL is a very aggressive lymphoma. Two-year overall survival rate for PBL patients was 43% in a recent study conducted in German [13]. Increased mortality in PBL patients is due to pathologic misdiagnosis, delayed initial presentation at an advanced stage (III or IV), and lack of optimal therapy [2]. Over 55% of PBL patients are at stage IV at the time of diagnosis in extra-oral as compared to oral sites, indicating more common dissemination in extra-oral PBL [18]. In our case, the primary PBL of the peripancreatic tissues had infiltrated adjacent lymph nodes, and resulting lymphadenopathy compressed the pancreas; accordingly a clinical stage III was assigned. Our patient demonstrated a dramatic response to CHOP treatment. However, standard therapeutic approach for PBL patients has not been reached so far. Previously employed chemotherapy regimens include cyclophosphamide, doxorubicin, vincristine, and prednisone (CHOP); dose-adjusted etoposide, prednisone, vincristine, cyclophosphamide, and doxorubicin (DA-EPOCH); and cyclophosphamide, vincristine, doxorubicin, high-dose methotrexate/ifosfamide, etoposide, and high-dose cytarabine (CODOX-M/IVAC) [22]. Recently, bortezomib and dose-adjusted EPOCH have demonstrated efficacy in untreated patients with HIV-positive PBL [23]. Future studies aiming at EBV antigens or/and *MYC* dysregulation in addition to autologous stem cell transplant may help to devise an effective treatment approach for PBL.

4. Conclusion

This paper implicates that plasmablastic lymphoma, albeit rare, should be included in the differential diagnosis of pancreatic and peripancreatic tumors. The diagnosis can be challenging due to complex cytomorphologic and immunophenotypic characteristics, particularly in extra-oral locations. Plasmablastic lymphoma follows an aggressive clinical course and associated with poor outcomes. Hence, the clinicians and pathologists should always maintain a high index of suspicion for this hard-to-diagnose and hard-to-treat disease.

Acknowledgment

The authors are highly indebted to Dr. Daniel Yoon for providing the radiology illustrations.

References

[1] H. J. Delecluse, I. Anagnostopoulos, F. Dallenbach et al., “Plasmablastic lymphomas of the oral cavity: a new entity associated with the human immunodeficiency virus infection,” *Blood*, vol. 89, no. 4, pp. 1413–1420, 1997.

[2] J. J. Castillo, M. Bibas, and R. N. Miranda, “The biology and treatment of plasmablastic lymphoma,” *Blood*, vol. 125, no. 15, pp. 2323–2330, 2015.

[3] J. J. Liu, L. Zhang, E. Ayala et al., “Human immunodeficiency virus (HIV)-negative plasmablastic lymphoma: a single institutional experience and literature review,” *Leukemia Research*, vol. 35, no. 12, pp. 1571–1577, 2011.

[4] D. J. Riedel, L. F. Gonzalez-Cuyar, X. F. Zhao, R. R. Redfield, and B. L. Gilliam, “Plasmablastic lymphoma of the oral cavity: a rapidly progressive lymphoma associated with HIV infection,” *The Lancet Infectious Diseases*, vol. 8, no. 4, pp. 261–267, 2008.

[5] T. Haramura, M. Haraguchi, J. Irie, S. Ito, H. Tokai, K. Noda et al., “Case of plasmablastic lymphoma of the sigmoid colon and

literature review," *World Journal of Gastroenterology*, vol. 21, no. 24, pp. 7598–7603, 2015.

[6] Y. Takahashi, I. Saiga, J.-I. Fukushima et al., "Plasmablastic lymphoma of the retroperitoneum in an HIV-negative patient," *Pathology International*, vol. 59, no. 12, pp. 868–873, 2009.

[7] K. L. Chuah, S. B. Ng, L. Poon, and W. M. Yap, "Plasmablastic lymphoma affecting the lung and bone marrow with CD10 expression and t(8;14)(q24;q32) translocation," *International Journal of Surgical Pathology*, vol. 17, no. 2, pp. 163–166, 2009.

[8] R. Yasuhara, T. Irié, E. Shiozawa et al., "Plasmablastic lymphoma of the maxillary sinus with intraoral manifestation caused by direct alveolar bone infiltration in an HIV-negative patient," *Pathology International*, vol. 64, no. 11, pp. 588–590, 2014.

[9] H. Metta, M. Corti, A. Maranzana, R. Schtirbu, M. Narbaitz, and M. De Dios Soler, "Unusual case of plasmablastic non-hodgkin's lymphoma located in the liver. First case reported in an AIDS patient," *Annals of Hepatology*, vol. 8, no. 3, pp. 242–245, 2009.

[10] P. A. R. Urrego, M. Smethurst, M. Fowkes et al., "Primary CNS plasmablastic lymphoma: report of a case with CSF cytology, flow cytometry, radiology, histological correlation, and review of the literature," *Diagnostic Cytopathology*, vol. 39, no. 8, pp. 616–620, 2011.

[11] J. J. Castillo, E. S. Winer, D. Stachurski et al., "Clinical and pathological differences between human immunodeficiency virus-positive and human immunodeficiency virus-negative patients with plasmablastic lymphoma," *Leukemia and Lymphoma*, vol. 51, no. 11, pp. 2047–2053, 2010.

[12] J. Morscio, D. Dierickx, J. Nijs et al., "Clinicopathologic comparison of plasmablastic lymphoma in HIV-positive, immunocompetent, and posttransplant patients: single-center series of 25 cases and meta-analysis of 277 reported cases," *American Journal of Surgical Pathology*, vol. 38, no. 7, pp. 875–886, 2014.

[13] P. Schommers, M. Hentrich, C. Hoffmann et al., "Survival of AIDS-related diffuse large B-cell lymphoma, Burkitt lymphoma, and plasmablastic lymphoma in the German HIV Lymphoma Cohort," *British Journal of Haematology*, vol. 168, no. 6, pp. 806–810, 2015.

[14] G. Elyamany, A. M. Alzahrani, M. Aljuboury et al., "Clinicopathologic features of plasmablastic lymphoma: single-center series of 8 cases from Saudi Arabia," *Diagnostic Pathology*, vol. 10, article 78, 2015.

[15] S. P. Perrine, O. Hermine, T. Small et al., "A phase 1/2 trial of arginine butyrate and ganciclovir in patients with Epstein-Barr virus-associated lymphoid malignancies," *Blood*, vol. 109, no. 6, pp. 2571–2578, 2007.

[16] A. Friis, B. Åkerlund, B. Christensson et al., "Epstein Barr virus DNA analysis in blood predicts disease progression in a rare case of plasmablastic lymphoma with effusion," *Infectious Agents and Cancer*, vol. 8, article 28, 2013.

[17] M. F. Law, W. L. Poon, K. S. Ng et al., "Quantification of plasma Epstein-Barr virus DNA for assessing treatment response in a patient with plasmablastic lymphoma," *Annals of Hematology*, vol. 91, no. 5, pp. 789–791, 2012.

[18] E. Campo, S. H. Swerdlow, N. L. Harris, S. Pileri, H. Stein, and E. S. Jaffe, "The 2008 WHO classification of lymphoid neoplasms and beyond: evolving concepts and practical applications," *Blood*, vol. 117, no. 19, pp. 5019–5032, 2011.

[19] F. Vega, C.-C. Chang, L. J. Medeiros et al., "Plasmablastic lymphomas and plasmablastic plasma cell myelomas have nearly identical immunophenotypic profiles," *Modern Pathology*, vol. 18, no. 6, pp. 806–815, 2005.

[20] A. Valera, O. Balagué, L. Colomo et al., "IG/MYC rearrangements are the main cytogenetic alteration in plasmablastic lymphomas," *American Journal of Surgical Pathology*, vol. 34, no. 11, pp. 1686–1694, 2010.

[21] H. Y. Dong, D. T. Scadden, L. de Leval, Z. Tang, P. G. Isaacson, and N. L. Harris, "Plasmablastic lymphoma in HIV-positive patients: an aggressive Epstein-Barr virus-associated extramedullary plasmacytic neoplasm," *The American Journal of Surgical Pathology*, vol. 29, no. 12, pp. 1633–1641, 2005.

[22] J. J. Castillo and J. L. Reagan, "Plasmablastic lymphoma: a systematic review," *TheScientificWorldJOURNAL*, vol. 11, pp. 687–696, 2011.

[23] J. J. Castillo, J. L. Reagan, W. M. Sikov, and E. S. Winer, "Bortezomib in combination with infusional dose-adjusted EPOCH for the treatment of plasmablastic lymphoma," *British Journal of Haematology*, vol. 169, no. 3, pp. 352–355, 2015.

53

Tumor Reduction with Pazopanib in a Patient with Recurrent Lumbar Chordoma

Maurício Fernando Silva Almeida Ribeiro,[1] Micelange Carvalho de Sousa,[1] Samir Abdallah Hanna,[1] Marcos Vinicius Calfat Maldaun,[1] Ceci Obara Kurimori,[1] Luiz Guilherme Cernaglia Aureliano de Lima,[1,2] Romulo Loss Mattedi,[1,2] and Rodrigo Ramella Munhoz[1,2]

[1]*Hospital Sírio Libanês, São Paulo, SP, Brazil*
[2]*Oncology Service, Instituto do Câncer do Estado de São Paulo, Universidade de São Paulo, São Paulo, SP, Brazil*

Correspondence should be addressed to Rodrigo Ramella Munhoz; rodrigo.rmunhoz@hsl.org.br

Academic Editor: Peter F. Lenehan

Introduction. Chordomas are rare malignancies of bone origin that occur in the axial skeleton, typically the skull base and lumbar/sacral regions. Although often classified as low-grade neoplasms, its locally infiltrative behavior may result in significant morbidity and mortality. Optimal surgical resection may be curative, but up to 50% of the cases relapse within 5 years, and currently there are no systemic treatments approved in this setting. A large proportion of these tumors express stem-cell factor receptor (c-KIT) and platelet-derived growth factor receptors (PDGFRs), providing a rationale for the use of tyrosine-kinase inhibitors (TKIs). *Case report.* A 27-year-old male presented with recurrent chordoma of the lumbar spine 4 years after initial diagnosis. Salvage therapies in the interval included repeat resections and radiation therapy. He ultimately developed multifocal recurrence not amenable to complete excision or reirradiation. A comprehensive genomic profiling assay was performed and revealed nondrugable alterations. Decision was made to proceed with systemic treatment with pazopanib 800 mg/day, resulting in tumor reduction (−23.1% reduction in size) and prolonged disease control. *Conclusion.* For this patient with a multiple recurrent chordoma and limited treatment options, pazopanib resulted in sustained clinical benefit following initial tumor reduction.

1. Introduction

Chordomas are uncommon neoplasms that originate from embryonic remnants of notochord and account for only 1–4% of all bone tumors. They predominate in men around the sixth decade of life, and have an approximate incidence of 0.1–0.8 per 1,000,000 individuals per year [1, 2]. Approximately 50% of the cases arise from the sacrum, 30% from skull base, and 20% from the vertebral column, most of which are diagnosed at advanced stages due to the presence of nonspecific symptoms (or their total absence) in early tumors. Three histological subtypes are described: conventional, chondroid, and dedifferentiated, the latter being the rarest and most aggressive subtype [3, 4]. Most chordomas present high levels of expression of brachyury, a key transcription factor for the development of notochord, being silenced after embryonic development. Reactivation of the brachyury gene, associated with its hyperexpression, is considered a driver alteration in the development and progression of these tumors. In addition, the presence of positive immunostaining for brachyury has aided in the differential diagnosis from other neoplasms with primary site and histologic similarities [5].

En bloc resection with negative margins remains the treatment of choice [1, 6]. However, in up to 50% of the cases, the magnitude of its extension makes radical surgery difficult. The use of radiation therapy for patients with chordomas is still a matter of debate, especially considering the need for high doses of radiation (60–80 Gy) in the tumor and the potential toxicities related to the treatment.

Nevertheless, adjuvant radiation therapy is often used for patients undergoing suboptimal surgical procedures or for those with recurrent disease; advanced radiation techniques, including stereotactic radiosurgery and proton therapy, are being explored. Local recurrence is the main adverse prognostic factor in chordomas, making regional control challenging, given the limited possibilities of salvage therapies. Increased toxicity in previously irradiated structures (i.e., rectum and spinal cord) may be a limiting factor for reirradiation, and even repeat surgical procedures of already irradiated regions may be problematic [1, 4, 5].

For patients with advanced disease or refractory to conventional therapeutic modalities, there are no systemic treatments approved for clinical use to date. It is estimated that approximately 75–90% of chordomas exhibit positive immunostaining for tyrosine kinase receptors involved in signaling pathways related to cell proliferation and angiogenesis, such as the stem-cell factor receptor (C-KIT), platelet-derived growth factor receptor α (PDGFR-α), platelet-derived growth factor receptor β (PDGFR-β), and vascular endothelial growth factor (VEGF) [7, 8]. Based on this rationale, several authors have interrogated the activity of tyrosine kinase inhibitors (TKIs) for the blockade of these signaling pathways (i.e., imatinib, sorafenib, and sunitinib) in previously treated patients, with variable rates of disease control [7, 9–14]. However, no randomized trials have been conducted, and conclusions are hampered by the lack of control arms and bias inherent to a disease that may exhibit an indolent course. Despite the widespread use in other sarcoma subtypes, the activity of pazopanib in chordomas is poorly characterized. Lipplaa et al. described disease control in 2/4 patients treated with pazopanib 800 mg daily, with PFS intervals of 14 and 15 months [15].

In this report, we describe the case of a 27-year-old male diagnosed with a lumbar spine conventional chordoma with multiple recurrences following surgery and radiotherapy, who presented an important clinical and radiological response to pazopanib.

2. Case Report

A 27-year-old white male presented in December 2015 for evaluation of a relapsed conventional chordoma arising from the lumber spine. His diagnosis dated back to August 2013, when he underwent additional evaluation due to a recurrent lower back pain. Magnetic resonance imaging (MRI) of the lumbar spine and sacrum revealed a solid expansive lesion on L2 topography, with an extensive epidural soft tissue component, infiltrating the bone marrow and determining compression of the dural sac. At that time, a core biopsy was performed, which revealed a lesion consistent with a grade 2 chordoma with positive immunostaining for pan-cytokeratin (AE1/AE3), S-100 protein, epithelial membrane antigen (EMA), and Ki-67 index of 20%. The immunohistochemical assessment of brachyury was not conclusive. Three months after the diagnosis, the patient underwent L2 vertebrectomy with negative microscopic margins that confirmed the diagnosis of chordoma of the lumbar spine.

Surgical treatment was followed by adjuvant intensity-modulated radiotherapy (IMRT) to the tumor bed (45 Gy in 25 fractions), and he was then managed expectantly until September/2015, when he presented with disease relapse. MRI of the lumbosacral spine showed multiple lesions of cystic appearance and of small dimensions distributed in paravertebral soft parts at the level of L2, in the right psoas muscle and in the vertebral bodies of T11 and T12, measuring up to 2.2 cm, the largest diameter, without significant contrast enhancement. A new biopsy was then performed and reviewed by a reference pathologist, with histological confirmation of atypical chordoma. The neoplasia showed an expansive and multilobulated pattern of invasion and aspect of chordoma, with epithelioid and eosinophilic cells in the chondromyxoid matrix background. The mitosis figures were observed up to 04/10 high-power fields (HPFs) (Figures 1(a) and 1(b)). There were no areas of dedifferentiation (INI-1 intact). Despite the morphological and immunoexpression of cytokeratins, EMA and vimentin in neoplastic cells, expression of brachyury in the neoplasia was not detected (Figures 1(c) and 1(d)). Of note, even though it is an unusual finding, negative brachyury can be observed in rare cases, predominantly solid chordomas comprising more atypical cells with mitoses and necrosis [16].

A repeat MRI performed after 1 month revealed an increase in previously existing lesions, compression of the dural sac and medullary cone by a lesion extending from T11 to T12, and additional noncontiguous lesions at the level of L2 and multiple nodules measuring up to 1 cm in the right posterior abdominal musculature. In view of the spinal cord compression, a new surgical approach was recommended, and the patient underwent a T11-T12 level partial resection/decompression.

Eight months later, disease progression was once again documented in the thoracolumbar transition and the patient underwent another surgical procedure, with partial resection of the epidural lesion between T11 and T12, as well as the additional lesions between L1-L2 and L3. One month later, the control MRI showed an increase in the dimensions of the preexisting lesions in the lumbar spine and in the abdominal musculature, without new foci. The patient was then treated with image-guided radiotherapy (IGRT) at the dose of 54 Gy in the surgical bed and in regions of gross disease (bilateral paravertebral between T10 and S1). One month after the end of the radiotherapy treatment, a new MRI was performed (Figures 2(a)–2(g)), which indicated disease progression outside the radiated area.

Considering the lack of salvage therapies available in this scenario, a FoundationOne®Heme genomic profiling assay was requested, which revealed 5 nondrugable genomic alterations: *ATM* Q2593* mutation, *ARID1A* S2149fs*47 mutation, *CDKN2A/B* loss, *EP300* L415P mutation (subclonal), and *MLL3* Y306* mutation. *INI-1/SMARCB1* was included in the panel and showed no mutations. Despite the rationale for the use of poly (ADP-ribose) polymerase (PARP) inhibitors in patients with loss-of-function *ATM* mutations, there were no ongoing clinical trials for those alterations at that time.

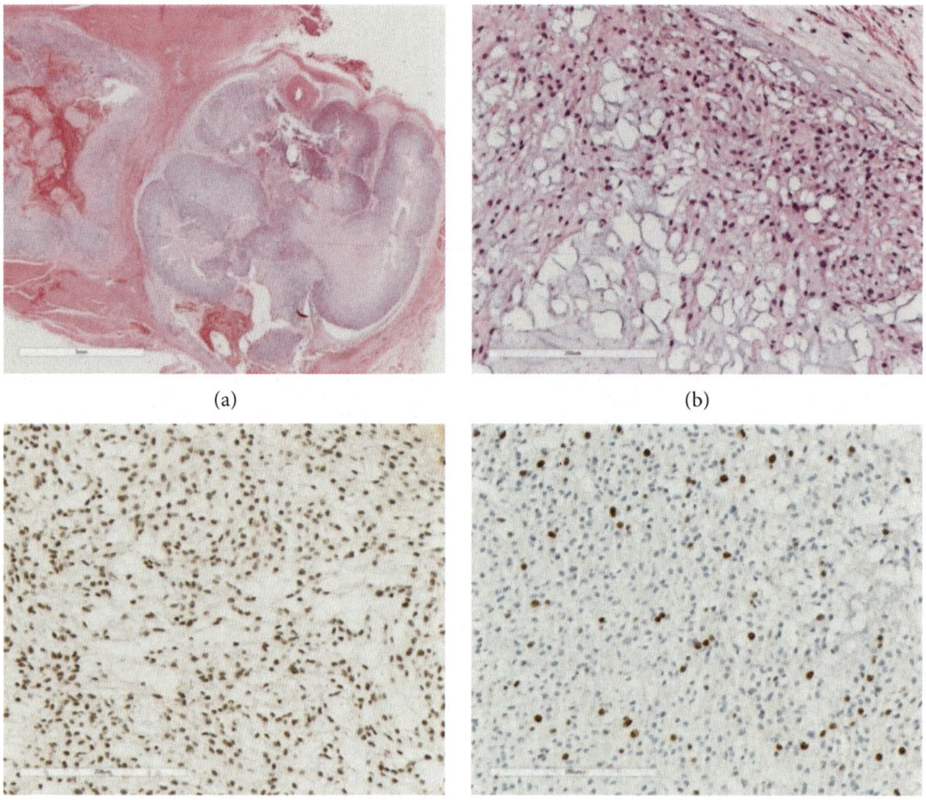

(a) (b) (c) (d)

Figure 1: Histopathologic and immunohistochemical evaluation. (a) Chordoma with expansive invasion (hematoxylin-eosin–HE, 10x). (b) Epithelioid eosinophilic cells in myxoid matrix (HE, 200x); (c) INI-1 positive/preserved expression in neoplastic cells (immunohistochemistry, 200x); (d) Ki-67 positive in neoplastic cells (immunohistochemistry, 200x).

Given the limited therapeutic options in the scenario, systemic treatment with pazopanib 800 mg/day was recommended. The patient developed grade 3 neutropenia, requiring dose reduction (400 mg daily, followed by 400 mg alternated with 800 mg per day), with subsequent good tolerance.

Restaging scans were performed following approximately 3 months of treatment with pazopanib, showing a reduction in size of previously described lesions in anterior paravertebral region, right psoas, and abdominal musculature, and stable dimensions of remaining foci of disease; no new lesions were characterized (Figures 2(b)–2(g)). The sum of the target lesions measurements showed a 23.1% reduction between baseline and posttreatment images (Table 1). Although reduction in target lesions was observed, accompanied by clinical improvement, we could not confirm a partial response according to the Response Evaluation Criteria in Solid Tumors 1.1 (RECIST 1.1). Focal growth in the form a paravertebral lesion was noted after 9 months of therapy, accompanied by sustained control of additional target lesions. Decision was made to proceed with salvage surgical resection of the area of progression. Due to the stability of nonexcised foci of disease, treatment with pazopanib was resumed after the surgery, and the patient continues to endure prolonged clinical benefit more than 15 months after treatment initiation.

3. Discussion

We report a case of a patient with a multiple recurrent lumbar spine chordoma initially treated with gross total resection with wide margins followed by adjuvant radiation therapy. Despite multimodal therapy, consisting of multiple surgical resections and reirradiation, the patient experienced locoregional disease progression and distant metastasis. Prolonged disease control following initial tumor reduction was achieved with the introduction of pazopanib, suggesting a role of this agent in the management of this challenging disease.

Although considered low-grade neoplasms that usually exhibit an indolent clinical course, conventional chordomas have a significant negative impact on patients' quality of life and may result in pronounced morbidity [17]. Complete *en bloc* surgical resection with wide margins remains the standard treatment; nevertheless, recurrences may develop in up to 50% of the cases. Radiotherapy is often used in patients presenting with locally advanced disease not amenable to complete excision or in scenarios in which surgery with negative margins is not feasible. For patients who fail standard approaches, treatment alternatives are limited to "salvage" re-resection with curative intent in a very small percentage of patients who present with isolated lesions, long disease-free interval, good performance status,

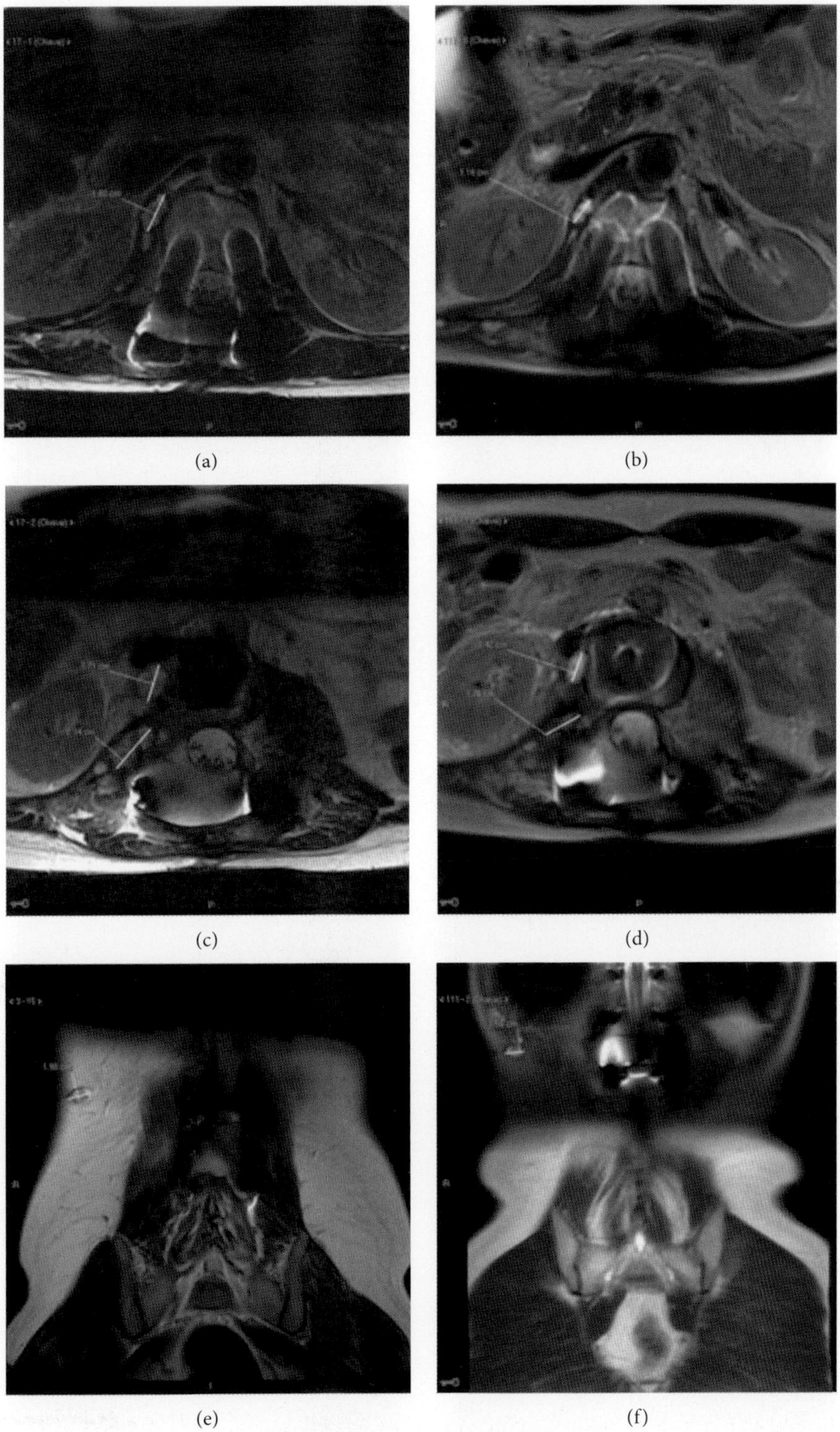

FIGURE 2: Continued.

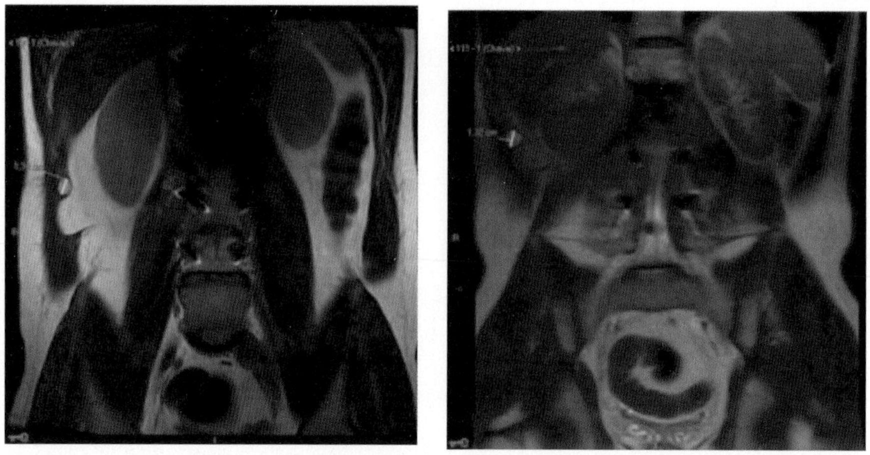

(g) (h)

Figure 2: Baseline and posttreatment imaging showing multifocal recurrence of spinal chordoma and tumor reduction following treatment with pazopanib. In the left column (a, c, e, and g): baseline lumbar spine MRI. In the right column (b, d, f, and h): follow-up abdominal MRI.

Table 1: Size of target lesions (measurements of the largest diameter).

	Baseline	Follow-up
	Target lesions	
T1 paravertebral	2.34 cm (Figure 2(c))	1.76 cm (Figure 2(d))
T2 abdominal wall	1.98 cm (Figure 2(e))	1.56 cm (Figure 2(f))
Sum	4.32 cm	3.32 cm (−23.1%)
	Nontarget lesions	
T3 paravertebral	1.80 cm (Figure 2(a))	1.18 cm (Figure 2(b))
T4 paravertebral	1.71 cm (Figure 2(c))	1.42 cm (Figure 2(d))
T5 abdominal wall	1.34 cm (Figure 2(g))	1.32 cm (Figure 2(h))

and acceptable morbidity; for those with multifocal recurrences, a history of piecemeal resection, tumor rupture, or prior treatment with high-dose RT, curative-intent therapies are definitely not recommended based on most recent guidelines from the Chordoma Global Consensus Group [18]. The lack of systemic agents capable of altering the course of the recurrent disease has made the management of these patients even more difficult [1, 3, 4].

Based on the frequent expression of markers associated with aberrant activation of signaling pathways related to cell proliferation and angiogenesis, including C-KIT, PDGFR-α/β and VEGF [7, 8], multiple attempts to use targeted therapies for this orphan disease are described in the literature. Casali et al. reported clinical benefit in 4/5 cases of imatinib-treated chordoma of the sacrum [9]. A prospective, multicenter, phase II, single-arm study evaluated the efficacy of imatinib 400 mg bid in 56 cases of chordomas with PDGFR-β overexpression, with clinical benefit demonstrated in 64% of patients and median PFS of 9 months [10]. In another phase II trial, which included several neoplasms (with positive immunostaining for imatinib-blocking receptors, despite the absence of activating mutations or rearrangements associated with PDGFR-β), stable disease was observed in 80% of the cases (4/5 cases) of the chordoma cohort [11]. The largest retrospective study evaluated 80 cases of recurrent chordomas treated with molecular target therapies (imatinib in 77% of the cases), showing median PFS and OS of 9.4 months and 4.4 years, respectively. Disease control rate was 78.8%, with only 6.3% of the patients achieving an objective response. Despite the low response rates observed, nearly 42% of the patients experienced symptomatic improvement, which was associated with longer PFS and duration of treatment [19].

In imatinib-pretreated patients, a study performed by Stacchiotti et al. comprising 10 cases of chordoma (9 arising in the sacrum and 1 in the skull-base) reported a PFS rate at 6 months of 87% with the combination of imatinib and sirolimus, supporting the role of the mammalian target of rapamycin (mTOR) pathway as a mechanism of resistance to imatinib in these tumors [7, 12]. The use of sunitinib 37.5 mg daily was also evaluated in a multicenter phase II trial that included non-GIST sarcomas. Among 9 cases of advanced chordoma, PFS rates of 20% and 12% at 16 and 24 weeks were observed, respectively, despite no objective responses [13]. A distinct TKI, sorafenib, was evaluated in a multicenter phase II study, coordinated by the French Sarcoma Group (GSF/GETO). Twenty-seven patients with chordoma were treated with sorafenib 800 mg daily, with 73% of patients being progression-free at 9 months and 86.5% alive at 12 months [14]. Using agents aiming at epidermal growth factor receptor (EGFR) blockade, Asklund et al. reported durable disease stability in 3 patients with recurrent chordomas treated with the combination of erlotinib and bevacizumab, with disease control intervals ranging from 24 to 54 months [2]. Based on the same rationale, the efficacy of lapatinib 1500 mg/day was interrogated in a phase II study in patients with chordoma with hyperexpression of EGFR and HER-2, which resulted in stable disease in 15 of the 18 patients, with median PFS and median OS of 8 and 25 months, respectively [20].

More recently, the development of a recombinant *Saccharomyces cerevisiae*-based vaccine encoding brachyury (GI-6301) brought a new insight into the treatment of chordomas [21]. In the phase I dose-escalation study, 34 patients with several solid tumors refractory to standard therapies, including 11 chordomas, were treated with GI-6301; objective response was observed in one patient within the chordoma cohort, with one being considered not available for RECIST 1.1 criteria, and the remaining 9 patients being progression-free in 5 months. A double-blind, phase II study testing the association of GI-6301 with radiotherapy in locally advanced and unresectable chordomas is currently ongoing (NCT02383498). There is also an ongoing phase I study aimed at evaluating the combination of nivolumab with stereotactic radiosurgery versus exclusive stereotactic radiosurgery in locally advanced, relapsed, or metastatic chordomas (NCT02989636). Still regarding the combined blockade of the PDGFR-β and mTOR pathways in advanced chordomas, we wait for the outcomes of the phase II study testing the efficacy of imatinib and everolimus combination therapy (EudraCT 2010-021755-34).

In conclusion, chordomas are challenging neoplasms with an unpredictable clinical course and a high chance of relapse. Patients presenting with multiple recurrent disease bring an unmet need for systemic therapies. Despite the lack of randomized trials, this case report adds to the available literature suggesting a role for the use of pazopanib.

References

[1] B. P. Walcott, B. V. Nahed, A. Mohyeldin, J. V. Coumans, K. T. Kahle, and M. J. Ferreira, "Chordoma: current concepts, management, and future directions," *The Lancet Oncology*, vol. 13, no. 2, pp. 69–76, 2012.

[2] T. Asklund, M. Sandström, S. Shahidi, K. Riklund, and R. Henriksson, "Durable stabilization of three chordoma cases by bevacizumab and erlotinib," *Acta Oncologica*, vol. 53, no. 7, pp. 980–984, 2012.

[3] S. Stacchiotti, P. G. Casali, S. Lo Vullo et al., "Chordoma of the mobile spine and sacrum: a retrospective analysis of a series of patients surgically treated at two referral centers," *Annals of Surgical Oncology*, vol. 17, no. 1, pp. 211–219, 2010.

[4] P. G. Casali and ESMO, "Bone sarcomas: ESMO clinical practice guidelines for diagnosis, treatment and follow-up," *Annals of Oncology*, vol. 25, no. 3, pp. iii113–iii123, 2014.

[5] S. Di Maio, S. Yip, G. A. A. Zhrani, F. E. Alotaibi, E. Kong, and R. C. Rostomily, "Novel targeted therapies in chordoma: an update," *Therapeutics and Clinical Risk Manegement*, vol. 11, pp. 873–883, 2015.

[6] A. T. Espariat, D. Bresson, M. Polivka et al., "Prognostic and therapeutic markers in chordomas: a study of 287 tumors," *Journal of Neuropathology & Experimental Neurology*, vol. 75, no. 2, pp. 111–120, 2016.

[7] S. Xin, F. Hornick, and J. H. Schwab, "Chordoma: an update on the pathophysiology and molecular mechanisms," *Current Reviews in Musculoskeletal Medicine*, vol. 8, no. 4, pp. 344–352, 2015.

[8] L. Lebellec, L. Aubert, F. Zaïri, T. Ryckewaert, B. Chauffert, and N. Penel, "Molecular targeted therapies in advanced or metastatic chordoma patients: facts and hypothesis," *Critical Reviews in Oncology/Hematology*, vol. 95, no. 1, pp. 125–131, 2015.

[9] P. G. Casali, A. Massina, S. Stacchiotti et al., "Imatinib mesylate in chordoma," *Cancer*, vol. 101, no. 9, pp. 2086–2097, 2004.

[10] S. Stacchiotti, A. Longhi, V. Ferraresi et al., "Phase II study of imatinib in advanced chordoma," *Journal of Clinical Oncology*, vol. 30, no. 9, pp. 914–920, 2012.

[11] M. C. Heinrich, H. Joensuu, G. D. Demetri et al., "Phase II, open-label study evaluating the activity of imatinib mesylate in treating life-threatening malignancies known to be associated with imatinib-sensitive tyrosine-kinases," *Clinical Cancer Research*, vol. 14, no. 9, pp. 2717–2725, 2008.

[12] S. Stacchiotti, A. Marrani, E. Tamborini et al., "Response to imatinib plus sirolimus in advanced chordoma," *Annals of Oncology*, vol. 20, no. 11, pp. 1886–1894, 2009.

[13] S. George, P. Merriam, R. G. Maki et al., "Multicenter phase II trial of sunitinib in the treatment of non-gastrointestinal stromal tumors sarcomas," *Journal of Clinical Oncology*, vol. 27, no. 19, pp. 3154–3160, 2009.

[14] E. Bompas, A. Le Cesne, E. Tresch-Bruneel et al., "Sorafenib in patients with locally advanced and metastatic chordomas: a phase II trial of the French Sarcoma Group (GSF/GETO)," *Annals of Oncology*, vol. 26, no. 10, pp. 2168–2173, 2015.

[15] A. Lipplaa, S. Dijkstra, and H. Gelderblom, "Efficacy of pazopanib and sunitinib in advanced axial chordoma: a single reference centre case series," *Clinical Sarcoma Research*, vol. 6, no. 1, p. 19, 2016.

[16] G. J. Oakley, K. Fuhrer, and R. R. Seethala, "Brachyury, SOX-9, and podoplanin, new markers in the skull-base chordoma vs chondrosarcoma differential: a tissue microarray-based comparative analysis," *Modern Pathology*, vol. 21, no. 12, pp. 1461–1469, 2008.

[17] J. S. Whelan and L. E. Davis, "Osteosarcoma, chondrosarcoma, and chordoma," *Journal of Clinical Oncology*, vol. 36, no. 2, pp. 188–193, 2018.

[18] S. Stacchiotti, A. Gronchi, P. Fossati et al., "Best practices for the management of local-regional recurrent chordoma: a position paper by the Chordoma Global Consensus Group," *Annals of Oncology*, vol. 28, pp. 1230–1242, 2017.

[19] L. Lebellec, B. Chauffert, and J. Blay, "Advanced chordoma treated by first-line molecular targeted therapies: outcomes and prognostic factors. A retrospective study of the French Sarcoma Group (GSF/GETO) and the Association des Neuro-Oncologues d'Expression Française (ANOCEF)," *European Journal of Cancer*, vol. 79, pp. 119–128, 2017.

[20] S. Stacchiotti, E. Tamborini, S. Lo Vullo et al., "Phase II study on lapatinib in advanced EGFR-positive chordoma," *Annals of Oncology*, vol. 24, no. 7, pp. 1931–1936, 2013.
[21] C. R. Heery, B. H. Singh, M. Rauckhorst et al., "Phase I trial of a yeast-based therapeutic cancer vaccine (GI-6301) targeting the transcription factor brachyury," *Cancer Immunology Research*, vol. 3, no. 11, pp. 1248–1253, 2015.

54

Small Cell Lung Cancer Patient with Profound Hyponatremia and Acute Neurological Symptoms: An Effective Treatment with Fludrocortisone

Jana Jaal,[1,2] Tõnu Jõgi,[1] and Alan Altraja[3,4]

[1] *Hematology and Oncology Clinic, Department of Radiotherapy and Oncological Therapy, Tartu University Hospital, 51014 Tartu, Estonia*
[2] *Department of Haematology and Oncology, University of Tartu, 51014 Tartu, Estonia*
[3] *Department of Pulmonary Medicine, University of Tartu, 51014 Tartu, Estonia*
[4] *Lung Clinic, Tartu University Hospital, 51014 Tartu, Estonia*

Correspondence should be addressed to Jana Jaal; jana.jaal@kliinikum.ee

Academic Editor: David Lindquist

Hyponatremia is a frequent electrolyte abnormality in patients with small cell lung cancer (SCLC). Being usually asymptomatic, hyponatremia may cause symptoms like nausea, fatigue, disorientation, headache, muscle cramps, or even seizures, particularly if severe and rapid decrease of serum sodium levels occurs. Here we report a case of SCLC patient with severe hyponatremia and acute neurological symptoms that developed 2 days after the first course of second-line chemotherapy, most probably due to the release of antidiuretic hormone (ADH, also known as arginine vasopressin) during lysis of the tumour cells. Initial treatment consisted of continuous administration of hypertonic saline that resulted in improvement of patient's neurological status. However, to obtain a persistent increase in serum sodium level, pharmacological intervention with oral fludrocortisone 0.1 mg twice daily was needed. We can therefore conclude that mineralocorticoids may be used to correct hyponatremia in SCLC patients when appropriate.

1. Introduction

Lung cancer is one of the most frequent and deadly types of cancer worldwide that causes more deaths than breast, colon, and prostate cancer combined [1]. Small cell lung cancer (SCLC) is a histologic subtype with a distinct biology and aggressive clinical course that comprises approximately 15–20% of all cases of lung cancer [2]. Although the overall incidence of SCLC is slightly declining, mainly due to the decrease in the percentage of smokers, it still remains a huge challenge in oncology [2]. Despite the decades of extensive research, the outcome of SCLC patients remains very poor, suggesting the need for more efficacious treatments and improved patient care [3].

Hyponatremia, defined as a serum sodium level of <136 mmol/L, is a frequent electrolyte abnormality in SCLC patients. In previous studies, rates of hyponatremia up to 44-45% have been reported with most cases caused by the paraneoplastic syndrome of inadequate antidiuretic hormone (ADH, also known as arginine vasopressin) secretion (SIADH) [4, 5]. Despite being prevalent in patients with SCLC, the influence of hyponatremia on the prognosis is largely underestimated in clinical practice. The emerging evidence, mainly from large scale retrospective studies, shows that hyponatremia is an independent factor of poor prognosis in patients with SCLC [6–8].

In the majority of cases, hyponatremia is asymptomatic in patients with SCLC. However, it may cause symptoms like nausea, fatigue, disorientation, headache, and muscle cramps or even seizures, particularly if a severe and rapid decrease of serum sodium levels occurs [4, 7]. Moreover, in some patients with SCLC, a delirious state might be the first neurological symptom of the paraneoplastic syndrome and the first sign of the underlying malignant lung disease [9].

Here, we report a case of SCLC patient with severe hyponatremia and acute neurological symptoms that developed 2 days after the first course of second-line chemotherapy, most probably due to the release of ADH during lysis of the tumour cells. Persistent increase in serum sodium levels of this patient was achieved only with fludrocortisone therapy.

2. Case Presentation

A 57-year-old male patient with a smoking history of more than 40 years and extensive stage SCLC was brought to The Emergency Department at the Tartu University Hospital due to acute neurological symptoms: the patient had suddenly become disoriented and did not recognize his family members and relatives. Severe hyponatremia was diagnosed at his admission, with the sodium level of 104 mmol/L.

The patient had first been admitted to the Tartu University Hospital approximately 7 months earlier with extensive stage SCLC (lymph node and liver metastases). Patient's serum sodium level at diagnosis was normal. Patient's initial treatment had consisted of 6 cycles of chemotherapy with cisplatin and etoposide that had resulted in stable disease. Afterwards, the patient had been followed up for 2 months. Subsequently, a progressive disease had been diagnosed in primary site and liver and second-line chemotherapy with topotecan started. First cycle of topotecan had ended 2 days prior to the patient's admittance to the emergency department with acute neurological symptoms (mainly disorientation) described above.

In parallel with the hyponatremia referred to above, other abnormal blood tests included slight increases in the levels of serum bilirubin (43 μmol/L) and liver enzymes (alanine aminotransferase 145 U/L, aspartate aminotransferase 107 U/L), as well as increased levels of alkaline phosphatase (460 U/L) and lactate dehydrogenase (798 U/L). Serum levels of potassium, glucose, creatinine, urea, and ammonia were normal. Serum osmolality was decreased (218 mOsm/L), which is a frequent finding in patients with hyponatremia. For unknown reasons, urine sodium and osmolality analyses were not ordered by first physicians taking care of the patient. Definitely, these latter analyses would have added valuable information in the management of this case. Patient was euvolemic.

The computed tomography with contrast media showed no brain metastases.

In the emergency department, treatment of hyponatremia was initiated according to the current guidelines by administration of hypertonic saline via continuous infusion that resulted in improvement of patient's general condition and neurological status [4, 10]. This treatment was continued for several days at the department of oncology. However, with hypertonic saline infusion, only minor correction of hyponatremia was achieved with an increase of the serum sodium level up to only 119 mmol/L. After this slight increase in blood sodium level, an aggravation of hyponatremia evolved (115 mmol/L) with a new episode of disorientation and mental confusedness that was compared to the first episode (at admission to the emergency department) much slighter and

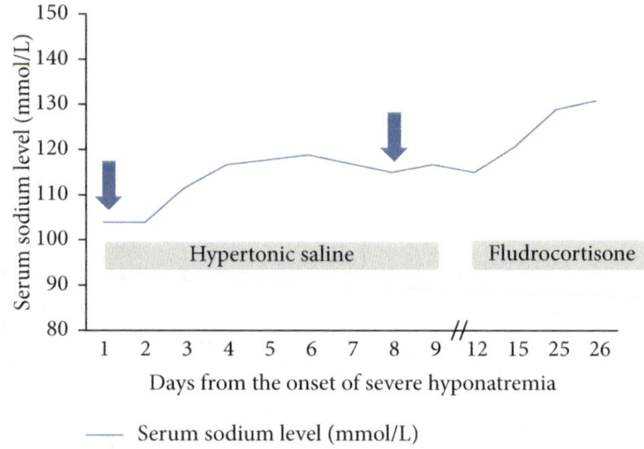

FIGURE 1: Changes in serum sodium levels during the treatment of hyponatremia in a patient with extensive stage SCLC. The figure illustrates changes in serum sodium levels in relation to the received treatment (hypertonic saline or fludrocortisone). The blue arrows indicate the onset of neurological symptoms. The first and relatively severe neurological symptoms (disorientation, mental confusedness) appeared 2 days after the completion of the first cycle of second-line chemotherapy with topotecan. Secondary, a slighter and less durable disorientation appeared during the treatment with hypertonic saline. Hypertonic saline treatment was given on days 1–9 after the onset of severe hyponatremia and fludrocortisone starting from day 12. In between (on days 10 and 11), patient received no treatment since the acquisition of the fludrocortisone from hospital pharmacy took 2 days. Quick increase of the serum sodium level into the steady normal range was achieved only with fludrocortisone 0.1 mg b.i.d.

shorter. Subsequently, the saline infusion therapy was discontinued and treatment with fludrocortisone (Florinef 0.1 mg b.i.d.) started. The treatment with fludrocortisone resulted in a quick increase in the serum sodium levels from 115 to 121 mmol/L within 3 days and subsequent persistent increase up to 131 mmol/L within the following 11 days. Changes in the serum sodium levels during the treatment of hyponatremia are illustrated in Figure 1.

The patient continued treatment with fludrocortisone (Florinef 0.1 mg b.i.d.) with no more episodes of severe hyponatremia and neurological symptoms. Eventually, due to pneumonia, second-line chemotherapy was postponed and terminated later on because of treatment brake that was long enough to allow the tumour to progress. The patient died of progressive SCLC approximately 2 months later.

3. Discussion

There are several conditions that result in decreased serum sodium levels in SCLC patients. Out of these, the paraneoplastic syndrome of inadequate antidiuretic hormone (ADH) secretion (SIADH, Schwartz-Bartter syndrome) is the most frequently described [4, 11]. Other possible causes of hyponatremia include ADH release during the initial lysis of the tumour cells after an effective chemotherapy, chronic heart failure, nephritic syndrome, volume depletion, and adrenal or hypophyseal deficiency [7, 12]. Also, in euvolemic patients, an increased release of ADH can be caused by several medications, such as diuretics, angiotensin-converting-enzyme (ACE) inhibitors, and selective serotonin reuptake inhibitors [7]. Our patient was euvolemic, did not have comorbidities, and was devoid of any medications that might have caused changes in his serum sodium levels. The most probable reason of severe hyponatremia in our patient was ADH release during the initial lysis of tumour cells after chemotherapy, since acute symptoms developed 2 days after the start of second-line therapy with topotecan. Similar "tumour lysis syndrome" and acute development of hyponatremia have been described in SCLC patient after the first course of chemotherapy with vindesine, ifosfamide, and cisplatin [12]. Also, in the review of 350 SCLC patients, the authors mentioned only one patient with normal sodium at the diagnosis, who subsequently developed a hyponatremia of as low as 101 mmol/L after one cycle of chemotherapy [11]. Although this phenomenon is very uncommon, it is important to be aware of this possibility because the occurrence of hyponatremia during SCLC chemotherapy could be interpreted as an increase in paraneoplastic expression reflecting tumour progression, which could in turn erroneously lead to discontinuation of the still effective chemotherapy [12].

In euvolemic patients, severely symptomatic hyponatremia should be initially corrected with continuous infusion or bolus of hypertonic saline [4]. The treatment with hypertonic saline should be stopped once the symptoms related to hyponatremia resolve, a safe blood sodium concentration is achieved, or the maximum sodium correction limits are approached [4]. In our patient, the initial acute neurological symptoms (disorientation, mental confusion) resolved; however, hyponatremia was corrected only to a maximum level of 119 mmol/L. This slight increase was followed by the secondary decrease in the sodium level (down to 115 mmol/L) and the new episode of disorientation. In such circumstances, pharmacological intervention was needed.

For the pharmacotherapy of hyponatremia, demeclocycline, a tetracycline analogue, can be administered at a dose of 100 mg to 300 mg for 3-4 times a day. Demeclocycline negates the effects of ADH at the level of renal tubules; however, the effect of this drug may be delayed for 1-2 weeks [4, 13]. Also, vasopressin receptor antagonists may be used. In particular, vasopressin receptor 2 (V2) is an attractive target of ADH, because ADH activates the V2 receptor to stimulate water reabsorption with the consequent dilution of serum sodium concentrations. Out of the vasopressin receptor antagonists, conivaptan, tolvaptan, and mozavaptan have been introduced into clinical practice, whereas newer drugs (e.g., lixivaptan, satavaptan) are in clinical testing [4]. Recently, the first report was published on a prospective case series showing an efficient management of hyponatremia with tolvaptan in patients with SCLC and severe SIADH (plasma sodium <125 mmol/L) [14]. Although tolvaptan is registered by the State Agency of Medicines of Estonia, it is not currently marketed. Therefore, we were not able to use this drug in our patient.

Out of all available medicines, we chose fludrocortisone for the treatment of severe hyponatremia in our SCLC patient. Fludrocortisone acetate is a mineralocorticoid that enhances renal tubular sodium absorption [13]. It has been used to treat several conditions that cause hyponatremia, such as adrenal insufficiency, cerebral salt wasting syndrome, and subarachnoid haemorrhage [15–17]. Moreover, successful management of hyponatremia with fludrocortisone has been reported in a patient with adrenal insufficiency caused by breast cancer bilateral adrenal metastases [18]. It has been found that oral or intravenous use of fludrocortisone at 0.2 mg b.i.d. reduces the frequency of a negative sodium balance and natriuresis and corrects thereby hyponatremia [13]. Oral fludrocortisone, at a slightly lower dose (0.1 mg b.i.d.), was also effective in the treatment of severe hyponatremia in our patient.

To the knowledge of the authors, there are no other reports that would have described the use of fludrocortisone to treat severe hyponatremia in SCLC patients. Since hyponatremia is an independent factor of poor prognosis in patients with SCLC, correction of this electrolyte abnormality should be always attempted, especially in acute situations as described in this report [6–8]. No prospective data from randomized clinical trials exist to show that correction of hyponatremia leads to prolonged survival of SCLC patients. Nevertheless, large scale retrospective study in 395 SCLC patients has shown that sodium supplementation restored normal sodium values in 91% of patients with severe hyponatremia (sodium <129 mmol/L) resulting in median survival time of 11 months [7]. In contrast, patients with falling sodium levels despite adequate treatment were prone to rapid disease progression with median survival below 3 months.

In summary, the present case demonstrated that fludrocortisone may be effectively used to correct serum sodium levels in appropriate SCLC patients. However, problems with the use of fludrocortisone, such as hypokalemia, fluid overload, and hypertension, must be carefully monitored [13].

References

[1] J. Ferlay, H.-R. Shin, F. Bray, D. Forman, C. Mathers, and D. M. Parkin, "Estimates of worldwide burden of cancer in 2008: GLOBOCAN 2008," *International Journal of Cancer*, vol. 127, no. 12, pp. 2893–2917, 2010.

[2] R. Govindan, N. Page, D. Morgensztern et al., "Changing epidemiology of small-cell lung cancer in the United States over the last 30 years: analysis of the surveillance, epidemiologic, and end results database," *Journal of Clinical Oncology*, vol. 24, no. 28, pp. 4539–4544, 2006.

[3] I. Oze, K. Hotta, K. Kiura et al., "Twenty-seven years of phase III trials for patients with extensive disease small-cell lung cancer: disappointing results," *PLoS ONE*, vol. 4, no. 11, Article ID e7835, 2009.

[4] J. J. Castillo, M. Vincent, and E. Justice, "Diagnosis and management of hyponatremia in cancer patients," *Oncologist*, vol. 17, no. 6, pp. 756–765, 2012.

[5] M. Zarzecka, P. Kubicki, and J. Kozielski, "Hyponatraemia—evaluation of prevalence in patients hospitalized in the pulmonary department and prognostic significance in lung cancer patients," *Pneumonologia i Alergologia Polska*, vol. 82, no. 1, pp. 18–24, 2014.

[6] O. Hansen, P. Sørensen, and K. H. Hansen, "The occurrence of hyponatremia in SCLC and the influence on prognosis: a retrospective study of 453 patients treated in a single institution in a 10-year period," *Lung Cancer*, vol. 68, no. 1, pp. 111–114, 2010.

[7] A. Hermes, B. Waschki, and M. Reck, "Hyponatremia as prognostic factor in small cell lung cancer—a retrospective single institution analysis," *Respiratory Medicine*, vol. 106, no. 6, pp. 900–904, 2012.

[8] M. Tiseo, S. Buti, L. Boni, R. Mattioni, and A. Ardizzoni, "Prognostic role of hyponatremia in 564 small cell lung cancer patients treated with topotecan," *Lung Cancer*, vol. 86, no. 1, pp. 91–95, 2014.

[9] A. Günther, M. Rauch, U. Krümpelmann, and M. Driessen, "Hyponatraemic delirium as an early symptom of small-cell lung cancer," *Nervenarzt*, vol. 74, no. 11, pp. 1016–1019, 2003.

[10] G. Spasovski, R. Vanholder, B. Allolio et al., "Clinical practice guideline on diagnosis and treatment of hyponatraemia," *European Journal of Endocrinology*, vol. 170, no. 3, pp. G1–G47, 2014.

[11] A. F. List, J. D. Hainsworth, B. W. Davis, K. R. Hande, F. A. Greco, and D. H. Johnson, "The syndrome of inappropriate secretion of antidiuretic hormone (SIADH) in small-cell lung cancer," *Journal of Clinical Oncology*, vol. 4, no. 8, pp. 1191–1198, 1986.

[12] S. L. Vanhees, R. Paridaens, and J. F. Vansteenkiste, "Syndrome of inappropriate antidiuretic hormone associated with chemotherapy-induced tumour lysis in small-cell lung cancer: case report and literature review," *Annals of Oncology*, vol. 11, no. 8, pp. 1061–1065, 2000.

[13] A. A. Onitilo, E. Kio, and S. A. R. Doi, "Tumor-related hyponatremia," *Clinical Medicine and Research*, vol. 5, no. 4, pp. 228–237, 2007.

[14] C. Petereit, O. Zaba, I. Teber, H. Lüders, and C. Grohé, "A rapid and efficient way to manage hyponatremia in patients with SIADH and small cell lung cancer: treatment with tolvaptan," *BMC Pulmonary Medicine*, vol. 13, no. 1, article 55, 2013.

[15] M. Quinkler, W. Oelkers, H. Remde, and B. Allolio, "Mineralocorticoid substitution and monitoring in primary adrenal insufficiency," *Best Practice and Research in Clinical Endocrinology and Metabolism*, vol. 29, no. 1, pp. 17–24, 2015.

[16] M. J. Choi, Y. S. Oh, S. J. Park, J. H. Kim, and J. I. Shin, "Cerebral salt wasting treated with fludrocortisone in a 17-year-old boy," *Yonsei Medical Journal*, vol. 53, no. 4, pp. 859–862, 2012.

[17] D. Hasan, K. W. Lindsay, E. F. M. Wijdicks et al., "Effect of fludrocortisone acetate in patients with subarachnoid hemorrhage," *Stroke*, vol. 20, no. 9, pp. 1156–1161, 1989.

[18] C. Bausewein, R. Kühnbach, and B. Haberland, "Adrenal insufficiency caused by bilateral adrenal metastases—a rare treatable cause for recurrent nausea and vomiting in metastatic breast cancer," *Onkologie*, vol. 29, no. 5, pp. 203–205, 2006.

55

Synchronous Orbital and Gastrointestinal Metastases from Breast Cancer: A Case Report

Ramawad Soobrah,[1] Fiona Tsang,[2] Veronica Grassi,[3] Hassan Hirji,[4] Sreelakshmi Mallappa,[2] and Robert Reichert[4]

[1] *Victoria Hospital, Ministry of Health & Quality of Life, Mauritius*
[2] *Ealing Hospital, Uxbridge Road, Southall, Middlesex UB1 3HW, UK*
[3] *King's College Hospital, Denmark Hill, London SE5 9RS, UK*
[4] *Northwick Park Hospital, Watford Road, Harrow HA13UJ, UK*

Correspondence should be addressed to Ramawad Soobrah; ritish@doctors.org.uk

Academic Editor: Jose I. Mayordomo

Breast cancer is the most common malignancy among women and is a significant cause of morbidity and mortality worldwide. With the advent of improved imaging techniques and screening programmes, only a small proportion of women present with metastatic disease. Metastases involving the gastrointestinal (GI) tract and orbit are rare occurrences. We describe the case of a woman with simultaneous GI and orbital metastases from breast cancer who initially presented with abdominal pain and blurred vision and also summarise a review of the literature.

1. Introduction

With 5.2 million cases diagnosed in 2008, breast cancer remains the most prevalent neoplasm in women after non-melanoma skin cancer [1] and is the second leading cause of cancer deaths in women [2]. Histologically, there are two main subtypes of breast cancer: invasive ductal carcinoma (IDC) and invasive lobular carcinoma (ILC). Invasive lobular carcinoma comprises approximately 10% to 15% of these cases and it is reported that its incidence has been increasing over the last several decades, especially in postmenopausal women [3–5]. ILCs have a distinctive growth pattern which can sometimes lead to vague findings on clinical breast examination making it difficult to diagnose; they fail to form palpable discrete nodules like IDC tumours [6]. Lobular carcinomas often do not have characteristic mammographic appearances and present with subtle abnormalities such as focal asymmetry or architectural distortion [7–10]. About 16% of cases are mammographically occult and the reported sensitivity of mammography to detect ILCs varies between 57% and 81% [11]. This makes early clinical and radiological detection of these tumours very challenging, particularly in women with dense breast tissue. Due to such limitations, other modalities such as ultrasonography and magnetic resonance imaging (MRI) are recommended to further evaluate known cases of ILC [12]. About 10% of breast cancers have already metastasized at the time of presentation and the metastatic patterns of IDC and ILC vary considerably [13]. Various studies have reported that ductal carcinomas tend to spread to the lungs, bones, and liver, whereas lobular carcinomas have a tendency to involve the GI tract, gynaecological organs, and the peritoneum/retroperitoneum [13–15]. Gastrointestinal metastases from ILC are rare and many large series have reported an incidence of less than 1% [13, 16, 17].

The first case of orbital metastasis from lung cancer was described by Horner in 1864 [18]. Around 2.5% to 13% of all orbital tumours are metastatic in nature [19]. Orbital tumours from metastatic breast cancer (MBC) are relatively uncommon. In a large observational case series involving 1264 patients, only 4% were found to be metastatic lesions from breast cancer [20]. However, this figure is likely to be an underestimate because smaller asymptomatic lesions are often undiagnosed [21]. Although orbital and GI metastases from lobular carcinomas are unusual, it is important to

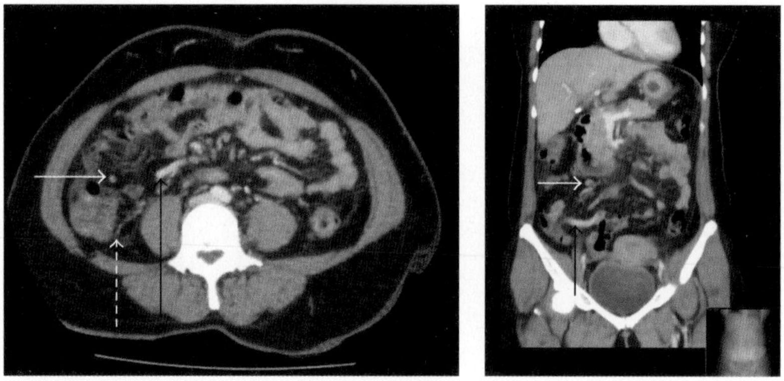

(a) (b)

Figure 1: (a) Axial CT with intravenous contrast. The appendix is seen anterior to the right psoas muscle belly and is with a little surrounding free fluid (solid black arrow). Increased attenuating soft tissue in the right paracolic gutter suggests free fluid or secondary peritoneal metastases (broken arrow). (b) Coronal section of the same patient demonstrating the enhancing appendix medial to the caecum. Mural enhancement is commonly seen in appendicitis. However, in this case, there is little surrounding fat stranding and no fluid filled lumen is seen; these features are more atypical. Enlarged lymph nodes are seen in the mesentery (solid white arrow).

recognise these entities to enable physicians to make prompt and accurate diagnosis and provide appropriate treatment. To our knowledge this is the only reported case of breast cancer with synchronous metastasis to the orbit and appendix.

2. Case Presentation

A 42-year-old lady presented to the emergency department with a three-day history of nausea, vomiting, fever, abdominal pain, and disturbed vision. She also complained of a three-week history of bilateral breast swelling and right-sided breast pain. On examination, she was apyrexial and had a pulse rate of 76 beats per minute. Both breasts were dense with no discrete palpable lumps; however, she was also noted to have enlarged left axillary lymph nodes. Her abdomen was very tender in the right lower quadrant. White cell count and C-reactive protein were within normal limits.

A contrast CT scan of the abdomen and pelvis found increased attenuation with mild thickening of the appendix and a small amount of free fluid in the right paracolic gutter; an enlarged lymph node was also seen in the right iliac fossa (Figure 1). A clinical diagnosis of appendicitis was made and the patient underwent an open appendicectomy. During the procedure, a morphologically inflamed appendix was found with abnormal thickening at the base; adjacent small bowel loops were also found to be adherent to the base. The postoperative recovery was uneventful and the patient was discharged home three days later with a planned outpatient breast clinic follow-up. Imaging of the left breast (mammograms and ultrasound scan) showed an ill-defined spiculate mass measuring 30 mm by 27 mm (Figure 2) and enlarged left axillary lymph nodes. Core biopsies of the breast mass and fine needle aspiration (FNA) cytology of the pathological nodes were performed.

Histology of the appendix showed extensive infiltration of the wall by a tumour which was present in sheets of cells sometimes showing an "Indian filing" pattern. The tumour infiltration also involved the lumen, mesoappendix, and peritoneum. Areas of angiolymphatic invasion were also present (Figure 3). These features were consistent with a metastatic adenocarcinoma of breast origin showing lobular differentiation. The breast core biopsies showed a grade 1 invasive ductal carcinoma with some lobular differentiation (Figure 4) and low grade ductal carcinoma in situ. The FNA of the left axillary lymph node confirmed the presence of metastatic carcinoma. Both tumours were CK7 positive, CK20 and CDX2 negative (the latter precluding a gastrointestinal origin). The tumours were also positive for GCDFP15 (which is consistent with a breast primary), ER positive (7/8), PR positive (8/8), and HER2 negative. Based on the immunohistochemistry results, a diagnosis of metastatic breast cancer was made.

During the postoperative recovery period the patient noted a worsening of diplopia and left-sided headache. A head CT and contrast-enhanced MRI of the orbits were therefore performed. The MRI scan showed a left retroorbital, intraconal soft tissue mass between the medial and inferior recti muscles, suggestive of a metastatic deposit (Figure 5: MRI orbits). No other significant brain lesions were noted.

The patient completed 6 cycles of chemotherapy (FEC: fluorouracil, epirubicin, and cyclophosphamide), each at 3-weekly interval, and was then started on tamoxifen 20 mg daily. Staging scans (CT and MRI) performed after the chemotherapy and endocrine therapy showed a partial response in all the tumour sites, with reduction of the size of the left breast mass, the axillary, peritoneal, and mesenteric nodes. The orbital metastasis had also reduced in size and the patient noticed an improvement in her vision. Repeat whole body staging CT scan 9 months later showed further marginal reduction of the previously noted left orbital mass and no overt intra-abdominal pathology. Given the noticeable improvement in her condition, she currently remains under close clinical follow-up with the oncology team.

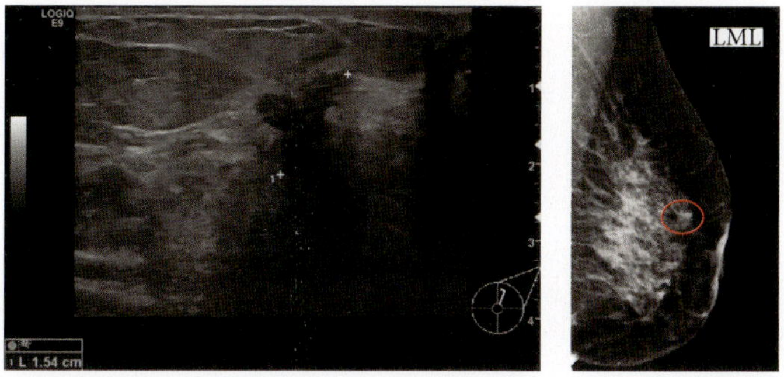

(a) (b)

FIGURE 2: (a) Ultrasound of the left breast showing a 15 mm ill-defined hypoechoic mass. (b) Mammogram of left breast (mediolateral view) demonstrates a spiculate mass (red circle).

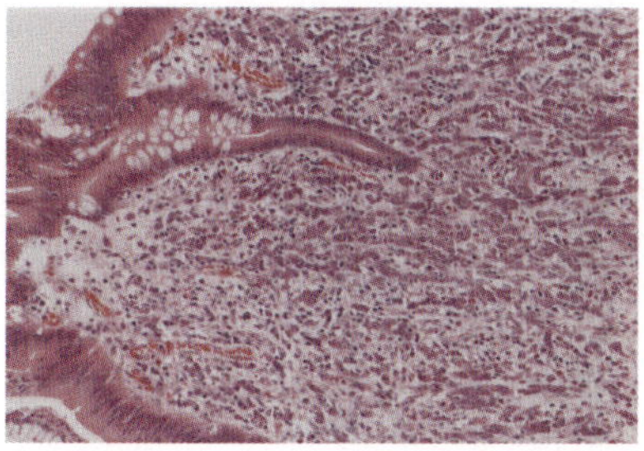

FIGURE 3: Submucosa shows diffuse infiltration by small to moderate sized malignant epithelial cells with prominent trabecular/Indian filing pattern and vesicular nucleolated nuclei. There is no evidence of glandular formation (H&E stain, magnification ×10).

3. Discussion

According to 2012 GLOBOCAN estimates, there were nearly 1.7 million new cases of breast cancer diagnosed worldwide [22] and this figure is expected to rise to 2.1 million by 2030 [1]. Extrahepatic gastrointestinal metastases are rare with the stomach reported as the most common site involved, followed by the small intestine and colon [3, 17, 23]. Several large studies have reported that less than 1% of patients with metastatic breast cancer have GI involvement [13, 16, 17]. On autopsy studies, however, this incidence varies between 8% and 35% [24–26]. This discrepancy can be explained by the fact that a large number of cases may be undiagnosed because of their nonspecific symptoms and late presentation. The most common presenting symptoms are abdominal pain followed by bloating, melena, GI hemorrhage, bowel obstruction, nausea and vomiting, early satiety, dysphagia, weight loss, anaemia or fatigue, and palpable mass [13]. Patients present with gastrointestinal metastases after an average of 7 years [13] and as long as 30 years from initial diagnosis of breast cancer [27]. Moreover, GI metastases can present as the first manifestation in clinically occult primary breast cancer [23]. In a large retrospective study, Iorfida et al. showed that independent risk factors for metastatic disease included positive axillary node status, tumours over 2 cm in size, and positive HER2 status [28]. Interestingly, our patient presented with two of these features.

Breast cancer metastasizing to the appendix is also a rare occurrence [23] and there are very few published reports of MBC presenting as appendicitis [29–31]. McLemore et al. [13] reported that 21% of patients presented with metastatic disease masquerading as an alternate disease process, thus making accurate diagnosis difficult. In our case, the patient presented initially with GI symptoms suggestive of possible appendicitis which made her seek medical advice, whilst disregarding her breast complaints. Breast carcinoma has the potential for widespread dissemination and virtually any organ can be involved. Among women, it is the most common primary malignancy to metastasize to the GI tract and is second only to melanoma [24, 32]. The metastatic patterns of lobular and ductal carcinoma vary significantly in terms of sites of distant metastases. Several studies have reported a greater tendency for lobular and mixed ductal-lobular carcinomas to metastasize to the GI tract and it usually occurs in association with spread to other sites [13, 17, 26, 33]. It has also been described that the lobular component of mixed tumours ultimately spread to the GI tract [17]; these findings were confirmed on radiological and histological examinations performed in this case.

Despite the fact that ILCs infrequently spread to the lower GI tract, it is important to differentiate them from other primary lesions as this will allow initiation of appropriate treatment and help prevent unnecessary operations. Our patient underwent an open appendicectomy nevertheless because there were some clinical and radiological signs suggestive of acute appendicitis. There were no histological features of appendicitis in the case described; however, the lumen of the appendix contained metastatic tumour deposits. Dirksen et al. [31] have suggested that metastatic adenocarcinoma to the appendix can often present as appendicitis at a late stage leading to a high incidence of perforation. Chemotherapy and endocrine therapy, often in combination, is the treatment of choice in these patients. Radiotherapy and palliative surgery (resection, GI bypasses, and debulking of metastatic disease) can be used in selected patients [13]. Some authors have also advocated closer GI follow-up for patients

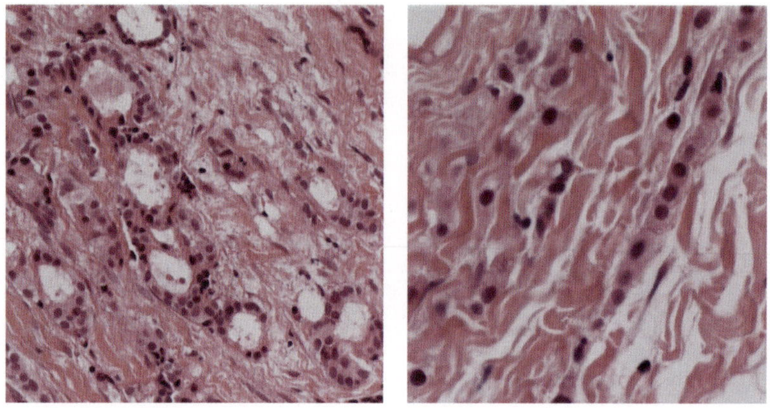

(a) (b)

FIGURE 4: (a) Several malignant ductal structures in a desmoplastic stroma (H&E stain, magnification ×20). (b) Breast biopsy shows typical lobular carcinoma pattern with Indian filing (H&E stain, magnification ×40).

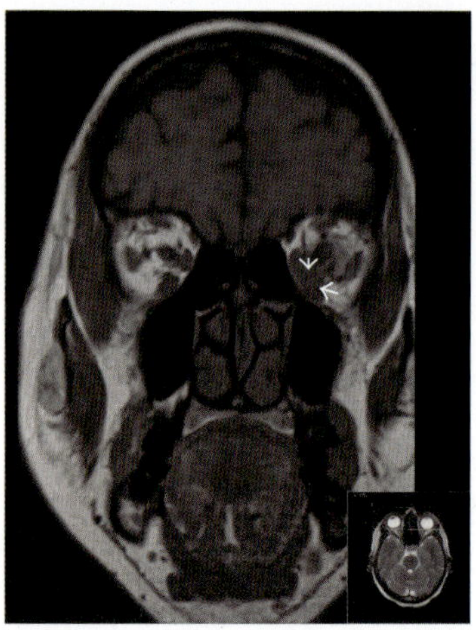

FIGURE 5: T1 weighted MRI orbits show soft tissue replacing fat in the medial left orbit is isointense with the adjacent recti and it is suggestive of a soft tissue deposit (white arrows).

diagnosed with ILC [3, 34]. In a recent review article looking at patients with MBC affecting the GI tract, Ambroggi et al. [17] reported that the median overall survival is 16 months with a range of 5–41 months.

Orbital metastases from breast cancer are relatively uncommon and affect between 2% and 6% of patients with MBC [35–37]. Of those, about 5% involve the extraocular muscles only [38]. However, these metastases occur more frequently than is clinically recognised because they may affect other major organ systems where the consequences are easily detectable or they may remain small and asymptomatic. Some studies suggest that the incidence can be up to 30% in asymptomatic patients with known MBC [21, 36]. Metastatic lesions are more commonly found in the uvea than the orbit, with a ratio of approximately one to eight [21, 37]. Several studies have shown that breast cancer is the most common source of orbital metastases and accounts for 29%–50% of cases [21, 37, 39, 40]. The most common orbital symptoms that patients present with include diplopia, proptosis, pain, and decreased vision [19, 36, 37, 40]. Several case reports have also described ocular metastasis as the initial manifestation of a previously undetected primary breast carcinoma [36, 41, 42]. MRI is the diagnostic tool of choice as it can better visualize soft tissue structures and more precisely evaluate tumour metastases involving the orbital structures [20, 43]. Patients usually present during the sixth decade of life and orbital involvement occurs on average 4.5–6.5 years after the primary tumour is diagnosed [21]. The presence of orbital metastasis usually indicates extensive haematogenous spread from the primary tumour and the majority of these patients will also have simultaneous nonorbital metastases at the time of presentation [19, 21, 40, 44]. Furthermore, breast cancer has a strong tendency to localize in the orbital fat and muscle [40], as is illustrated in our case. Treatment for orbital metastases often requires a multidisciplinary approach and modalities include radiotherapy, chemotherapy, hormone therapy, surgery, and immunotherapy; however, the mainstay treatment is orbital irradiation because it can offer significant symptomatic improvement of orbital signs and symptoms [20, 40, 43]. Despite the fact that short-term visual prognosis after radiotherapy can be good, the systemic prognosis of these patients remains poor; mean survival time is reported to vary between 10 and 20 months [37, 44, 45].

4. Conclusion

Breast cancer has the potential to disseminate via the lymphatic or haematogenous routes and hence virtually any anatomical site can be affected with metastatic deposits [19]. Extrahepatic GI and orbital metastases from breast cancer are unusual in clinical practice. Both of these conditions can be asymptomatic or present with nonspecific symptoms, thus making their diagnosis difficult. Physicians need to recognise the different metastatic patterns of lobular and ductal carcinomas; they also need to have a high index of suspicion for metastatic disease especially in patients with a known history of breast cancer who present with new gastrointestinal complaints or orbital symptoms. For lesions in the gastrointestinal tract, it is important to distinguish a primary carcinoma from a metastatic one in order to initiate appropriate treatment in such patients and help prevent unnecessary surgical procedures. Similarly, early recognition and treatment of patients affected by ocular metastases can help preserve their vision and maximize their quality of life.

Acknowledgments

The authors would like to thank Dr. Nayef Aqel (consultant histopathologist) for providing the histopathology images and Dr. Sanjay Mugon (consultant pathologist) for describing those images.

References

[1] F. Bray, J.-S. Ren, E. Masuyer, and J. Ferlay, "Global estimates of cancer prevalence for 27 sites in the adult population in 2008," *International Journal of Cancer*, vol. 132, no. 5, pp. 1133–1145, 2013.

[2] R. Siegel, D. Naishadham, and A. Jemal, "Cancer statistics, 2012," *CA: A Cancer Journal for Clinicians*, vol. 62, no. 1, pp. 10–29, 2012.

[3] P. Carcoforo, M. T. Raiji, R. C. Langan et al., "Infiltrating lobular carcinoma of the breast presenting as gastrointestinal obstruction: a mini review," *Journal of Cancer*, vol. 3, no. 1, pp. 328–332, 2012.

[4] C. I. Li, B. O. Anderson, P. Porter, S. K. Holt, J. R. Daling, and R. E. Moe, "Changing incidence rate of invasive lobular breast carcinoma among older women," *Cancer*, vol. 88, no. 11, pp. 2561–2569, 2000.

[5] J. V. Alvarez, D. Perez, and L. A. Chodosh, "mILC-ing the mouse mammary gland: a model for invasive lobular carcinoma," *Cancer Cell*, vol. 10, no. 5, pp. 347–349, 2006.

[6] K. J. Dedes and D. Fink, "Clinical presentation and surgical management of invasive lobular carcinoma of the breast," *Breast Diseases*, vol. 30, pp. 31–37, 2008-2009.

[7] W. P. Evans, L. J. W. Burhenne, L. Laurie, K. F. O'Shaughnessy, and R. A. Castellino, "Invasive lobular carcinoma of the breast: mammographic characteristics and computer-aided detection," *Radiology*, vol. 225, no. 1, pp. 182–189, 2002.

[8] M. A. Helvie, C. Paramagul, H. A. Oberman, and D. D. Adler, "Invasive lobular carcinoma: imaging features and clinical detection," *Investigative Radiology*, vol. 28, no. 3, pp. 202–207, 1993.

[9] K. N. Krecke and J. J. Gisvold, "Invasive lobular carcinoma of the breast: mammographic findings and extent of disease at diagnosis in 184 patients," *The American Journal of Roentgenology*, vol. 161, no. 5, pp. 957–960, 1993.

[10] E. A. Sickles, "The subtle and atypical mammographic features of invasive lobular carcinoma," *Radiology*, vol. 178, no. 1, pp. 25–26, 1991.

[11] J. K. Lopez and L. W. Bassett, "Invasive lobular carcinoma of the breast: spectrum of mammographic, US, and MR imaging findings," *Radiographics*, vol. 29, no. 1, pp. 165–176, 2009.

[12] W. A. Berg, L. Gutierrez, M. S. NessAiver et al., "Diagnostic accuracy of mammography, clinical examination, US, and MR imaging in preoperative assessment of breast cancer," *Radiology*, vol. 233, no. 3, pp. 830–849, 2004.

[13] E. C. McLemore, B. A. Pockaj, C. Reynolds et al., "Breast cancer: presentation and intervention in women with gastrointestinal metastasis and carcinomatosis," *Annals of Surgical Oncology*, vol. 12, no. 11, pp. 886–894, 2005.

[14] S. Ferlicot, A. Vincent-Salomon, J. Médioni et al., "Wide metastatic spreading in infiltrating lobular carcinoma of the breast," *European Journal of Cancer*, vol. 40, no. 3, pp. 336–341, 2004.

[15] M. Harris, A. Howell, M. Chrissohou, R. I. Swindell, M. Hudson, and R. A. Sellwood, "A comparison of the metastatic pattern of infiltrating lobular carcinoma and infiltrating duct carcinoma of the breast," *British Journal of Cancer*, vol. 50, no. 1, pp. 23–30, 1984.

[16] M. J. Borst and J. A. Ingold, "Metastatic patterns of invasive lobular versus invasive ductal carcinoma of the breast," *Surgery*, vol. 114, no. 4, pp. 637–642, 1993.

[17] M. Ambroggi, E. M. Stroppa, P. Mordenti et al., "Metastatic breast cancer to the gastrointestinal tract: report of five cases and review of the literature," *International Journal of Breast Cancer*, vol. 2012, Article ID 439023, 8 pages, 2012.

[18] F. Horner, "Carcinoma der dura mater exophthalmus," *Klin Monatsbl Augenheilkd*, vol. 2, pp. 186–190, 1864.

[19] K. K. Toller, J. W. Gigantelli, and M. J. Spalding, "Bilateral orbital metastases from breast carcinoma. A case of false pseudotumor," *Ophthalmology*, vol. 105, no. 10, pp. 1897–1901, 1998.

[20] J. A. Shields, C. L. Shields, and R. Scartozzi, "Survey of 1264 patients with orbital tumors and simulating lesions: the 2002 Montgomery Lecture, part 1," *Ophthalmology*, vol. 111, no. 5, pp. 997–1008, 2004.

[21] S. Fenton, E. G. Kemp, and A. N. Harnett, "Screening for Ophthalmic involvement in asymptomatic patients with metastatic breast carcinoma," *Eye*, vol. 18, no. 1, pp. 38–40, 2004.

[22] International Agency for Cancer Research. World Health Organization, *GLOBOCAN 2012: Estimated Cancer Incidence, Mortality and Prevalence Worldwide in 2012*, 2012, http://globocan.iarc.fr/Pages/fact_sheets_cancer.aspx.

[23] C. B. Winston, O. Hadar, J. B. Teitcher et al., "Metastatic lobular carcinoma of the breast: patterns of spread in the chest, abdomen, and pelvis on CT," *American Journal of Roentgenology*, vol. 175, no. 3, pp. 795–800, 2000.

[24] K. Washington and D. McDonagh, "Secondary tumors of the gastrointestinal tract: surgical pathologic findings and comparison with autopsy survey," *Modern Pathology*, vol. 8, no. 4, pp. 427–433, 1995.

[25] E. Caramella, J. N. Bruneton, P. Roux, D. Aubanel, and P. Lecomte, "Metastases of the digestive tract. Report of 77 cases and review of the literature," *European Journal of Radiology*, vol. 3, no. 4, pp. 331–338, 1983.

[26] G. Cervi, N. Vettoretto, A. Vinco et al., "Rectal localization of metastatic lobular breast cancer: report of a case," *Diseases of the Colon & Rectum*, vol. 44, no. 3, pp. 453–455, 2001.

[27] A. Benfiguig, M.-L. Anciaux, C. Eugene, G. Benkémoun, and J.-C. Etienne, "Gastric metastasis of breast cancer occurring after a cancer-free interval of 30 years," *Annales de Gastroenterologie et d'Hepatologie*, vol. 28, no. 4, pp. 175–177, 1992.

[28] M. Iorfida, E. Maiorano, E. Orvieto et al., "Invasive lobular breast cancer: subtypes and outcome," *Breast Cancer Research and Treatment*, vol. 133, no. 2, pp. 713–723, 2012.

[29] K. S. Latchis and J. W. Canter, "Acute appendicitis secondary to metastatic carcinoma," *The American Journal of Surgery*, vol. 111, no. 2, pp. 220–223, 1966.

[30] R. E. Burney, N. Koss, and I. S. Goldenberg, "Acute appendicitis secondary to metastatic carcinoma of the breast: a report and review of two cases," *Archives of Surgery*, vol. 108, no. 6, pp. 872–875, 1974.

[31] J. L. Dirksen, M. G. Souder, and A. J. Burick, "Metastatic breast carcinoma presenting as perforated appendicitis," *Breast Care*, vol. 5, no. 6, pp. 409–410, 2010.

[32] A. Ciulla, G. Castronovo, G. Tomasello et al., "Gastric metastases originating from occult breast lobular carcinoma: diagnostic and therapeutic problems," *World Journal of Surgical Oncology*, vol. 6, article 78, 2008.

[33] S. Dhar, M. N. Kulaylat, K. Gordon, P. Lall, and R. J. Doerr, "Solitary papillary breast carcinoma metastasis to the large bowel presenting as primary colon carcinoma: case report and review of the literature," *The American Surgeon*, vol. 69, no. 9, pp. 799–803, 2003.

[34] J. Nazareno, D. Taves, and H. G. Preiksaitis, "Metastatic breast cancer to the gastrointestinal tract: a case series and review of the literature," *World Journal of Gastroenterology*, vol. 12, no. 38, pp. 6219–6224, 2006.

[35] J. A. Shields, C. L. Shields, H. K. Brotman, C. Carvalho, N. Perez, and R. C. Eagle Jr., "Cancer metastatic to the orbit: the 2000 Robert M. Curts Lecture," *Ophthalmic Plastic and Reconstructive Surgery*, vol. 17, no. 5, pp. 346–354, 2001.

[36] S. Wickremasinghe, K. K. Dansingani, P. Tranos, S. Liyanage, A. Jones, and C. Davey, "Ocular presentations of breast cancer," *Acta Ophthalmologica Scandinavica*, vol. 85, no. 2, pp. 133–142, 2007.

[37] D. H. Char, T. Miller, and S. Kroll, "Orbital metastases: diagnosis and course," *British Journal of Ophthalmology*, vol. 81, no. 5, pp. 386–390, 1997.

[38] R. W. Arnold, B. A. Adams, J. K. Camoriano, and J. A. Dyer, "Acquired divergent strabismus: presumed metastatic gastric carcinoma to the medial rectus muscle," *Journal of Pediatric Ophthalmology and Strabismus*, vol. 26, no. 1, pp. 50–51, 1989.

[39] C. F. Merrill, D. I. Kaufman, and N. V. Dimitrov, "Breast cancer metastatic to the eye is a common entity," *Cancer*, vol. 68, no. 3, pp. 623–627, 1991.

[40] A. A. Valenzuela, C. W. Archibald, B. Fleming et al., "Orbital metastasis: clinical features, management and outcome," *Orbit*, vol. 28, no. 2-3, pp. 153–159, 2009.

[41] P. J. Vlachostergios, I. A. Voutsadakis, and C. N. Papandreou, "Orbital metastasis of breast carcinoma," *Breast Cancer: Basic and Clinical Research*, vol. 3, no. 1, pp. 91–97, 2009.

[42] M. Kadivar, A. Joulaee, M. B. Kashkouli, H. H. Kharazi, M. Kalantari, and P. V. Kumar, "Orbital metastasis as the first presentation of nonpalpable invasive lobular carcinoma of the breast," *The Breast Journal*, vol. 12, no. 1, pp. 75–76, 2006.

[43] S. M. Ahmad and B. Esmaeli, "Metastatic tumors of the orbit and ocular adnexa," *Current Opinion in Ophthalmology*, vol. 18, no. 5, pp. 405–413, 2007.

[44] E. Ng and P. F. Ilsen, "Orbital metastases," *Optometry*, vol. 81, no. 12, pp. 647–657, 2010.

[45] D. Holland, S. Maune, G. Kovács, and S. Behrendt, "Metastatic tumors of the orbit: a retrospective study," *Orbit*, vol. 22, no. 1, pp. 15–24, 2003.

56

The Case of an Elderly Male Patient with Unknown Primary Mucinous Adenocarcinoma within Presacral Teratoma (Teratoma with Malignant Transformation)

Ozgur Tanriverdi,[1] Ayca Ersen,[2] Suna Cokmert,[3] Emine Koca,[4] Naki Bulut,[5] Suha Gul,[6] and Nevin Yilmaz[7]

[1] *Department of Medical Oncology, Sitki Kocman University Faculty of Medicine, 48000 Mugla, Turkey*
[2] *Department of Pathology, Dokuz Eylul University Faculty of Medicine, 35010 Izmir, Turkey*
[3] *Department of Medical Oncology, Kent Hospital, 35010 Izmir, Turkey*
[4] *Department of Internal Medicine, Sitki Kocman University Faculty of Medicine, 48000 Mugla, Turkey*
[5] *Department of General Surgery, Sitki Kocman University Education and Research Hospital, 48000 Mugla, Turkey*
[6] *Department of Radiodiagnostics, Sitki Kocman University Education and Research Hospital, 48000 Mugla, Turkey*
[7] *Department of Internal Medicine and Gastroenterohepatology, Sitki Kocman University Faculty of Medicine, 48000 Mugla, Turkey*

Correspondence should be addressed to Ozgur Tanriverdi; mugla.medicaloncology@gmail.com

Academic Editor: Cesar V. Reyes

Teratomas are rarely seen in adults, and presacral region is an area where they rarely settle in. Similarly, only about 1% of teratomas show malignant transformation. Malignant transformation is often associated with the area where teratoma settles in. Malignant transformation of mediastinal teratomas is more frequent than the ones located in retroperitoneal area and gonad. They most commonly show rhabdomyosarcoma, primitive neuroectodermal tumor, enteric adenocarcinoma, and leukemia transformation. In teratomas showing malignant transformation, the clinical course is aggressive; and survival of patients with metastatic disease is very low. The primary treatment of teratomas with malignant transformations is surgical. Effect of radiotherapy and chemotherapy is not clear in patients, to whom surgical operation cannot be applied, or those who are with residual tumor, even if surgical operation can be applied to them, or those who are at metastatic stage. In this paper, we presented a 76-year-old male patient due to the histologic diagnosis of mucinous adenocarcinoma within teratoma, in whom approximately 7 cm presacral mass was found during the radiographic examination made by the reason of low back pain and pelvic pain.

1. Introduction

Tumors settled in presacral region are highly rare [1–3]. Such tumors may have developed congenitally or by acquisition. Additionally, the frequency of tumors settled in presacral area was reported to be 1/10000. Only 10% of such tumors are seen in adults, which develop usually in newborns or infants. In addition, 80% of adults with presacral tumor are women. These tumors are usually benign, and only 1-2% of them shows malignant character [1–4].

Teratomas are the tumors most commonly seen in presacral area in infants and newborns. The rate of teratoma incidence in infants and newborns was 1/35,000–40,000, with the dominance of male gender, while the ratio was determined to be 1/40,000–63,000 in adults, with a higher incidence in women [1–3]. In adults, malignant transformation rate of primary teratomas settled in presacral region was about 1%. Adult teratomas may be transformed into squamous cell carcinoma, adenocarcinoma, sarcoma, and other malignancies [4–9].

While there were numerous reports on malignant transforming, including mucinous, adenocarcinoma, or squamous, from teratomas of ovary and testicle, no case of unknown primary mucinous adenocarcinoma within presacral teratoma in an adult male was found in English literature. In this paper, we presented the case of mucinous

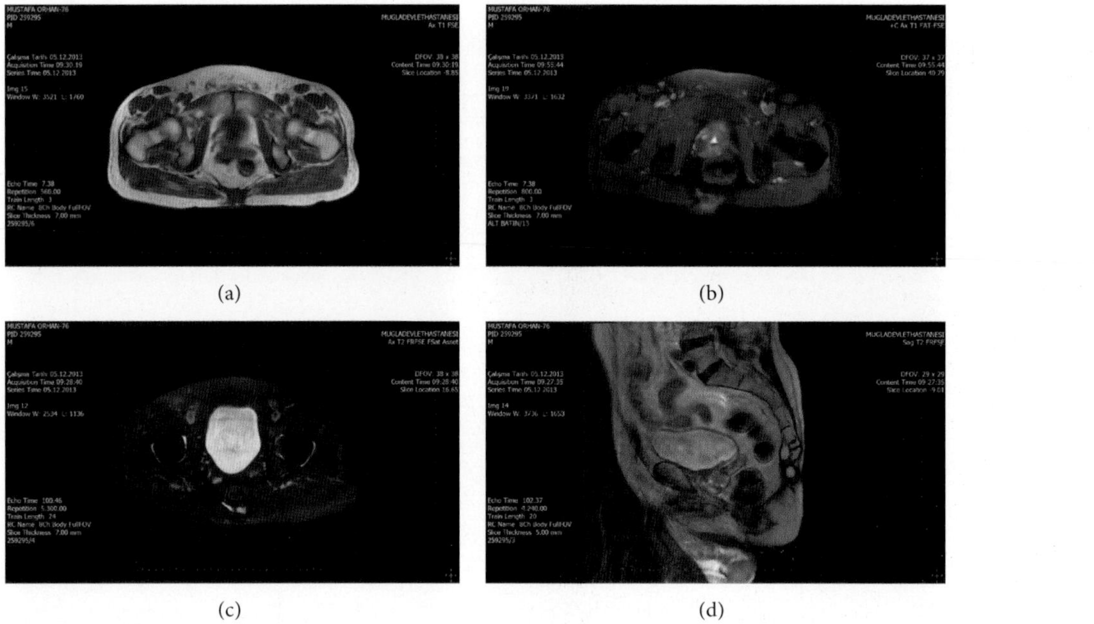

FIGURE 1: Magnetic resonance imaging. (a)–(d) A mass lesion was observed, which was separated with thin septations in the dimension of approximately 7 × 5.5 cm at *os coccyx* level, a part of which shines both in T1 and in T2, a part of which gives high signals in T1, and which had intense involvement of peripheral and septal heterogeneous contrast from postcontrast study.

carcinoma that developed on the basis of presacral teratoma, which we diagnosed in a 76-year-old male patient, for the purpose of emphasizing the fact that both the settlement area and the type of malignant transformation were rare.

2. Case

The 76-year-old male patient presented to the outpatient clinic of general surgery, with the complaints of increasing and intensifying low back pain and pelvic pain, as well as constipation, suffered for the last two months. The history obtainedfrom the patient enabled us to ascertain that he had no different symptom related to other systems, especially weight loss, rectal bleeding, and abdominal pain; and he had no systemic disease history. No lymphadenopathy, organomegaly, abdominal mass symptom, skin lesion, abnormal pulmonary, or cardiovascular finding was detected during his physical examination. The patient's blood biochemistry and complete blood count were normal. There was no peculiarity in the rectal touch, except for presacral sensitivity and swelling detected during the examination.

In the pelvic magnetic resonance imaging, a mass lesion was observed, which was separated with thin septations in the dimension of approximately 7 × 5.5 cm at *os coccyx* level, a part of which shines both in T1 and in T2, a part of which gives high signals in T1, and which had intense involvement of peripheral and septal heterogeneous contrast from postcontrast study (Figure 1). No other findings suggestive of malignancy were observed in his thorax and abdominal computed tomography. Total excision of the presacral mass was made (Figure 2). The histopathological diagnosis of the patient, in whom no postoperative complication was observed, was reported as teratoma containing mucinous adenocarcinoma.

Lymphadenopathy and organomegaly were not detected in the patient, who applied to the oncology outpatient department with his pathology result. His blood biochemistry and complete blood count were normal. The patient's alpha-fetoprotein, human chorionic gonadotropin hormone, cancer antigen (CA) 19-9, CA 125, carcinoembriogenic antigen, and prostate specific antigen levels were within normal limits. Any finding related to malignancy was observed in the esophagus, stomach, and the colorectal during the endoscopic examination of the upper and lower gastrointestinal systems. The testicular ultrasonography was normal. No primary tumor or metastatic lesion was detected in terms of mucinous adenocarcinoma, by the performed positron-emission tomography/computerized tomography. Adjuvant systemic chemotherapy was recommended to the patients with negative surgical margins. The therapy was commenced with the biweekly application of the regimen containing irinotecan 185 mg/m^2/day, d1, 400 mg/m^2/day, d1 and 2800 mg/m^2, d1-d2 infusional fluorouracil. The patient is still under treatment and the metastasis is being monitored for 10 months.

2.1. Histopathological Examination. On microscopically examination the mass was located in the subcutaneous area and it had an appearance of a multiloculated cyst with some areas being more solid. The cystic areas were lined by either ciliated columnar epithelium with serous nature or mucinous epithelium. There were some large mucin pools. Some of these mucin pools contained some atypical cell groups which were considered malignant based on the morphological and immunohistochemical staining (diffuse MIB-1 staining and

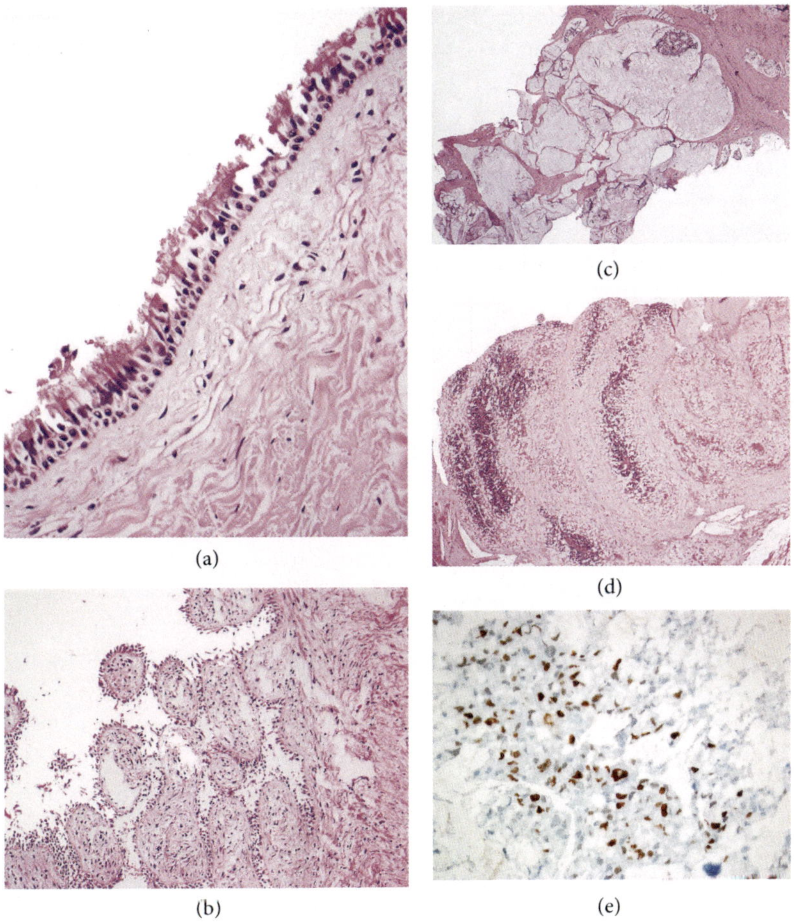

FIGURE 2: (a) The lining of some cysts was composed of ciliated columnar. (b) There were papillary structures with hyalinized stroma and ciliated columnar epithelium. (c) In some areas, there was a multiloculated cystic appearance of the tumor, most of which were filled with mucinous matrix. (d) Inside the mucin pools, there were atypical and mitotically active cells, with increased nuclear/cytoplasmic ratio; (e) the MIB-1 staining was high in these cells which were considered as malignant.

p53 positivity). The tumor was reported as a sacrococcygeal subcutaneous teratoma with malignant mucinous adenocarcinoma (Figure 2). Status of isochromosome 12 could not be tested due to technical problems.

3. Discussion

In this paper, we discussed our 76-year-old male patient diagnosed with mucinous carcinoma developing on teratoma, as a result of total presacral mass excision.

Teratomas are tumors containing different types of cells developing from multiple germinal layers. Most of teratomas are seen in testicles and ovaries of adolescents [4, 7, 9]. However, it may also develop in sacrococcygeal, presacral, retroperitoneal, postanal or mediastinal, and pineal gland, which are also known as midline structures. Different hypotheses were proposed, in regard to the development of teratomas. "Germ cell theory" is the most widely accepted one proposing that primitive totipotential cells act as a "wandering germ cell," arisen from cells left behind during migration of embryonic germ cells from yolk sac to the gonads [9].

Primary presacral teratomas are highly rare in adults. Its malignant transformation rate is about 1% [9]. In the literature, we did not find any case of presacral teratoma that showed malignant transformation, in older adults. Our case gains importance due to this rare situation.

Presacral teratomas are often asymptomatic in adults, and they are usually detected during clinical or radiological examination. Although 90% of sacrococcygeal teratomas are externally visible in neonatal period, most of the teratomas in this region are presented as pelvic mass in adults [1–4, 10]. The most frequent symptom was reported to be pain. The pain is severe increasing with movement, in the back, lower back, and pelvic area. However, the other symptoms are mild and they are considered as nonspecific [1–4, 10]. Symptoms related to compression of organs located around presacral mass may occur [8, 11]. Constipation, sensation of incomplete evacuation, narrowed stools, or incontinence is among the possible symptoms. Frequent urine, dysmenorrhea, vomiting, nausea, edema, and paresthesia in the lower extremities are the other possible symptoms [12]. Our patient applied to the general surgery polyclinic, with the complaints of low back pain, pelvic pain, and constipation.

Presacral cystic teratomas should be distinguished from ependymomas in men and from ovarian cancer in women. However, in both sexes, meningocele, rectal duplication, tail-gut cyst, neurogenic tumors, osseous lesions, renal cysts, the Mullerian ducts cysts, and epidermal cysts are the reasons for benign disorders that they may encounter. Besides these, also lymphangioma, sarcoma, mucinous adenocarcinoma, cystic mesothelioma, metastatic lymphadenopathy, ovaries or uterus metastatic tumors listed as Wilms tumor, and soft tissue malignancies should be distinguished [4, 9, 13–17]. In addition, sometimes perirectal abscess, granulomata, fistulas, and sometimes tuberculosis cases, and so forth, may arise [13–17]. And extraneural myxopapillary ependymoma thought to be derived from embryological residues that can be seen in sacrococcygeal area should be considered during the definitive diagnosis, as well. Particularly teratomas in mucinous content may create a diagnosis difficulty, with myxopapillary ependymoma [4–8, 13, 15, 17].

Our patient was diagnosed with adenocarcinoma on the teratoma surface, during the histopathological examination. Malignant tumor finding was not observed in the testicle, colon, stomach, and pancreas during the radiological and endoscopic examinations intended for primer. Tumor markers were not guiding. Our patients was evaluated to be a patient with unknown primary cancer.

No case of mucinous adenocarcinoma transformation in teratoma was found in the literature. However, two cases with retroperitoneal adenocarcinoma transformation have been reported [9, 16]. Metastasis frequency is high, and clinical course is highly aggressive. Previous studies reported that prognosis is poor in metastatic patients and that the average survival time is limited to 28 months [10, 14].

Altman et al. [18] have classified sacrococcygeal teratomas in 4 categories. In Type 1 patients, predominant external tumor accompanied with minimal presacral component is detected, whilst Type 2 patients are presented externally—however, their intrapelvic extension is explicit. In Type 3 patients, externality is still explicit but pelvic mass extending into the abdomen is predominant. Type 3 is the category most frequently seen in adults. On the other hand, Type 4 patients are presacral masses without external presentation [18]. Our patient was evaluated to be a Type 4 patient.

Histological features of teratomas showing malignant transformation have been very well defined. They are considered to be somatic components of histological features of a tumor with nonseminomatous germ cell, which cannot be distinguished from a somatic malignancy [13–17]. Malignant transformation often includes rhabdomyosarcoma, primitive neuroectodermal tumor, enteric adenocarcinoma, and leukemia. Malignant transformations may occur in any primary area, where mature or immature teratomas develop. On the other hand, mediastinal teratomas and other tumors with nonseminomatous germ cell are more likely to show malignant transformation, compared to gonadal or retroperitoneal primary tumors [9]. Although some chromosomal abnormalities such as isochromosome 12p are associated with malignant transformation and carcinogenesis has yet to be clarified [9, 17, 19, 20]. Similarly, although surgical treatment of operable patients by means of total excision is considered to be a standard, systemic chemotherapy of such patients is still complex. It is because they are resistant to standard chemotherapy [14]. However, there are a limited number of studies and case presentations showing that a significant ratio of response and survival advantages can be obtained in a group of patients through a chemotherapy regimen to be selected depending on the cell, into which the transformation will occur [9, 14]. It has been reported that cisplatin-based chemotherapy regimens are likely not to be effective enough but fluorouracil-based regimens may produce good results especially in adenocarcinoma transformation arising from retroperitoneal or presacral teratomas [20].

In conclusion, it should be remembered that teratomas can be seen in presacral spaces in adults and may develop malignant transformation even though rarely; and histopathological examination should be carried out in detail, based on this thought. No standard systemic treatment intended for teratomas showing malignant transformation is clear yet; and therefore, sharing such rare cases may create an important database.

Disclosure

The authors certify that all of their affiliations with or without financial involvement within the past 5 years and foreseeable future and any organization or entity with a financial interest in or financial conflict with the subject matter or materials discussed in the paper are completely disclosed (e.g., employment, consultancies, honoraria, stock ownership or options, expert testimony, grants or patents received or pending, and royalties).

References

[1] R. O. Valdiserri and E. J. Yunis, "Sacrococcygeal teratomas: a review of 68 cases," *Cancer*, vol. 48, no. 1, pp. 217–221, 1981.

[2] J. Ghosh, T. Eglinton, F. A. Frizelle, and A. J. M. Watson, "Presacral tumours in adults," *Surgeon*, vol. 5, no. 1, pp. 31–38, 2007.

[3] I. M. Audet, R. T. Goldhahn Jr., and T. L. Dent, "Adult sacrococcygeal teratomas," *American Surgeon*, vol. 66, no. 1, pp. 61–65, 2000.

[4] E. W. Ng, P. Porcu, and P. J. Loehrer, "Sacrococcygeal teratoma in adults: case reports and a review of the literature," *Cancer*, vol. 86, no. 7, pp. 1198–1202, 1999.

[5] K. Szyllo and N. Lesnik, "Sacrococcygeal teratoma—case report and review of the literature," *The American Journal of Case Reports*, vol. 14, pp. 15–19, 2013.

[6] O. O. Afuwape, O. O. Ogundoyin, D. I. Ogunlana, and A. O. Adeleye, "Adult sacrococcygeal teratoma: a case report," *Ghana Medical Journal*, vol. 43, no. 1, pp. 40–42, 2009.

[7] J. Bull Jr., K. A. Yeh, D. Mcdonnell, P. Caudell, and J. Davis, "Mature presacral teratoma in an adult male: a case report," *American Surgeon*, vol. 65, no. 6, pp. 586–591, 1999.

[8] M. M. Golas, B. Gunawan, B.-W. Raab, L. Füzesi, and B. Lange, "Malignant transformation of an untreated congenital sacrococcygeal teratoma: a amplification at 8q and 12p detected by comparative genomic hybridization," *Cancer Genetics and Cytogenetics*, vol. 197, no. 1, pp. 95–98, 2010.

[9] J. Wang and S. A. J. Kazmi, "Teratoma with malignant transformation: a case report with pathological, cytogenetic, and immunohistochemistry analysis," *Sarcoma*, vol. 2011, Article ID 450743, 5 pages, 2011.

[10] C. V. Comiter, A. S. Kibel, J. P. Richie, M. R. Nucci, and A. A. Renshaw, "Prognostic features of teratomas with malignant transformation: a clinicopathological study of 21 cases," *Journal of Urology*, vol. 159, no. 3, pp. 859–863, 1998.

[11] P.-Y. Chu, T.-H. Teng, C.-C. Lee, and Y.-Y. Chou, "Adenocarcinomas arising from primary retroperitoneal teratoma in an adult female patient," *International Journal of Urology*, vol. 13, no. 10, pp. 1352–1354, 2006.

[12] D. Paramythiotis, T. S. Papavramidis, A. Michalopoulos et al., "Chronic constipation due to presacral teratoma in a 36-year-old woman: a case report," *Journal of Medical Case Reports*, vol. 4, article 23, 2010.

[13] A. Mazreku, A. Karaj, I. Avdia, and S. Bilali, "The presentation and management of presacral tumors.," *Acta chirurgica Iugoslavica*, vol. 57, no. 2, pp. 55–59, 2010.

[14] A. C. Donadio, R. J. Motzer, D. F. Bajorin et al., "Chemotherapy for teratoma with malignant transformation," *Journal of Clinical Oncology*, vol. 21, no. 23, pp. 4285–4291, 2003.

[15] N. Omezzine, C. Khouatra, S. Larivé et al., "Rhabdomyosarcoma arising in mediastinal teratoma in an adult man: a case report," *Annals of Oncology*, vol. 13, no. 2, pp. 323–326, 2002.

[16] T. Ahmed, G. J. Bosl, and S. I. Hajdu, "Teratoma with malignant transformation in germ cell tumors in men," *Cancer*, vol. 56, no. 4, pp. 860–863, 1985.

[17] N. Zeh, P. J. Wild, P. K. Bode et al., "Retroperitoneal teratoma with somatic malignant transformation: a papillary renal cell carcinoma in a testicular germ cell tumour metastasis following platinum-based chemotherapy," *BMC Urology*, vol. 13, pp. 9–13, 2013.

[18] R. P. Altman, J. G. Randolph, and J. R. Lilly, "Sacrococcygeal teratoma: American academy of pediatrics surgical section survey—1973," *Journal of Pediatric Surgery*, vol. 9, no. 3, pp. 389–398, 1974.

[19] G. T. Gurda, C. J. Vandenbussche, R. Yonescu et al., "Sacrococcygeal teratomas: clinico-pathological characteristics and isochromosome 12p status," *Modern Pathology*, vol. 27, no. 4, pp. 562–568, 2014.

[20] S. P. Ho, J. S. Wang, H. H. Tseng, and T. M. King, "Presacral teratocarcinoma presenting as anal fistula and rectal adenocarcinoma: a unique case presentation and literature review," *Case Reports in Oncology*, vol. 5, no. 1, pp. 84–90, 2012.

Effective Downsizing of a Large Oesophageal Gastrointestinal Stromal Tumour with Neoadjuvant Imatinib Enabling an Uncomplicated and without Tumour Rupture Laparoscopic-Assisted Ivor-Lewis Oesophagectomy

Kyriakos Neofytou,[1] Mafalda Costa Neves,[1] Alexandros Giakoustidis,[1] Charlotte Benson,[2] and Satvinder Mudan[1]

[1]*Royal Marsden Hospital, Department of Academic Surgery, Upper GI/HPB Unit, Fulham Road, London SW3 6JJ, UK*
[2]*Royal Marsden Hospital, Sarcoma Unit, Fulham Road, London SW3 6JJ, UK*

Correspondence should be addressed to Kyriakos Neofytou; kneophy2@gmail.com

Academic Editor: Raffaele Palmirotta

Neoadjuvant imatinib for gastrointestinal stromal tumours (GISTs) is increasingly used nowadays. As oesophagectomy is associated with high morbidity and mortality, a preoperative downsizing of an oesophageal GIST to limit the extent of resection would be ideal. Because these tumours are rare and neoadjuvant treatment with imatinib is recent, there is limited literature available regarding neoadjuvant administration of imatinib in patients with oesophageal GISTs. A 50-year-old woman presented with total dysphagia. An upper endoscopy and biopsy revealed a large submucosal KIT-positive GIST obstructing the mid oesophagus. CT confirmed a lesion measuring 99 mm × 50 mm × 104 mm. Because the size and location of the tumour increased the risk of intraoperative rupture, it was decided to administer preoperative imatinib. The patient had an excellent clinical and radiological response. Her dysphagia gradually resolved and the follow-up CT scans of the first 10 months showed a gradually reducing tumour size to 54 mm × 33 mm × 42 mm. The patient underwent an uneventful laparoscopic-assisted Ivor-Lewis oesophagectomy. Postoperatively, the patient continued with adjuvant imatinib. At the last follow-up, 1 year from operation and 38 months from the diagnosis, the patient is disease free.

1. Introduction

Gastrointestinal Stromal Tumours (GISTs) are mesenchymal neoplasms located primarily in the gastrointestinal (GI) tract and represent 80% of all GI sarcomas [1]. Surgery is the only potentially curative option, and for approximately 60% of patients, the successful surgical removal of the tumour would represent cure [2].

A benchmark in dealing with these chemotherapy-insensitive tumours was the introduction of treatment with imatinib and later of sunitinib, two tyrosine-kinase inhibitors [3, 4]. The indications for imatinib use are locally advanced inoperable disease, metastatic disease, and adjuvant therapy in patients at high risk for relapse [3].

Although 80% of newly diagnosed cases are resectable at presentation, the high efficacy of imatinib in the metastatic and adjuvant setting quickly made way for its usage also in the neoadjuvant setting [4–6].

The main indications for preoperative imatinib are (1) unresectable or metastatic disease with an aim of tumour downsizing and conversion of patient to candidate for radical resection and (2) resectable metastatic or nonmetastatic disease with an aim of downsizing of disease as well, thus reducing the extent of surgery and postoperative morbidity and mortality (e.g., laparoscopic removal avoiding the need for multivisceral resection, local excision versus more radical interventions for tumours in difficult anatomical locations such as the rectum, duodenum, and oesophagus). In this

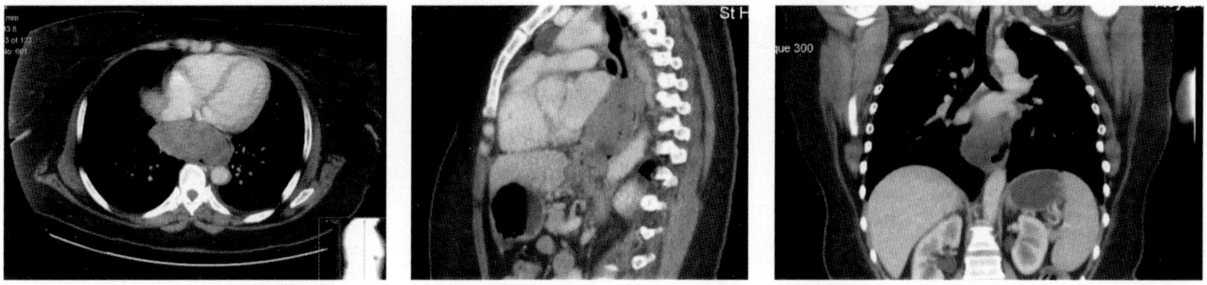

(a) (b) (c)

FIGURE 1: CT scan at presentation: (a) axial view, (b) sagittal view, and (c) coronal view.

second group of patients, with resectable disease at presentation, preoperative administration of imatinib also aims to improve the oncological outcome by reducing the likelihood of intraoperative tumour rupture, which has been identified as being an independent predictor of disease recurrence and is currently included in systems assessing the likelihood of postoperative relapse [2, 7].

Oesophageal GISTs are very rare, representing less than 2% of GISTs [8]. Because of the high morbidity/mortality associated with oesophagectomy, preoperative downsizing of oesophageal GIST is ideal, in an attempt to reduce the extent of surgery and consequently the risk of perioperative complications. Due to the rarity of these tumours and the fact that neoadjuvant treatment with imatinib is a recent development, there is limited literature available regarding neoadjuvant administration of imatinib in patients with oesophageal GISTs [9–12].

We report a case of large oesophageal GIST in a 50-year-old woman who underwent laparoscopic-assisted Ivor-Lewis oesophagectomy after 26 months of neoadjuvant imatinib therapy.

2. Case Report

A 50-year-old lady presented to our hospital with a 4-month history of progressive dysphagia. Her symptoms worsened progressively resulting in total dysphagia, pain mainly in the epigastric and lower chest area radiating to her back, and one recent episode of haematemesis. At presentation, she was unable to swallow even her saliva. She had no associated medical comorbidities, except for being an ex-smoker and having a BMI of 41. The physical examination was unremarkable. Standard laboratory test results were within normal range, with haemoglobin of 11 mg/dL. An oesophagogastroscopy revealed a large submucosal obstructing oesophageal mass, partially ulcerated, situated 42 mm above diaphragmatic hiatus, and extending over a distance of at least 10 cm. Biopsy revealed a GIST with diffuse positivity for CD117 and CD34 and a mitotic index of 3/22 hpf (insufficient material to count mitoses/50 fields). Gene analysis with direct sequencing revealed a 6 bp deletion in exon 11 of the KIT gene [mutation details: c.1670_1675del p.Trp557_Val559delinsPhe (reference cDNA sequence: NM_000222.2)].

A computed tomography (CT) scan of chest and abdomen revealed an annular polypoidal mass, 99 mm × 50 mm × 104 mm in diameter in the mid oesophagus, arising 42 mm above the diaphragmatic hiatus and extending cranially over a distance of 10 cm to the subcarinal level (Figure 1). There was evidence of extension through the oesophageal wall over a distance of at least 10 mm but without lymphadenopathy or metastatic disease. The tumour was classified as high risk according to Fletcher's classification [13].

The patient was admitted to our hospital for pain and symptoms of total dysphagia and an 8F nasogastric tube was inserted endoscopically.

Her case was further discussed in the sarcoma Multidisciplinary Team (MDT) meeting. Despite the tumour being resectable at presentation, its size and location rendered it to an increased risk of intraoperative rupture. Furthermore, GIST with mutations in exon 11 of KIT is generally associated with sensitivity to imatinib. Therefore, the MDT decided on preoperative administration of imatinib 400 mg daily.

She had an excellent clinical response with dysphagia gradually improving, and 12 days later, she was able to tolerate solid food once again.

The first follow-up CT scan two months after initiating treatment showed an excellent partial response, with the mass measuring 65 mm × 42 mm × 51 mm and reduction of tumour mass to 27% of the initial volume. New CT three months after showed further response, with mass reduction to 53 mm × 33 mm × 42 mm (Figures 2 and 3). During this period, she had been tolerating treatment very well, apart from Grade 1 fatigue.

After ten months of treatment, the tumour had been stabilized at 54 mm × 33 mm × 42 mm, suggesting plateau response. According to our policy, this would be the correct timing for surgery. However, because the patient was considered high risk for operation, as indicated by her cardiopulmonary exercise testing (CPX) revealing an anaerobic threshold of 9.3, the MDT decided the patient should continue treatment with imatinib and further take up an exercise program in an attempt to reduce her risks of perioperative complications.

Unfortunately, the next CT scan after 13 months of treatment demonstrated localized but progressive disease (90 mm × 42 mm × 60 mm) (Figures 2 and 3). Although

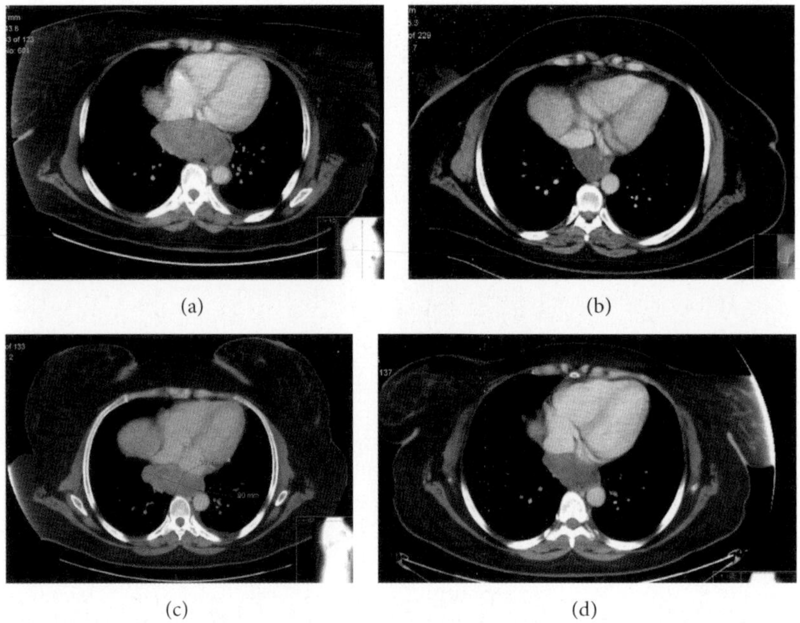

FIGURE 2: (a) CT scan at diagnosis, Longest Axial Diameter (LAD) 99 mm; (b) CT scan after 10 months of imatinib therapy, partial response LAD 54 mm; (c) CT scan after 13 months of imatinib therapy, disease progression LAD 90 mm; and (d) CT scan after 26 months of imatinib therapy, partial response LAD 44 mm.

disease progression under treatment with imatinib is a well described phenomenon, the previous excellent response in combination with the very fast disease progression raised the question of drug compliance [6]. On further questioning, the patient admitted not being compliant with drug therapy because of side effects of dry skin and periorbital oedema.

Further management of this patient was challenging. On one hand, we were not keen to lose the surgical window of opportunity for a bulky but localised tumour of the oesophagus, but on the other hand, the risk of intraoperative tumour rupture was similar to that prior to treatment.

After extensive discussion with the patient regarding the advantages and disadvantages of continuing imatinib therapy, the patient agreed to restart treatment.

She received her treatment regularly, and the follow-up CTs during the next year showed progressive reduction of the tumour size (Figures 2 and 3). 26 months after diagnosis, and with the latest CT demonstrating the oesophageal tumour measuring 44 mm × 36 mm × 35 mm, equal to 13.84% of the volume at diagnosis, the patient underwent an uncomplicated and without tumour rupture laparoscopic-assisted Ivor-Lewis oesophagectomy and was discharged 12 days after surgery.

Histopathology revealed a GIST with extensive areas of hypocellularity with hyalinised stroma and haemosiderin deposition, consistent with therapy effect, and viable tumour was estimated at approximately 30–50%. There was mucosal ulceration and the lesion extended from the mucosa to the adventitia. The tumour margins measured 10 mm from the oesophageal resection margin, >30 mm from gastric resection margin, and <1 mm from the serosal surface. Nine lymph nodes were identified, with no evidence of metastatic tumour. The mitotic index was 14/50 hpf.

Both the original size of the tumour and the mitotic index (14/50 hpf) classified the tumour as "high risk" and the decision was taken for further adjuvant imatinib, according to the Scandinavian Sarcoma Group Trial [14].

At the last follow-up, 1 year after operation and 38 months from the diagnosis, the patient remained disease free.

3. Discussion

We present a patient with a large oesophageal GIST who underwent radical surgical resection following neoadjuvant administration of imatinib for 26 months. Despite the fact that the plateau response to imatinib was reached 10 months after initiating treatment, the combination of high operative risk and noncompliance with therapy prolonged the neoadjuvant administration of imatinib. The lack of compliance to daily dosage imatinib resulted in the rapid enlargement of the tumour. The subsequent improved drug compliance resulted in a new response to treatment, with a better radiological response than the one seen on plateau phase before. Finally, the patient underwent an uneventful laparoscopic-assisted Ivor-Lewis oesophagectomy without tumour rupture. Postoperatively, the patient continued imatinib treatment and remained disease free at 1 year follow-up.

The discovery that the vast majority of GISTs have characteristic activating mutations in c-KIT (75–80%) or PDGFRA (5–15%) radically changed the management of these tumours by the approval of the use of tyrosine-kinase inhibitors [4, 15]. Imatinib, the first approved drug in this category, is an adenosine triphosphate, competitive inhibitor of KIT, PDGFRA, BCR-ABL, and ABL tyrosine kinases, which was already used in the treatment of patients with chronic myeloid leukemia (CML) who bear the BCR-ABL

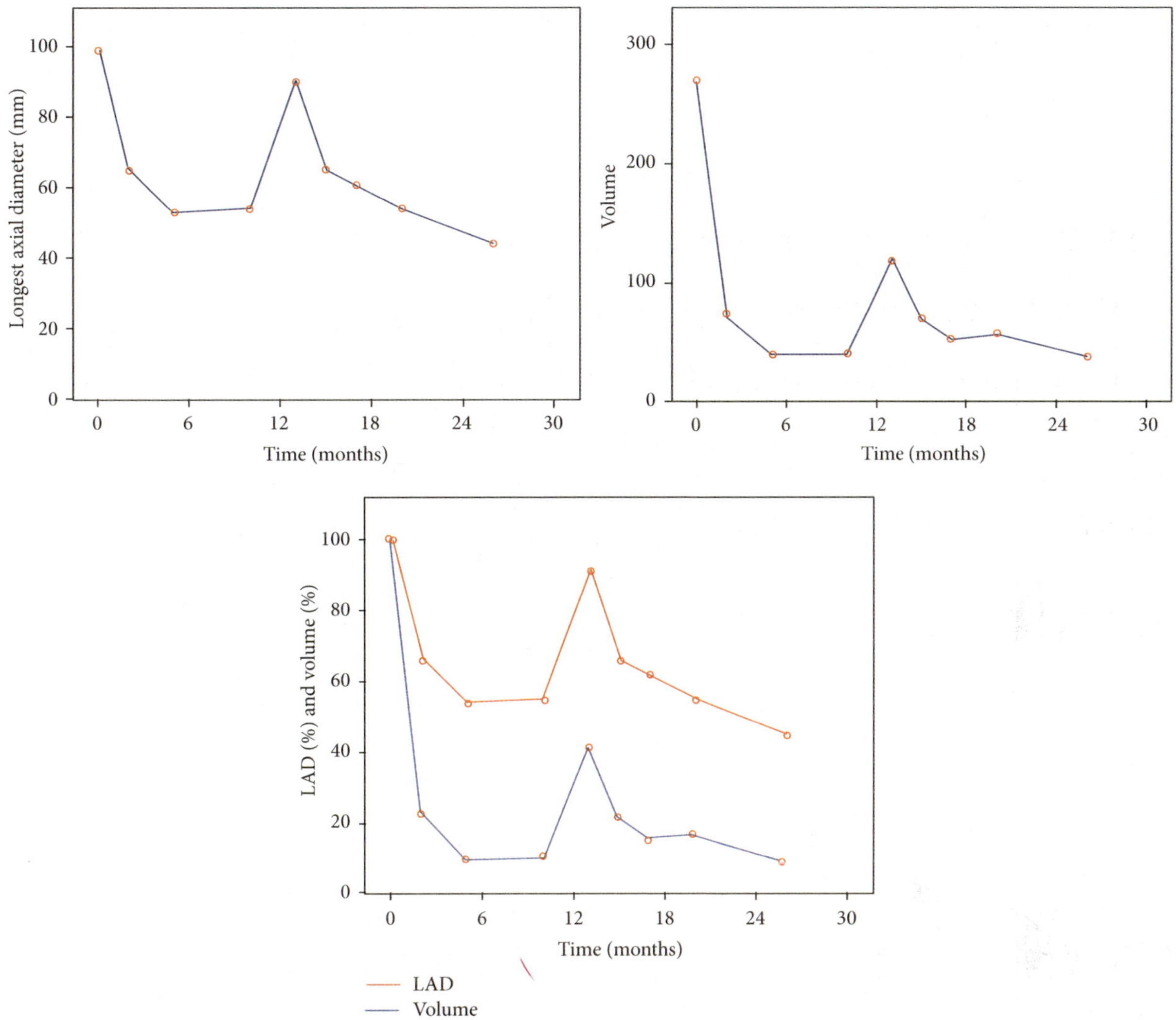

FIGURE 3: Changes of Longest Axial Diameter and volume (cm^3) during imatinib therapy.

fusion gene [3, 16]. The approval of sunitinib followed, which is another inhibitor of several tyrosine kinases, including KIT, PDGFR, and VEGFR for the treatment of patients with imatinib-resistant GIST or patients who do not tolerate imatinib [4].

Although preoperative downsizing of oesophageal GIST in an attempt to reduce the high morbidity/mortality associated with oesophagectomy seems ideal, literature available regarding neoadjuvant administration of imatinib in patients with oesophageal GISTs is very limited as oesophageal GISTs are rare and also neoadjuvant treatment with imatinib is a recent development [9–12]. Yanagawa et al. reported the successful downsizing of a large GIST of lower oesophagus after 6 months of neoadjuvant imatinib administration, allowing for a complete resection of the tumour without rupture [9]. Tirumani et al., in a recent study regarding the timing of earliest, best, and plateau response to neoadjuvant imatinib in patients with GIST, reported that one of the 20 patients who were enrolled in this study was diagnosed with oesophageal GIST and underwent Ivor-Lewis oesophagectomy after 20 weeks of neoadjuvant administration of imatinib with stable disease [10]. Fiore et al. studied the efficacy of preoperative administration of imatinib for unresectable or locally advanced primary GIST, and the authors included in their study one patient with locally advanced oesophageal GIST (9 cm) who had partial response according to RECIST after 9 months of imatinib administration and who then underwent an uncomplicated Ivor-Lewis oesophagectomy [11]. Shinagare et al. have also reported a patient with oesophageal GIST who underwent esophagectomy after 4 months of neoadjuvant administration of imatinib [12]. As we can see from the above mentioned cases, the experience regarding the preoperative administration of imatinib in patients with oesophageal GIST is limited, and experience from dealing with such cases could give way to answering questions regarding the benefit of patients related to the oncological outcome and also the optimal duration of the preoperative administration of imatinib.

The accurate prediction of recurrence is very important for the decision of administration of adjuvant imatinib.

The existing risk stratification systems (Fletcher's classification, Joensuu liner-model, AFIP criteria, and modified NIH criteria) are based on tumour size, mitotic activity, tumour rupture prior to or at surgery, and tumour location [2, 7, 13, 17].

Regarding oesophageal GISTs, despite the fact that these can be classified according to the risk stratification systems mentioned above, the contribution of oesophageal GISTs to the creation of these systems was very small. This fact raises concerns about the accuracy of these systems regarding the prognosis of patients with oesophageal GISTs. For example, only 8 of the 1625 patients (0.49%) who validated for the creation of Joensuu liner-model had oesophageal GIST [2]. Also, it is worth noting that none of these systems include patients who received neoadjuvant imatinib. A similar lack of information is observed regarding the effectiveness of adjuvant administration of imatinib in patients with oesophageal GISTs. Although Joensuu et al. demonstrated the superiority of administration of adjuvant imatinib for 3 years when compared to 1 year with regard to disease free and overall survival for patients with KIT-positive GISTs, once again the number of patients with oesophageal GISTs included in this study was very small [14].

The optimal duration of preoperative imatinib administration is not fully documented. NCCN states that the treatment should be continued until the tumour stops responding to imatinib or if PD appears unresponsive even to increased dose of imatinib [18]. Interruption of preoperative imatinib despite continuous tumour response is also acceptable, with the assumption that any further reduction in volume will not affect the type and extent of surgery [6, 10]. There are published studies about the duration of preoperative administration of imatinib ranging from a few days to more than one year [6, 19, 20].

Disease progression during neoadjuvant imatinib has been reported as a rare phenomenon for primary tumours, which has been attributed in part to the emergence of secondary mutations following prolonged treatment [6, 21]. Moreover, the increased understanding of mutational status with respect to KIT and pDGFRA mutations has meant that patients with truly imatinib insensitive disease (e.g., PDGFRA D842V mutations) are not considered for treatment. The hypothesis of the emergence of secondary mutations was considered when our patient demonstrated progressive disease after 13 months of imatinib. However, the explanation was much simpler, as the patient had not been fully compliant with the treatment.

The rarity of oesophageal GISTs explains the lack of clear recommendations regarding their optimal surgical management. As oesophageal segmental and wedge resections are not feasible, the surgical options include the high morbidity/mortality associated oesophagectomy and the much less invasive surgical tumour enucleation [8, 22–25]. The oncological outcome of these two procedures is similar, providing proper selection of patients (enucleation indicated for smaller tumours and with no evidence of mucosal ulceration) [8, 22–25]. An alternative approach for lower oesophageal GISTs is the Merendino procedure, which is utilized in our hospital providing that the tumour is accessible transhiatally [26]. This technique bears a low morbidity and mortality due to the avoidance of thoracotomy, provides a good functional outcome, and can also be applied to patients with tumours with mucosal ulceration (unpublished observations). Although our patient's comorbidities were favourable for a less invasive approach, both enucleation and Merendino procedure were not feasible. On one hand, enucleation was rejected because of the mucosal ulceration, and on the other hand, Merendino procedure in a patient with a high upper margin tumour would increase the possibility of an incomplete transhiatal tumour resection. Under these circumstances, we proceeded to a laparoscopic-assisted Ivor-Lewis oesophagectomy.

4. Conclusions

In the absence of clear guidelines for the optimal treatment of oesophageal GISTs, preoperative administration of imatinib in an attempt to downsizing, particularly in patients with large tumours, presented as an attractive approach aiming to (1) decrease the risk of intraoperative tumour rupture, thus achieving a better oncological outcome, and (2) reduce the extent of surgery and therefore the risks of perioperative morbidity and mortality. Compliance with drug therapy is essential for the success of this approach.

References

[1] M. Miettinen and J. Lasota, "Gastrointestinal stromal tumors: review on morphology, molecular pathology, prognosis, and differential diagnosis," *Archives of Pathology and Laboratory Medicine*, vol. 130, no. 10, pp. 1466–1478, 2006.

[2] H. Joensuu, A. Vehtari, J. Riihimäki et al., "Risk of recurrence of gastrointestinal stromal tumour after surgery: an analysis of pooled population-based cohorts," *The Lancet Oncology*, vol. 13, no. 3, pp. 265–274, 2012.

[3] P. Reichardt, H. Joensuu, and J.-Y. Blay, "New fronts in the adjuvant treatment of GIST," *Cancer Chemotherapy and Pharmacology*, vol. 72, no. 4, pp. 715–723, 2013.

[4] H. Joensuu, P. Hohenberger, and C. L. Corless, "Gastrointestinal stromal tumour," *The Lancet*, vol. 382, no. 9896, pp. 973–983, 2013.

[5] B. L. Eisenberg, J. Harris, C. D. Blanke et al., "Phase II trial of neoadjuvant/adjuvant imatinib mesylate (IM) for advanced primary and metastatic/recurrent operable gastrointestinal stromal tumor (GIST): early results of RTOG 0132/ACRIN 6665," *Journal of Surgical Oncology*, vol. 99, no. 1, pp. 42–47, 2009.

[6] B. K. Bednarski, D. M. Araujo, M. Yi et al., "Analysis of prognostic factors impacting oncologic outcomes after neoadjuvant tyrosine kinase inhibitor therapy for gastrointestinal stromal tumors," *Annals of Surgical Oncology*, vol. 21, no. 8, pp. 2499–2505, 2014.

[7] H. Joensuu, "Risk stratification of patients diagnosed with gastrointestinal stromal tumor," *Human Pathology*, vol. 39, no. 10, pp. 1411–1419, 2008.

[8] H. J. Lee, S. I. Park, D. K. Kim, and Y. H. Kim, "Surgical resection of esophageal gastrointestinal stromal tumors," *The Annals of Thoracic Surgery*, vol. 87, no. 5, pp. 1569–1571, 2009.

[9] S. Yanagawa, K. Tanabe, T. Suzuki, N. Tokumoto, K. Arihiro, and H. Ohdan, "A large esophageal gastrointestinal stromal tumor that was successfully resected after neoadjuvant imatinib treatment: case report," *World Journal of Surgical Oncology*, vol. 12, no. 1, article 47, 2014.

[10] S. Tirumani, A. Shinagare, J. Jagannathan, K. Krajewski, N. Ramaiya, and C. Raut, "Radiologic assessment of earliest, best, and plateau response of gastrointestinal stromal tumors to neoadjuvant imatinib prior to successful surgical resection," *European Journal of Surgical Oncology*, vol. 40, no. 4, pp. 420–428, 2014.

[11] M. Fiore, E. Palassini, E. Fumagalli et al., "Preoperative imatinib mesylate for unresectable or locally advanced primary gastrointestinal stromal tumors (GIST)," *European Journal of Surgical Oncology*, vol. 35, no. 7, pp. 739–745, 2009.

[12] A. B. Shinagare, K. A. Zukotynski, K. M. Krajewski et al., "Esophageal gastrointestinal stromal tumor: report of 7 patients," *Cancer Imaging*, vol. 12, no. 1, pp. 100–108, 2012.

[13] C. D. M. Fletcher, J. J. Berman, C. Corless et al., "Diagnosis of gastrointestinal stromal tumors: a consensus approach," *Human Pathology*, vol. 33, no. 5, pp. 459–465, 2002.

[14] H. Joensuu, M. Eriksson, K. S. Hall et al., "One vs three years of adjuvant imatinib for operable gastrointestinal stromal tumor: a randomized trial," *Journal of the American Medical Association*, vol. 307, no. 12, pp. 1265–1272, 2012.

[15] P. A. Cassier, E. Fumagalli, P. Rutkowski et al., "Outcome of patients with platelet-derived growth factor receptor alpha-mutated gastrointestinal stromal tumors in the tyrosine kinase inhibitor era," *Clinical Cancer Research*, vol. 18, no. 16, pp. 4458–4464, 2012.

[16] The ESMO/European Sarcoma Network Working Group, "Gastrointestinal stromal tumors: ESMO Clinical Practice Guidelines for diagnosis, treatment and follow-up," *Annals of Oncology*, vol. 23, supplement 7, pp. vii49–vii55, 2012.

[17] M. Miettinen and J. Lasota, "Gastrointestinal stromal tumors: pathology and prognosis at different sites," *Seminars in Diagnostic Pathology*, vol. 23, no. 2, pp. 70–83, 2006.

[18] M. von Mehren, R. S. Benjamin, M. M. Bui et al., "Soft tissue sarcoma, version 2.2012 featured updates to the NCCN guidelines," *Journal of the National Comprehensive Cancer Network*, vol. 10, no. 8, pp. 951–960, 2012.

[19] J. C. McAuliffe, K. K. Hunt, A. J. F. Lazar et al., "A randomized, phase II study of preoperative plus postoperative Imatinib in GIST: evidence of rapid radiographic response and temporal induction of tumor cell apoptosis," *Annals of Surgical Oncology*, vol. 16, no. 4, pp. 910–919, 2009.

[20] R. Tielen, C. Verhoef, F. van Coevorden et al., "Surgery after treatment with imatinib and/or sunitinib in patients with metastasized gastrointestinal stromal tumors: is it worthwhile?" *World Journal of Surgical Oncology*, vol. 10, article 111, 2012.

[21] P. Rutkowski, A. Gronchi, P. Hohenberger et al., "Neoadjuvant imatinib in locally advanced gastrointestinal stromal tumors (GIST): the EORTC STBSG experience," *Annals of Surgical Oncology*, vol. 20, no. 9, pp. 2937–2943, 2013.

[22] W. B. Robb, E. Bruyere, D. Amielh et al., "Esophageal gastrointestinal stromal tumor: is tumoral enucleation a viable therapeutic option?" vol. 261, no. 1, pp. 117–124, 2015.

[23] M. G. Blum, K. Y. Bilimoria, J. D. Wayne, A. L. de Hoyos, M. S. Talamonti, and B. Adley, "Surgical considerations for the management and resection of esophageal gastrointestinal stromal tumors," *Annals of Thoracic Surgery*, vol. 84, no. 5, pp. 1717–1723, 2007.

[24] P. Jiang, Z. Jiao, B. Han et al., "Clinical characteristics and surgical treatment of oesophageal gastrointestinal stromal tumours," *European Journal of Cardio-Thoracic Surgery*, vol. 38, no. 2, pp. 223–227, 2010.

[25] B. H. A. von Rahden, H. J. Stein, H. Feussner, and J. R. Siewert, "Enucleation of submucosal tumors of the esophagus: minimally invasive versus open approach," *Surgical Endoscopy and Other Interventional Techniques*, vol. 18, no. 6, pp. 924–930, 2004.

[26] C. Zapletal, C. Heesen, J. Origer et al., "Quality of life after surgical treatment of early Barrett's cancer: a prospective comparison of the Ivor-Lewis resection versus the modified Merendino resection," *World Journal of Surgery*, vol. 38, no. 6, pp. 444–452, 2014.

Permissions

All chapters in this book were first published in CROM, by Hindawi Publishing Corporation; hereby published with permission under the Creative Commons Attribution License or equivalent. Every chapter published in this book has been scrutinized by our experts. Their significance has been extensively debated. The topics covered herein carry significant findings which will fuel the growth of the discipline. They may even be implemented as practical applications or may be referred to as a beginning point for another development.

The contributors of this book come from diverse backgrounds, making this book a truly international effort. This book will bring forth new frontiers with its revolutionizing research information and detailed analysis of the nascent developments around the world.

We would like to thank all the contributing authors for lending their expertise to make the book truly unique. They have played a crucial role in the development of this book. Without their invaluable contributions this book wouldn't have been possible. They have made vital efforts to compile up to date information on the varied aspects of this subject to make this book a valuable addition to the collection of many professionals and students.

This book was conceptualized with the vision of imparting up-to-date information and advanced data in this field. To ensure the same, a matchless editorial board was set up. Every individual on the board went through rigorous rounds of assessment to prove their worth. After which they invested a large part of their time researching and compiling the most relevant data for our readers.

The editorial board has been involved in producing this book since its inception. They have spent rigorous hours researching and exploring the diverse topics which have resulted in the successful publishing of this book. They have passed on their knowledge of decades through this book. To expedite this challenging task, the publisher supported the team at every step. A small team of assistant editors was also appointed to further simplify the editing procedure and attain best results for the readers.

Apart from the editorial board, the designing team has also invested a significant amount of their time in understanding the subject and creating the most relevant covers. They scrutinized every image to scout for the most suitable representation of the subject and create an appropriate cover for the book.

The publishing team has been an ardent support to the editorial, designing and production team. Their endless efforts to recruit the best for this project, has resulted in the accomplishment of this book. They are a veteran in the field of academics and their pool of knowledge is as vast as their experience in printing. Their expertise and guidance has proved useful at every step. Their uncompromising quality standards have made this book an exceptional effort. Their encouragement from time to time has been an inspiration for everyone.

The publisher and the editorial board hope that this book will prove to be a valuable piece of knowledge for researchers, students, practitioners and scholars across the globe.

List of Contributors

Inaya Ahmed
Rutgers Robert Wood Johnson Medical School, New Brunswick, NJ 08901, USA

Kavita Dharmarajan, Sheryl Green and Richard L. Bakst
Department of Radiation Oncology, Icahn School of Medicine at Mount Sinai Hospital, New York, NY 10029, USA

Amy Tiersten
Department of Medical Oncology, Icahn School of Medicine at Mount Sinai Hospital, New York, NY 10029, USA

Ira Bleiweiss
Department of Pathology, Icahn School of Medicine at Mount Sinai Hospital, New York, NY 10029, USA

Hank Schmidt
Department of Surgery, Icahn School of Medicine at Mount Sinai Hospital, New York, NY 10029, USA

James R. Stier
Department of Pediatrics, Tulane University School of Medicine, New Orleans, LA 70112, USA
Department of Pediatrics, Ochsner Health System, New Orleans, LA 70112, USA

Robert J. Vasquez
Department of Pediatrics, Tulane University School of Medicine, New Orleans, LA 70112, USA
Department of Pediatric Hematology-Oncology, Ochsner Health System, New Orleans, LA 70121, USA
University of Queensland School of Medicine, Brisbane, QLD 4006, Australia

Basnet Alina
Trinitas Regional Medical Center, Seton Hall University of Health and Medical Sciences, Elizabeth, NJ 67202,USA
Department of Internal Medicine, Trinitas Regional Medical Center, Elizabeth, NJ 67202, USA

Jofre A. Sebastian
Trinitas Regional Medical Center, Seton Hall University of Health and Medical Sciences, Elizabeth, NJ 67202,USA
Touro College of Osteopathic Medicine, 230W125th Street No. 1, New York, NY 10027, USA

Capo Gerardo
Trinitas Regional Medical Center, Seton Hall University of Health and Medical Sciences, Elizabeth, NJ 67202,USA
Department of Hematology and Oncology, Trinitas Comprehensive Cancer Center, Elizabeth, NJ 07202, USA

Pashtoon Murtaza Kasi, Gita Thanarajasingam, Heidi D. Finnes, Jose C. Villasboas Bisneto, Joleen M. Hubbard and Axel Grothey
Division of Medical Oncology, Mayo Clinic, Rochester, MN 55905, USA

Nouritza M. Torossian
Institut Universitaire du Cancer de Toulouse Oncopole, Toulouse, France

Roy T. Wallace
Retina Consultants of Nashville, Nashville, TN, USA

Wen-Jen Hwu and Agop Y. Bedikian
MD Anderson Cancer Center, Houston, TX, USA

Irappa Madabhavi, Pritam Kataria, Apurva Patel, Asha Anand, Harsha Panchal, Sonia Parikh, Gaurang Modi, Rahul Kulkarni and Sandip Shah
GCRI, Civil Hospital Complex, Asarwa, Ahmedabad, Gujarat 830016, India

Swaroop Revannasiddaiah
Department of Radiotherapy and Clinical Oncology, Swami Rama Cancer Hospital and Research Institute, Haldwani, Uttarakhand, India

Malay Sarkar
Department of Pulmonary Medicine, IGMC, Shimla, Himachal Pradesh, India

Christos Nikolaou, Alexios Matikas, Dimitris Mavroudis and Lampros Vamvakas
Department of Medical Oncology, University Hospital of Heraklion, Voutes, P.O. Box 1352, Heraklion, 71110 Crete, Greece

Maria Papavasilopoulou
Olympion General Clinic, Volou and Meilichou, 26443 Patra, Greece

Ahmet Turan Aydın
Orthopaedics and Trauma Department, Antalya Memorial Hospital, 07020 Antalya, Turkey

Kemal Gökkuş
Private Memorial Antalya Hospital, Zafer Mahallesi, Yildirim Beyazit Caddesi, No. 91, Kepez, 07020 Antalya, Turkey
Orthopaedics and Trauma Department, Antalya Memorial Hospital, 07020 Antalya, Turkey

Tolgay Akin
General Surgery Department, Antalya Memorial Hospital, 07020 Antalya, Turkey

Ergin Sagtas
Radiodiagnostic Department, Antalya Memorial Hospital, 07020 Antalya, Turkey

Murat Saylik
Orthopaedics and Trauma Department, Ozel Bahar Hospital, 16100 Bursa, Turkey

Asad Jehangir, Kim Aderhold, Priya Rajagopalan and Oluwaseun Shogbesan
Department of Internal Medicine, Reading Health System, Spruce Street/6th Avenue, West Reading, PA 19610, USA

Sharon Swierczynski
Department of Pathology, Reading Health System, Spruce Street/6th Avenue, West Reading, PA 19610, USA

Anam Qureshi
King Edward Medical University, Mayo Hospital Road, Nelagumbad, Anarkali, Lahore 54000, Pakistan

Qasim Jehangir
Rawalpindi Medical College, Tipu Road, Rawalpindi 46000, Pakistan

Christian Espana Schmidt
Reading Health System, Spruce Street/6th Avenue, West Reading, PA 19610, USA

Seongseok Yun and Iyad Mansour
Department of Medicine, University of Arizona, Tucson, AZ 85721, USA

Nicole D. Vincelette
Molecular Pharmacology and Experimental Therapeutics, Mayo Clinic, Rochester, MN 55905, USA

Dana Hariri
Department of Pathology, University of Arizona, Tucson, AZ 85721, USA

Sara Motamed
Midwestern University, Arizona College of Osteopathic Medicine, Glendale, AZ 85308, USA

Clarissa Groberio Borba, Rafael Loch Batista, Nina Rosa de Castro Musolino, Vanielle Carvalho Machado, Ana Elisa Evangelista Alcantara and Malebranche Berardo Carneiro da Cunha Neto
Neuroendocrinology Unit, Functional Neurosurgery Division, Hospital das Clinicas, Faculdade de Medicina, Universidade de São Paulo, Brazil

Gilberto Ochman da Silva and Valter Angelo Sperling Cescato
Pituitary Neurosurgery Unit, Functional Neurosurgery Division, Hospital das Clinicas, Faculdade de Medicina, Universidade de São Paulo, Brazil

Shinya Sakata, Sho Saeki, Sayuri Hirooka, Susumu Hirosako, Hidenori Ichiyasu and Hirotsugu Kohrogi
Department of Respiratory Medicine, Kumamoto University Hospital, 1-1-1 Honjo, Chuo-ku, Kumamoto 860-8556, Japan

Kyu Chan Lee, Seung Heon Lee, KiHoon Sung, So Hyun Ahn, Jinho Choi and Seok Ho Lee
Department of Radiation Oncology, Gil Medical Center, School of Medicine, Gachon University, Incheon 405-760, Republic of Korea

Jae Hoon Lee and Junshik Hong
Department of Internal Medicine, Gil Medical Center, School of Medicine, Gachon University, Incheon 405-760, Republic of Korea

Sang Hui Park
Department of Pathology, Ewha Womans University School of Medicine, Seoul 158-710, Republic of Korea

Khin Thway, Dirk C. Strauss, Myles J. Smith and Cyril Fisher
Sarcoma Unit, Royal Marsden Hospital, London SW3 6JJ, UK

Lauren Chiec
University of Cincinnati College of Medicine, Cincinnati, OH 45267, USA

Sadhna Verma
Division of Radiology, University of Cincinnati College of Medicine, Cincinnati, OH 45267, USA

Ady Kendler
Division of Pathology, University of Cincinnati College of Medicine, Cincinnati, OH 45267, USA

Nagla Abdel Karim
The Vontz Center for Molecular Studies, 3125 Eden Avenue, RM 1312, ML 0562, Cincinnati, OH 45267, USA

Carsten Nieder
Department of Oncology and Palliative Medicine, Nordland Hospital, 8092 Bodø, Norway
Department of Clinical Medicine, Faculty of Health Sciences, University of Tromsø, 9038 Tromsø, Norway

Khalid Al-Shibli
Department of Pathology, Nordland Hospital, 8092 Bodø, Norway

Terje Tollåli
Department of Pulmonology, Nordland Hospital, 8092 Bodø, Norway

Deepak Ravindranathan
Department of Medicine, Emory University School of Medicine, Atlanta, GA, USA

Emilie Elise Hitron, Greta Anne Russler and Mehmet Asim Bilen
Department of Hematology and Medical Oncology, Winship Cancer Institute of Emory University, Atlanta, GA, USA

Yue Xue
Department of Pathology, Emory University School of Medicine, Atlanta, GA, USA

Ali Zakaria and Bayan Al Share
Department of Internal Medicine, Providence-Providence Park Hospital, Michigan State University College of Human Medicine, Southfield, MI, USA

Sri Kollepara and Cynthia Vakhariya
Division of Hematology and Oncology, Providence-Providence Park Hospital, Michigan State University College of Human Medicine, Southfield, MI, USA

Christina F. Marlow
Department of Internal Medicine, George Washington University School of Medicine, USA

Shailendra Sharma and Faizan Babar
Division of Kidney Diseases and Hypertension, George Washington University School of Medicine, USA

Jianqing Lin
Division of Hematology and Oncology, George Washington University School of Medicine, USA

Tomoko Takagishi, Yuta Niimi, Goshi Matsuki, Shinta Nagano, Junsuke Hinami, Masaaki Kajiwara, Kiyoshi Kaneko, Yoshihiro Kubota and Osamu Nakai
Department of Surgery, Uji Tokushukai Medical Center, Uji, Kyoto 611-0041, Japan

Janelle Gyorffy and Samuel M. Philbrick
Department of Internal Medicine, SAUSHEC, San Antonio, TX, USA

Adrian R. Bersabe and Alexander Brown
Department of Hematology Oncology, SAUSHEC, San Antonio, TX, USA

Richard J. Upton and Derek A. Mathis
Department of Pathology, SAUSHEC, San Antonio, TX, USA

Austin Peters
Department of Radiology, SAUSHEC, San Antonio, TX, USA

Frank S. Fan
Section of Hematology and Oncology, Department of Medicine, Changhua Hospital, Ministry of Health and Welfare, Chang-Hua County, Taiwan

Chung-Fan Yang
Department of Pathology, Changhua Hospital, Ministry of Health and Welfare, Chang-Hua County, Taiwan

Yi-Fen Wang
Department of Radiology, Changhua Hospital, Ministry of Health and Welfare, Chang-Hua County, Taiwan

Sassine Ghanem
Department of Medicine, Staten Island University Hospital, Northwell Health, 475 Seaview Avenue, Staten Island, NY 10305, USA

Gwenalyn Garcia and Marcel Odaimi
Department of Hematology/Oncology, Staten Island University Hospital, Northwell Health, 475 Seaview Avenue, Staten Island, NY 10305, USA

Liu Ying and Matthew Hurford
Department of Pathology, Staten Island University Hospital, Northwell Health, 475 Seaview Avenue, Staten Island, NY 10305, USA

Jila Agah
Department of Obstetrics and Gynecology, Faculty of Medicine, Sabzevar University of Medical Sciences, Sabzevar, Iran

Sedighe Karimzadeh and Fateme Moharrer Ahmadi
School of Medicine, Sabzevar University of Medical Sciences, Sabzevar, Iran

Paul Gonzales and Seth Klusewitz
Department of Internal Medicine, San Antonio Military Medical Center, Fort Sam Houston, San Antonio, TX 78234, USA

Johanna Marowske and John Gancayco
Gastroenterology Service, San Antonio Military Medical Center, Fort Sam Houston, San Antonio, TX 78234, USA

Michael B. Osswald and Robert Setlik
Hematology/Oncology Service, San Antonio Military Medical Center, Fort Sam Houston, San Antonio, TX 78234, USA

Mohammad Saud Khan
Department of Internal Medicine, University of Toledo Medical Center, Toledo, OH 43614, USA

Veena Balakrishnan Iyer
Department of Hematology and Oncology, Rhode Island Hospital, Providence, RI, USA
Department of Oncology, University of Toledo Medical Center, Toledo, OH 43614, USA

Neha Varshney
Department of Pathology, University of Toledo Medical Center, Toledo, OH 43614, USA

Chieko Yoshida
Department of Respiratory Medicine, Kumamoto University Hospital, 1-1-1 Honjo, Chuo-ku, Kumamoto 860-8556, Japan

Jhong-You Li, Chung-Liang Li and Chun-Kuan Lu
Kaohsiung Medical University Hospital, No. 100 Tzyou 1st Road, Kaohsiung 807, Taiwan

Mali Him and Vikas Mehta
Mount Sinai Hospital, Chicago, IL, USA

Maggie Meier
St. Luke's Hospital St. Louis, MO, USA

Laura E. Zyczynski and Scott M. Schuetze
Department of Internal Medicine, University of Michigan Health System, 1500 E. Medical Center Drive, Ann Arbor, MI 48109,USA

Jonathan B. McHugh
Department of Pathology, University of Michigan Health System, 1500 E. Medical Center Drive, Ann Arbor, MI 48109, USA

Thomas E. Gribbin
Mercy Health Lacks Cancer Center, 250 Cherry Street SE, Grand Rapids, MI 489503, USA

Anna Koumarianou
Hematology-Oncology Unit, Fourth Department of Internal Medicine, National and Kapodistrian University of Athens, Attikon University Hospital, Rimini 1, Haidari, 12462 Athens, Greece

Christina Kontopoulou
Second Radiology Department, Attikon University Hospital, National and Kapodistrian University of Athens, Rimini 1, Haidari, 12462 Athens, Greece

Vassilis Kouloulias
Radiotherapy Unit, Second Radiology Department, Attikon University Hospital, National and Kapodistrian University of Athens, Rimini 1, Haidari, 12462 Athens, Greece

Christina Tsionou
Maternity-Health, 30 Papanikoli Street, Halandri, 15232 Athens, Greece

Kazuyuki Yusa and Mitsuyoshi Iino
Department of Dentistry, Oral and Maxillofacial, Plastic and Reconstructive Surgery, Yamagata University Faculty of Medicine, Yamagata, Japan

Hideyuki Yamanouchi and Ayako Sugano
Department of Dentistry and Oral Surgery, Shinjo Tokushukai Hospital, Yamagata, Japan

Jason Hew, Fauzia Rana and Louise Zhou
Department of Internal Medicine, Division of Medical Oncology, University of Florida COM, Jacksonville, FL, USA

Anirban Das
Department of Pulmonary Medicine, Murshidabad Medical College, Berhampore, West Bengal 742101, India

Abhishek Pratap
Department of Pulmonary Medicine, Medical College, Kolkata, West Bengal 700 073, India

Ali Altalhy, Yazid Maghrabi and Saleh S. Baeesa
Division of Neurosurgery, Department of Surgery, Faculty of Medicine, King Abdulaziz University, Jeddah, Saudi Arabia

Zuhoor Almansouri
Department of Pathology and Laboratory Medicine, King Faisal Specialist Hospital and Research Center, Jeddah, Saudi Arabia

Jong An and Russell Baur
Department of Hematology and Oncology Service, San Antonio Military Medical Center, Fort Sam Houston, San Antonio, TX 78234, USA

Jason Brownell
Department of Internal Medicine, San Antonio Military Medical Center, Fort Sam Houston, San Antonio, TX 78234, USA

Darrell Barker
Department of Gastroenterology, San Antonio Military Medical Center, Fort Sam Houston, San Antonio, TX 78234, USA

Theresa Stockinger, Robert Brady and Katherine Cebe
Department of Pathology, San Antonio Military Medical Center, Fort Sam Houston, San Antonio, TX 78234, USA

Georgia Mitropoulou
Pathology Department, "Agia Sofia" Children's Hospital, Athens, Greece

Adamantia Zizi-Sermpetzoglou, Athanasios Kountourogiannis and Despoina Myoteri
Pathology Department, "Tzaneion" General Hospital, Piraeus, Greece

Hippokrates Moschouris
Radiology Department, "Tzaneion" General Hospital, Piraeus, Greece

Dionysios Dellaportas
2nd Department of Surgery, University Hospital "Aretaieion", Athens, Greece

Reiko Ideguchi, Saori Akashi, Michiko Shindo, Kazunori Minami and Toshio Fukuda
Department of Radiology, Nagasaki Harbor Medical Center City Hospital, Nagasaki, Japan

Kazuto Ashizawa
Department of Clinical Oncology, Nagasaki University Graduate School of Biomedical Sciences, Nagasaki, Japan

Junji Irie
Department of Pathology, Nagasaki Harbor Medical Center City Hospital, Nagasaki, Japan

Minoru Fukuda
Department of Internal Medicine, Nagasaki Harbor Medical Center City Hospital, Nagasaki, Japan

Masataka Uetani
Department of Radiological Sciences, Nagasaki University Graduate School of Biomedical Sciences, Nagasaki, Japan

Ashraf Abugroun, Ahmed Chaudhary and Gabriel Rodriguez
Advocate Illinois Masonic Medical Center, Chicago, IL, USA

Rubens Barros Costa, Jason B. Kaplan, Maureen Sadim and Aparna Kalyan
Developmental Therapeutics Program, Feinberg School of Medicine and Robert H. Lurie Comprehensive Cancer Center of Northwestern University, 233 East Superior Street, Chicago, IL 60611, USA
Division of Hematology and Oncology, Robert H. Lurie Comprehensive Cancer Center, Northwestern University, 676 North Clair Street, Chicago, IL 60611, USA

Al Benson
Division of Hematology and Oncology, Robert H. Lurie Comprehensive Cancer Center, Northwestern University, 676 North Clair Street, Chicago, IL 60611, USA

Vahid Yaghmai
Department of Radiology, Northwestern University Feinberg School of Medicine, 676 North Saint Clair Street, Chicago, IL 60611, USA

Ricardo L. B. Costa
Department of Breast Oncology, Lee Moffitt Cancer Center, Moffitt McKinley Outpatient Center, 10920 North McKinley Drive, BR-Program, Tampa, FL 33612, USA

Haijun Zhou and Amir Behdad
Department of Pathology, Northwestern University Feinberg School of Medicine, 251 East Huron Street, Chicago, IL 60611, USA

Sarah Talamantes
Northwestern University Feinberg School of Medicine, 420 East Superior Street, Chicago, IL 60611, USA

Dearbhaile Catherine Collins and Derek Gerard Power
Department of Medical Oncology, Cork University Hospital, Wilton, Co. Cork, Ireland

Ruben Yela
Department of Histopathology, Cork University Hospital, Wilton, Co. Cork, Ireland

Noel Horgan
Department of Ophthalmology, Royal Victoria Eye and Ear Hospital, Dublin 2, Ireland

Kristian Larson
Early Phase Clinical Trial Program, The University of Arizona Cancer Center, 1515 N. Campbell Ave., Tucson, AZ 85724, USA

Andrew Kovoor
Division of Hematology and Oncology, University of Arizona College of Medicine, 1515 N. Campbell Ave., Tucson, AZ 85724, USA

Emad Elquza
Early Phase Clinical Trial Program, e University of Arizona Cancer Center, 1515 N. Campbell Ave., Tucson, AZ 85724, USA
Division of Hematology and Oncology, University of Arizona College of Medicine, 1515 N. Campbell Ave., Tucson, AZ 85724, USA

Hani M. Babiker
Early Phase Clinical Trial Program, e University of Arizona Cancer Center, 1515 N. Campbell Ave., Tucson, AZ 85724, USA
Translational Genomics Research Institute (TGen), 445 N. 5th Street, Phoenix, AZ 85004, USA
Division of Hematology and Oncology, University of Arizona College of Medicine, 1515 N. Campbell Ave., Tucson, AZ 85724, USA

Joy Liau
Department of Medical Imaging, University of Arizona, 1501 N. Campbell Ave., Tucson, AZ 85712, USA

Jordan Eldersveld
Department of Pathology, University of Arizona, 1501 N. Campbell Ave., Tucson, AZ 85712, USA

Sapna Vinit Amin, Sunanda Bharatnur and Akhila Vasudeva
Department of OBG, Kasturba Medical College, Manipal University, Manipal 576104, India

Aswathy Kumaran
IVF and Reproductive Biology Centre, Maulana Azad Medical College, New Delhi 110002, India

Kartik Udupa
Department of Medical Oncology, Kasturba Medical College, Manipal University, Manipal 576104, India

Dinesh Bangalore Venkateshiah
Department of Surgery, Kasturba Medical College, Manipal University, Manipal 576104, India

Shaila T. Bhat
Department of Pathology, Melaka Manipal Medical College, Manipal University, Manipal 576104, India

Pei-Yuu Yang
Department of Traditional Chinese Medicine, Taipei Medical University Hospital, Taipei 11031, Taiwan

Chen-Jei Tai
Department of Traditional Chinese Medicine, Taipei Medical University Hospital, Taipei 11031, Taiwan
Department of OB/GYN, School of Medicine, College of Medicine, Taipei Medical University, Taipei 11031, Taiwan

Keiki Nagaharu
Department of Hematology and Oncology, Suzuka General Hospital, Yamanohana, Yasuzuka, Suzuka, Mie Prefecture 1275-53, Japan

Kenji Ikemura
Department of Pharmacy, Mie University Hospital, Edobashi 2-174, Tsu, Mie Prefecture 514-8507, Japan

Yoshiki Yamashita, Hiroyasu Oda, Mikiya Ishihara, Yumiko Sugawara, Satoshi Tamaru, Toshiro Mizuno and Naoyuki Katayama
Department of Hematology and Oncology, Mie University Graduate School of Medicine, Edobashi 2-174, Tsu, Mie Prefecture 514-8507, Japan

Tiffany A. Pompa, Michael Styler and Chetan Jeurkar
Department of Medicine, Division of Hematology/ Oncology, Drexel University College of Medicine, Philadelphia, PA 19102, USA

William F. Morano and Wilbur B. Bowne
Department of Surgery, Division of Surgical Oncology, Drexel University College of Medicine, Philadelphia, PA 19102, USA

Hui Li and Suganthi Soundararajan
Department of Pathology and Laboratory Medicine, Drexel University College of Medicine, Philadelphia, PA 19102, USA

Jaganmohan Poli
Department of Radiation Oncology, Drexel University College of Medicine, Philadelphia, PA 19102, USA

A. Vennepureddy and V. Motilal Nehru
Department of Internal Medicine, Staten Island University Hospital, 475 Seaview Avenue, Staten Island, NY 10305, USA

Y. Liu
Department of Pathology, Staten Island University Hospital, 475 Seaview Avenue, Staten Island, NY 10305, USA

F. Mohammad and J. P. Atallah
Division of Hematology and Oncology, Staten Island University Hospital, 475 Seaview Avenue, Staten Island, NY 10305, USA

Udit Bhaskar Bhatnagar and Daulath Singh
Internal Medicine, University of Missouri-Kansas City School of Medicine, 2301 Holmes Street, Kansas City, MO 64108, USA

Alexy Glazyrin
Department of Pathology, University of Missouri-Kansas City School of Medicine, 2301 Holmes Street, Kansas City, MO 64108, USA

Jill Moormeier
Department of Medicine, Hematology/Oncology, University of Missouri-Kansas City School of Medicine, 2301 Holmes Street, Kansas City, MO 64108, USA

Jan Van Keer
Nephrology, Dialysis and Renal Transplantation, University Hospitals Leuven, 3000 Leuven, Belgium

Björn Meijers
Nephrology, Dialysis and Renal Transplantation, University Hospitals Leuven, 3000 Leuven, Belgium
Laboratory of Nephrology, Department of Microbiology and Immunology, KU Leuven, 3000 Leuven, Belgium

Michel Delforge
Hematology, University Hospitals Leuven, 3000 Leuven, Belgium
Laboratory for Stem Cell Biology and Embryology, Department of Development and Regeneration, KU Leuven, 3000 Leuven, Belgium

Gregor Verhoef
Hematology, University Hospitals Leuven, 3000 Leuven, Belgium
Laboratory for Experimental Hematology, Department of Oncology, KU Leuven, 3000 Leuven, Belgium

Koen Poesen
Laboratory Medicine, University Hospitals Leuven, 3000 Leuven, Belgium
Laboratory for Molecular Neurobiomarker Research, Department of Neurosciences, KU Leuven, 3000 Leuven, Belgium

Mushegh A. Sahakyan
The Intervention Centre, Oslo University Hospital, Rikshospitalet, 0027 Oslo, Norway
Institute of Clinical Research, Medical Faculty, University of Oslo, 0318 Oslo, Norway
Department of Surgery No. 1, Yerevan State Medical University after M. Heratsi, 0025 Yerevan, Armenia

Airazat M. Kazaryan
The Intervention Centre, Oslo University Hospital, Rikshospitalet, 0027 Oslo, Norway
Department of Gastrointestinal Surgery, Akershus University Hospital, 1478 Lørenskog, Norway

Ewa Pomianowska, Bjørn Atle Bjørnbeth and Bård Ingvald Røsok
Department of HPB Surgery, Oslo University Hospital, Rikshospitalet, 0407 Oslo, Norway

Bjørn Edwin
The Intervention Centre, Oslo University Hospital, Rikshospitalet, 0027 Oslo, Norway
Institute of Clinical Research, Medical Faculty, University of Oslo, 0318 Oslo, Norway
Department of HPB Surgery, Oslo University Hospital, Rikshospitalet, 0407 Oslo, Norway

Andreas Abildgaard
Department of Radiology, Oslo University Hospital, Rikshospitalet, 0027 Oslo, Norway

Pål-Dag Line
Department of Transplantation Medicine, Oslo University Hospital, Rikshospitalet, 0424 Oslo, Norway

Sammy G. Nakhla
Department of Medicine, Southern Arizona VA Health Care System, Tucson, AZ 85723, USA

Srinath Sundararajan
Department of Hematology/Oncology, University of Arizona Cancer Center, Tucson, AZ 85724, USA

Faisal Inayat
Department of Medicine, New York-Presbyterian Hospital, Weill Cornell Medical College, New York, NY 10065, USA

Hafeez Ul Hassan Virk and Ahmad R. Cheema
Department of Medicine, Mount Sinai St. Luke's and Mount Sinai Roosevelt Hospitals, Icahn School of Medicine, New York, NY 10019, USA

Muhammad Wasif Saif
Department of Hematology/Oncology, Tufts Medical Center, Tufts University School of Medicine, Boston, MA 02111, USA

Maurício Fernando Silva Almeida Ribeiro, Micelange Carvalho de Sousa, Samir Abdallah Hanna, Marcos Vinicius Calfat Maldaun and Ceci Obara Kurimori
Hospital Sírio Libanês, São Paulo, SP, Brazil

Luiz Guilherme Cernaglia Aureliano de Lima, Romulo Loss Mattedi and Rodrigo Ramella Munhoz
Hospital Sírio Libanês, São Paulo, SP, Brazil
Oncology Service, Instituto do Câncer do Estado de São Paulo, Universidade de São Paulo, São Paulo, SP, Brazil

Jana Jaal
Hematology and Oncology Clinic, Department of Radiotherapy and Oncological Therapy, Tartu University Hospital, 51014 Tartu, Estonia
Department of Haematology and Oncology, University of Tartu, 51014 Tartu, Estonia

Tõnu Jõgi
Hematology and Oncology Clinic, Department of Radiotherapy and Oncological Therapy, Tartu University Hospital, 51014 Tartu, Estonia

Alan Altraja
Department of Pulmonary Medicine, University of Tartu, 51014 Tartu, Estonia
Lung Clinic, Tartu University Hospital, 51014 Tartu, Estonia

Ramawad Soobrah
Victoria Hospital, Ministry of Health and Quality of Life, Mauritius

Fiona Tsang and Sreelakshmi Mallappa
Ealing Hospital, Uxbridge Road, Southall, Middlesex UB1 3HW, UK

Veronica Grassi
King's College Hospital, Denmark Hill, London SE5 9RS, UK

Hassan Hirji and Robert Reichert
Northwick Park Hospital, Watford Road, Harrow HA13UJ, UK

Ozgur Tanriverdi
Department of Medical Oncology, Sitki Kocman University Faculty of Medicine, 48000 Mugla, Turkey

Ayca Ersen
Department of Pathology, Dokuz Eylul University Faculty of Medicine, 35010 Izmir, Turkey

Suna Cokmert
Department of Medical Oncology, Kent Hospital, 35010 Izmir, Turkey

Emine Koca
Department of Internal Medicine, Sitki Kocman University Faculty of Medicine, 48000 Mugla, Turkey

Naki Bulut
Department of General Surgery, Sitki Kocman University Education and Research Hospital, 48000 Mugla, Turkey

Suha Gul
Department of Radiodiagnostics, Sitki Kocman University Education and Research Hospital, 48000 Mugla, Turkey

Nevin Yilmaz
Department of Internal Medicine and Gastroenterohepatology, Sitki Kocman University Faculty of Medicine, 48000 Mugla, Turkey

Kyriakos Neofytou, Mafalda Costa Neves, Alexandros Giakoustidis and Satvinder Mudan
Royal Marsden Hospital, Department of Academic Surgery, Upper GI/HPB Unit, Fulham Road, London SW3 6JJ, UK

Charlotte Benson
Royal Marsden Hospital, Sarcoma Unit, Fulham Road, London SW3 6JJ, UK

Index